Disability at the Dawn of the 21st Century

and
The State of the States

DAVID BRADDOCK
EDITOR

AAMR
AMERICAN ASSOCIATION ON MENTAL RETARDATION

Disability at the Dawn of the 21st Century

and
The State of the States

Edited
by
David Braddock, PhD
Coleman-Turner Chair in Cognitive Disability
and Professor of Psychiatry
Coleman Institute for Cognitive Disabilities
and Department of Psychiatry
University of Colorado

American Association on Mental Retardation
Washington, DC

Published by

American Association on Mental Retardation
Research Monographs and Book Publication Program
444 N. Capitol Street, NW, Suite 846
Washington, DC 20001-1512

Printed in the United States of America

Library of Congress Cataloging-in-Publication Data

Braddock, David L.
    Disability at the dawn of the 21st century and the state of the states /
David Braddock.
        p. cm.
    Rev. ed. of: The state of the states in developmental disabilities / by David Braddock.
[et al.]. 5th ed. c1998.
    Includes index.
    ISBN 0-940898-85-3
    1. Developmentally disabled--Services for--United States--States.2. Developmentally
disabled--Services for--United States--States--Finance. 3. Developmentally
disabled--Government policy--United States--States. 4. People with disabilities--Services
for--History. I. State of the states in developmental disabilities. II. Title.

HV 1570.5.U65 B73 2002
362.1'968--dc21

                                                                    2002066472

Contents

TABLES AND FIGURES viii

PREFACE x

ACKNOWLEDGMENTS xii

PART I: CROSS DISABILITY PERSPECTIVES

CHAPTER 1: An Institutional History of Disability 1
David Braddock & Susan Parish

   IMPAIRMENT AND DISABILITY 3

   FOREVIEW OF THE CHAPTER 4

   ANTIQUITY 5

      Prehistory 5

      The Old Testament 5

      Ancient Greece and Rome 6

   MIDDLE AGES 8

      Demonology 8

      Compassion and Support 9

      Residential Institutions Emerge 10

   EARLY MODERN PERIOD THROUGH THE 18TH CENTURY 12

      Renaissance and the Scientific Method 12

      Poverty and Disability 13

      Philosophical Enlightenment 14

      Distinguishing Between Intellectual Disability and Mental Illness 15

      Institutions for People With Mental Illness Established 15

      Developments in the American Colonies and Early United States 16

      Schools for the Deaf and Blind Persons Opened in Europe 18

   THE 19th CENTURY 19

      Educational Developments 19

      First North American Mental Hospitals and Residential Schools 21

      Overcrowding and the Demise of the Moral Treatment 23

      Deaf Community Organizing 25

      First U.S. Institution for People With Intellectual Disability 26

      From Training Schools to Custodial Asylums 26

      Freak Shows 27

      Threat of the Eugenicists 28

   THE 20th CENTURY 29

      Segregation and Expansion of the Institutional Model 29

      Developments for Persons With Physical Disabilities 32

      Emergence of Family, Community, and Consumer Models 33

      The Social Model of Disability 33

      Organizational Developments 34

      Beginnings of Deinstitutionalization 34

      Political Activism and the Right to Treatment 35

      Independent Living and Self-Advocacy 37

      International Disability Rights Initiatives 39

   CONCLUSION 41

   REFERENCES 45

PART I: CROSS DISABILITY PERSPECTIVES
CHAPTER 2: PUBLIC FINANCIAL SUPPORT FOR DISABILITY AT THE DAWN
OF THE 21st CENTURY 63
David Braddock
    METHOD 65
    RESULTS 66
        Public Sector Spending for Disability Programs in the US 66
        Income Maintenance 67
        General Health Care 67
        Long-Term Care 67
        Special Education 68
        Institutional Versus Community Services Spending 68
        Medicaid Long Term Care Spending 68
        Assessing Fiscal Effort in the States 70
    DISCUSSION AND CONCLUSION 72
    REFERENCES 75
    APPENDICES 77
        1. Public Financial Support for Disability Services in the United States 78
        2. Public Spending for Medicaid Long-Term Care Services 79
        3. Recipients of Disability Services, Payments, and Benefits 80
        4. Long Term Care Spending and Participants 81

PART II: THE STATE OF THE STATES IN DEVELOPMENTAL DISABILITIES
SUMMARY OF THE STUDY 83
David Braddock, Richard Hemp, Mary C. Rizzolo, Susan Parish, & Amy Pomeranz
    INTRODUCTION 85
    COMMUNITY RESIDENTIAL SERVICES 87
        Cost by Setting 88
        Community Staff Wage Initiatives 89
    PUBLIC AND PRIVATE INSTITUTIONS 89
        Public Institutions 91
            Census Trends 91
            Public Institutional Closures 91
            Average Costs of Care 92
        Privately Operated Institutions and Nursing Facilities 95
            Nursing Facility Utilization 95
    GENERAL TRENDS IN SYSTEM FINANCING 96
        Impact of Economic Recession in the States 98
    COMMUNITY SERVICES TRENDS 99
        Sources of Revenue 99
        The HCBS Waiver 101
            Leveraging Federal Funds 103
        Local Funding 103
        Variations in State Commitments for MR/DD Services 104
        Individual and Family Support 112
        Family Support Services 112
        Supported Employment 115
        Supported Living and Personal Assistance 117
    SIGNIFICANCE OF MEDICAID 119
    ASSESSING FISCAL EFFORT IN THE STATES 120

State Spending Patterns 121
CONCLUSION 121
    Aging Caregivers and the Growing Demand for Services 121
    Increased Longevity of Persons with Developmental Disabilities 125
    Waiting Lists in the States 126
    Civil Rights and Advocacy 127
    Litigation in the States 128
REFERENCES 131
NOTES ON DATA SOURCES 137

STATE PROFILES 141
    ALABAMA 143
    ALASKA 147
    ARIZONA 151
    ARKANSAS 155
    CALIFORNIA 159
    COLORADO 163
    CONNECTICUT 167
    DELAWARE 171
    DISTRICT OF COLUMBIA 175
    FLORIDA 179
    GEORGIA 183
    HAWAII 187
    IDAHO 191
    ILLINOIS 195
    INDIANA 199
    IOWA 203
    KANSAS 207
    KENTUCKY 211
    LOUISIANA 215
    MAINE 219
    MARYLAND 223
    MASSACHUSETTS 227
    MICHIGAN 231
    MINNESOTA 235
    MISSISSIPPI 239
    MISSOURI 243
    MONTANA 247
    NEBRASKA 251
    NEVADA 255
    NEW HAMPSHIRE 259
    NEW JERSEY 263
    NEW MEXICO 267
    NEW YORK 271
    NORTH CAROLINA 275
    NORTH DAKOTA 279
    OHIO 283
    OKLAHOMA 287
    OREGON 291
    PENNSYLVANIA 295
    RHODE ISLAND 299
    SOUTH CAROLINA 303

SOUTH DAKOTA 307
TENNESSEE 311
TEXAS 315
UTAH 319
VERMONT 323
VIRGINIA 327
WASHINGTON 331
WEST VIRGINIA 335
WISCONSIN 339
WYOMING 343
UNITED STATES 347

PART III: FORCES SHAPING DEVELOPMENTAL DISABILITIES SERVICES IN THE STATES: A COMPARATIVE STUDY 351
Susan Parish

    INTRODUCTION 353
        Background 353
        Statement of the Problem 353
    LITERATURE REVIEW 354
        The Deinstitutionalization Movement and Related Research ... 354
        Determinants of State Policy 355
        Variables 356
        Conceptual Framework 358
    METHODS 359
        Overview 359
        Data Collection Procedures 360
            Sample 360
            Document Evaluation 363
        Interview Phase 363
            Instrument Development 364
            Sample 365
        Data Analysis 366
        Credibility of Findings 367
            Internal Validity 367
            External Validity 368
            Reliability 369
            Study Strengths 370
    MICHIGAN CASE STUDY 370
        Trends and Developments in Residential Services 371
        Adminstrative Overview 384
        Scandals 385
        Politics 387
        Federal Influences 388
        Public Officials and Bureaucratic Leadership 392
            The Governors 392
            The Legislature 394
            The Judiciary 396
            The Department of Mental Health 397
            Advocacy Groups 399
            Conclusions 402
    ILLINOIS CASE STUDY 404

Trends and Developments in Residential Services 405

Adminstrative Overview 414

Scandals 417

Politics 420

    The Illinois Constitution and Home Rule Powers 420

    Structure of the Legislature 421

    Campaign Finance and the Consolidation of Legislative Power 421

    The Emergence of AFSCME as a Political Power 422

    Political Patronage 423

    Politics and Developmental Disabilities: Conclusions 424

Federal Influences 424

Public Officials and Bureaucratic Leadership 426

    The Governors 426

    The Legislature 428

    The Department of Mental Health and Developmental Disabilities 431

Advocacy Groups 431

Conclusions 434

DISCUSSION AND CONCLUSIONS 435

Sociopolitical Factors and the Development of the States' DD Residential Systems 436

    Economic Factors 436

    Prisons 437

    Governmental Structure and Politics 438

    Federal Policy Influences 439

Leadership 440

    Dimensions of Leadership 440

    Policy Entrepeneurs 442

Legislation 443

Litigation 443

Limitations of the Study 444

Implications for Advocates 445

DEVELOPMENTS IN MICHIGAN AND ILLINOIS: 1990-2000 447

General Trends 448

    Types of Residential Settings 448

    Financial Trends 451

    Family Support 452

Michigan 453

    Reduced Reliance on Institutions and the Ongoing Transformation to Community 453

    Changes in Elected Leadership 453

    Innovations 454

Illinois 455

Advocacy Efforts 456

Federal Influences 457

Conclusions 459

REFERENCES 461

AUTHOR INDEX 477

SUBJECT INDEX 487

TABLES AND FIGURES

PART I: CHAPTER 2
PUBLIC FINANCIAL SUPPORT FOR DISABILITY PROGRAMS AT THE
DAWN OF THE 21st CENTURY

Table 1.1   Percentage of Public Spending for Long-Term Care
                Allocated to Community Care Services in the States,1997 69
Table 1.2   Public Spending for Community Long-Term Care Services for Persons With
                Disabilities in the States per $1,000 of Personal Income, 1997 71

Figure 1.1   Public-Sector Spending for Disability Programs in the United States, 1997 66
Figure 1.2   Income Maintenance Spending, 1997 67
Figure 1.3   Long -Term Care Spending, 1997 68
Figure 1.4   Medicaid Long-Term Care Spending, 1997 70

PART II
THE STATE OF THE STATES IN DEVELOPMENTAL DISABILITIES: STUDY SUMMARY

Table 2.1   Individuals Served by Residential Setting, FY 2000 86
Table 2.2   Community Residences for 1 to 15 Persons:
                Growth in Per Capita Placements, FY2000 87
Table 2.3   Annual Cost of Care Per Average Daily Resident, FY 2000 88
Table 2.4   Public Institution Census, FYs 1977, 1996, & 2000 90
Table 2.5   Completed and In-Progress Closures of Public Institutions 93
Table 2.6   State Institution Daily Costs, 1996 & 2000 95
Table 2.7   Nursing Facility Residents With Developmental Disabilities, FYs 1996 & 2000 96
Table 2.8   Inflation-Adjusted Change in GSP & Total MR/DD Spending, 1996-1999 98
Table 2.9   Federal HCBS Waiver Expenditures, FY 2000 102
Table 2.10   State Funds Potentially Available to Match Additional Federal
                Medicaid Funding, FY 2000 104
Table 2.11   Percentage of Total MR/DD Spending Allocated for Community Services, FY 2000 111
Table 2.12   Family Support Programs, FY 2000 114
Table 2.13   Supported Employment, FY 2000 116
Table 2.14   Supported Living and Personal Assistance, FY 2000 118
Table 2.15   Fiscal Effort, FYs 2000, 1996, & 1977 122
Table 2.16   Fiscal Effort Rankings, FYs 2000, 1996, & 1977 123
Table 2.17   Individuals with Developmental Disabilities Living in Households with
                Caregivers Aged 60+ Years, 2000 126
Table 2.18   Fiscal Effort for People with Developmental Disabilities and
                Right to Habilitation Class-Action Litigation 128
Table 2.19   Community Services Litigation 129

Figure 2.1   United States: Distribution of Residential Services by Setting, 1996 & 2000 85
Figure 2.2   United States: Persons Served in Public and Private Institutions
                & Nursing Facilities, FYs 1990-2000 89
Figure 2.3   United States: Institutional Closures by Decade 91
Figure 2.4   United States: Daily Costs Per Resident in Public Institutions, FYs 1977-2000 92

TABLES AND FIGURES CONTINUED

Figure 2.5   United States: Trends in MR/DD Spending, FYs 1977-2000 97

Figure 2.6   United States: Trends in Spending for Community Services
by Level of Government, FYs 1977-2000 99

Figure 2.7   United States: Community Services Revenue Sources, FY 2000 100

Figure 2.8   United States: Components of Federal MR/DD Medicaid Spending: FYs 1977-2000 103

Figure 2.9   Public Spending for Developmental Disabilities by State, FYs 1977-2000 105

Figure 2.10   United States, FYs 1990-2000: Spending for Family Support,
Number of Families Supported 113

Figure 2.11   United States: Fiscal Effort for Developmental Disabilities: FYs 1977-2000 120

Figure 2.12   Growing Numbers of Americans Aged 65+ Years, 1980-2050 124

Figure 2.13   United States: Distribution of Individuals with MR/DD
by Living Arrangement, FY 2000 124

Figure 2.14   United States: Distribution of Individuals with MR/DD
Living with Family Caregivers, FY 2000 125

PART III
FORCES SHAPING DEVELOPMENTAL DISABILITIES SERVICES IN THE STATES: A COMPARATIVE STUDY

Table 3.1   Documentary Sources of Data, by Author or Publisher 364

Table 3.2   Affiliation of Interviewees 366

Table 3.3   Resources and Contributions of Influential Factors in Michigan 403

Table 3.4   Major Factors Related to the Development of Community Services 436

Table 3.5   Potential Coalition Participants in Illinois 446

Figure 3.1   Conceptual Framework of the Investigation 360

Figure 3.2   Public DD Institutions in Michigan, 1960-90 372

Figure 3.3   Residential Service Recipients in Michigan by Setting, 1977 & 1990 384

Figure 3.4   Sources of Funding for Michigan's Total DD Service System, 1977-90 389

Figure 3.5   Sources of Funding for Community Services in Michigan, 1977-90 390

Figure 3.6   Conceptual Framework of Influence in Michigan, 1970-1990 404

Figure 3.7   Public DD Institutions in Illinois, 1960-90 407

Figure 3.8   Residential Service Recipients in Illinois by Setting, 1977 & 1990 414

Figure 3.9   Sources of Funding for Illinois' Total DD Services, 1977-90 424

Figure 3.10   Sources of Funding for Community Services in Illinois, 1977-90 425

Figure 3.11   Conceptual Framework of Influence in Illinois, 1970-90 435

Figure 3.12   State Prisoners per 100,000 of General Population, 1970-90 438

Figure 3.13   Public Institutional Residential Populations, Michigan and Illinois, 1970-1990 440

Figure 3.14   Michigan Residential Service Recipients by Setting Size, 1990-2000 448

Figure 3.15   Illinois Residential Service Recipients by Setting Size, 1990-2000 449

Figure 3.16   Residential Service Recipients by Setting, Michigan and Illinois, 2000 449

Figure 3.17   Supported Living Spending, Michigan and Illinois, 1992-2000 450

Figure 3.18   Sources of MR/DD Services Funds, Michigan, 1990-2000 451

Figure 3.19   Sources of MR/DD Services Funds, Illinois, 1990-2000 451

Figure 3.20   Family Support Spending, Michigan and Illinois, 1992-2000 452

PREFACE

This is the most extensive edition of The State of the States published since the first volume was completed two decades ago. This is as it should be since the growth of programs for persons with disabilities in the states and at the federal level has itself been so extensive over the past 20 years.

Part I of the book--Cross Disability Perspectives-- explores the historical basis of contemporary disability services from antiquity to the present day across the spectrum of mental, physical, and sensory disability. The utilization of a "cross-disability" approach reveals the often closely interconnected histories of people with disabilities, particularly with respect to the adoption of social and public policies toward such individuals.

Is it naive to hope that greater awareness and appreciation of this history might promote more collaboration among the various disability constituencies on the issues of the day in long-term care, education, technology, civil rights, scientific research and in other areas? Perhaps so; but persons with disabilities, their families, and advocates and professionals as well, are insufficiently numerous to be a truly important social force in our society unless we do bind together on common cross-disability goals. It is only in this manner that a future can be forged in which disability emerges as a significant international priority for the 21st century.

Part I also presents a cross-disability empirical study of public financial support for disability in the United States. This is the first study, to my knowledge, which attempts to integrate the analysis of such data across federal, state, and local levels of government and across the broad categories of mental and physical disability. Each of the 50 states is the focus of this study, which is particularly timely given the recent U.S. Supreme Court ruling promoting community services in *Olmstead v. L.C.* (1999). One of the findings of the study is that the majority of the nation's $109 billion commitment to long-term care for people with disabilities in the states supports institutional settings, including nursing facilities.

Part II of the book presents the 2002 study update of the "State of the States in Developmental Disabilities." Part II begins with an analytical overview of the study and concludes with state-by-state profiles for each of the states and the District of Columbia. The profiles examine the programmatic structure and financing of mental retardation/ developmental disabilities services. The profiles cover the 1977-2000 period and the analysis identifies emerging trends and issues in the states in areas such as aging family caregivers, the rise of a new wave of class action litigation associated with waiting lists for residential services, and the growth of the Medicaid Home and Community Based Services Waiver. The Waiver is the principal financial engine driving the growth of community services across the country today.

Part III is an in-depth comparative study of the development of institutional and community services in two states: Michigan and Illinois. These states were selected for study to illustrate the complex interplay of forces at work in shaping how long term care service system priorities are formulated and implemented in one component of the disability field: developmental disabilities. Michigan and Illinois are similar on many dimensions such as demography, personal income, and general midwestern moderate conservatism, but they differ dramatically from one another in that Michigan has emphasized extensive innovation in the community over the past two decades, while Illinois retained a substantial and more traditional commitment to public and private residential institutions. This study is a compelling "tale of two states"--rich in detailed documentation from interview, archival, and statistical sources.

The overarching theme across all three parts of the book is that the provision of services to people with disabilities in the United States today is the product of a complex interplay of historical and contemporary forces. Contemporary forces include the often competing interests of consumers with disabilities and family constituencies, unions, service providers and professionals along with elected political leaders, agency officials, and the dynamic economies of the states and the nation. Historical forces shaping current attitudes, interventions, and social policies toward people with disabilities include centuries of oppression, stigma, marginalization, and institutionalization interspersed with recurring and compelling examples of compassion and love, community and family support, scientific achievement and very recently, by the rising crescendo of voices of people with disabilities speaking for themselves.

David Braddock
Boulder, Colorado
April 16, 2002

ACKNOWLEDGMENTS

We acknowledge with appreciation the support of the Administration on Developmental Disabilities (ADD) and the National Institute on Disability and Rehabilitation Research (NIDRR). ADD supported, in part, the research leading to Parts II and III of the book--specifically the analysis of trends in the structure and financing of mental retardation and developmental disabilities services in the states. We especially appreciate the support of former ADD Commissioner Sue Swenson, current Commissioner Dr. Patricia Morrissey, and project officer Gretchen Menn. We are grateful to ADD for assisting us in the Project's transition from the University of Illinois at Chicago to the University of Colorado. We also gratefully acknowledge our productive collaboration on data collection with the state officials in each of the 50 states and the District of Columbia. These individuals are listed by name in an appendix to Part II of the book (pp. 137-140).

The NIDRR provided financial assistance to develop and pilot test a methodology to implement the collection of public sector financial and programmatic data from several states across the entire spectrum of mental and physical disability. This assistance, which led to the study reported in Part I, Chapter 2, was initially provided by the Distinguished Research Fellowship Program to the editor of this volume. The ADD subsequently supported a larger scale effort to implement the study on a nationwide basis.

Part III of the book is a condensation of Susan Parish's doctoral dissertation at the University of Illinois at Chicago's School of Public Health. This study has been honored nationally with a dissertation award by the American Academy on Mental Retardation. Members of the Parish dissertation committee included Professors David Braddock (chair), Glenn Fujiura, Carol Gill, Tamar Heller, and Christopher Keys.

Dr. Parish was a research associate on the State of the States in Developmental Disabilities Project from 1996-2001. Mary Kay Rizzolo worked closely with Susan in the condensation and editing of Part III along with Richard Hemp and Amy Pomeranz. Rick and Mary Kay both tirelessly proofread the entire manuscript and contributed in many other ways to the book's completion.

This volume of the State of the States is the first one produced in our new academic home at the University of Colorado. We are particularly appreciative of the support for our work provided by the Coleman Institute for Cognitive Disabilities, which is a component of the University of Colorado System's Office of the Vice President for Academic Affairs and Research. We are equally grateful for the support we received from the Department of Psychiatry at the University's Health Sciences Center campus in Denver. We specifically thank Dr. Robert Freedman and Anna John for their departmental support.

Peggy Seiter of Seiter-Vaughn Communications has, as always, been a pleasure to work with on the myriad editing and bookmaking tasks associated with the creation of the present volume. We appreciate the opportunity to be part of the publication program at the American Association on Mental Retardation, and always enjoy working with Executive Director Doreen Croser and Bruce Appelgren, the director of the Association's publication program.

PART I
Cross Disability Perspectives
Chapter 1

An Institutional History of Disability

David Braddock & Susan L. Parish

The primary objective of this chapter is to describe the history of disability in Western society, establishing explicit connections between the social context in which people have lived, and the ways in which disability has or has not been identified and addressed as a social problem. Our central thesis is that changing social and political perspectives on poverty during the 17th and 18th centuries, coupled with the development of increasingly medical interpretations of disability during the 19th and 20th centuries, contributed to the increasing segregation and stigmatization of persons with disabilities. However, a related thesis is that the congregation of people with similar disabilities for treatment and services also made possible the development of group identities, which ultimately facilitated the rise of political activism in the modern era. This chapter is a revision and update of a paper which previously appeared in the *Handbook of Disability Studies* (Braddock & Parish, 2001).

IMPAIRMENT AND DISABILITY

Throughout Western history disability has existed at the intersection between the particular demands of a given impairment, society's interpretation of that impairment, and the larger political and economic context of disability. The contrast between disability and impairment informs a key underlying premise of this chapter: disability exists as it is situated within the larger social context while impairment is a biological condition. Lennard Davis (2000) has succinctly described the relationship between disability and impairment as follows:

> Disability is not so much the lack of a sense or the presence of a physical or mental impairment as it is the reception and construction of that difference. . . An impairment is a physical fact, but a disability is a social construction. For example, lack of mobility is an impairment, but an environment without ramps turns that impairment into a disabil-

ity. . . a disability must be socially constructed; there must be an analysis of what it means to have or lack certain functions, appearance and so on. (p. 56)

Davis notes that disability was not constituted as a social category prior to the 18th century, even though impairments were no doubt quite prevalent in the general population.

Writing a history of disability in the West is a challenging undertaking. We will comment briefly on just three of the key problems facing researchers. First, the utilization of primary source evidence, the gold standard of historical research (Brundage, 1989; Schafer, 1980), is extremely limited in the literature, especially for periods preceding the 19th century (Brockley, 1999). Recent historical accounts of disability have relied more heavily on primary source documentation but have generally limited their focus to the institutional nature of service delivery in the United States beginning in the 19th century (Bredberg, 1999; Brockley, 1999; Ferguson, 1994; Trent, 1995; Wright & Digby, 1996). While the constraints of writing a disability history within the confines of a concise book chapter have forced us to utilize secondary sources frequently, primary sources have been utilized when possible to reveal the rich historical fabric of a diverse and varied existence.

A second limitation of many published historical accounts is that the archive mainly describes formal services and treatment approaches from the standpoint of the professionals who controlled the delivery of services (e.g., Barr, 1904; Earle, 1898; Obermann, 1968; Scheerenberger, 1983; Sheldon, 1921); this institutional perspective has often eclipsed the perspectives of persons with disabilities and even their families. The reliance on professionals' records has reflected and legitimated professional behavior (Hirsch, 1995). Historians, for example, have tended to rely on the public record of residential institutions, while largely ignoring lay perspectives toward disability (Jackson, 1998). Such a practice has occurred even though only a small fraction of the entire disabled population has ever been institutionalized, particularly prior to the 20th century. Moreover, people with disabilities have only infrequently recorded accounts of their experiences, so historians are left to interpret "lived experience" vicariously through the filter of professionals who did leave extensive records (Porter, 1987; Rushton, 1988). Historians, thus, are often put in the perilous position of interpreting the history of people with disabilities based on the claims of professionals, although this posture has been soundly rejected in recent years by the disability movement (Anspach, 1979; Carabello & Siegel, 1996; Shapiro, 1993; Ward & Schoultz, 1996), which today advances the philosophy of "nothing about us without us" (Charlton, 1998).

The third limitation is that histories of disability are rarely representative of a broad cross-disability perspective that depicts the historical interconnections across the full spectrum of mental, physical, and sensory disability. In this chapter, we will address disability history across this broad spectrum, but we will also explicitly examine the history of mental disability in greater depth.

FOREVIEW OF THE CHAPTER

The chapter begins with a discussion of the extensive presence of people with impairments in ancient times and moves forward chronologically to the present day. Ancient Western notions of impairment in Greece and Rome accepted the belief that persons with congenital impairments embodied the wrath of the gods and should be killed. Yet this view coexisted with the fact that those who acquired their disabilities later in life were often integrated into society as workers, citizens, and soldiers. During the Middle Ages, widespread belief in demonology as an etiology of impairment was counterbalanced by religious movements preaching compassion and support toward persons with disabilities. Development of the first residential institutions for persons with disabilities is traced to the Middle Ages as well.

In the early modern period through the close of the 18th century, disability was strongly influenced by the rise of the scientific method during the Renaissance and by changing public perceptions toward poverty and disability. The radical intellectual revolution born

of the Enlightenment, including scientists' subsequent emphasis on distinguishing mental illness from intellectual disability, is considered in some depth in this section of the chapter. Enlightenment thinking transformed fundamental concepts about the essential relationships among humans, nature, and God. This transformation involved the increasing legitimacy of science in society, and led to the ascendancy of physicians, educators, and caretakers in the lives of persons with disabilities. Scientific inquiry into the medical aspects of impairment has been characterized by the development and application of increasingly complex diagnostic and etiological classification schemes. This process of categorizing persons with disabilities into the minutiae of their impairments resulted in the development of specialized treatments and residential and educational services, but also established and reinforced notions of the boundaries between normalcy and aberrance in Western society.

Disability in the American colonies during the 17th and 18th centuries is examined along with the subsequent development and proliferation across Europe of institutions for persons with mental disabilities and schools for the deaf and blind. In the American colonies, and later in the United States, persons with impairments were often perceived to menace the economic well-being of the community. The practices of auctioning off the care of disabled persons to the highest bidder or running them out of town with threatened or real violence reflected an intimate connection between poverty and disability in this period of history.

Our discussion of disability history in the 19th century acknowledges the significance of political organization by deaf advocates--the first rumblings of activism by people with disabilities. That nascent movement sharply contrasted with the contemporaneous exploitation of people with disabilities as freak show attractions and the ascendancy of the eugenics era. The onset of the 20th century was marked by a dramatic expansion of residential institutions for persons with mental disabilities and by the rapidly increasing segregation of children and youth with disabilities in public schools. We trace developments for persons with physical disabilities, independent living, and the emergence of family, community, and consumer advocacy, and discuss litigation that forged a constitutional right to treatment for persons with mental disabilities in the United States. The chapter also discusses international disability rights initiatives such as the United Nation's Standard Rules, the Americans with Disabilities Act, and various European anti-discrimination legislation such as Great Britain's Disability Discrimination Act of 1995. The chapter concludes with a consideration of disability priorities in the 21st century.

ANTIQUITY

Prehistory

Individuals with physical impairments have been part of the social order since well before the evolution of humans. There is also anthropological evidence of impaired members living in prehistoric subhuman primate groups. Berkson (1993,1974) argues persuasively that:

> …Monkey and ape groups include individuals who have fallen from trees or who have been injured by predators. [They] may survive in natural animal groups when their injury does not actually interfere with foraging or escape from predators. In other words, the injury may not be handicapping.

Injured animals may survive and live in a group because group living itself can provide aid to adaptation. Mother monkeys provide care that compensates for even severe injuries, and other members of the group may "baby sit" injured babies, as they do other young of the group…where predation pressure is low and food is plentiful, handicapped animals may live to be adults. (1993, pp. 5-6)

Citing work by Solecki (1971) and Stewart (1958), Berkson (1993) describes a published description of an adult Neanderthal male with severe arm and head injuries incurred at an early age. He accommodated the injury by using his teeth to hold objects. Berkson also uncovered research documenting the fact that disabling arthritis and other chronic impairments were common in Neanderthals (Goldstein, 1969; Straus & Cave, 1957). He concludes that individuals with both minor and even highly significant impairments were part of primate societies "even before the evolu-

tion of modern Homo sapiens" (p. 6). Thus, the presence of impairments among subsequent prehistoric Homo sapiens should not surprise us.

The Old Testament

Documentation of the treatment and life experiences of people with impairments during the earliest periods of recorded history is extremely limited. Edicts about disability offer some insight into prevailing attitudes, but the messages that they convey are mixed. The Old Testament commanded "Thou shalt not curse the deaf nor put a stumbling block before the blind, nor maketh the blind to wander out of the path" (Leviticus 19:14). Daniels (1997) argues that this Hebraic command in Leviticus is the first attempt by any nation to legislate for the protection of the deaf. Daniels further asserts that deaf persons without speech were viewed as children under Hebrew law and provided with the same protections as children.

People were also reminded about their responsibilities toward one another with the injunction that "There will always be poor people in the land. Therefore, I command you to be openhanded toward your brothers and toward the poor and needy in your land" (Deuteronomy 15:11).

In contrast, the Old Testament also warned that:

> If you do not carefully follow His commands and decrees. . . all these curses will come upon you and overtake you: the Lord will afflict you with madness, blindness and confusion of mind. At midday, you will grope around like a blind man in the dark. (Deuteronomy 28:15, 28-29)

These paradoxical statements reflect competing attitudes toward disability. While society seems to have recognized a charitable obligation to people with disabilities, disability was also perceived as a punishment meted out by God. The belief that illness was inflicted by an angry deity or by a supernatural power was widespread among ancient peoples (Rosen, 1968). The Old Testament also supports the notion that people with disabilities were classified with prostitutes and menstruating women as unclean and were thereby prohibited from making sacrifices as priests. According to Stiker (1997), people with disabilities were allowed to otherwise participate in religious observances. The early Christian church, however, held that faith came from hearing (Romans 10:17), and therefore the deaf were necessarily without faith in the eyes of the church (Daniels, 1997).

In records dating back to 2000 BCE, the births of children with congenital impairments were used to predict future events for a community. In the Babylonian region, ancient Semitic Chaldean diviners of the future maintained a list of birth deformities and the specific prophetic meanings each foretold. The manifestation of disability was viewed as a portent of things to come (Warkany, 1959).

Ancient Greece and Rome

Average life expectancy in ancient Greece and Rome didn't generally exceed 37 and 44 years, respectively, for women and men. Due to the omnipresence of disease, war, poor prenatal care, malnutrition, and injury sustained during the hard work performed by most people, impairments and deformities were doubtless prevalent. Even such minor injuries as broken limbs would have produced disabling impairments in a majority of the population who were too poor to obtain medical care (Garland, 1995). As Garland has noted, "Life in the ancient world was nasty, brutish, and short. The most privileged were those who happened to be freeborn, well-to-do males in perfect health. But the overwhelming majority did not, of course, belong to that ideal category" (p.11).

In the midst of this society beset by endemic impairment, the Greeks and Romans had varied interpretations of persons with such conditions. Babies born with congenital deformities were often regarded as signs that their parents had displeased the gods. However, public support was available to individuals whose impairments precluded them from working. In some exceptional situations, having an impairment was not a barrier to attaining power. The Roman Emperor Claudius had significant congenital deformities, and Spartans elected a short-statured man as their king. In any case, care for persons with impairments would have been reserved for those few who were wealthy enough to afford it--disability for the vast majority of Greeks and Romans would have increased the extent to which they were marginalized and excluded from society and living in deprived economic conditions (Garland, 1995).

The notion that Greeks practiced infanticide of children with disabilities has been widely accepted (e.g., Mackelprang & Salsgiver, 1996; Scheerenberger, 1983; Woodill & Velche, 1995). However, this practice was not as widespread as has been believed (Garland, 1995). In ancient Greece and Rome, infanticide was practiced for economic reasons when there were too many children. In Sparta, however, children born with obvious physical deformities were put to death regardless of a family's means (Stiker, 1997; Warkany, 1959). Spartan law mandated the practice of killing newborns who had been born with deformities, while there is some limited evidence that Athenians may have been more inclined to raise such children (Garland, 1995). Infants with deformities were sometimes perceived to represent the anger of the gods, and murdering such babies was a sacrifice intended to mollify the gods.

> Aberrancy within the species not only threatens the future and continuation of this species, but also announces, threatens, signifies a condemnation by the gods: a condemnation of the group. . . an aberrancy within the corporeal order is an aberrancy in the social order. (Stiker, 1997, p. 40)

Stiker (1997) further notes that the subjection of infants with deformities to death by exposure was specifically for infants we would today say have physical disabilities. Infants with hearing impairments, vision impairments, and mental retardation were not categorized as "deformed," and were not put to death, except perhaps for those most profoundly limited intellectually who could have been "diagnosed" early on.

It is likely, however, that many children with physical impairments survived even in Sparta, because their impairments would not have been evident until they passed the age at which killing them would have been contemplated (Gaw, 1906b). Furthermore, adults with congenital disabilities were a presence in ancient Greece (Stiker, 1997). M.L. Edwards' (1996, 1997) reviews of the scant documentary records from ancient Greece indicates that deformity was not perceived as absolutely negative by the Greeks, but that this perspective was developed by historians during the 19th century, who applied contemporary contempt for people with disabilities to their assessment of the ancient world. She further concludes that the assumption that deformity in a child was automatically associated with economic burden is not appropriate, since many people with disabilities had jobs and earned income. It is difficult to determine from these conflicting records the extent to which the infanticide of children with disabilities was practiced; what is clear is that people with congenital disabilities, broadly defined, existed in society, indicating that infants with disabilities were not uniformly put to death.

Given high rates of disease and war, there was likely a higher prevalence of disability in ancient communities. Greeks who sustained injuries on the battlefield would often be expected to continue to fight, as mobility was not always a requisite for combat participation. Existing court records provide compelling evidence that the linkage between disability and entitlement to monetary support from the government was not absolute. Individuals with disabilities in Greece would have had to prove that they truly were economically needy, and not just physically disabled, in order to receive a small food grant (M.L. Edwards, 1997).

Greek records also substantiate a public acknowledgment of providing support for those who were classified as unable to work. Dating from at least the sixth century BCE, Athens offered modest public support for those individuals who were unable to work due to their impairments. The Constitution of Athens provides information regarding the process of providing this support:

> The Council inspects those who are disabled. For there is a law which bids those who possess less than three minai and who are incapacitated and incapable of work to undergo inspection by the Council, which is to give them two obols per day each at public expense. (Garland, 1995, p. 35)

Military medicine was in widespread use in ancient Greece as was public support of men disabled by war (Stiker, 1997). Pensions were granted to sol-

diers who had been injured in battle, and food was provided to others with disabilities who could prove their economic need. The conclusion that Edwards (1997) draws regarding the status of people with disabilities during ancient Greek times is telling:

> The consequences of physical handicaps varied according to the context and to the individual. Without a codified notion of 'able-bodied' on one hand and 'disabled' on the other, people were not automatically assigned to one category or the other on the basis of medical diagnosis or appearance. . . We see very few instances in which people with physical handicaps were banned a priori from certain roles. . .people with disabilities in Greek society were integral to the society. There is no indication that people with physical handicaps in the ancient Greek world identified themselves or were identified as a distinct minority group. (pp. 43-44)

Surviving historical and literary accounts have indicated that prosthetic devices were used by persons who sustained injuries during battle or had congenital limb malformations (Bliquez, 1983). Herodotous recounts a warrior amputating his own foot in order to free himself and escape his impending execution. In 479 BCE, this warrior supported himself fighting on the battlefield by using a wood prosthesis. In a tomb dating to 300 BCE, a skeleton was found with an artificial lower right leg. This prosthesis was made of bronze, indicating that its owner was a person of some wealth.

Early Roman law chiefly protected the property rights of people with disabilities. Persons who were designated as intellectually deficient in early Roman times were provided with guardians to assist in the management of their affairs (Winzer, 1993). Deaf persons capable of speech were granted authority to discharge legal obligations such as marriage and property ownership. Deaf persons without speech were classified alongside persons with intellectual disabilities, mental illness, and infants, and were forbidden to perform any legal acts (Gaw, 1906a, 1906b, 1907; Hodgson, 1953).

In the Roman Empire, short-statured slaves and

slaves with intellectual disabilities were often maintained by wealthy men for entertainment purposes. "Keeping" such individuals was considered good luck. The earliest records of court jesters date from Egyptian pharaohs of the Fifth Dynasty who kept short-statured people (Welsford, 1966/1935). Both ancient China and pre-Columbian American civilizations had short-statured people serve as court jesters as well (Willeford, 1969).

Later Roman law enumerated the specific rights of people with disabilities. In the sixth century CE, the Justinian Code classified persons with disabilities in detail and delineated rights pertaining to different types and degrees of disability; for example, people with mental disabilities were not permitted to marry. Drawing on the Jewish discrimination between degrees of deafness (Daniels, 1997), the Justinian Code identified five classes of deafness (Gaw, 1906a, 1906b, 1907). The Code became the basis of law in most European countries from the 6th to the 18th centuries.

Writings from the New Testament offer insight into attitudes about disability shortly after the time of Christ. Mark records Jesus' healing of a blind man by spitting and laying hands on the man's eyes (Marcus, 1999; Mark 8:22-26). Mark and Matthew also record Jesus' healing of a man with paralysis (Black, 1996; Mark 2:1-12; Matthew 8:5-13). The New Testament relates other stories of people with leprosy, epilepsy, mental illness, deafness, and blindness being healed by Christ (Black, 1996). These healing tales may be interpreted to mean that people "have disabilities... to show the power of God" (p. 29). When asked whether a blind man's sin or his parents' sin had caused the man's blindness, Jesus replied that it was neither, but rather a mechanism for "God's work [to be] revealed in him" (John 9:3). However, the fact that the disciples believed that the man's blindness was caused by sin may be indicative of prevailing wisdom regarding the supernatural etiology of this condition at the time.

Interpreting disability in antiquity is difficult in that the timespan considered is vast and competing attitudes toward disability are evident at many points. Writings from the Old Testament suggest paradoxical attitudes, which exhorted society to be generous and kind toward individuals with impairments, while also declaring that impairment was a mark of the wrath of God. Ancient Greece and Rome offer similarly com-plex interpretations of impairment. The killing of new-borns with congenital impairments existed in some form throughout Greece and Rome, and society clearly perceived the birth of a child with congenital anomalies as the mark of the anger of the gods. However, the provision of pensions to soldiers injured on the battlefield was also a part of ancient Athenian life, and citizens with impairments were widely known to have worked at different trades. Impairment at the time of Christ was similarly fraught with different meanings, offering both redemption opportunities for kind strangers and signifying superstition. In the ancient world, impairment was accepted, at least in part, as an aspect of the course of life.

MIDDLE AGES

In the fourth to sixth centuries CE, monastically inspired hospices for blind persons were established in what is now Turkey, Syria, and France. These hospices were organized as refuges for people with disabilities within existing religious enclaves (Winzer, 1993). Bishop Nicholas cared for persons with intellectual disabilities in a hospice in southern Turkey during the fourth century and the Belgian village of Gheel initiated the support of persons with mental disabilities in family-care settings in the 13th century (Stevens, 1858; Roosens, 1979). The latter community provided vocational opportunities in a community setting which included an infirmary and a church centered around the shrine of St. Dymphna (Kroll, 1973; Pollock, 1945; Rumbaut, 1972). By the sixth century CE, institutions to segregate people with Hansen's disease (leprosy) were developing sporadically. Germany and Italy had hundreds of these facilities by the Early Middle Ages (Weymouth, 1938; Howard, 1789).

Demonology

Many disabling conditions, including intellectual disability, mental illness, deafness, and epilepsy were thought to have supernatural or demonological causes during the Medieval period. The devil was believed to cause epilepsy (Alexander & Selesnick, 1964). Belief in demonic possession as a primary etiology of mental illness led to attempted cures based on religious ideas about exorcism (Clay, 1966; Neaman, 1978). Attempts to cure people with disabilities from early Medieval times reflect supernatural beliefs in the abilities of magic and religious elements. For instance, Anglo-Saxons offered the following antidote to mental illness:

> A pleasant drink against insanity. Put in ale hassock, lupine, carrot, fennel, radish, betony, water-agrimony, marche, rue, wormwood, cat's mint, elecampane, enchanter's nightshade, wild teazle. Sing twelve Masses over the drink, and let the patient drink it. He will soon be better. (Russell, 1980, p. 45)

Interest in persecuting witches developed gradually, culminating in the craze that began in 1450 (Russell, 1980). During the Middle Ages, the first heresy executions occurred in France in 1022, and thousands of so-called witches were subsequently executed (Russell, 1972). Persecution was frequently led by the Catholic Church, although Protestant European countries also followed Papal orders regarding the execution of witches. Pope Innocent IV authorized the seizure of heretics' goods, their imprisonment, torture, and execution (Russell, 1980). In 1484, Pope Innocent VIII declared war on witches (Russell, 1980). While it is acknowledged that disabled persons were among those who were persecuted, the extent to which this occurred is not known. It seems likely that persons whose impairments were not amenable to contemporary treatment, and particularly those with mental illness, would have been disproportionately affected by the witch craze (Winzer, 1993).

Some of those individuals later persecuted for witchcraft in colonial New England would have had mental illness, even given the crude understanding of mental illness at the time. Erikson (1966) recounts instances of clearly mentally disabled colonial women being put to death for their various crimes. American psychiatrists of the mid-19th century described colonial New England's witchcraft as manifestations of mental illness. These psychiatrists interpreted the persecution of people with mental illness as pitiable, but not necessarily peculiar. They expressed surprise that physicians misapplied the label "witch" to women who had mental illness ("Witchcraft and insanity," 1849).

Compassion and Support

In spite of the negative impact that widespread superstition had on people with disabilities during Medieval times, there is evidence that other attitudes about disabilities, and particularly mental illness, were also common (Kroll, 1973; Neugebauer, 1979; Rosen, 1968). Kroll (1973) argues that the absence of demonology in medical texts from the Medieval era, scattered advocates for the natural causes of mental illness, and town's assumption of responsibility for people with mental disabilities are strong evidence that demonological beliefs were only a part of the picture. However, views toward disability were complex and apparently included "elements of empirical rationality and humane interest" (Rosen, 1968, p. 139). Further evidence of positive, or at least sympathetic attitudes toward people with disabilities is manifested in the fact that some towns actually funded pilgrimages to distant religious sites for people with epilepsy and mental illness to seek cures (Rosen, 1968).

The relationship between poverty and disability during the Medieval period is also significant. Malnutrition and infectious diseases were endemic, doubtless contributing to significantly higher rates of impairment, making persons quite visible in their communities. The chances of living to adulthood averaged just 50% during the Medieval period (Jankauskas & Urbanavicius, 1998). In 13th-century France, Italy, and England, tax records indicate that as much as 75% of the population was too poor to pay taxes and was particularly susceptible to dire consequences if they became disabled (Farmer, 1998). This profound poverty meant that adults not capable of working were often a tremendous burden to their families. Even in families where both spouses worked, women often supplemented their low wages with begging (Farmer, 1998). In this context, begging by people with disabilities seems more related to their poverty than to their disability. Begging during the early Middle Ages was not stigmatized as it later would be. The existence of the poor was accepted as part of the natural order, and the poor were perceived to offer opportunities for wealthier citizens to do good by providing alms (Spierenburg, 1984). In this context, persons with disabilities doubtless had more widespread acceptance as part of the poor.

Evaluating records from the canonization of St. Louis provides extensive evidence that people with disabilities sought cures for their disabilities at his tomb, and that during the Medieval period people with disabilities survived by relying on a variety of supports: family members, neighbors, employers, charitable institutions, and begging (Farmer, 1998). Charitable institutions appear to have been the least likely source of support for people with disabilities, often only providing assistance until an individual was sufficiently recovered to leave the hospital and beg for alms. There is also evidence that family, friends, and neighbors, in addition to providing material support as they were able, would assist people with disabilities to beg in the streets even by carrying them if necessary (Farmer, 1998). The networks of support that appeared to exist, even for women who were recent immigrants, provide evidence that Medieval attitudes toward disability were more complex than is often believed, and not entirely negative.

Examining court records between the 13th and 17th centuries in England, Neugebauer (1978, 1979, 1996) found that demonological beliefs about the origins of brain disorders were not the only etiological beliefs held by society. The Crown's legal incompetency jurisdiction differentiated between intellectual disability (termed "natural fools" and later "idiots") and mental illness (termed "non compos mentis" and later "lunacy") (Neugebauer, 1996). The Prerogativa Regis in the latter half of the 13th century endowed the Crown with specific responsibilities for protecting the person and property of individuals whose mental disabilities rendered them legally incompetent. Differentiation of "idiots" and "lunatics" by the Prerogativa Regis enabled the Crown to take custody and profits generated from lands owned by "idiots." In the case of individuals with mental illness, the Crown had the responsibility to ensure the safekeeping of lands held by "lunatics." The Crown, however, was not entitled to profits generated by "lunatics'" lands that it supervised (Neugebauer, 1996).

Perhaps even more significantly, verbatim transcripts of custody hearings indicate that the means used to determine the presence of mental disability relied on tests of literacy, numerical ability, reasoning, knowledge as to place and kin, etc. (Neugebauer, 1996). The records of these examinations indicate that the essential questions utilized to determine the presence of mental disability were relatively constant from the 13th through the 17th centuries, indicating relative stability in the understanding of mental disability during this prolonged period (Neugebauer, 1996; Swinburne, 1590).

Residential Institutions Emerge

During the Middle Ages, Greek and Roman medical and philosophical traditions were introduced into Europe by the Arabs, who had conquered much of the continent and penetrated Spain and France. Asylums for people with mental disabilities had previously been established by the Arabs in Baghdad, Fez (Morocco) and Cairo in the eighth century and subsequently in Damascus and Aleppo in 1270 (Alexander & Selesnick, 1964). Since the Arabs held the general belief that mental disability was divinely inspired and not demonic in origin, care in these facilities was generally benevolent.

In England, the Priory of St. Mary's of Bethlehem was founded in 1247 in London with the explicit purpose of supporting the Order of Bethlehem by gathering alms to provide a base for members of the Order visiting from abroad (MacDonald, 1981). Although the Order may have begun supporting physically ill persons as a hospital as early as 1330, it didn't begin caring for mentally disabled persons, except perhaps incidentally and temporarily, until 1403. After this date mentally disabled persons gradually displaced the physically sick as the primary focus of the facility, but "…it was nearly a hundred years later before there is evidence that London's magistrates thought that only the mad should be admitted" (Andrews et al., 1997, p. 90). Today, Bethlehem Hospital is the longest continually operating mental hospital in Europe.

In Spain, a hospital dedicated exclusively to mental disability was founded by Father Joffre in Valencia in 1409 (Rumbaut, 1972). Other asylums also opened in 15th century Spain in Zaragoza (1425), Seville (1436), Valladolid (1436), Palma Majorca (1456), Toledo (1480), and in Granada in 1527 (Bassoe, 1945). A general hospital known to have housed persons with mental disabilities was also opened in Barcelona in 1412. No less an authority than France's great psychiatrist Phillipe Pinel believed Spain's asylums to be the world's most humanely and wisely administered mental hospitals from the 15th through the 18th centuries. In Traité Médico-Philosophique sur l'alienation Mentale (1809), he specifically cited the excellence of the Zaragoza asylum, "the founders of which aimed to construct mental disorder by charm inspired by the cultivating of fields, the instinct which prompts people to render the earth fertile and secure the fruits of their industry" (Pinel, 1809, p. 238).

A madhouse was constructed as part of the Georghospital in Elbing in 1326, in what is modern-day Germany. The Grosse Hospital in Erfurt, Germany included a "mad hut" when it was constructed in 1385. Prior to the building of separate facilities for people with mental illness, general hospitals or infirmaries accepted people with mental disorders (Rosen, 1968). However, given the lack of care institutions during the Medieval era, people with mental disabilities must have been a relatively common presence in their communities (Digby, 1996).

It has become part of the lore that people with mental disabilities were cast out to sea in so-called Ships of Fools during the Middle Ages (Maher & Maher, 1982). The notion of the ship of fools was created in 1494 with the publication in German of a book of the same name by Brant (Swain, 1932). There is no evidence that these ships actually existed, however (Maher & Maher, 1982). Brant was a preacher who used the fool as a metaphorical device to rebuke his congregation to be pious (Swain, 1932).

During the 12th century, institutions for the quarantine of people with Hansen's disease (leprosy) became prolific (MacArthur, 1953). Howard (1789) chronicles the existence of numerous facilities, termed "leprosariums," throughout Europe, many of which evolved as part of the charitable work done by religious orders (Kipp, 1994). This confinement experience with leprosy represents the first time that institutional, segregated facilities were systematically utilized in Europe to address the issues presented by people with disabilities. Isolation of lepers was a harbinger of the perceived merits of segregation and confinement of other disabled populations, although institutional treatments for people with disabilities other than leprosy were slower to develop. As leprosy virtually disappeared in Europe by the 16th century (Weymouth, 1938), many converted leprosariums became privately operated madhouses for people with mental illness, and in some cases, for persons with intellectual disabilities (Alexander & Selesnick, 1964). Leprosy, however, subsequently spread to the Americas and had a substantial impact. De Souza-Araujo (1937, 1946, 1948) has described in great detail the spread of leprosy from Portugal, Spain, France, Holland, and Africa to Brazil beginning in the 15th century. The first Brazilian leprosarium opened in Rio de Janeiro in 1766, followed by the establishment of scores of such facilities nationwide.

During the Middle Ages, begging was a common way for people with disabilities to support themselves when their families were unable or unwilling to do so. Guilds and brotherhoods of blind beggars were organized to address issues of competition and conflict (Covey, 1998; French, 1932). One of the strongest guilds was developed in 1377 in Padua, Italy. This guild regulated begging and organized pensions for elderly blind beggars (Covey, 1998; Gowman, 1957). As the active role of the Catholic Church in promoting charity diminished following the Reformation, "little of the medieval fabric of hospices, almshouses and refuges" was left for care of "unfortunates" (Porter, 1987, p. 121). Since monastic institutions were seized by the government during the Reformation, and charity concomitantly diminished, the number of beggars increased dramatically. The passage of the Elizabethan Poor Law in England in 1601 was enacted partly in response to the large number of beggars (Covey, 1998). And in 1657, Paris outlawed begging within its city limits (Foucault, 1965).

In summary, the Middle Ages were notable for the contradictory beliefs held about disability. One common conception of disability was that some disabilities, particularly deafness, epilepsy, and mental disabilities, had demonological origins. This point of view contributed to the persecution of people with disabilities as witches and the use of magic to attempt to cure the disabling condition. A second conception of disability was also widespread — that persons with disabilities were part of the natural order, situated with other poor people and subject to the random havoc occasioned by the plagues in Europe. Stiker (1997) argues that the widespread nature of the plagues actually de-emphasized difference (impairment) more than in any epoch. There is significant evidence that people with disabilities used networks of support in their communities to survive in times that were harsh for nearly everyone. These two competing aspects of disability in Medieval society appear to have coexisted, lending credence to the claim that there wasn't a universal definition or interpretation of disability through this period.

EARLY MODERN PERIOD THROUGH THE 18th CENTURY

Renaissance and the Scientific Method

In the 14th through 16th centuries, beginning primarily in Italy, humanism in art was accompanied by advances in the anatomical and physiological study of hearing, vision, and the human body by Versalius, Da Vinci, William Harvey, and others (P. Edwards, 1996). In the mid-16th century, Girolamo Cardano pioneered instructional approaches for people with hearing and visual impairments. He also attacked the prevailing practice of witch hunting (Gannon, 1981; Wright, 1969). While the last witchcraft execution in England took place in 1684, English laws halting the persecution of witches were not repealed until 1736 (Russell, 1980).

In spite of the advances in human understanding that were secured during the Renaissance, beliefs in the bestial nature of, and possession by, people with mental disabilities continued during the early modern period. During the 16th century, Reformation leaders John Calvin and Martin Luther independently preached that persons with mental disabilities were possessed or created by Satan (Colon, 1989; Kanner, 1964).

During the Renaissance, voluntary beatings of the head were employed to treat people with many mental diseases, including depression, paralysis, and intellectual disability (Bromberg, 1975). Physicians would also bore holes in the head or purge persons with mental disabilities to release the "stones" or "black bile" thought to cause illness (Gilman, 1982). Treatment for epilepsy included the ingestion of a mountain goat's brain or the still-warm gall of a dog killed at the moment of the seizure (Tuke, 1878, 1968/1882). One treatment of deafness consisted of frying earthworms

with goose-grease and dropping the solution into the ears (Winzer, 1993). While these endeavors to cure illness and disability seem fantastic by today's standards, they focused on biological etiologies and treatments, and therefore signified a change in the prevailing beliefs that the causes of disability and illness were supernatural. Cures during this period were related to primitive understandings of anatomical functions, and to physicians' abilities to intervene to address bodily difference and dysfunction.

Analysis of an array of legal records in England during the early modern period indicates that society perceived two groups of people with mental disabilities, the "safe" and the "dangerous." The safe would have included most people with intellectual disabilities and many people with mental illness who weren't perceived to be violent (Fessler, 1956; Rushton, 1988; Suzuki, 1991). These individuals were cared for largely by their families, with an unclear and diverse amount of assistance from their local communities. The "dangerous" of the mentally ill were either cared for by their relatives, by local constables, or by sending them to a house of correction (Suzuki, 1991).

In early modern England, there is further evidence that the general understanding of intellectual disability was understood to arise from birth and to be relatively fixed, whereas people understood that mental illness often had an onset in later life and could be quite transitory. While there were ambiguities in philosophical, medical, and legal interpretations of intellectual disability, fundamental aspects of differentiation clearly existed (Andrews, 1998). The perceived need to differentiate between mental illness and intellectual disability seems to be more related to the application of property law than to treatment, which was essentially non-existent at this time.

An important development of the 16th century was the initiation of education of deaf persons, which began in Spain and the Turkish Ottoman Court. In Spain, instruction began with deaf aristocratic children who had been hidden in monasteries and convents by their wealthy families. This education was undertaken by the monks with whom they lived (Plann, 1997). During the next century, deaf education in Spain was still limited to the wealthy classes, but it moved beyond the monasteries. In 1620, Juan Pablo Bonet of

Madrid published the first treatise on the education of the deaf (Gannon, 1981; Whitney, 1949; Wright, 1969). Sixty years later, George Dalgarno published the first finger alphabet designed specifically for deaf persons (Wright, 1969).

Miles (2000) found that deaf persons employed in the Turkish Ottoman court were actually training one another in the use of sign language as early as 1500 and for the next two centuries. Their signing system became popular and was used regularly by hearing people including Sultans and diplomats. Miles (2000) observed that:

> The use of this language, and the training of deaf people by deaf people for responsible employment in a highly privileged but risky environment, was evidently developing from the early sixteenth century at a time when Western Europeans very seldom thought deaf people could be educated or could make any useful contribution to society. (p.129)

The English statesman and philosopher Francis Bacon (1900/1605) believed that the supernatural and speculative philosophies of the Middle Ages and Renaissance had contributed nothing to the advancement of knowledge. He was impressed with the revolutionary discoveries of Copernicus and Galileo, who, for the first time, had proven certain characteristics of the universe. He was impressed with Marco Polo's travels and with the invention of gun powder. Bacon introduced the notion of science as systematic study. He called for experiments to be conducted based on the collection of empirical data (Bacon, 1900/1605; Park & Daston, 1981). The secrets of nature could be revealed, he argued, by the systematic observation of its regularities. In 1605, Bacon published *Advancement of Learning, Divine and Humane*. In it, he refuted the notion of divine punishment as a cause of mental illness. He suggested four lines of inquiry that would guide psychological research for the next 300 years: studies of mental faculties and the interaction of body and mind; individual case studies; anatomical inquiry and postmortem studies; and the interaction between society and the individual.

Poverty and Disability

A profound change in attitudes toward poverty occurred across Europe during the 13th through 17th centuries that would have an impact on people with disabilities. Poverty had traditionally been associated with followers of Jesus in the Christian European countries, and beggars represented a means for almsgivers to please God (Spierenburg, 1984). Ideas about the changing perception of poverty, from a necessary and even blessed state to a curse, began to slowly evolve from the 13th century. By the 16th century, this transformation was more or less complete and poor people were deemed suspect. This metamorphosis of attitudes resulted in the eventual development of incarcerating facilities for the poor, and particularly for people with mental illness (Spierenburg, 1984). As previously noted, begging was outlawed in the streets of Paris in 1657, further marginalizing people with disabilities and separating them from what had been an important source of income for centuries.

England's Poor Law of 1601 was a watershed that specifically designated responsibility for poor and other people unable to provide for themselves. If a person was unable to procure a living for him or herself, the first line of responsibility was his or her family. Barring the possibility of family provision of support, local communities were charged with providing for such persons in need (Rushton, 1988, 1996). "[C]ompetent sums of money for and towards the necessary relief of the lame, impotent, old, blind, and such other among them" were to be set aside by the local community (43 Elizabeth 1601, cited in Axinn & Levin, 1982, p. 10). These laws became the general model in the American colonies, and local responsibility for people with disabilities who were unable to provide their own care was the common practice (Axinn & Levin, 1982).

During the early modern and Renaissance periods, a complex relationship existed between community support, religious and medical institutions, and family resources in coping with mental disability (Adair et al., 1997). While the implementation of English Poor Law was distinguished by the provision of relief in the community, on the Continent the provision of public welfare "was usually within the context of structures likely to produce a sense of social stigma and alien-ation. Continental institutions are thus seen as com-pulsory and segregated from the outside world, and characterized by day-to-day procedures inherently de-humanizing" (Cavallo, 1998, p. 91). During the early modern period in Italy, for example, there is evidence that people with disabilities sought admission to hos-pitals for the poor in large numbers, and were thereby subject to stigmatization.

English administrative records of the overseers of the poor indicate that people with intellectual dis-ability were widely supported through the Poor Law, and policies of relief were relatively well-organized during the early modern period (Rushton, 1996). People with mental illness fared differently from those with intellectual disability. While most people with dis-abilities remained in the community with their families, there is evidence that people with mental illness were more likely to be incarcerated in gaols and houses of correction than their peers with intellectual disability (Rushton, 1996). What is particularly important about the administration of welfare at this time is that it "marked a shift from the predominantly familial sys-tem that dominated the medieval period" (Rushton, 1988, p. 34). Examining welfare records in England, Rushton found that custodial care was virtually never contemplated for people with intellectual disability or mental illness, but families sought relief when their pov-erty was related to the impairment of a family mem-ber.

The first almshouse in the United States was es-tablished in Boston in 1662 and served a heteroge-neous population including persons with physical and mental disabilities, blind persons, deaf persons, the poor, the elderly, and orphans. However, the devel-opment of institutions for disabled persons was slow in the United States until the 1820s (Rothman, 1990). Privately operated "madhouses" also began to spread across Britain during the Enlightenment period (Parry-Jones, 1972). The first English workhouse was estab-lished in Bristol in 1697. By the end of the 18th cen-tury, there were 127 workhouses in England alone. Contagious invalids were turned away from work-houses but people with mental disabilities were not. Workhouses spread rapidly across Europe by the beginning of the 19th century (Foucault, 1965). In spite of the spread of institutional care for people with men-tal illness in England between 1650-1850, families re-mained the main source of support during this period for poor people with mental illness (Suzuki, 1998).

Philosophical Enlightenment

The "Enlightenment" or "Age of Reason" is a cul-tural historian's term for revolutionary changes in think-ing that began in Europe in the 17th century. The En-lightenment represented the intellectual platform for the rise of contemporary Western civilization, and drew heavily from the contributions of Francis Bacon, Isaac Newton, and John Locke. Two themes in Enlighten-ment thinking are related to changes in the care and treatment of people with disabilities. First, a "sensa-tionalist" theory of knowledge laid the foundation for bold new psychological and educational interventions by arguing that experience and reason – rather than innate ideas – were the sources of all knowledge, and that social and environmental modification could thus improve humans and society by manipulating society and the environment (Condillac, 1930/1754; Locke, 1690). The second Enlightenment idea of importance to people with disabilities was the growing belief in the merits of natural science to advance the species (P. Edwards, 1996).

The Enlightenment's sensationalist school of phi-losophy spawned changes in attitudes, new institutions, voluntary charitable societies, interest groups, and lit-erary work. In 1656 in Paris, the great "Hôpital Gen-eral," France's charitable hospital, was formed as a single, semi-judicial administrative entity out of sev-eral existing establishments including the Salpêtriere and the Bicêtre (mental hospitals for women and men, respectively), and several smaller general hospitals (Andrews et al., 1997). The first public charity hospi-tal in France had opened in Lyons in 1612 and func-tioned in an analogous manner (Foucault, 1965). Con-finement no doubt accelerated in Paris with the enact-ment of the aforementioned edict in 1657 that prohib-ited begging.

Thus, poverty, disability, and the inability to work came to rank prominently among the major problems of the city. The soon to emerge "sensationalist" phi-losophies of the Enlightenment, however, provided the moral imperative and the tools for new and construc-tive interventions with the interconnected problem of disability and poverty (Winzer, 1986).

Distinguishing Between Intellectual Disability and Mental Illness

While English property law differentiated between intellectual disability and mental illness beginning in the 13th century, John Locke's 1690 *Essay Concerning Human Understanding* presented the most influential distinction to date between "idiots and madmen":

> . . . the defect in [idiots] seems to proceed from want of quickness, activity, and motion in the intellectual faculties, whereby they are deprived of reason: whereas mad men seem to suffer by the other extreme. For they do not appear to me to have lost the faculty of reasoning: but having joined together some ideas very wrongly . . . they argue right from wrong principles. . . But there are degrees of madness as of folly; the disorderly jumbling [of] ideas together, is in some more, and some less. In short, herein seems to lie the difference between idiots and mad men, that mad men put wrong ideas together, and so make wrong propositions, but argue and reason right from them: but idiots make very few or no propositions, but argue and reason scarce at all. (p. 236)

Although Rushton (1996) argued that Locke merely "provides a gloss on the pre-existing legal concepts rather than a critical challenge to them" (p. 50), he also acknowledges that Locke had a significant influence on Blackstone's later legal interpretations of intellectual disability. Goodey (1996) credits Locke with establishing the dichotomy between mental illness and intellectual disability that ultimately influenced social policy doctrine for people with intellectual disability. Even before Locke, in 1614, the Portuguese physician Montalto wrote a major medical work in which he distinguished mental illness from intellectual disability, and described the diagnosis, prognosis, and treatment for intellectual disability (Woolfson, 1984). This work, written while Montalto was personal physician to Italian Grand Duke Ferdinand I, has been largely ignored by historians.

Swinburne's definition of intellectual disability, published a century earlier, in 1590, is important as well, in that it points to the importance of basic reasoning ability and suggests the elements of an assessment test to evaluate the provenance of "idiocy":

> An idiote or a naturall foole is he who notwithstanding he bee of lawfull age, yet he is so witlesse, that he can not number to twentie, nor can tell what age he is of, nor knoweth who is his father, or mother, nor is able to answer to any such easie question. Whereby it may plainelye appeare that he hath not reason to discerne what is to his profite or damage, though it be notorious, nor is apt to be informed or instructed by anie other. Such an Idiote cannot make any testament nor may dispose either of his lands, or goodes. (p. 39)

Shortly after Locke penned his 1690 essay, Daniel Defoe, journalist and the author of Robinson Crusoe, recommended, to no avail, creating government-sponsored residential institutions for persons with intellectual disabilities, to be paid for with an author's tax (Defoe, 1894/1694; Goodey, 1996). In 1720, Defoe also made a real deaf-mute person the hero in his book *The Life and Adventures of Mr. Duncan Campbell*, and he described sign language and approaches to deaf education in considerable detail.

Institutions for People With Mental Illness Established

In 1700, county asylums for "idiots, blind, and cripples" were proposed in England (Anonymous, 1700). Parliament enacted a law in 1714 authorizing confinement, but not treatment, for the "furiously mad," and exempted them from the whippings routinely applied to rogues, beggars, and vagabonds. In 1704, Bethlem Hospital had 130 residents. There were 64 admissions and 50 persons were cured and discharged that year (Strype, 1720). Bethel and St. Luke's Mental Hospitals opened in Norwich in 1724 and in London in 1751, respectively. British Parliament repealed the witchcraft acts in 1736, and pressure mounted to improve conditions in the private madhouses. A statute was enacted regulating madhouses in 1774, and this was followed by a major Parliamentary inquiry in 1815-1816 covering England, Scotland, and Ireland. According to one noted British authority, glaring deficiencies were noted between the best practices delineated in books about mental disability and actual conditions found in such facilities (Parry-Jones, 1972).

In the 18th century, madhouses and criminal prisons were combined facilities in what is modern-day Germany. In these facilities, inmates were expected to work to contribute to the upkeep and expenses of the facility, particularly women through spinning (Spierenburg, 1984). In Holland and Germany, private confinement was sought by wealthier families for their relatives with mental illness, frequently to avoid dishonor to the family by the person's behavior (Spierenburg, 1984).

While the institutionalization of people with mental illness who were violent began during the 15th century, by the 18th century, facilities accepted people with mental illness who were not violent (Spierenburg, 1984). This was the case in England, Germany, Holland, France, and Spain as well as in the New Spain (Mexico).

Developments in the American Colonies and Early United States

In colonial America, the first petition to secure payment for the guardianship of a person with intellectual disability was submitted to England's King Charles I in 1637. Support was sought for custody of Benoni Buck of Virginia (Harris, 1971; Hecht & Hecht, 1973; Neugebauer, 1987). However, Puritans in colonial America still believed that disability was a result of God's divine displeasure (Covey, 1998). Increase Mather, president of Harvard and father of witchcraft zealot Cotton Mather, wrote about the birth of children with disabilities as evidence of God's retribution. His son Cotton Mather later preached and wrote the same (Covey, 1998; Winship, 1994).

The American colonies largely appropriated English laws for their governance, including the Poor Law initially passed in 1601 under Queen Elizabeth. Since towns had ultimate responsibility for the poor under the law, communities took steps to discourage "vagabonds, beggars, or idle persons" (Peterson, 1982, p.

109) from settling therein. People who were considered likely to become a public charge would be "warned out" of town, with public whipping — the penalty for not leaving. People with mental illness were particularly susceptible to being warned out; however, there is also evidence that they received public support. The earliest provision for the maintenance of a mentally disabled individual in the Pennsylvania colony, for example, dates to 1676. In that year, the Upland Court in Delaware County, Pennsylvania, ordered that "a small Levy be Laid to pay for the buildings of ye house and the maintaining of ye said madman according to the laws of ye government" (Morton, 1897, p. 4).

In 1752, with leadership from the physician Thomas Bond and Benjamin Franklin, the first general hospital was established in the American colonies in Philadelphia. Care for persons with mental illness was a major motive in the founding of this hospital. The principal argument expressed in the petition filed with the Pennsylvania Provincial Assembly and subsequently embodied in the authorizing legislation of May 11, 1751, was to address the growing problem of mental disability in the colony. The petition read as follows:

To the honourable House of Representatives of the Province of Pennsylvania, The Petition of sundry Inhabitants of the said Province, Humbly showeth,

THAT with the Numbers of People, the number of Lunaticks or Persons distempered in Mind and deprived of their rational Faculties, hath greatly encreased in this Province.

That some of them going at large are a Terror to their Neighbours, who are daily apprehensive of the Violences they may commit; And others are continually wasting their Substance, to the great Injury of themselves and Families, ill disposed Persons wickedly taking Advantage of their unhappy Condition, and drawing them into unreasonable Bargains, &c.

That few or none of them are so sensible of their Condition, as to submit voluntarily to the Treatment their respective Cases require, and therefore continue in the same deplorable State during their Lives; whereas it has been found, by the Experience of many Years, that above two Thirds of the Mad People received into Bethlehem Hospital, and there treated properly have been perfectly cured.

Your Petitioners beg Leave farther to represent, that tho' the good Laws of this Province have made many compassionate and charitable Provisions for the Relief of the Poor, yet something farther seems wanting in Favour of such, whose Poverty is made more miserable by the additional Weight of a grievous Disease, from which they might easily be relieved, if they were not situated at too great a Distance from regular Advice and Assistance; whereby many languish out their Lives tortur'd perhaps with the Stone, devour'd by the Cancer, deprived of Sight by Cataracts, or gradually decaying by loathsome Distempers; who, if the Expense in the present manner of Nursing and Attending them separately when they come to Town were not so discouraging, might again, by the judicious Assistance of Physic and Surgery, be enabled to taste the Blessings of Health, and be made in a few Weeks, useful Members of the Community, able to provide for themselves and Families.

The kind Care our Assemblies have heretofore taken for the Relief of sick and distempered Strangers, by providing a Place for their Reception and Accommodation, leaves us no Room to doubt their showing an equal tender Concern for the Inhabitants. And we hope they will be of Opinion with us, that a small Provincial Hospital, erected and put under proper Regulations, in the Care of Persons to be appointed by this House, or otherwise, as they shall think meet, with Power to receive and apply the charitable Benefactions of good People towards enlarging and supporting the same, and some other Provisions in a Law for the Purposes above mentioned, will be a good Word, acceptable to God and to all the good People they represent. (Morton, 1897, p. 8)

Initially, cells in the basement of the hospital's temporary quarters were set aside for persons with mental disabilities. Four years later, a special wing in the hospital was utilized for this purpose and in 1836, the cornerstone of a separate building was laid for the Pennsylvania Hospital for the Insane ("A sketch," 1845). In its first years, the treatment of persons with mental disabilities in the Pennsylvania Hospital consisted of an assault on the body and the senses. Morton's (1897) comprehensive history of the hospital describes the treatment of "phrenze" in 1791 as consisting of being:

> …drenched or played upon, alternately with warm and cold water (which may have accounted for some of the pulmonary fatalities elsewhere mentioned). Their scalps were shaved and blistered; they were bled to the point of snycope; purged until the alimentary canal failed to yield anything but mucous, and, in the intervals, they were chained by the wrist, or the ankle to the cell wall. (p.125)

The noted American psychiatrist Benjamin Rush may have introduced some improvements in care during his nearly 30 years of continuous service at the hospital between 1783-1813, but he is most widely remembered for introducing two mechanical contrivances for treatment (Rush, 1812). One, called a gyrator or revolving machine, was used in cases of "torpid madness" to spin the body and raise the heart rate to 120 beats per minute. A second device, the tranquilizing chair, was intended to reduce sensorimotor activity and reduce the pulse. Rush, the only physician signee of the Declaration of Independence, also prescribed bloodletting, a common medical practice he learned in his studies at Edinburgh University, along with low diet, purges, emetics, cold and shower baths (Morton, 1897, p. 164).

Veterans of the Revolutionary War were the first people with disabilities in the new United States to receive a pension, providing compensation for war-related impairments. In 1776, the first national pension law was adopted, and the sentiment of the Continental Congress reveals compassionate and concerned attitudes regarding those men whose impairments were sustained during the war:

> Permit not him, who, in the pride and vigor of youth, wasted his health and shed his blood in freedom's cause, with desponding heart and palsied limbs to totter from door to door, bowing his yet untamed soul, to meet the frozen bosom of reluctant charity (Glasson, as cited in Obermann, 1968, p. 137).

One of the first American states to establish provisions for people with intellectual disability and mental illness was Kentucky. In 1793, the state passed legislation authorizing payment to families too poor to continue caring for members with either mental illness or intellectual disability without assistance (Estabrook, 1928). A trial system for determining the person's identity as an "idiot" or "lunatic," as well as the person's need for such support, was established. This pension system continued throughout the 19th century, and was still in existence in 1928. Annual payments remained at $75 from 1870 to 1928 (Estabrook, 1928). It is noteworthy that professionals felt that the use of this pension encouraged idleness in people with intellectual disabilities, and that the only appropriate form of support was institutionalization (Estabrook, 1928).

Another American response to meeting the need for care of people with mental disabilities that could not be met by their families was the practice of "bidding out." In this system, a person with mental illness or intellectual disabilities was auctioned off to the lowest bidder, who would receive the bid amount to provide care for a year. This practice of "bidding out" was administered by counties in many states for people with intellectual disability and mental illness until about the 1820s, when it was perceived to become too expensive (Breckinridge, 1939). Bidding out was a common form of welfare throughout the nation (Peterson, 1982).

Schools for Deaf and Blind Persons Opened in Europe

The 18th century saw the gradual proliferation of residential schools for both deaf and blind persons. Schools for the deaf began in Spain and France and gradually spread to other European countries and the United States. The roots of deaf education began in North Central Spain with Pedro Ponce de León, a Benedictine monk working in the monastery of San Salvador de Oña in the province of Burgos. He is credited with being the first teacher of the deaf in the Western world. The exact date he began his work is not known, but by the mid-16th century he had initiated a school within the monastery for his students, many of whom were the children of wealthy Spanish families. He apparently utilized a manual alphabet and conventional signing and instructed about 20 students (Daniels, 1997). After de León's death in 1584, Juan Pablo Bonet further disseminated de León's methods, publishing in 1620 in Spanish *The Art of Teaching the Deaf to Speak*. This book is recognized as fully derivative of de León's work; however, no original manuscripts of de León's earlier contributions have been located to date (Daniels, 1997).

Ponce de León's methods appeared in mid-18th century France carried forward by Charles Michael de l'Epée. De l'Epée, a Paris priest, established the world's first public residential school for deaf persons in Paris in 1755 (Gannon, 1981; Minski, 1957; Wright, 1969). By 1783 the School had 68 pupils (Daniels, 1997). Signs were the communication technique preferred by de l'Epée (instead of the oral communication championed by his rival Péreiere), and the support provided for his school by the king had a lasting influence on deaf communication (Lane, 1989; Sacks, 1989).

In 1760, Thomas Braidwood established the first British school in Edinburgh, Scotland (Gannon, 1981; Minski, 1957; Wright, 1969). The first school for deaf persons in Germany was opened in 1778 in Leipzig by Samuel Heinicke. Abba Silvestri opened the first Italian school for deaf persons in Rome in 1784 (Gannon, 1981). Germany's Heinicke favored "pure oralism", in the belief that articulation was necessary for deaf people to obtain respected status in society (Gannon, 1981; Minski, 1957; Wright, 1969).

Abbé de l'Epée believed that deaf persons were representative of primordial ancestors, not unlike Rousseau's (1991/1762) notion of "man in the state of nature," and that their silence made them extremely similar to the first people on earth. He invited the public to visit his school, with the intent that doing so facilitated insight into the "natural path of human mental and linguistic development" (Rosenfeld, 1997, p. 157). Scientists and statesmen from Europe and the United States visited his school and Enlightenment philosophers were intrigued with his educational methods and the unique opportunity represented by studying deaf persons and their sign language.

Although de l'Epée believed that sign language was a primitive form of communication, he believed that it was effective for deaf people. De l'Epée died in 1789 and was succeeded by the Abbé Sicard, who had previously headed a school for the deaf founded in the Bordeaux region of France in 1786. Sicard subsequently hosted Thomas Gallaudet of the United States during the latter's visit to Paris in 1816, and assisted Gallaudet in establishing the first school for the deaf in the United States (in Hartford, Connecticut) the following year.

In 1784, Valentin Haüy opened the first residential school for blind students in Paris (Allen, 1899; Farrell, 1956; Roberts, 1986). He developed the first embossed print and used it to teach reading. The first school for blind students in England was opened in Liverpool in 1791 by Edward Rushton. Between 1804-1820, schools for blind children and youth opened in Vienna, Steglitz (Germany), Milan, Amsterdam, Prague, Stockholm, St. Petersburg, Dublin, Copenhagen, Aberdeen, Brussels, Naples, and Barcelona (Farrell, 1956). The first U.S. institutions for blind students were opened in Boston (Perkins Institute) and in New York City in 1832. Pennsylvania followed one year later and Ohio opened a public school for blind students in 1837 (Allen, 1899, 1914; French, 1932).

The Early Modern period through the 18th century was a time of far-reaching change for persons with disabilities. Systematic differentiation between people with mental illness and intellectual disability was established to ensure correct adjudication of property laws. Comprehensive education of deaf and blind children began in Spain and France, respectively. This period saw the first manifestations of criminalizing and regulating idleness and poverty, which had a direct impact on people with disabilities who were usually poor. Institutional solutions to the problems ostensibly posed by poverty and disability — houses of correction, workhouses, asylums, and madhouses — be-

came more common as the 18th century ended. The intellectual revolution of the Renaissance and Enlightenment contributed to fundamental changes in the relationships between humans, society, and God. For the first time, people were deemed to be capable of intervening in what had been perceived to be the immutable natural order: a belief that society and human beings could be perfected. This revolution in thinking stimulated extensive efforts to develop treatment interventions for people with disabilities, including the deaf, blind, and people with mental disabilities, and it led to the ascendancy of a professional class of physicians, educators, and caretakers. The medicalization and professionalization of disability reinforced the development and proliferation of institutions and schools across Europe and subsequently in North America. The trend toward institutionalization would gain greater momentum during the 19th and 20th centuries.

THE 19th CENTURY

Educational Developments

Residential schools for deaf and blind students grew rapidly during the 19th century, as did institutionalized segregation of people with mental illness and intellectual disability. Therapeutic advances occurred for people with speech impairments, and controversy developed regarding two competing philosophies for educating deaf persons — oralism and manualism.

Schools for children with physical disabilities opened somewhat later in Europe than did those for deaf and blind students. The first school designed exclusively for children with physical disabilities was opened in 1832 in Bavaria by John Nepinak. Schools subsequently opened in other parts of Germany, France, England, Switzerland, and Italy. Denmark established the first program of industrial training for children with physical disabilities. A program of segregation in workshops became common in European schools by the middle of the 19th century (Obermann, 1968).

In 1829, Louis Braille published an explanation of his embossed dot code which was an improvement on a system developed by Barbier in 1808 (French, 1932; Roberts, 1986). Competing systems of communication would exist until 1932 when American and

British committees finally signed an agreement to adopt Standard English Braille as the uniform type (Roberts, 1986). In 1858, the American Printing House for the Blind was chartered in Louisville, Kentucky. This organization would become the premier printer of materials for blind persons in the United States, and in 1879, Congress legislated an annual appropriation of $10,000 for the printing of educational materials for blind persons (Allen, 1914; American Printing House for the Blind, 1999).

An intimate link between the fields of deafness and intellectual disability developed at the dawn of the 19th century. In 1800, Jean Itard (1775-1850) joined the medical staff at Sicard's National Institution for Deaf Mutes in Paris in order to study speech and hearing. The previous summer, a feral child was discovered in southern France and scholars in Paris were anxious to examine him in the belief that the boy approximated "man in the state of nature." Thus, basic philosophical questions about human learning and development prominent in French Enlightenment thinking of the day could be systematically studied. Since the "wild boy" was mute, he was placed in the school for deaf persons in Paris. Pinel, who first examined the boy at the Bicêtre, was initially convinced that the boy, later named Victor, was unteachable. However, Itard committed the next five years of his life to instructing Victor, utilizing educational approaches pioneered during the mid-18th century by one of the first professional French teachers of deaf persons, Jacob Péreiere. Péreiere's teaching methods drew heavily on Rousseau's interpretation of Locke's "sensationalist" empirical psychology (Winzer, 1993). Itard's approach emphasized individualization of instruction in five areas: sensory stimulation, speech, socialization, concept development, and transfer of learning (Itard, 1802).

Itard initially believed Victor suffered from early social and educational deprivation, and he thought his teaching had failed because Victor developed only minimal speech and wasn't fully restored to a useful life in society. Nevertheless, Itard's work subsequently stimulated highly successful interventions for children with intellectual disabilities by his pupils Edward Seguin and Maria Montessori. Itard is also known for his early contributions to the oral education of deaf persons, the medical specialty otolaryngology, the use of behavior modification with children with disabilities, and the special education of persons with mental and physical disabilities (Itard, 1821a, 1821b; Lane, 1989). One of Itard's greatest contributions to his age's understanding of intellectual disability stemmed from his rejection of overly inclusive diagnoses of "idiocy." Also, in an under-acknowledged paper he published in 1828 ("Mutism Caused by a Lesion of the Intellectual Functions"), Itard described how to distinguish between children with intellectual disability and those with pervasive developmental disorders such as autism (Carrey, 1995).

Seguin expanded Itard's sensory techniques into what he termed the "physiological method," emphasizing sensory-motor training, intellectual training (including academics and speech), and moral training or socialization (Simpson, 1999; Talbot, 1967). Early in his career, Seguin (1846) acknowledged his debt to Péreiere and noted that intellectual disability, deafness, and congenital blindness shared two key characteristics, early age of onset and permanence of the condition. It followed that there would be similarities in remedial techniques. Seguin's work was embraced by the French Academy of Sciences in 1844 and subsequently became the standard worldwide reference. After heading schools for children with intellectual disabilities at the Bicêtre and in private schools for 20 years, Seguin left Paris for the United States in 1848 to escape political instability (Simpson, 1999; Talbot, 1967). Elsewhere in Europe, special residential schools for persons with intellectual disabilities were established by Guggenbuhl in Switzerland in 1842, by Saegert in Germany in 1842, and by Connolly and Reid in England in 1846 (Barr, 1904; Bucknill, 1873; Fernald, 1893). It was common during this period for superintendents of facilities in one nation to visit Paris' facilities and report on the methods observed (Anonymous, 1847a, 1847b, 1847c).

The 19th century also witnessed dynamic changes in the education of other people with disabilities. In 1810, John Thelwall published the first book to be concerned solely with speech disability, *Letter to Henry Cline* (Rockey, 1980). Thelwall is regarded as England's first speech therapist, and the 19th century marks the beginning of the differential diagnosis, evaluation, and treatment of speech disorders (Rockey, 1980). The development of speech correction techniques in continental Europe was largely the province of educators of deaf persons, while in England, orators, clergymen, actors, and singing teachers were principally involved (Rockey, 1980).

In Spain, deaf educator Tiburcio Hérnandez at the Royal School decreed a return to oralism following the 1814 opening of the school after Spain's War of Independence. While Hérnandez adopted the subordinate use of signs, borrowed from Frenchmen Abbé de l'Epée and Sicard, he advocated the primacy of oralism (Plann, 1997). Hérnandez held derogatory views of deaf students, believing them to be essentially defective and unintelligent. Students were thus encouraged to learn manual trades, because of persistent beliefs in their intellectual deficits. The domination of oralism in Spanish education of deaf students did not end with Hérnandez' 1823 execution during a period of political upheaval. Students were subjected to considerable physical abuse, which led to an uprising by some of the pupils against the teachers. For the rest of the 19th century in Spain, there was a marked rejection of teachers who were deaf, and education of deaf students became entrenched as the domain of experts who could hear.

In France during the 19th century, society continued to perceive deaf people negatively, often as a stereotype of naïve, incompetent children. The Deaf Institute in Paris, a state-sponsored facility for deaf persons, served both educational and social welfare purposes. Two professors at the Institute (Bébian and Paulmier), however, advocated the use of sign language, and fostered a belief in the existence of deaf culture (Quartararo, 1995).

First North American Mental Hospitals and Residential Schools

The first mental hospital established on the North and South American continents was opened in Mexico City two centuries before similar initiatives were undertaken in the United States and Canada. San Hipólito Hospital was established in 1566 near San Hipólito Chapel in Mexico City by the Spanish philanthropist Bernadino Alvarez. Alvarez was joined in the effort by several clergymen from an order which subsequently come to be known as Los Hipólitos. New hospital structures were erected in 1739 and 1777 and the

administration of the facility was taken over by the municipal government in 1821. The facility was closed in 1910 when all patients were transferred from this facility and from a second asylum for women which opened in 1700 to a new institution called La Casteñada Asylum. The women's asylum, La Canoa Hospital for Mental Disease, also known as the Divino Salvador Hospital, was a product of the efforts of a local carpenter José Sayago and his wife, who provided shelter, food, and care for poor mentally disabled women who were an everyday sight on the streets in the capital of the New Spain (Ramirez-Moreno, 1937, 1942).

The first American almshouse was constructed in Boston in 1662, and the first mental asylum was constructed in Virginia in 1773. However, such institutions did not begin to become common in the American landscape until the Jacksonian era, beginning in the 1820s. At this time, the nation was faced with increasing urbanization and manufacturing, and changing demographics that included the first major influx of immigrants. These changing conditions led to social turmoil and institutional solutions for social problems were sought for the first time in the United States. There is widespread disagreement among historians and social scientists as to the reasons for the appearance of institutions in the United States beginning in the 1820s (Mora, 1992). Rothman (1990) contends that it was absolutely not inevitable for institutions to develop in the U.S., but that they represented an innovative solution to pressing social problems and profound changes in the economic and social structure of the country. He argues that the concurrent development of orphanages, asylums for people with mental illness, prisons, almshouses, and reformatories was the result of a nation grappling with tremendous social upheaval and a desire to manage the social order by controlling deviant members. Others have argued that the development of institutions followed the European example and were the product of American interest in solving social problems by adhering to the natural course established by Europe (Mora, 1992; Grob, 1990). Symonds (1995) has argued that mental institutions developed in England during the 19th century as a sociological response to perceptions of the threat of deviance, which is consistent with Rothman's (1990) conclusions about the development of such facilities in the

United States.

During this period, residential schools in the U.S. began for deaf persons with the 1817 opening of the American Asylum for the Education of the Deaf and Dumb in Hartford, Connecticut, by Thomas Gallaudet and Laurent Clerc (Fay, 1893). Within two years, this first school for deaf students in the United States was accepting students from 11 states (Ely, 1893). The national character of the school stemmed in part from the fact that in 1819 the federal government granted the school an endowment of 23,000 acres of land in Alabama Territory (Breckinridge, 1927).

The state of New York established the second U.S. school in 1818 in New York City (Gannon, 1981). Many of the first schools in the United States were initially begun as day schools and later evolved into residential schools (Gordan, 1885).

The first separate schools for blind students in the United States began instruction within months of one another in 1832 in New York City and at the Perkins Institute in Boston (Allen, 1899; Farrell, 1956; Frampton & Kerney, 1953).

The Bishop of Québec erected the first building in Canada exclusively dedicated to the confinement of mentally disabled individuals in 1714 (Hurd, 1910). The building was located adjacent to the Québec General Hospital. However, people with mental illness and intellectual disability had been cared for in two general hospitals in Québec since at least 1694 (Griffin & Greenland, 1981).

As previously noted, the colonial government of Virginia opened the first mental hospital in the U.S. exclusively dedicated to mental disability in 1773 in Williamsburg (Eastern State Hospital). The opening of this facility had virtually no impact as a model on other states. The impulse to establish this facility stemmed from Virginia's English colonial governor, Francis Fauquier, who was motivated through a sense of noblesse oblige to establish similar institutions abroad (Grob, 1973). The establishment of this first facility in the U.S. was not preceded by a public campaign as would become the common practice for subsequent American facilities. The Virginia facility's capacity was 24-36 persons and the governing authorities "never publicized the work of the hospital, and thereby reinforced its essentially local character" (Grob, 1973, p. 29). The facility shut down for four years beginning in

1782 due to the American Revolution. The state of Maryland then opened the fledgling nation's second state mental institution in 1798—fully 25 years after the opening of the first facility in Virginia. The third state institution for people with mental illness opened 25 years later, in Kentucky in 1824 (Grob, 1973).

Private initiatives in the northeastern United States led to the creation of several mental hospitals modeled after the York Retreat in England. York was a private facility opened by the Quaker William Tuke in 1792. Between 1817 and 1847, private institutions opened in Philadelphia, Boston, New York, Connecticut, Vermont, and Rhode Island (Earle, 1845; Hamilton, 1944; Kirkbride, 1845; Wood, 1853). By the time the Butler Hospital opened in Providence in 1847 (Rochefort, 1981), however, it had become clear that the exclusiveness and higher costs of private hospitals rendered them inadequate to meet the needs of the poorer classes, particularly the growing populations of urban poor in America's developing cities (Grob, 1973; Hamilton, 1944).

The development of mental asylums accelerated following Dorothea Dix' advocacy beginning in the 1840s (Brown, 1998; Grob, 1994; Rothman, 1990). Dix traveled across the country, inspecting conditions of people with mental illness kept in prisons, living with their families, and in "bidded out" contracts. She lobbied individual state legislatures for the construction of asylum facilities for the mentally disabled by writing memorials that described her findings (Brown, 1998). In her first memorial, written after canvassing conditions in Massachusetts, Dix (1843) described:

> The present state of Insane Persons confined within this Commonwealth, in cages, closets, cellars, stalls, pens! Chained, naked, beaten with rods, and lashed into obedience!... Irritation of body, produced by utter filth and exposure, incited [one woman] to the horrid process of tearing off her skin by inches; her face, neck, and person, were thus disfigured to hideousness. (p. 7)

Institutions for people with mental illness continued to be constructed, frequently due to Dix' agitation. During the 1840s-1870s, she was involved in the construction or expansion of more than 30 such facilities across the US and in Britain (Brown, 1998). Mental asylums of the earliest period were generally designed to house fewer than 300 people and were organized under the leadership of psychiatrist-superintendents. These men adhered to the moral treatment method pioneered by Pinel and Tuke (Grob, 1966). However, the first institutions were marked by specific divisions in the care and treatment of the poor from the privileged classes (Tuke, 1815). This initial segregation within public facilities between the middle class and the poor was the beginning of practices that would eventually become a hallmark of American institutions (Rothman, 1990; Trent, 1995). During the first half of the 19th century, physician-superintendents of the first mental asylums in the U.S. believed that mental illness was curable (Grob, 1966; Kirkbride, 1973/1880). Kirkbride (1973/1880), superintendent of the Pennsylvania asylum, argued that in cases where uncomplicated insanity was "properly and promptly treated, and having this treatment duly persevered in, may be regarded as curable…80%" of the time (p. 23).

Overcrowding and the Demise of the Moral Treatment

Beginning almost immediately after they were constructed, mental institutions experienced severe overcrowding as prisons sought to release their most dangerous and disturbed inmates to the newly available facilities (Grob, 1966). Overcrowding and expansion soon made the superintendents' attempts at moral treatment impossible as the management of large facilities became paramount. In the later decades of the 1800s, as treatment gave way to confinement and custodial care in larger facilities, cure rates concomitantly dropped and psychiatrists reported that mental illness was largely incurable (Earle, 1877; Grob, 1966; Rothman, 1990; Scull, 1991).

As populations in these asylums swelled, conditions of overcrowding became serious by the end of the 19th century. The sheer number of inmates in most facilities, along with growing administrative responsibilities in increasingly complex institutions, translated into less time with patients for the superintendent. The moral treatment subsequently faded, along with beliefs in the curability of mental illness as custodial functions of the asylums became primary (Grob, 1966;

Rothman, 1990).

By the late 1800s, the earlier optimism of rehabilitating patients with mental illness and sending them back to their home communities had been replaced with a rigid pessimism that decried the possibility of cure and demanded the lifelong custody of patients reported as extremely dangerous to their home communities (Earle, 1877; Grob, 1966; Rothman, 1990). Grob (1966) argues that superintendents gave way to the inevitability of poor conditions given severe overcrowding and limited contact with patients. Rothman (1990) and Scull (1991) contend that superintendents used the opportunities presented by expanding demand for mental asylum space to legitimate their own existence and secure their power. Our review of the *American Journal of Insanity* from its 1844 inception to 1900, reveals extensive discussions of the architecture of asylums and the management of such facilities. However, there were fewer than 10 articles that dealt with patient treatment or care. This lends credence to Rothman (1990) and Scull's (1991) claims that superintendents were more interested and absorbed in the management of their facilities than in therapeutic issues.

Writing of his experiences of incarceration in the New York Asylum at Utica, a patient with mental illness recounts extraordinary abuse, patient overcrowding, and horrific conditions at the facility during the mid-19th century (Anonymous, 1849). Elizabeth Packard (1868) wrote of being physically abused at the Illinois State Insane Asylum at Jacksonville, and after her eventual release she campaigned for the civil rights of mental patients in Illinois and other states. Lydia Button (1878) wrote an autobiography recounting abusive conditions she and other inmates endured while institutionalized at the State Asylum in Kalamazoo, Michigan. By all accounts, Packard and Button were not mentally ill but were victimized by a legal system that permitted husbands to institutionalize their wives during the 19th century (Peterson, 1982). However, the treatment of these individuals is representative of the institutional experiences of many other people with mental illness during the mid-19th century in the United States. Conditions in English mental asylums during the beginning of the 19th century were equally severe. Visitors related stories of seeing people with mental illness confined in rooms without heat or clothing, chained, and physically abused (Browne, 1837).

Before the first distinct residential institution for persons with intellectual disabilities had opened in the U.S. in 1848, 31 institutions for persons with mental illness had been established (Hamilton, 1944). There were 4,730 residents, a small percentage of whom had intellectual disabilities; 27 of the facilities were public, four were private.

The psychiatrist Phillipe Pinel was the major figure in the care of people with mental illness at the close of the 18th century. He is most popularly known for his bold act in 1792 of simultaneously unchaining 50 patients in a Paris mental hospital. The act echoed the "liberty, equality, and fraternity" spirit of the French Revolution popularized by Rousseau (1991/1762). Pinel's *Treatise on Insanity* (1977/1801) had worldwide influence on the developing field of psychology and psychiatry. Nearly 50 years after its publication, the editors of the *American Journal of Insanity* noted that "we know not of any work on insanity superior to this...none more worthy of our daily study" ("The moral treatment," 1847, p. 4). In Belgium a generation later, psychiatrist Joseph Guislain similarly unchained mental patients at the asylum in Ghent, earning the nickname of the "Belgian Pinel" (Brierre de Boismont, 1867). In spite of Pinel, Guislain, and, in Italy, Chiarugi's notoriety in promulgating the moral treatment (Alexander & Selesnick, 1964), there is evidence that it did not originate with them; rather, changing therapeutic philosophies were emerging before Pinel wrote his treatise and even before Chiarugi's works were known in England. English physician William Pargeter wrote *Observations on Maniacal Disorders* in 1792, prior to Pinel's arrival at the Bicêtre (Jackson, 1988). Pargeter advocated for humane care of people with mental illness by arguing against the use of restraints, beatings, and forced remedies in advance of Pinel and Tuke (Jackson, 1988; Pargeter, 1988/1792). Like Pinel and Chiarugi, he emphasized the importance of the management of insanity in lieu of medicine and punishment:

> The chief reliance in the cure of insanity must be rather on management than medicine. The government of maniacs is an art, not to be acquired without long experience, and frequent and attentive observation. Although it has been of late years much advanced, it is still capable of improvement. (p. 49)

The emphasis that Pargeter, Pinel, Chiarugi, Guislain, and Tuke placed on management has been interpreted by later analysts as an emphasis on social control and coercion. Thomas Szasz (1973) has argued that involuntary institutionalization of persons with mental illness established a relationship between doctor and patient during the rise of psychiatric power in the 17th and 18th centuries that is akin to that of master and slave. Szasz further argues that this relationship between doctor and patient still exists in contemporary Western society.

In 1790, only six U.S. cities had more than 8,000 people and the population of the U.S. was 3.9 million. By 1850, there were 85 such metropolises, 26 cities had more than 25,000 persons, and the total U.S. population was 23.2 million people (Hamilton, 1944). Between 1824, when the nation's third state mental institution opened, and 1851, 19 state-operated facilities were established in 15 states including New York (3), Virginia, South Carolina, Massachusetts (2), Tennessee, Maine, New Hampshire, Georgia, Indiana, New Jersey, Louisiana, Pennsylvania (2), Missouri, Illinois, and California (Hamilton, 1944). All of these state facilities, which collectively housed 4,730 persons in 1850, were opened before the first separate and distinct U.S. institution was constructed for people with intellectual disabilities.

Between 1850 and 1890, 55 state psychiatric institutions were opened in the U.S. and the census of patients with mental illness in mental hospitals grew dramatically to 40,942 (Hamilton, 1944, p. 86). It would nearly double by 1890 to 74,028 and double again to 187,791 in 1910. Overcrowding in mental institutions became pronounced during the latter half of the 19th century in the United States. During this time, facilities essentially abandoned their therapeutic capacities in favor of custodial arrangements designed to protect society from the perceived threat posed by people with mental illness (Rothman, 1990; Scull, 1991). However, one innovative response to overcrowding was family care, a program of placing people with mental illness in the homes of unrelated families. In the United States, family care was initiated first in Massachusetts in 1885 (Pollock, 1945). A similar program had been in place in Scotland dating back to at least the 1860s (Pollock, 1945). The use of family care for people with mental illness represents the first efforts to provide state-sponsored services in community settings. While a few other states followed Massachusetts' lead, family care for people with mental illness never became widespread in the U.S. (Pollock, 1945). Large-scale community-based services would not develop for people with mental illness until late in the 20th century (Grob, 1994).

Growing concern about the number of people with disabilities in the United States resulted in their enumeration by the census. Beginning in 1830, counts were taken of deaf and blind persons, and in 1840 the census began counting people labeled "idiotic" and "insane" (Gorwitz, 1974). The 1840 census reflected pervasive racism. All black residents in some towns were classified as insane (Gorwitz, 1974). Between 1870 and 1880, the proportion of the population counted as insane rose from 97 to 183 per 100,000, while the proportion of the population counted as intellectually disabled rose from 64 to 153 per 100,000 (Gorwitz, 1974). This dramatic increase can be attributed, at least in part, to the fact that census enumerators received extra compensation in 1880 for each person with mental illness or intellectual disability that they counted (Gorwitz, 1974). The rapid increase in the mentally disabled population was seen as evidence that society needed to take drastic measures to address mental disability (Knight, 1895). These concerns ultimately fueled the agenda of the eugenics movement. The publication and dissemination of the results of such "scientific inquiry" was widely used in propaganda campaigns to catalyze public support for sterilization and marriage restriction laws (Pernick, 1996). By 1912, numerous states prohibited the marriage of persons with mental disabilities and epilepsy, or allowed such marriages only after age 45 (Smith, Wilkinson, & Wagoner, 1914).

Historians and advocates have argued that the professionals involved with the operation of institutions for people with mental illness (Rothman, 1990; Scull, 1979) and intellectual disability (Blatt, 1977;

Trent, 1995; Tyor, 1972; Tyor & Bell, 1984) were personally invested in perpetuating the life of these institutions, often at the expense of the residents. Social historians studying leprosy have made similar claims (Navon, 1998). Cochrane (1963), Gussow (1989), and MacArthur (1953) argued that Christian missionaries supported the need for segregation and the negative images toward people with leprosy in order to continue to receive funding for their missionary efforts.

Deaf Community Organizing

During the mid-19th century, the number of schools for deaf and blind students grew rapidly both in the United States and in Europe. In 1856 in the United States, a donated estate in Washington, DC, was used to establish a residential school for 12 deaf and 6 blind students, the Columbia Institution for the Instruction of the Deaf and Dumb and the Blind (Gallaudet, 1983; Lane, 1989). In 1864, President Lincoln signed legislation authorizing Columbia to confer college degrees. Columbia later became Gallaudet University (Gallaudet, 1983; Lane, 1989).

Suppression of sign language was championed by Alexander Graham Bell in the United States at the end of the 19th century. In 1872, he opened a speech-based school for teachers in Boston intending to banish the use of sign and encouraging deaf persons to "pass" as hearing individuals (Gannon, 1981; Lane, 1989). In 1880, at the International Congress on Education of the Deaf which met in Italy, a resolution passed that banned the use of sign language in the education of deaf children (Gannon, 1981; Gallaudet, 1983). Also in 1880, the National Association of the Deaf was organized by deaf people. This organization would become the leading association fighting the oralists for manual instruction of deaf people in the United States (Baynton, 1996).

One of the first self-advocacy organizations by people with disabilities was the British Deaf and Dumb Association (BDDA), now the British Association of the Deaf. The BDDA initially organized in 1890 in direct response to the International Congress' sign language ban and the view that deaf persons did not need to be involved in matters that concerned them. The 1880 International Congress on the Deaf had only two deaf teachers in attendance (British Association of the Deaf, 1999).

First U.S. Institution for People With Intellectual Disability

Superintendents of asylums for the mentally ill were among the first in the United States to call for separate provisions for people with intellectual disabilities. Reflecting on the path-breaking developments in Europe, Samuel Woodward, superintendent of the Worcester State Hospital in Massachusetts, and Amariah Brigham, of New York's Bloomingdale facility, both recommended in their 1845 annual state hospital reports that their states make a public educational provision for children and youth with intellectual disabilities (Brigham, 1845; Woodward, 1845).

In 1846, the noted reformer, leader of the education of blind students, and committed oralist in the education of deaf students, Samuel Gridley Howe, was appointed to chair an epidemiological committee regarding intellectual disabilities appointed by the Massachusetts legislature. Howe carried out the nation's first investigation of the prevalence of intellectual disabilities and presented recommendations to establish an experimental school. Howe's report is replete with purported connections between the etiology of intellectual disability and the immoral behavior of one's parents (Howe, 1848). His perspective was no doubt indicative of attitudes of the day that disability was a punishment for violating natural law.

The residential school that Howe recommended opened in October 1848 in South Boston in a wing of the Perkins Institute for the Blind (Howe, 1851). A few months earlier, in July 1848, Hervey Wilbur had opened a small private school in his own home for the instruction of children with mental retardation in Barre, Massachusetts (Elm Hill Private School and Home, 1911). A few years later, Wilbur left Barre to superintend the new institution at Syracuse, site of the first institution for people with intellectual disabilities constructed specifically for that purpose in the U.S. The Syracuse institution opened in 1855 (Fernald, 1893; FitzGerald, 1900).

It became common for states to initially open experimental schools (Kerlin, 1877), and other states followed Massachusetts and New York's lead. Penn-

sylvania opened a private school in 1852 that was incorporated in 1853 as the Pennsylvania Training School for Idiotic and Feebleminded Children. In 1855, this school was moved to its present site at Elwyn, Ohio. Connecticut, Kentucky, and Illinois established residential schools in 1857, 1858, 1860, and 1865, respectively (Fernald, 1917). The Illinois school was administered for its first decade under the auspices of the Illinois School for the Deaf. Twenty-six years after Howe opened the United States' first school for 10 children, seven states had established publicly operated or assisted institutions for 1,041 residents, and there were two private facilities in Massachusetts (Fernald, 1917). Although the national census of institutions for people with intellectual disabilities was now growing steadily, almshouses housed more people with intellectual disabilities until 1906 (U.S. Bureau of the Census, 1914).

From Training Schools to Custodial Asylums

Institutions for people with intellectual disabilities, similar to those for people with mental illness, grew rapidly both in size and number following their initial construction in the mid-1800s. Early training efforts were quite successful, and many of the children with intellectual disabilities were returned to their communities as "productive workers" (Stewart, 1882; Trent, 1995). Economic hardship hit the nation following the Civil War and severe recessions occurred in the 1870s and again in the 1880s. Due to extensive unemployment, it became increasingly difficult for superintendents to discharge trained residents who couldn't compete for already scarce jobs in their home communities. Superintendents also noted the value of using unpaid resident labor to offset the costs of running the institutions (Fenton, 1932; Knight, 1891). The exploitation of resident labor, or peonage, prevailed in both institutions for people with mental illness and intellectual disability (Bartlett, 1964; Bonsall, 1891; Fenton, 1932; Johnson, 1899; Knight, 1891; MacAndrew & Edgerton, 1964) until the late 1960s (Scheerenberger, 1983).

By 1880, the training schools envisioned by Howe and Seguin had evolved into custodial asylums with reduced emphasis on educating residents and returning them to community life (Trent, 1995; Wolfensberger, 1976). The optimism of the 1840-1870 "amelioration" period confronted two difficult realities including negative attitudes toward persons with mental retardation held by the general public and the lack of supportive social services, family support, and work opportunities in the community. Wilbur (1888), at the 15th annual gathering of the National Conference of Charities and Corrections, observed that institutions would offer lifelong protective custodial care. Other professionals in the field joined Wilbur in calling for lifelong institutionalization of people with intellectual disabilities (Barr, 1902; Bicknell, 1895; Fish, 1892; Fort, 1892; Johnson, 1896). Samuel Gridley Howe had strongly opposed this trend, arguing in an 1866 speech that people with disabilities "should be kept diffused among sound and normal persons. Separation, and not congregation, should be the law of their treatment." The states, he said, should "gradually dispense with as many [custodial institutions] as possible" (cited in Wolfensberger, 1976, p. 26).

But the states did not dispense with custodial institutions. They continued to build them, expand them, and stress self-sufficiency and economical management in all aspects of facility operation. In 1900, the census of mental retardation institutions in the United States was 11,800 persons (Fernald, 1917). Many institutions were located in remote areas and farmed extensive lands. Residents worked laundries, farms, and workshops, not so much to develop skills for community out-placement, but rather to contribute to the self-sustaining economy of the institution. While most superintendents championed the growth of large institutions during this period (Trent, 1995), Seguin (1870) warned against this phenomenon. He wrote, "let us hope that the State institutions for idiots will escape that evil of excessive growth. . . in which patients are so numerous that the accomplished physicians who have them in charge cannot remember the name of each" (p. 21).

At the dawning of the 20th century, institutions for persons with intellectual disabilities were firmly established in the developed nations of the world. Barr (1904), who wrote the first U.S. textbook on intellectual disability, completed an international survey and reported that 21 nations were operating 171 institutions for people with intellectual disability. There were

25 institutions in the United States by 1900 (Kuhlmann, 1940). Barr also noted that "following the experiments worked out in the continental cities and in England, the special classes for backward children opened first in Providence, Rhode Island, and [are] now part of the educational systems of New York, Philadelphia, Chicago, and Boston" (p. 71).

In the United States, the course of the initial development of institutions for people with mental illness and intellectual disabilities had numerous similarities. Superintendents of both types of facilities utilized existing social and economic issues to develop secondary goals for their facilities after their initial goals of training failed. Both sets of leaders aggressively agitated for the next phase of institutional development -- custodial care (Rothman, 1990; Scull, 1991; Trent, 1995).

Freak Shows

Institutions were not the only manifestation of society's attitudes toward people with disabilities during the 19th century. So-called freak shows displayed people with physical and mental disabilities throughout the 19th century in the United States and Europe (Bogdan, 1988; Rothfels, 1996; Thomson, 1996, 1997). People with intellectual disabilities were among those exhibited, their "abnormal" characteristics exaggerated into caricatures of the grotesque (Bogdan, 1988; Thomson, 1997). These exhibits were extremely popular at circuses, fairs, and expositions. People with disabilities who were displayed at freak shows were frequently "sold" to the show organizers, who maintained the right to display them for the duration of their lives (Bogdan, 1988).

In displaying people with disabilities in these shows, exotic stories of wild and far-flung origins of the exhibited people were fabricated by the show organizers (Bogdan, 1988; Thomson, 1997). Thomson argues that the exploitation of people with disabilities in the United States served to reinforce average Americans' notions of their own normality, by emphasizing disability and often race as profound and monstrous difference. Freak shows served to institutionalize notions of disability as the ultimate deviance, thus solidifying Americans' needs to perceive themselves as normal (Thomson, 1997). Freak shows reached the height of their popularity at the end of the 19th century, at a time when eugenic beliefs in the superiority of the white middle class were crystallizing. In the United States, freak shows continued until the 1940s, when competing forms of entertainment, as well as economic hard times, led to their demise (Bogdan, 1986).

While freak shows were at their zenith during the mid- to late-19th century, there is evidence that they had been popular for centuries in England (Park & Daston, 1981; Semonin, 1996). Semonin (1996) describes the "taste for monsters" as "an almost universal craze among English citizens of all ranks" (p. 69). In Medieval and modern England, people with disabilities, racial and ethnic minorities, and people with unusual attributes were termed "monsters," and their display in markets for profit was commonplace (Semonin, 1996). It was common for people to visit Bethlem during the Medieval and later periods for the "entertainment" provided by the inmates (MacDonald, 1981).

Threat of the Eugenicists

The period from 1880 to 1925 was a time in which persons with intellectual disabilities were viewed as deviant social menaces, and intellectual disability was seen as an incurable disease (Barr, 1902; Butler, 1907; East, 1917; Fernald, 1915; Gosney & Popenoe, 1929; Kerlin, 1887; Scheerenberger, 1983; Sloan & Stevens, 1976; Switzky et al., 1988; Trent, 1995; Watkins, 1930; Winspear, 1895). The eugenic belief widely held during this period was that intellectual disability was inherited as a Mendelian characteristic that degraded the species (Barr, 1902; Fernald, 1915; Galton, 1883; Rafter, 1988; Roberts, 1952). Intellectual disability was linked in numerous studies to criminality, immoral behavior, and pauperism (Dugdale, 1910/1877; Evans, 1926; Fernald, 1915; Goddard, 1912; Rafter, 1988). Intelligence tests, developed shortly after the turn of the century, were employed widely in the major cities of the United States to identify children with intellectual disabilities and place them in segregated special classes. Intelligence tests were also used to support ethnocentric and class biases against immigrants in the United States (Davenport, 1921; Fernald, 1915). Subsequent to the implementation of intelligence testing at ports of entry, deportations for mental deficiency in-

creased 350% in 1913, and 570% in 1914 (Gould, 1981). Rampant abuse existed in the classification of both immigrants and poor Americans as mentally deficient. Workers were "trained" to classify people as mentally deficient by sight (Gould, 1981).

Economic problems occurred at the same time that Galton's ideas of social Darwinism were beginning to take hold in the United States and abroad. Superintendents' writings reflect changing attitudes toward their charges as their institutional populations soared; the menace and burden of people with intellectual disabilities was frequently discussed (Barr, 1895; Bicknell, 1895; Fernald, 1912; Kerlin, 1887). Society needed protection from these menaces, and institutional care became the way to achieve these goals. Trent (1995) argues that the superintendents readily espoused the new social Darwinism and its messages of fear about deviant persons because it offered a way for them to legitimate and consolidate their authority.

The eugenics movement in the United States was accompanied by extensive instances of physicians refusing to treat, and thereby facilitating the death of infants born with disabilities and birth defects (Pernick, 1996). Newspaper accounts publicized the withholding of lifesaving treatment of babies with disabilities during the decade after 1915, and movies propagating the eugenics agenda became quite common (Pernick, 1996).

In England, concern about people termed "mental defective" led to the 1886 passage of the "Idiots Act," which called for further clarification of the distinction between "idiots" and "lunatics" (Gladstone, 1996), and preceded the eugenics movement in that country (Carpenter, 1996). Passage of the 1899 Education Act led to the growth of institutions for people with intellectual disability and epilepsy in England (Carpenter, 1996; Koven, 1994).

Social Darwinism had an impact on the deaf community in the United States as well. At the end of the century, the debate between manualists and oralists intensified. Oralists claimed that people who used sign language were less evolved than people who spoke, and were like apes, or racial minorities (Baynton, 1993; Porter, 1894). This debate eventually resulted in the near eradication of manual education of deaf students, which was supplanted by oral education, a trend that was strongly opposed by deaf adults but which continued well into the mid-20th century (Semi-deaf lady, 1908; Baynton, 1996). Zealously opposed to signed instruction, hearing teachers and other oralists used physical abuse of students to suppress sign language (Baynton, 1996; Lane, 1989; Porter, 1894). In 1920, 82% of the 13,917 deaf students in school were taught speech ("Statistics of Speech," 1920).

The deaf movement that began in the United States in the late 19th century expressed a desire for independence and an evolving commitment to the emergence of deaf culture (de Saint-Loup, 1996). The foundation of this movement was use of sign language, which had been opposed by such notable figures as Alexander Graham Bell. Bell even explicitly rejected marriage among deaf people (Bell, 1969/1883). Deaf culture was further facilitated by the printing and circulation of newspapers among deaf residential schools across the nation. By 1893, at least 29 schools had 35 newspapers (Haller, 1993). It is a testament to the strength of the deaf community that sign language survived and thrived during nearly a century of repression, and it is now a primary communication strategy in educating deaf children.

In summary, the 19th century is best characterized as the century of institutions and interventions. Schools and institutions for persons with physical disabilities, deafness, blindness, mental illness, and intellectual disability took root throughout Europe and North America. Professionals developed differential diagnosis to particularize disability, and devised treatment interventions and educational schemes focused on specific impairments. The medical model of defining and classifying disability became thoroughly accepted in this century. However, the segregation of individuals with similar impairments also afforded people with disabilities opportunities to begin to develop group identities. By the close of the 19th century, deaf persons advocating for manual education and control of their own schools had begun to coalesce into the first disability political action groups.

THE 20th CENTURY

Segregation and Expansion of the Institutional Model

At the opening of the 20th century the eugenics era was gaining momentum, and social reformers sought segregation and prohibitions on marriage and procreation by people with disabilities. Conditions in facilities for people with mental disabilities were deteriorating, and deaf persons were fighting to be able to use sign language in their schools.

In spite of the rapid expansion of institutions for people with mental disabilities after the turn of the century, poorfarms or almshouses were also a significant aspect of state provision for people with intellectual disabilities and mental illness. By the 1920s, poorfarms were "dumping grounds" for all undesirables, including people with disabilities and the poor. In 1922, Ohio reported that 70% of poorfarm inmates had "feeblemindedness," or what is today known as intellectual disability. North Carolina estimated that 85% of inmates were "mentally abnormal." Iowa reported that, in 1924, 45% of its poorfarm inmates were mentally ill (Evans, 1926, pp. 7-8). In a nationwide study of inmates of poorhouses, 36% were found to be "feebleminded, borderline defective, psychopathic, psychoneurotic, epileptic, or suffering from mental disease" (Haines, 1925, p. 138).

The sterilization of institutional residents with intellectual disabilities was commonplace in some states (Ferster, 1966; Watkins, 1930). Between 1907 and 1949, there were more than 47,000 recorded sterilizations of people with mental disabilities in 30 states (Woodside, 1950). Of particular interest was the sterilization of people with intellectual disability who would eventually be discharged into the community (Popenoe, 1927). Sterilization of women with epilepsy and mental illness was also widely believed by physicians to have therapeutic benefits in spite of overwhelming empirical evidence to the contrary (Church, 1893). In the face of evidence that removal of the ovaries and Fallopian tubes was wholly ineffective, physicians continued to perform such surgery on women with an array of conditions, including hysteria, depression, epilepsy, insanity related to childbirth, and nymphomania. Surgery was also deemed appropriate to "prevent the prospect of illegitimate and defective children" (Church, 1893, p. 496).

The U.S. Supreme Court's 1927 *Buck v. Bell* decision affirmed the states' right to sterilize people with intellectual disabilities and propelled the eugenics movement to further lobby for its agenda (Kevles,

1985; Radford, 1994; Reilly, 1991). In 1933, using California's program as a model, Nazi Germany enacted its own eugenic sterilization law (Reilly, 1991). This legislation led to the forced sterilization of between 300,000 and 400,000 persons, a majority on the grounds of "feeblemindedness." Most were institutional residents. This unprecedented oppression against disabled persons culminated in the murder by euthanasia of between 200,000 and 275,000 individuals with mental and physical disabilities between 1939 and 1945 in Germany. The eugenics movement had reached its zenith (Friedlander, 1997; Gallagher, 1995; Reilly, 1991; U.S. Holocaust Memorial Museum, undated; Wolfensberger, 1981). Justification for the killing of people with disabilities in Nazi Germany was made on the basis of utilitarian arguments, and German health professionals and psychiatrists were among those who accommodated themselves to these policies (Burleigh, 1994). Psychiatrists, particularly, had been responsible for identifying the pool of potential victims, and in some cases, participated in victim selection and murder (Burleigh, 1994).

The United States and Germany were not the only nations to sterilize people with disabilities. Denmark had an active program of sterilization between 1930 and 1954, sterilizing at least 8,627 persons over this period. Sweden's program operated throughout the 1930s and 1940s, with 2,278 persons being sterilized in 1948 alone (Trombley, 1988).

Contemporaneous with zealous agitation by eugenicists, evidence began to emerge that questioned the assumptions of deviance in people with intellectual disabilities. In Massachusetts, Fernald's (1919) Waverly studies demonstrated that with proper support from their families, individuals with intellectual disabilities could function well in the community. Fernald (1919) also concluded that only about 8% of a sample of 5,000 schoolchildren with intellectual disabilities in Massachusetts exhibited behavioral problems of any type. In addition, Wallace (1929) presented a compelling paper discrediting the link between intellectual disability and criminality. Also, the "parole plan," which could lead to permanent institutional discharge, was devised in the first decade of the 20th century as an early release program for institutional residents with milder impairments. Paroled residents were cared for in the community by relatives, employers, or support-

ive volunteers (Bernstein, 1917, 1918, 1921; Davies, 1930; Fernald, 1902; Hoakley, 1922; Mastin, 1916; Matthews, 1921).

In 1908, with the publication of former mental patient Clifford Beers' *A Mind That Found Itself*, the mental hygiene movement began in the United States (Felix, 1957). Beers' autobiographical account of his two-year institutionalization presents chilling details of life for those hospitalized at the turn of the century (Beers, 1908; Peterson, 1982). Describing constant physical abuse, Beers' narrative resembles those of earlier inmates of the 19th century. Like Elizabeth Packard, Beers was interested in reform and established an agenda to promote humane care (Peterson, 1982). Influenced by Beers, leaders in psychiatry supported the reform agenda, and psychiatric hospitals began offering clinics in their communities to treat and prevent chronic mental illness (Grob, 1983, 1994). In 1909, as a result of Beers' advocacy and leadership, the National Committee for Mental Hygiene was established (Felix, 1957).

Shock therapies were developed and implemented in the 1920s, including the use of insulin, metrazol, and malaria to induce shock and hopefully cure patients with mental illness. Electroshock began to be used on people with mental illness in Europe in the 1830s, and a few late 18th-century physicians experimented with electroshock on people with epilepsy, blindness, and mental illness (Harms, 1955). However, the widespread acceptance and use of electroshock didn't occur until the 1930s, when the Italian Ugo Cerletti invented and publicized modern electroshock therapy. Electroshock involved the application of electricity to induce improvements in psychiatric conditions (Cerletti, 1950; Harms, 1955).

While psychosurgery had been performed by the Swiss surgeon Gottlieb Burkhardt in 1890, his contemporaries rejected its use (Ramsey, 1952; Swayze, 1995). The Portuguese neuropsychiatrist Egas Minoz developed modern psychosurgery in 1933, and from its initial use until the 1950s, nearly 20,000 patients were lobotomized (Grob, 1994; Ramsey, 1952; Swayze, 1995; Valenstein, 1986). Psychosurgery involved the severing of the frontal lobe from the rest of the brain, and frequently left patients with changed personalities, diminished intellectual faculties, and other severe problems (Ramsey, 1952; Swayze, 1995).

Recent advocates with mental illness have rejected the use of shock therapy and psychosurgery as barbaric attempts to control people with mental illness (Lefley, 1996; MadNation, 1999; Peterson, 1982). Litigation in the United States has resulted in determinations that patients in mental hospitals have the right to refuse electroshock treatment (Levy & Rubenstein, 1996; Parry, 1995).

The repression and social control of people classified as deviant is an important aspect of the discussion of the history of disability, and particularly, the history of mental illness. Historians and social scientists have offered extensive critiques of psychiatry as a social control device. Thomas Szasz (1970), one of the most vocal and articulate critics of psychiatry, has argued that society has scapegoated people with mental illness and severely abused them. Elliot Valenstein (1986) has argued that the use of psychosurgery and the shock therapies so popular during the first half of the 20th century were vehicles for ambitious psychiatrists to pursue their own career agendas at the cost of individuals with mental illness.

The census of American psychiatric hospitals continued to increase during the first half of the 20th century, reaching 461,358 persons in 1940 and peaking at over 550,000 persons in 1955 (Braddock, 1981; Hamilton, 1944). The size of many of the public facilities was truly immense, even by American standards. In 1941, Hamilton reported that 10 public facilities housed over 5,000 residents (one had 9,177 residents); 22 had over 4,000; 40 housed over 3,000 individuals and 102 of the nation's 475 mental hospitals on December 31, 1941, contained more than 2,000 patients.

In 1880, there were 1,382 persons with intellectual disability in insane asylums. By 1940, the number of persons with intellectual disabilities living in psychiatric hospitals peaked at nearly 29,000 persons (U.S. Bureau of the Census, 1939, 1940). The census of separate state institutions for people with intellectual disabilities swelled to 55,466 persons by 1926 (Lakin, 1979). Switzky et al. (1988) described several common practices in institutions of this era. Residents were "patients" who lived on "wards" in a facility, often called a "hospital," which was governed by a hierarchical medical structure. Resident programs were termed "treatments" or "therapy," e.g., recreational therapy,

industrial therapy, educational therapy. Living units were locked, windows barred, and the institution became increasingly structured "like a hospital for the care of sick animals rather than as a place for the special education of human children and adults" (p. 28). Prolonged institutionalization exacted a price from residents by promoting excessive conformity to the institutional culture at the expense of personal spontaneity, excessive fantasizing, fear of new situations, and excessive dependency on the institution (Sarason & Gladwin, 1958).

Because of widespread unemployment and poverty during the Great Depression, families sought institutional care for their relatives with intellectual disabilities in increasing numbers (Noll, 1996). Institutional facility censuses continued to swell and overcrowding became commonplace (Noll, 1996; Trent, 1995; Tyor & Bell, 1984; Watkins, 1930). The Depression also brought relief with President Roosevelt's economic recovery programs. Passed in 1935, Title X of the Social Security Act provided specific relief for blind persons, but no other disability groups (Axinn & Levin, 1982; Braddock, 1987; Lende, 1941; Scotch & Berkowitz, 1990). By 1940, approximately 50,000 blind people across the United States were receiving this aid (Lende, 1941). While Title V of the Social Security Act authorized Crippled Children's Services grants of $2.85 million (Braddock, 1986a), minutes of the 1936 Crippled Children's Services National Advisory Committee stated that "children with incurable blindness, deafness, or mental defect. . . and those requiring permanent custodial care" were beyond the intended scope of the new program (Social Security Board, 1946, p. 1).

The widespread segregation of people with intellectual disabilities in institutions made them targets for medical experiments. At the Wrentham and Fernald facilities in Massachusetts, institutional residents with intellectual disabilities were subjected to tests with foods that had been laced with radioactive elements. Neither the individuals with disabilities who served as subjects in these experiments, nor their parents, were ever apprised of the nature of the foods that were ingested. This illegal research spanned the period between 1946-73 (Moreno, 1999). Residents at the Willowbrook institution in New York were similarly exposed to hepatitis-B without their knowledge or informed consent (Rothman & Rothman, 1984).

Developments for Persons With Physical Disabilities

Religious charity, as has been previously discussed, had been part of the landscape of support provided to people with disabilities and the poor for centuries. However, numerous secular charitable societies organized in the United States during the period between the 1840s and the 1880s. For example, Clara Barton founded the American Red Cross in 1881, an affiliate of an endeavor already in existence in Europe. The predecessor of the original European Red Cross had been founded to prevent death and disability on an Italian battlefield in 1859 (Obermann, 1968).

Secular charitable organizations began to make an impact on persons with disabilities, and in some instances, became forerunners of the vocational rehabilitation movement in the early 20th century. Among the most important of these was the Red Cross' establishment of the Institute for Crippled and Disabled Men in 1917. This organization was an experimental school for the rehabilitation of veterans, one of the first in the United States. Borrowing on ideas learned from visits to France, Germany, Italy, and England, the Institute developed retraining programs for veterans with disabilities that were later used in U.S. Army hospitals as well. The predecessor of the Easter Seal Society, the National Society for Crippled Children and Adults, was established in 1907 in Ohio (Obermann, 1968).

Legal protections for laboring men were among the first formal provisions enacted for persons with physical disabilities. Germany and Austria legislated compensation for men disabled while working in 1884 and 1887, respectively. In the United States, Maryland enacted the first "workmen's compensation" law in 1902, which specifically provided a stated schedule of benefits to persons who became disabled while they were working (Obermann, 1968). During the opening decades of the 20th century, many other states followed Maryland's lead and established similar laws of their own.

Developments in worker's compensation laws led to discussions about rehabilitating disabled workers, and thus providing them with the training neces-sary to successfully reenter the workforce. The U.S. Congress passed Pub. L. 66-236 in 1920, which was the first civilian vocational rehabilitation law in the country (Braddock, 1986a; Obermann, 1968). Two years earlier the Congress had authorized rehabilitation services for disabled soldiers returning from World War I. While the 1920 law primarily targeted industrially injured persons, services were to be provided to "any person, who, by reason of a physical defect or infirmity, whether congenital or acquired by accident, injury, or disease" (Obermann, 1968, p. 161). Persons with mental disabilities were not, however, eligible for rehabilitation services at this time.

Goodwill Industries was established in 1902 in Boston. Goodwill initially collected and distributed clothing and other contributions for the poor. Unemployed persons were subsequently hired to repair and renovate donations before they were sold with the intention that the income generated would pay the workers. This program was later expanded to provide rehabilitation and sheltered work to persons with disabilities who were perceived as otherwise unable to support themselves (Obermann, 1968). Goodwill Industries expanded across the United States and into other countries by the 1940s.

Charitable organizations often involved themselves in the monitoring of physical disability after the turn of the 20th century. These organizations would conduct surveys to determine the extent of physical disability, and then promulgate recommendations to address the needs of those found to have disability. A typical survey was one conducted in New York City in 1919, following a polio epidemic in 1916. The committee sent orthopedic surgeons to the homes of individuals that the survey had identified who had not received treatment, and proposed that a system of services be developed that included the following components: education, vocational training, medical treatment, convalescent care, custodial care, social services, home treatment, summer outings, employment placement, braces and appliances, and work in the home (Wright, 1920). The result of collaboration among 41 social service agencies in New York, this comprehensive plan for people with physical disabilities reported on nearly every aspect of life with disability and recommended greater access to education and employment opportunities as the central issues of concern.

A similar survey was conducted in Cleveland in 1916 by the Welfare Federation of Cleveland. This survey included numerous interviews with working men with physical disabilities. Their attitudes and advice are insightful. One locksmith stated that, "If you have something to offer, you can usually get a job, but you must be sure that what you have to offer is of real value" (Anonymous, as cited in Wright & Hamburger, 1918, p. 237). This man reported stories of being harassed about his disability by others, but he also told of his ability to persevere and succeed in the working world. Other men with disabilities described similar successes in maintaining employment, albeit in the face of difficult conditions.

Advances in orthopedic treatment and prosthetic devices for people who lost limbs during wartime or in industry were made during World War I. While primitive forms of artificial limbs had been used for centuries, technological advances subsequent to World War I resulted in the development of more comfortable and effective prosthes. These advances enabled greater numbers of men with disabilities to return to work after sustaining impairments. During this period, an understanding of the importance of individually fitting each person, as opposed to mass-producing devices, developed (Martin, 1924).

Emergence of Family, Community, and Consumer Models

Although the Depression and World War II inhibited innovation in service delivery for people with intellectual disability in the United States (Noll, 1996; Trent, 1995), some progress was de. New York State, for example, introduced foster family care in the 1930s, authorizing payment for the care of persons with intellectual disabilities in family homes (Vaux, 1935). Research subsequently confirmed the beneficial effects of placement in foster or adoptive homes (Skeels & Harms, 1948; Speer, 1940) and the benefits of preschool intervention programs (Lazar & Darlington, 1982; Skeels et al., 1938).

The 1940s witnessed greater public awareness of conditions in mental hospitals brought on by another autobiographical account of institutionalization. Publication of Mary Jane Ward's *The Snake Pit* (1946), which was subsequently made into an Acad-

emy Award-winning movie, heightened awareness of brutal conditions in American mental hospitals (Peterson, 1982). The perceived need for enhanced research efforts in mental illness led to the 1946 creation of the National Institute of Mental Health (NIMH), which also led to increased community services for people with mental illness in the United States (Braddock, 1986a; Felix, 1957). In 1946, when the National Mental Health Act that created the NIMH was enacted, 24 states had community-based mental health programs. By 1957, every state had at least some community-based mental health services stimulated in part by the NIMH (Felix, 1957).

In 1940, the National Federation of the Blind was founded, the first consumer-advocacy organization for blind persons in the U.S. This group opposed the non-blind leadership in the American Foundation for the Blind, which had formed in 1921 (Koestler, 1976; Matson, 1990). The split between organizations for blind persons and those led by blind people was international as well. In 1964, blind persons decided to separate from the World Council for the Welfare of the Blind and form their own organization (Driedger, 1989).

The Social Model of Disability

While some people with disabilities at mid-century wrote about their experiences as a tragedy to be overcome (e.g., Walker, 1950), writings of blind Americans in the mid-20th century describe not blindness, but the social and physical environment, as the essential problem of disability. "Not blindness, but the attitude of the seeing to the blind is the hardest burden to bear" (Keller, as cited in Gowman, 1957, p. 5). "All too frequently the great tragedy of a blind person's life is not primarily his blindness, but the reactions of the family and social group toward him as a non-typical member" (Maxfield, as cited in Gowman, 1957, p. 5). Chevigny (1946) writes:

> The tragic aspect of blindness does not inhere in the condition nor can it do so. In nature it is absent. It is an entirely civilized idea. The world in which a man finds himself creates the tragedy for him and in him. If I found blindness more of a major nuisance than a

tragedy, therefore, it was because of the world in which I moved and had my being. (p. ix)

The intellectual basis for these ideas regarding the interaction between disability and society was powerfully advanced in Berger and Luckmann's (1967) sociological treatise on the social nature of knowledge. Their social-constructivist view was a harbinger of the social model of disability that would later emerge in the research of Saad Nagi (1970), and in disability studies and the independent living movement of the 1970s (Bowe, 1978; Davis, 1997; Linton, 1998; Oliver, 1983, 1990; Scott, 1968). The World Health Organization's (1980) definitions of impairment, disability, and handicap, which proposed a distinction between the socially constructed disadvantages that accrue to persons with impairments and the physical realities of impairment, were grounded in the writings of these early theorists and advocates (Lupton, 2000). Explaining the significance of this distinction, Bickenbach (1993) has argued that:

> Handicaps are thus socially created disadvantages that arise from the social reception of impairments and disabilities. The explicit focus of this dimension of disablement is social valuations of physical states (or perceived physical states); there is no question here of normative neutrality. Moreover, nearly every aspect of the conceptual structure of the notion is shaped by and so relative to social and cultural forces. (p. 48)

Organizational Developments

Beginning in the 1950s, friends and parents of people with disabilities began organizing for more extensive services for people with disabilities in many parts of the world. At that time, schools and activity centers were established, and ultimately international associations were founded, comprising national organizations interested in the prevention of disability.

Parents of people with intellectual disabilities in Washington State had actually organized to advocate for services for their children as early as the 1930s (Jones, 1987); however, larger-scale organizing by such groups didn't occur until the 1950s. During the 1950s, local groups of parents from many states joined forces and formed the group that became the National Association for Retarded Children (now The Arc). These families organized to advocate for services for their children including better conditions in institutions and the development of schools and workshops (Goode, 1999). A similar nationwide organization of families of people with mental illness would not be developed until the 1979 founding of NAMI, the National Alliance for the Mentally Ill (Grob, 1994; Lefley, 1996).

In 1953, the Council of World Organizations Interested in the Handicapped (CWOIH, now the International Council on Disability) was formed (Driedger, 1989). The constituent organizations of the World Council generally did not include people with disabilities as active leaders, however (Driedger, 1989). In the United States, the 1950s and 1960s saw the formation of organizations directed by people with disabilities, a departure from organizations led by the able-bodied for people with disabilities (Roberts, 1989). Single-disability-focused international organizations led by consumers with those disabilities were subsequently established including the World Federation of the Deaf, International Federation of the Blind, and the Fédération Internationale des Mutilés, des Invalides du Travail et des Invalides Civils (Driedger, 1989).

Beginnings of Deinstitutionalization

The introduction of anti-psychotic drugs in the 1950s coupled with public commitments to a community treatment approach, resulted in a rapid decline in the average daily resident population of state and county-operated psychiatric hospitals (Grob, 1994). The aggregate census began declining for two additional reasons. Penicillin, which was utilized to cure syphilis, led to a decrease in the number of persons with this disease in public mental hospitals. Also, following implementation of the Social Security Act of 1935, many elderly residents were moved to nursing homes (Holstein & Cole, 1995; Hughes, 1986). Between 1955-75, the census in psychiatric hospitals dropped by 200,000 persons from a high of 559,000 (Braddock, 1981; National Association of State Mental Health Program Directors Research Institute, 1996). However, the declining overall census of such facilities during this period tells only part of the story. While psychiatric hospitals continued to be exceedingly overcrowded, admissions and discharges operated like a revolving door for many patients. In a typical one-year period, there were more than 147,000 admissions and nearly 188,000 discharges and deaths (Grimes, 1964). Homelessness has also been a serious consequence of the deinstitutionalization movement for persons with mental illness (Grob, 1994; Lefley, 1996). However, the community movement for persons with intellectual disabilities has been considerably more successful in developing services and support programs, and avoiding homelessness to the degree experienced by persons with mental illness (Braddock, 1992).

The census in public facilities for persons with intellectual disabilities peaked at 194,650 in 1967 (U.S. Department of Health, Education, and Welfare, 1972). More than 20,000 additional persons with intellectual disabilities resided in state and county psychiatric hospitals at the time. The average facility population of institutions for people with intellectual disabilities was 1,422 residents in 1962 (Survey and Research Corporation, 1965). Several facilities, such as Willowbrook in New York and Lincoln in Illinois, housed 4,000-8,000 residents. In the 1960s, despite growing evidence to the contrary, American society still treated persons with intellectual disabilities as a group that needed to be controlled by segregation, sterilization, and isolation.

Political Activism and the Right to Treatment

In light of deplorable conditions in institutions for people with mental illness, discussion began to take shape within the legal community about the right to treatment for people who were incarcerated in these facilities. Morton Birnbaum led this initiative with the 1960 publication of his paper, "The Right to Treatment" (Birnbaum, 1965; Levy & Rubenstein, 1996). The first case in which an American court recognized the right to treatment was the landmark 1966 case of *Rouse v. Cameron*, which held that if an individual was involuntarily committed to a facility, at a minimum,

he or she had the right to receive treatment, because the purpose of confinement was treatment and not punishment (Levy & Rubenstein, 1996). Subsequent cases upheld this right, which was extended in the 1970s to include people with intellectual disability as well (Levy & Rubenstein, 1996; Parry, 1995).

The election of John F. Kennedy to the United States presidency in 1960 ushered in the modern era of intellectual disability services in the United States and an expanded concern for people with mental illness as well. On October 11, 1961, President Kennedy issued an unprecedented statement regarding the need for a national plan in the field of mental retardation. "We as a nation," he said, "have for too long postponed an intensive search for solutions to the problems of the mentally retarded. That failure should be corrected" (p.196). Kennedy appointed the President's Panel on Mental Retardation. The Panel's 95 recommendations, released in 1962, were broad and far-reaching. They extended from issues of civil rights to the need for scientific research on etiology and prevention. The panel called for a substantial downsizing of institutional facilities, an expansion of community services, and most importantly, it clearly embraced the principle of normalization (Nirje, 1976; Wolfensberger, 1972) as a guide to future innovation in service delivery.

Many of the 95 recommendations of the President's Panel (1962) were enacted into law by the 88th Congress as Pub. L. 88-156 and 88-164. Pub. L. 88-156, the Maternal and Child Health and Mental Retardation Planning Amendments of 1963, doubled the spending ceiling for the existing Maternal and Child Health State Grant Program, and established a new mental retardation planning grant program in the states. The planning effort was unique in the history of the field in that federal legislation required all 50 participating states to produce comprehensive plans for the development of improved residential, community, and preventive services.

President Kennedy also signed into law the Community Mental Health Centers Act of 1963, which stimulated the development of such centers across the country (Grob, 1994). While these centers were never funded at a level consistent with the desires of their supporters (Braddock, 1987), they did develop into a network of community support for people with mental illness (Grob, 1994).

The 1970s was a decade of considerable progress in public policy for people with disabilities in the United States (Silverstein, 2000). There were four major, catalytic events: (a) the 1971 passage of the ICF/MR (Intermediate Care Facilities/Mental Retardation) program as part of Title XIX (Medicaid) of the Social Security Act; (b) Judge Frank M. Johnson's landmark 1972 right to treatment ruling in the Alabama case of *Wyatt v. Stickney*; (c) the political organizing which led to the 1973 passage of Section 504 of the Rehabilitation Act prohibiting discrimination against disabled individuals in any program receiving federal financial assistance; and (d) the 1975 passage of the Education of All Handicapped Children Act (now known as IDEA) (Braddock, 1986b; Scotch, 1984).

The passage of the ICF/MR law in 1971 enabled the states to obtain federal funding for institutional services for people with intellectual disabilities if the care provided met minimal federal standards of treatment and space. Insofar as the federal government would reimburse states for 50-78% of the costs of institutional care, states had great incentives to change their services to conform to federal standards. This led to a tremendous push to deinstitutionalize as the minimum space requirements were well beyond the overcrowded capacities of nearly all the nation's institutions (Rothman & Rothman, 1984). Peaking in 1967 at more than 194,000 people, the population of the nation's public institutions for persons with mental retardation and developmental disabilities has declined steadily to 47,374 persons in 2000 (Braddock, Hemp, Rizzolo, Parish, & Pomeranz, 2002). Advances in applied behavioral interventions have facilitated community, employment, and social integration (Jacobson, Burchard, & Carling, 1992; Koegel, Koegel, & Dunlap, 1996; Thompson & Grabowski, 1977).

The *Wyatt v. Stickney* (1971) decision in regard to people with intellectual disability was built upon the principle of right to treatment developed for people with mental illness. Judge Johnson found that people in Alabama's institutions had a constitutional right to treatment (Levy & Rubenstein, 1996; Parry, 1995). This case began a tidal wave of federal class-action cases related to conditions in institutions for people with intellectual disabilities, culminating in more than 70 cases in 41 states (Braddock et al., 2000; Hayden,

1997; Levy & Rubenstein, 1996). Similar litigation was also filed on the right to education (Martin, Martin, & Terman, 1996; *Pennsylvania Ass'n. Retarded Child. v. Commonwealth of PA*, 1971).

In 1973, the U.S. Congress enacted Section 504 of the Rehabilitation Act, which prohibited discrimination against people with disabilities by any entity that received federal funds (National Council on Disability, 1997; Percy, 1989; Scotch, 1984). The promulgation of regulations that would clarify the operating provisions of Section 504 were delayed by Secretary David Mathews of the U.S. Department of Health, Education, and Welfare (HEW), and then by his successor, Secretary Joseph Califano (National Council on Disability, 1997; Scotch, 1984). Disabled advocates organized to force promulgation of the regulations, first by suing Secretary Mathews and then by organizing sit-ins and demonstrations in HEW offices in San Francisco, New York, and Washington (Fleischer & Zames, 1998). For the first time, American television audiences saw people with disabilities occupying federal buildings to secure their rights (Roberts, 1989). These demonstrations resulted in the 1977 promulgation of regulations four years after the law was signed. Judy Heumann, a leader in the fight for release of the regulations, stated, "I don't think the regulations would have been signed without the demonstrations, as they were. I am totally convinced of that. I mean the political pressure was really getting to be heavy. They had to sign those regulations" (as cited in Scotch, 1984, p. 116). Highlights of Section 504 included a mandate for new construction to be barrier-free, mandating accessibility in programs and activities in existing facilities, and supporting reasonable accommodations for the employment of people with disabilities (Scotch, 1984).

The coalition-building and advocacy by disability groups during the Section 504 political action activities was one of the first times in American history that cross-disability advocacy groups had successfully worked together on a unified disability rights agenda. This cross-disability advocacy has been instrumental in gaining passage of other legislation such as the Technology Related Assistance for Individuals with Disabilities Act (Pub. L. 100-407), recently amended in 1998 (Pub. L. 105-394). Coalition-building and advocacy helped establish the foundation for the passage of the Americans with Disabilities Act in 1990 (Fleischer & Zames, 1998; National Council on Disability, 1997).

In 1980, after years of seeking equal representation within the professional organization Rehabilitation International (RI), disabled people broke with RI, and formed Disabled Peoples' International. Since 1922, RI had been the only international cross-disability organization that addressed the needs of people with a variety of mental, physical, and sensory disabilities (Driedger, 1989). In 1980, at a World Congress of RI, a resolution was defeated that would have mandated the equal participation of people with disabilities in each country's RI organization. In response, disabled advocates then established Disabled Peoples' International (DPI), indicating no tolerance for patronizing behavior by professionals. Disabled people would direct their own destiny. DPI worked energetically to establish the presence of people with disabilities on the world stage. By 1983, it had achieved consultative status with several United Nations organizations, and by 1985, organizations of disabled people had been established in nearly every country in the world (Driedger, 1989).

The fourth watershed civil rights event in the 1970s in the United States was passage of the Education for All Handicapped Children's Act of 1975, which guaranteed children and youth with disabilities the right to a free, appropriate, public education. For the first time in the history of compulsory education in the United States, parents had a federally enforced right to education for their children with disabilities. Beyond the obviously important changes in education for children with disabilities, this legislation also created a generation of parents who believed that their children were entitled to related community services. Many of these parents would become strong advocates for community services and inclusive education. In the 1995-96 school year, 46% of children with disabilities in the U.S. were educated in regular classroom settings, while the remainder were educated in a combination of other settings including resource rooms, separate classrooms, and separate schools (U.S. Department of Education, 1998).

The education for deaf and blind students in the U.S., however, has traditionally been provided in special residential schools that began in the 19th century.

Some have objected to the segregated education provided in such schools. For example, research conducted with women with visual impairments in England has demonstrated that the women educated in special schools felt that their experiences had been detrimental to their growth and that dependence was fostered in such settings (French, 1996).

Recent analysis of educational data for blind and deaf students indicated that the number of blind students educated in residential schools has declined. Kirchner, Peterson, and Suhr (1988) found that between 1963 and 1978, the percent of blind students educated in public and private residential schools declined from 45% to 24%. By 1996, the latest school year for which data are available, 11% of deaf children were being educated in residential schools (U.S. Department of Education, 1998). In 1998, the number of blind children being educated in residential schools had fallen to 8% (American Printing House for the Blind, 1999). The total number of deaf and blind children being educated in residential schools in 1996 were 7,311 and 2,179, respectively (U.S. Department of Education, 1998).

Independent Living and Self-Advocacy

The 1970s was also the decade of the rise of independent living in the United States (DeJong, 1979a, 1979b; Stewart et al., 1999). As previously noted, this movement gathered strength from the advocacy needed to force the promulgation of the Vocational Rehabilitation Act of 1973's Section 504 rules. Such legislation was predicated on the notion that people with disabilities need supports to live independently in their communities, not only because of their impairments, but because society is constructed in such a way as to preclude their full participation (Bowe, 1978). The initial catalysts for the independent living movement in the United States were drawn from a critical analysis of the processes of medicalization and professionalization in the rehabilitation system (Lysack & Kaufert, 1994; Zola, 1979). In Canada, the independent living movement emerged in the early 1980s, also driven by the advocacy efforts of people with disabilities (Boschen & Krane, 1992).

The independent living movement embraced the

notion that the barriers which confront people with disabilities are less related to individual impairment than to social attitudes, interpretations of disability, architectural barriers, legal barriers, and educational barriers (Bowe, 1978; Americans Disabled for Attendant Programs Today, 1995). The creation in the early 1970s of the nation's first Independent Living Center in Berkeley, California, served as a model for the development of such centers across the country (DeJong, 1979a; Roberts, 1989). This first center, and hundreds of others that followed it, offered an array of services including peer counseling, advocacy services, van transportation, training in independent living skills, wheelchair repair, housing referral, and attendant care referral, among others (DeJong, 1979a; Roberts, 1989). Central to the independent living movement is the notion that people with disabilities themselves must set the agenda for research and political action in disability policy (DeJong, 1981). Ed Roberts (1989), one of the founders of the Independent Living Movement, identified the four core principles of independent living as self-determination, self-image and public education, advocacy, and service to all (pp. 238-239). In the year 2000, there were 336 Centers for Independent Living and 253 subordinate sites operating in the U.S. They served 212,000 persons in approximately 60% of the nation's 3,141 counties (Innes et al., 2000).

Self-determination in the United States has focused on the independent living center as a primary coordinating organization by which disabled people engage in the advocacy and education activities needed to meet their individual and collective goals. In the Netherlands, the independent living needs of people with disabilities have been embraced by the country's mainstream entitlement programs, wedding a system of residential care and independent living to the country's general health and social welfare systems (DeJong, 1984). Denmark and Germany, nations similar to the Netherlands in welfare policy, also have connected programs for people with disabilities to their mainstream entitlement programs (Fröhlich, 1982; Jørgensen, 1982). In Britain, housing has been a pivotal advocacy and policy concern of the independent living movement (Stewart et al., 1999).

The advocacy organization Disabled in Action was founded in 1970 by Judy Heumann to address barriers faced by people with disabilities and by 1972 it

had 1,500 members. The group engaged in activities ranging from a march on Washington protesting President Nixon's veto of the Vocational Rehabilitation Act Amendments of 1973 to the staging of protests at inaccessible buildings and at Jerry Lewis telethons. The telethons utilized paternalistic, pity-oriented depictions of people with disabilities to raise funds. These initial political advocacy efforts led to the formation in 1974 of the American Coalition of Citizens with Disabilities, which became an umbrella organization for disability advocacy groups across the nation (Scotch, 1989).

In America, states' efforts to "reform" institutions for people with intellectual disabilities in the 1970s gave way to efforts to reallocate institutional resources to community services activities. States began closing institutions in significant numbers for the first time in the early 1980s (Braddock & Heller, 1985). In 1991, New Hampshire closed the Laconia Developmental Center and became the first state in the United States to provide all of its services to people with intellectual disability in the community (Covert et al., 1994). By 2000, 37 states had closed 125 state institutions for people with intellectual disabilities (Braddock et al., 2002). In addition to New Hampshire, all public institutions for people with intellectual disabilities have also been closed in Alaska, the District of Columbia, Hawaii, Minnesota, New Mexico, Rhode Island, Vermont, and West Virginia (Braddock et al., 2002).

Institutional phase-downs and closures have been accompanied by a growing emphasis on supported community living for individuals with intellectual disabilities. Between 1977 and 1998, the number of persons living in community-based settings for 1 to 6 persons expanded from 20,409 to 263,359 persons, a more than 12-fold increase. Much of this tremendous expansion in community services was fueled by the federal-state partnership in the Medicaid Home and Community Based Services (HCBS) Waiver Program (Braddock et al., 2002).

The reduction in reliance on residential institutions for people with intellectual disability occurred in Great Britain and across Western Europe as well (Keith & Schalock, 2000). In England, for example, the census of public hospitals for people with intellectual disability (those operated by the National Health Service) declined 83%, from 44,400 in 1980 to 7,400 persons in 1996. Similarly significant declines were noted in other U.K. countries. In Wales, Scotland, and Northern Ireland, census reductions of 70%, 51%, and 48%, respectively, were noted during the same 1980-96 period (Emerson et al., 2000).

Organized self-advocacy is an important manifestation of the emergence of autonomy and self-determination for people with intellectual disability (Dybwad & Bersani, 1996; Longhurst, 1994). Membership in local and statewide self-advocacy groups like People First has grown rapidly. Hayden and Senese (1996) identified over 1,000 self-advocacy groups, some in every state. This represented almost a three-fold expansion in the number of groups since 1990 (Longhurst, 1994). In 1995, self-advocacy groups established a national organization called Self Advocates Becoming Empowered (SABE). SABE has developed an advocacy agenda calling for the phase down and closure of all state operated mental retardation institutions in the United States (Dybwad & Bersani, 1996).

Self-advocacy by people with mental illness has included people completely opposed to organized psychiatry, psychotropic medication, and institutional treatment (Lefley, 1996). The first group of ex-patients devoted to the "liberation from psychiatry" formed in Portland, Oregon, in 1969. Advocacy by this group has included litigation to combat involuntary, uninformed use of electroconvulsive therapy (ECT), litigation against ECT manufacturers, and pressing for consumer advisory functions at the state level of mental illness service administration (MadNation, 1999).

Deaf students at Gallaudet University gained national attention in 1988 by advocating for a deaf president. In addition to initiating the Deaf President Now movement, the students sought a deaf majority on the university's board of directors. The university's first deaf president, I. King Jordan, was subsequently appointed, and the first deaf chair of the board, Philip Bravin, was selected (Gallaudet University, 1997).

International Disability Rights Initiatives

The 1990 passage of the Americans with Disabilities Act (ADA) in the United States was a watershed event for disability rights on the international stage. This law recognized that discrimination against people with disabilities in the form of purposeful unequal treatment and historical patterns of segregation and isolation was the major problem confronting people with disabilities and not their individual impairments (National Council on Disability, 1997; Parry, 1995). The ADA also stated that people with disabilities have been relegated to powerless positions based on stereotypical assumptions about their disabilities. As such, the ADA bars discrimination against people with disabilities in employment, public services, public accommodations, and telecommunications (Parry, 1995). The ADA was enacted after a concerted effort by a coalition of mental, physical, and sensory disability rights groups to work together to secure its passage (National Council on Disability, 1997). As noted, the cross-disability coalition that advocated for enactment of the ADA was built in part on the foundation initially developed by advocates pushing for the enactment and subsequent promulgation of rules for the Vocational Rehabilitation Act Amendments of 1973 (Scotch, 1989).

In Britain, a similar law protecting the rights of people with disabilities, the Disability Discrimination Act, was enacted in 1995 (Doyle, 1996; Gooding, 1996). This law mandated reasonable adjustments to the policies and physical environments of employers with 20 or more employees, compelling the removal of barriers facing people with disabilities (Gooding, 1996). The law also mandated accessibility in public transportation (Doyle, 1996; Gooding, 1996). While the law has been hailed as an advance in civil rights for people living in Scotland, England, Wales, and Ireland, disability advocates have expressed disappointment that the law did not go as far as it should have in protecting and facilitating enforcement of the rights of people with disabilities (Doyle, 1996; Gooding, 1996).

At the international level, the United Nations General Assembly unanimously adopted in 1994 the *Standard Rules on the Equalization of Opportunities for Persons With Disabilities* (United Nations, 1994). The *Standard Rules* are not legally enforceable internationally, but they do provide basic international standards for programs, laws, and policy on disability. The *Standard Rules* grew out of earlier pressure from international disability interests to promote greater participation by people with disabilities in society. This philosophy was initially expressed in the 1971 Declaration of the Rights of Mentally Retarded Persons (United Nations, 1971), the 1975 Declaration of the Rights of Disabled Persons (United Nations, 1975), and the more comprehensive statement expressed in the 1982 World Program of Action Concerning Disabled Persons (United Nations, 1982).

The purpose of the World Program of Action (WPA) is to:

> Promote effective measures for prevention of disability, rehabilitation and the realization of the goals of 'full participation' of disabled persons, in social life and development, and of 'equality'. This means opportunities equal to those of the whole population and an equal share in the improvement in living conditions resulting from social and economic development. These concepts should apply with the same scope and with the same urgency to all countries, regardless of their level of development.
>
> The WPA requires member states to plan, organize and finance activities at each level; create, through legislation, the necessary legal bases and authority for measures to achieve the objectives; ensure opportunities by eliminating barriers to full participation; provide rehabilitation services by giving social, nutritional, medical, educational and vocational assistance and technical aids to disabled persons; establish or mobilize relevant public and private organizations; support the establishment and growth of organizations of disabled persons; and prepare and disseminate information relevant to the issues of the World Programme of Action. (Metts, 2000, p. 20)

The United Nation's 1994 *Standard Rules* was predicated on the principles embodied in the World Program of Action which focuses on the equalization of opportunities for people with disabilities. This commitment to disabled persons goes well beyond traditional international anti-discrimination protections of property, political, and judicial rights by seeking to convey rights to rehabilitation, special education, and access to public and private facilities and programs.

The European Union (1996) has also adopted general disability policies similar to the U.N.'s World Program of Action.

In addition to Great Britain and the United States, a number of nations adopted legislation in the 1990s prohibiting discrimination against persons with disabilities. Australia adopted the Disability Discrimination Act of 1993 outlawing discrimination on the basis of disability and the constitutions of Germany, Austria, Finland, and Brazil have been similarly amended. Constitutional changes have also been adopted in South Africa, Malawi, Uganda, and the Philippines. These actions are representative of the recent flurry of legislative activity on a worldwide basis to promote the rights of people with disabilities (Metts, 2000).

In the United States, the growth of public spending for disability programs during the past 30 years has paralleled the rise of parent and consumer advocacy, and of the "disability business" (Albrecht, 1992). In fiscal year 1997, $108.8 billion was allocated for long-term care services and rehabilitation, housing and veterans activities by federal, state and local governments in the United States. General health care commanded $52.9 billion and $36.4 billion was allocated for special education activities. An additional $95.8 billion was spent for disability-related income maintenance in 1997, primarily through the Supplemental Security Income and Social Security Disability Insurance programs (Braddock, 2000; following chapter, this volume).

Thus, at the close of the 20th century the public sector in the United States was spending $293.3 billion for disability services and income supports for over 41.5 million recipients. This spending level was 12.2% of the country's total public expenditure for all purposes from combined federal and state sources in 1997. However, a large percentage of the $108.8 billion financial commitment for disability services long-term care — approximately 52% of the funds — supported the placement of hundreds of thousands of persons with disabilities in segregated settings such as nursing homes, sheltered workshops, and mental institutions. Furthermore, a large percentage of the 5.7 million students with disabilities in special education, particularly those with significant disabilities, received services in separate classes, separate educational facilities, or public or private institutions. Sixty-one percent of students with intellectual disabilities ("mental retardation"), for example, were served in segregated educational settings in 1996 (U.S. Department of Education, 1998). While it is clear that the United States has made enormous strides in the implementation of disability assistance programs over the past few decades (Silverstein, 2000), the basic funding priorities in many programs, such as Medicaid and special education, have not kept pace with contemporary consumer support models based on choice, self-determination, home care, family support, and inclusive education.

CONCLUSION

After the 17th century, medical science and the rise of custodial residential institutions undermined the self-determination of people with disabilities during a period of rapid and continuous urbanization and industrialization in the West. It did this by over-medicalizing what was, in large measure, a social, educational, and economic problem, separating many disabled people from their families, communities, and society at large. This socially sanctioned segregation reinforced negative societal attitudes toward human difference. However, the segregation of disabled people in one geographic place — in residential schools for deaf and blind persons, mental institutions for those with emotional problems and intellectual limitations and, eventually, in special public school classes and rehabilitation centers — also facilitated the development of empowered group identities that ultimately led to political activism.

Assertive political activism by people with disabilities and their families is primarily a late 20th century phenomenon that, in the United States, draws considerable strength from the example of the civil rights movement for people of color (Birnbaum & Taylor, 2000). It is, in fact, an often repeated general truism in the disability field today that prejudicial and exclusionary practices are greater barriers to social participation for disabled people than their particular mental, physical, or sensory impairments (Scotch, 1989).

People with disabilities have shared a history that has often been oppressive and included abuse, neglect, sterilization, stigma, euthanasia, segregation, and institutionalization. Disabled people, who have survived by relying on tenacity and resourcefulness and on support provided in different measures by family, friends, and local communities, are currently struggling to claim identity (Anspach, 1979; Gill, 1997; Linton, 1998) and political power (Hahn, 1985). While the deaf community has a history of struggling collectively to preserve their culture for more than a century, people with mental and physical disabilities have only emerged to champion their own interests collectively within the last three or four decades.

Advocacy by specific, single-disability groups in the United States began to evolve into cross-disability coalition-building in the 1970s, 1980s, and 1990s. Cross-disability advocacy, for example, secured passage of the Americans with Disabilities Act (National Council on Disability, 1997). The paternalism of non-disabled 19th century figures such as Howe, Pinel, Gallaudet, and Rushton has been replaced, at least in part, with leadership and self-determination by people with disabilities themselves. Thus, at the close of the 20th century, the foundation is gradually being established in the West for a new era based on civil rights, social participation, and a cross-disability perspective.

Achieving inclusive societies, however, will require persons with mental, physical, and sensory disabilities to learn more about one another and, on common ground, to construct more powerful community, state, national, and international cross-disability coalitions than have been developed in the past. In this chapter we argued that people across the spectrum of disability have a good deal in common historically, and that recognizing and celebrating this shared history is an important step in building stronger and more effective cross-disability coalitions in the future.

The potential strength of cross-disability coalitions should grow as societies age since the prevalence of impairment in a society is directly correlated with aging. Over the course of the next 30 years, the number of persons aged 65 and over will double in the United States, triple in Germany and Japan, and advance rapidly in virtually every developed nation of the world (U.S. Bureau of the Census, 1997; Janicki & Ansello, 2000). As more developing countries make significant economic advances, these nations will experience a concomitant rise in political advocacy by and for people with disabilities. Albrecht and Verbrugge (2000) refer to this growing phenomenon of disability across the developed and developing nations of the world as the global emergence of disability. "With or without anyone's attention," they argue, "global disability will be on the rise for many decades to come, fueled by population aging, environmental degradation, and social violence" (p. 305). The key disability issues for developing societies include controlling infectious diseases that lead to disability, reducing unsafe occupational conditions, managing drought and the environment, limiting ethnic, religious, and regional wars and launching thoughtful innovations in income support, health promotion, special education, rehabilitation, and the promotion of self-determination (Hoffman & Field, 1995). By adopting programs that stress consumer, family, and community values, many developing nations will hopefully be able to avoid replicating the developed world's self-destructive preoccupations with segregation, institutionalization, and eugenics.

The principal disability issues currently facing the developed nations in Europe, North America, and Australasia, according to Albrecht and Verbrugge (2000), include fashioning reasonable eligibility standards for income maintenance and service programs for persons with disabilities, advancing civil rights, creating access to employment, public accommodations and society at large and minimizing regional, state, and sub-state differences in public welfare benefits and service programs. To these critically important contemporary issues, we would add that developed nations also must confront (a) ethical and cost-benefit dilemmas accompanying advances in gene therapy, biotechnology, and neuroscience research; (b) the potential for assisted suicide to lead to the widespread euthanasia of persons with disabilities; (c) the continuing segregation of millions of persons with disabilities in nursing homes, institutions, and other segregated settings throughout the world; and, (d) developing productive and reciprocally valued working relationships between consumers with disabilities seeking greater self-determination and political power and the professionals who provide and study services to people with disabilities (Barnes, 1996; Humphrey, 2000; Oliver, 1992; Oliver & Barnes, 1999). The United States in particular must also confront the growing inequality in the distribution of the wealth of its citizenry and the profound health care and educational disparities between rich and poor (Galbraith, 1998).

The disability rights struggle of the first half of the 21st century will fundamentally be a struggle to de-link the enduring and oppressive relationship between poverty and disability. Even in the most economically developed nations of the world today, unemployment rates for disabled persons frequently approach 80% and average personal income is in the bottom decile.

As researchers, we need to mount a series of rigorous, comparative, recurring empirical studies to monitor the growth of public sector resource and service commitments for disability programs in every country of the world in which it is possible to do so. These recurring studies need to assess the allocation of resources on a nationwide basis for disability programs so that all the nations of the world can be held accountable for their commitments to disabled people and their families. Such studies would permit the priority which a nation assigns to disability to be evaluated over time and to be compared to other nations with similar levels of wealth. The information generated in such studies would be useful in program planning and, by identifying the leaders and the laggards among the nations of the world, it would be immensely useful to disability advocates seeking to influence public policy on behalf of their constituencies. Several international organizations should be approached to sponsor this research including the World Bank, the United Nations, the European Union, the Pan American Health Organization, and the World Health Organization. In the United States, the National Institute on Disability and Rehabilitation Research (NIDRR) should also consider launching one or more "International Rehabilitation Research and Training Centers." These Centers would focus on significantly expanding educational and research links on disability between and among the developed and developing nations of the world.

Albrecht and Verbrugge (2000) are right: disability is emerging globally. The number of disabled people in 175 nations of the world today was recently estimated to range from 235 to 549 million people. The lost Gross Domestic Product due to unemployment, underemployment, and services/support costs associated with disability was determined to range from $1.4 to $1.9 trillion per annum in current dollars (Metts, 2000). Disability research institutions such as NIDRR and international development organizations like the World Bank need to acknowledge the global emergence of disability by establishing and funding new strategies for international research leadership and action on disability in the 21st century.

One final point is in order. At the outset of this chapter we noted that the paucity of primary source evidence in most written histories of disability was a significant weakness. It is lamentable indeed that most existing records and publications have inevitably described disability history from the perspective of professionals who controlled the delivery of services. We endeavored in this chapter to use primary sources extensively when possible. However, in evaluating the strengths and weaknesses of this chapter, it is clear that we have barely touched on the potential of one very useful type of primary source material — literary and artistic archives — to complement the institutionally oriented history presented here. Studying the representation of disability in literature and art is an important and relatively unexplored research frontier in disability studies. It is a frontier with the potential to yield a richer understanding of the history of disability, with lived experience and perspective at the center of analysis rather than at the periphery. The work of Allen Thiher (1999), Robert Garland (1995), Rosemarie Garland Thomson (1997), David Mitchell (2000), and Sander Gilman (1988, 1995) exemplifies this approach and significant growth in research on disability and the humanities can be expected over the next decade. This scholarship will contribute greatly to the developing knowledge base on the history of disability and human diversity.

REFERENCES

Adair, R., Melling, J., & Forsythe, B. (1997). Migration, family structure, and pauper lunacy in Victorian England: Admissions to the Devon County Pauper Lunatic Asylum, 1845-1900, *Continuity & Change, 13*, 373-401.

Albrecht, G. L. (1992). *The disability business: Rehabilitation in America.* Newbury Park, CA: Sage.

Albrecht, G. L., & Verbrugge, L. M. (2000). The global emergence of disability. In G.L. Albrecht, R. Fitzpatrick, & S.C. Scrimshaw (Eds.), *The handbook of social studies in health and medicine* (pp. 293-307). London: Sage Publications.

Alexander, F. G., & Selesnick, S. T. (1964). *The history of psychiatry: An evaluation of psychiatric thought and practice from prehistoric times to the present.* New York: Harper & Row.

Allen, E. E. (1899). Education of defectives. In N.M. Butler (Ed.), *Monographs on education in the United States, 15.* New York: Department of Education for the United States Commission for the Paris Exposition of 1900.

Allen, E. E. (1914). *Progress of the education of the blind in the United States in the year 1912-1913: Chapter XXII, Volume I, 1913.* Washington, DC: U.S. Government Printing Office.

American Printing House for the Blind. (1999, February 1). *Distribution of eligible students based on the federal quota census of January 5, 1998.* Louisville, KY: Author. Available at: http://sun1.aph.org/dist98.htm

Americans Disabled for Attendant Programs Today. (1995). *Long-term care policy. It's good to have the facts when you choose (Statistics, sources, a call to action).* Rochester, NY: Free Hand Press.

Andrews, J. (1998). Begging the question of idiocy: The definition and socio-cultural meaning of idiocy in early modern Britain: Part I. *History of Psychiatry, 9*, 65-95.

Andrews, J., Briggs, A., Porter, R., Tucker, P., & Waddington, K. (1997). *The history of Bethlem.* New York: Routledge.

Anonymous. (1700). County asylums proposed. In R. Hunter & I. Macalpine (Eds., 1982), *Three hundred years of psychiatry: 1535-1860* (p. 277). Hartsdale, NY: Carlisle.

Anonymous. (1847a). A visit to the Bicêtre, first article. *Chambers's Edinburgh Journal, 7*(158), 20-22.

Anonymous. (1847b). A visit to the Bicêtre, second article. *Chambers's Edinburgh Journal, 7*(161), 71-73.

Anonymous. (1847c). A visit to the Bicêtre, third article. *Chambers's Edinburgh Journal, 7*(163), 105-107.

Anonymous. (1849). Five months in the New York State Lunatic Asylum. In D. Peterson (Ed., 1982), *A mad people's history of madness* (pp. 108-122). Pittsburgh: University of Pittsburgh Press.

Anspach, R. R. (1979). From stigma to identity politics: Political activism among the physically disabled and former mental patients. *Social Science & Medicine, 13A*, 765-773.

Axinn, J., & Levin, H. (1982). *Social welfare: A history of the American response to need.* New York: Longman.

Bacon, F. (1900). *The advancement of learning.* Oxford, England: Clarendon Press. (Original work published 1605)

Barnes, C. (1996). Disability and the myth of the independent researcher. *Disability & Society, 11*, 107-110.

Barr, M. W. (1895). Moral paranoia. *Proceedings of the Association of Medical Officers of American Institutions for Idiotic and Feeble-minded Persons, 20*, 522-531.

Barr, M. W. (1902). The imbecile and epileptic versus the taxpayer and the community. *Proceedings of the National Conference of Social Work,* pp. 161-165.

Barr, M. W. (1904). *Mental defectives.* Philadelphia: P. Blakiston's Sons.

Bartlett, F. L. (1964). Institutional peonage: Our exploitation of mental patients. *The Atlantic Monthly, 214*, 116-119.

Bassoe, P. (1945). Spain as the cradle of psychiatry. *American Journal of Psychiatry*, 731-738.

Baynton, D. C. (1993). "Savages and deaf-mutes":
Evolutionary theory and the campaign against sign
language in the 19th century. In J.V. Van Cleve
(Ed.), *Deaf history unveiled: Interpretations
from the new scholarship* (pp. 92-112). Washington, DC: Gallaudet University Press.

Baynton, D. C. (1996). *Forbidden signs: American culture and the campaign against sign
language.* Chicago: University of Chicago Press.

Beers, C. (1908). *A mind that found itself.* New
York: Longmans, Green.

Bell, A. G. (1969). *Upon the formation of deaf
variety of the human race.* Washington, DC:
Alexander Graham Bell Association for the Deaf.
(Original work published 1883)

Berger, P., & Luckmann, T. (1967). *The social
construction of reality: A treatise in the sociology of knowledge.* London: Allen Lane.

Berkson, G. (1974). Social responses of animals to
infants with defects. In M. Lewis & L.E.
Rosenblum (Eds.), *The effect of the infant on
its caregivers* (pp. 239-249). New York: Wiley.

Berkson, G. (1993). *Children with handicaps: A
review of behavioral research.* Hillsdale, NJ:
Lawrence Erlbaum.

Bernstein, C. (1917). Self-sustaining feebleminded.
Journal of Psycho-Asthenics, 22, 150-161.

Bernstein, C. (1918). Rehabilitation of the mentally
defective. *Journal of Psycho-Asthenics, 23,* 92-
103.

Bernstein, C. (1921). Colony care for isolation of
defective and dependent cases. *Proceedings of
the American Association on Mental Defect,
26,* 43-59.

Bickenbach, J. E. (1993). *Physical disability and
social policy.* Toronto: University of Toronto.

Bicknell, E. (1895). Custodial care of the adult
feebleminded. *Charities Review, 5,* 76-88.

Birnbaum, J., & Taylor, C. (2000). Introduction:
Where do we go from here? In J. Birnbaum & C.
Taylor (Eds.), *Civil rights since 1787: A reader
on the black struggle.* New York: New York
University Press.

Birnbaum, M. (1965). Some comments on "the right
to treatment." *Archives of General Psychiatry,
13,* 33-45.

Black, K. (1996). *Healing homiletic: Preaching
and disability.* Nashville, TN: Abingdon.

Blatt, B. (1977). The family album. *Mental Retardation, 15,* 3-4.

Bliquez, L. J. (1983). Classical prosthetics. *Archae-
ology, 36,* 25-29.

Bogdan, R. (1986). Exhibiting mentally retarded
people for amusement and profit, 1850-1940.
American Journal of Mental Deficiency, 91,
120-126.

Bogdan, R. (1988). *Freak show: Presenting
human oddities for amusement and profit.*
Chicago: University of Chicago Press.

Bonsall, A. (1891). Discussion on the care of
imbeciles. *Proceedings of the National Conference of Social Work,* 331-332.

Boschen, K. A., & Krane, N. (1992). A history of
independent living in Canada. *Canadian Journal
of Rehabilitation, 6,* 79-88.

Bowe, F. G. (1978). *Handicapping America:
Barriers to disabled people.* New York: Harper
& Row.

Braddock, D. (1981). Deinstitutionalization of the
retarded: Trends in public policy. *Hospital &
Community Psychiatry, 32,* 607-615.

Braddock, D. (1986a). Federal assistance for
mental retardation and developmental disabilities:
I. A review through 1961. *Mental Retardation,
24,* 175-182.

Braddock, D. (1986b). Federal assistance for
mental retardation and developmental disabilities:
II. The modern era. *Mental Retardation, 24,*
209-218.

Braddock, D. (1987). *Federal policy toward
mental retardation.* Baltimore: Brookes.

Braddock, D. (1992). Community mental health and
mental retardation services in the American states:
A comparative study of resource allocation.
American Journal of Psychiatry, 149, 175-
183.

Braddock, D. (2000). *Disability in the United
States: A comparative analysis of public
spending.* Chicago: University of Illinois at
Chicago, Department of Disability and Human
Development.

Braddock, D., & Heller, T. (1985). The closure of

mental retardation institutions: II. Implications. *Mental Retardation, 23,* 222-229.

Braddock, D., Hemp, R., Parish, S., & Rizzolo, M. C. (2000). *The state of the states in developmental disabilities: 2000 study summary.* Chicago: University of Illinois at Chicago, Department of Disability and Human Development.

Braddock, D., Hemp, R., Parish, S., & Westrich, J. (1998). *The state of the states in developmental disabilities* (5th ed.). Washington, DC: American Association on Mental Retardation.

Braddock, D., Hemp, R., Rizzolo, M. C., Parish, S., & Pomeranz, A. (2002). *The state of the states in developmental disabilities: 2002 study sumary.* Boulder: University of Colorado, Coleman Institute for Cognitive Disabilities and Department of Psychiatry.

Braddock, D. L., & Parish, S. L. (2001). An institutional history of disability. In G. Albrecht, K. Seelman, & M. Bury (Eds.), *Handbook of disability studies* (pp. 11-68). New York: Sage.

Breckinridge, S. P. (1927). *Public welfare administration in the United States: Select documents.* Chicago: University of Chicago Press.

Breckinridge, S. P. (1939). *The Illinois Poor Law and its administration.* Chicago: University of Chicago Press.

Bredberg, E. (1999). Writing disability history: Problems, perspectives, and sources. *Disability & Society, 14,* 189-201.

Brierre de Boismont, A. J. F. (1867). *Joseph Guislain, sa vie et ses ecrits [Joseph Guislain, his life and writings].* Paris: Bailliere.

Brigham, A. (1845). *Annual report of the Bloomingdale Insane Asylum.* Bloomingdale, NY: Bloomingdale Insane Asylum.

British Association of the Deaf. (1999). *Our history.* London: Author. Available at: http://www.bda.org.uk/index1.htm

Brockley, J. A. (1999). History of mental retardation: An essay review. *History of Psychology, 2,* 25-36.

Bromberg, W. (1975). *From shaman to psychotherapist: A history of the treatment of mental illness.* Chicago: Henry Regnery.

Brown, T. J. (1998). *Dorothea Dix: New England reformer.* Cambridge, MA: Harvard University Press.

Browne, W. A. F. (1837). *What asylums were, are, and ought to be: Being the substance of five lectures delivered before the managers of the Montrose Royal Lunatic Asylum.* Edinburgh: Adam & Charles Black.

Brundage, A. (1989). *Going to the sources: A guide to historical research and writing.* Arlington Heights, IL: Harlan Davidson.

Bucknill, J. C. (1873). Address on idiocy. *Journal of Mental Science, 19,* 167-83.

Burleigh, M. (1994). Psychiatry, German society, and the Nazi 'euthanasia' programme. *Social History of Medicine, 7,* 213-228.

Butler, A. W. (1907). The burden of feeble-mindedness. *Proceedings of the National Conference of Social Work,* 1-10.

Button, L. A. (1878). *Behind the scenes; or, life in an insane asylum.* Chicago: Culver, Page, Hoyne.

Carabello, B.J., & Siegel, J.F. (1996). Self-advocacy at the crossroads. In G. Dybwad & H. Bersani (Eds.), *New voices: Self-advocacy by people with disabilities* (pp. 237-239). Cambridge, MA: Brookline Books.

Carpenter, J. (1996). Rev. Harold Nelson Burden and Katherine Mary Burden: Pioneers of inebriate reformatories and mental deficiency institutions. *Journal of the Royal Society of Medicine, 89,* 205-209.

Carrey, N. J. (1995). Itard's 1828 memoire on "Mutism caused by a lesion of the intellectual functions": A historical analysis. *Journal of the American Academy of Child and Adolescent Psychiatry, 34,* 1655-1661.

Cavallo, S. (1998). Family obligations and inequalities in access to care in northern Italy, 17th to 18th centuries In P. Horden & R. Smith (Eds.), *The locus of care: Families, communities, institutions, and the provision of welfare since antiquity* (pp. 90-110). London: Routledge.

Cerletti, U. (1950). Old and new information about electroshock. *American Journal of Psychiatry, 107,* 87-94.

Charlton, J. I. (1998). *Nothing about us without*

us: *Disability, oppression, and empowerment.* Berkeley: University of California Press.

Chevigny, H. (1946). *My eyes have a cold nose.* New Haven, CT: Yale University Press.

Church, A. (1893). Removal of ovaries and tubes in the insane and neurotic. *American Journal of Obstetrics and Diseases of Women and Children, 28,* 491-498.

Clay, R. M. (1966). *The mediaeval hospitals of England.* London: Frank Cass.

Cochrane, R. G. (1963). *Biblical leprosy: A suggested interpretation* (2nd ed.). London: Tyndale Press for The Christian Medical Fellowship.

Colon, D. M. (1989). Martin Luther, the devil, and the Teufelchen: Attitudes toward mentally retarded children in 16th century Germany. *Proceedings of the PMR (Patristic, Medieval, and Renaissance) Conference, 14,* 75-84.

Condillac, (1930). *Treatise on the senses.* (G. Carr, Trans.). Los Angeles: University of Southern California. (Original work published 1754)

Covert, S. B., MacIntosh, J.D., & Shumway, D.L. (1994). Closing the Laconia state school and training center: A case study in system change. Iin V.J. Bradley, J.W. Ashbaugh, & B.C. Blaney (Eds.)*, Creating individual supports for people with developmental disabilities: A mandate for change at many levels* (pp. 197-211). Baltimore: Brookes.

Covey, H. C. (1998). *Social perceptions of people with disabilities in history.* Springfield, IL: Charles C. Thomas.

Daniels, M. (1997). *Benedictine roots in the development of deaf education: Listening with the heart.* Westport, CT: Bergin & Garvey.

Davenport, A. B. (1921). Selecting immigrants. *Proceedings and addresses of the American Association for the Study of the Feebleminded, 25,* 178-179.

Davies, S. P. (1930). *Social control of the mentally deficient.* New York: Thomas Y. Crowell.

Davis, L. (1997). *The disability studies reader.* New York: Routledge.

Davis, L. (2000). Dr. Johnson, Amelia, and the discourse of disability in the 18th century. In H.

Deutsch & F. Nussbaum (Eds.), *"Defects": Engendering the modern body* (pp. 54-74). Ann Arbor: University of Michigan Press.

de Saint-Loup, A. (1996). A history of misunderstandings: The history of the deaf. *Diogenes, 44,* 1-25.

Defoe, D. (1720). *The history of the life and adventures of Mr. Duncan Campbell.* London: E. Curll.

Defoe, D. (1894). *An essay upon projects.* London: Cassel. (Original work published 1694)

DeJong, G. (1979a). *The movement for independent living: Origins, ideology, and implications for disability research.* East Lansing: University Center for International Rehabilitation, Michigan State University.

DeJong, G. (1979b). Independent living: From social movement to analytic paradigm. *Archives of Physical Medicine and Rehabilitation, 60,* 435-446.

DeJong, G. (1981). *Environmental accessibility and independent living outcomes: Directions for disability policy research.* East Lansing: University Center for International Rehabilitation, Michigan State University.

DeJong, G. (1984). *Independent living and disability policy in the Netherlands: Three models of residential care and independent living.* New York: International Exchange of Experts and Information in Rehabilitation, World Rehabilitation Fund.

De Souza-Araujo, H. C. (1937). The origin of leprosy in Brasil and its present situation. *Leprosy Review, 8*(1), 12-16.

De Souza-Araujo, H. C. (1946). *História Da Lepra No Brasil, Vol. I.* Rio De Janeiro: Impresa Nacional.

De Souza-Araujo, H. C. (1948). *História Da Lepra No Brasil, Vol. II.* Rio De Janeiro: Impresa Nacional.

Digby, A. (1996). Contexts and perspectives. In D. Wright & A. Digby (Eds.), *From idiocy to mental deficiency: Historical perspectives on people with learning disabilities* (pp. 1-21). London: Routledge.

Dix, D. (1843). *Memorial: To the Legislature of*

Massachusetts. Boston: Munroe & Francis.

Doyle, B. (1996). *Disability discrimination: The new law*. Bristol, Great Britain: Jordans.

Driedger, D. (1989). *The last civil rights movement: Disabled Peoples' International*. London: Hurst.

Dugdale, R. L. (1910). *The Jukes*. New York: G. P. Putman. (Original work published 1877)

Dybwad, G., & Bersani, Jr., H. (Eds.). (1996). *New voices: Self-advocacy by people with disabilities*. Cambridge, MA: Brookline.

Earle, P. (1845). Historical and descriptive account of the Bloomingdale Asylum for the Insane. *American Journal of Insanity, 2*, 1-13.

Earle, P. (1877). *The curability of insanity*. Bloomingdale, NY: Bloomingdale Asylum for the Insane.

Earle, P. (1898). *Memoirs*. Boston: Damrell & Upham.

East, E. M. (1917). Hidden feeblemindedness. *Journal of Heredity, 8*, 215-217.

Edwards, M. L. (1996). The cultural context of deformity in the ancient Greek world. *Ancient History Bulletin, 10*, 79-92.

Edwards, M. L. (1997). Deaf and dumb in ancient Greece. In L. Davis (Ed.), *The disability studies reader* (pp. 29-51). New York: Routledge.

Edwards, P. (1996). *Encyclopedia of philosophy*. New York: Macmillan.

Elm Hill Private School and Home. (1911). *Elm Hill: Private School and Home*. Barre, MA: Author.

Ely, C. W. (1893). *History of the Maryland School for the Deaf and Dumb*. Frederick City: Maryland School for the Deaf and Dumb.

Emerson, E., Robertson, J., Gregory, N., Hatton, C., Kessissoglou, S., Hallam, A., Knapp, M., Järbrink, Walsh, P. N., & Netten, A. (2000). Quality and costs of community-based residential supports, village communities and residential campuses in the United Kingdom. *American Journal on Mental Retardation, 105*(2), 81-102.

Erikson, K. I. (1966). *Wayward Puritans: A study in the sociology of deviance*. New York: John Wiley.

Estabrook, A. H. (1928). The pauper idiot pension in Kentucky. *Journal of Psycho-Asthenics, 33*, 59-61.

European Union. (1996). *Resolution of the Council and the Representatives of the Governments of the Member States on Equality of Opportunity for People with Disabilities*. Official Journal C 12, 13.01.1997. Brussels.

Evans. H. C. (1926). *The American poorfarm and its inmates*. Mooseheart, IL: Loyal Order of Moose.

Farmer, S. (1998). Down and out and female in 13th-century Paris. *American Historical Review, 103*, 344-372.

Farrell, G. (1956). *The story of blindness*. Cambridge, MA: Harvard University Press.

Fay, E. A. (1893). *Histories of American schools for the deaf, 1817-1893*. Washington, DC: Volta Bureau.

Felix, R. H. (1957). Evolution of community mental health concepts. *American Journal of Psychiatry, 113*, 673-679.

Fenton, R. (1932). The Pacific Colony Plan. *Journal of Juvenile Research, 16*, 298-303.

Ferguson, P. M. (1994). *Abandoned to their fate: Social policy and practice toward severely retarded people in America, 1820-1920*. Philadelphia: Temple University Press.

Fernald, W. E. (1893). The history of the treatment of the feebleminded. *Proceedings of the National Conference of Social Work*, 203-221.

Fernald, W. E. (1902). The Massachusetts farm colony for the feebleminded. *Proceedings of the National Conference on Charities and Correction, 487-491*.

Fernald, W. E. (1912). The burden of feeblemindedness. *Journal of Psycho-Asthenics, 17*, 87-99.

Fernald, W. E. (1915). State care of the insane, feebleminded, and epileptic. *Proceedings of the National Conference of Charities and Correction*, 289-297.

Fernald, W. E. (1917). The growth of provision for the feebleminded in the United States. *Mental Hygiene, 1*, 34-59.

Fernald, W. E. (1919). A state program for the care

of the mentally defective. *Mental Hygiene, 3,* 566-574.

Ferster, E. Z. (1966). Eliminating the unfit: Is sterilization the answer? *Ohio State Law Journal, 27,* 591-633.

Fessler, A. (1956). The management of lunacy in 17th century England: An investigation of Quarter-Session records. *Proceedings of the Royal Society of Medicine, 49,* 901-907.

Fish, W. B. (1892). Custodial care of adult idiots. *Proceedings of the National Conference of Social Work, 17,* 203-218.

FitzGerald, J. F. (1900). The duty of the state towards its idiotic and feebleminded. *Proceedings of the New York State Conference of Charities, 1,* 172-189.

Fleischer, D. Z., & Zames, F. (1998). Disability rights. *Social Policy, 28,* 52-55.

Fort, S.J. (1892). What shall be done with the imbecile? *Maryland Medical Journal, 27,* 1057-1063.

Foucault, M. (1965). *Madness and civilization.* (R. Howard, Trans.) London: Tavistock.

Frampton, M. E., & Kerney, F. (1953). *The residential school: Its history, contributions, and future.* New York: Edwin Gould Printery, New York Institute for the Education of the Blind.

French, R. S. (1932). *From Homer to Helen Keller: A social and educational study of the blind.* New York: American Foundation for the Blind.

French, S. (1996). Out of sight, out of mind: The experience and effects of a 'special' residential school. In J. Morris (Ed.), *Encounters with strangers: Feminism and disability* (pp. 17-47). London: The Women's Press.

Friedlander, H. (1997). *The origins of Nazi genocide: From euthanasia to the final solution.* Chapel Hill: University of North Carolina Press.

Fröhlich, A. (1982). Movements toward greater independence of the handicapped in West Germany. In D. G. Tate & L. M. Chadderdon (Eds.), *Independent living: An overview of efforts in five countries* (pp. 35-70). East Lansing: Center for International Rehabilitation, Michigan State

University.

Galbraith, J. K. (1998). *Created unequal: The crisis in American pay.* New York: The Free Press.

Gallagher, H. G. (1995). *By trust betrayed: Patients, physicians, and the license to kill in the Third Reich.* Arlington, VA: Vandamere Press.

Gallaudet University. (1997, December 8). *History of Gallaudet.* Washington, DC: Author. Available at: http://www.gallaudet.edu/~pubreweb/visitor/history/page6.html

Gallaudet, E. M. (1983). *History of the College for the Deaf, 1857-1907.* Washington, DC: Gallaudet College Press.

Galton, F. (1883). *Inquiry into human faculty and its development.* London: Macmillan.

Gannon, J.R. (1981). *Deaf heritage: A narrative history of deaf America.* Silver Spring, MD: National Association of the Deaf.

Garland, R. (1995). *The eye of the beholder: Deformity and disability in the Graeco-Roman world.* Ithaca, NY: Cornell University Press.

Gaw, A. C. (1906a). The development of the legal status of the deaf: A comparative study of the rights and responsibilities of deaf-mutes in the laws of Rome, France, England, and America. *American Annals of the Deaf, 51,* 269-275.

Gaw, A. C. (1906b). The development of the legal status of the deaf: A comparative study of the rights and responsibilities of deaf-mutes in the laws of Rome, France, England, and America. *American Annals of the Deaf, 51,* 401-423.

Gaw, A. C. (1907). The development of the legal status of the deaf: A comparative study of the rights and responsibilities of deaf-mutes in the laws of Rome, France, England and America. *American Annals of the Deaf, 52,* 1-12.

Gill, C. J. (1997). Four types of integration in disability identity development. *Journal of Vocational Rehabilitation, 9,* 39-46.

Gilman, S. L. (1982). *Seeing the insane.* New York: Wiley-Interscience.

Gilman, S. L. (1988). *Disease and representation: Images of illness from madness to AIDS.* Ithaca, NY: Cornell University Press.

Gilman, S. L. (1995). *Picturing health and illness: Images of identity and difference.* Baltimore: Johns Hopkins University Press.

Gladstone, D. (1996). Western counties idiot asylum 1864-1914. In D. Wright & A. Digby (Eds.), *From idiocy to mental deficiency: Historical perspectives on people with learning disabilities* (pp. 134-160). London: Routledge.

Goddard, H. H. (1912). *The Kallikak family: A study in the heredity of feeblemindedness.* New York: Macmillan.

Goldstein, M. S. (1969). Human paleopathology and some diseases in living primitive societies: A review of recent literature. *American Journal of Physical Anthropology, 31,* 285-294.

Goode, D. (1999). *History of the Association for the Help of Retarded Children of New York City.* New York: AHRC.

Goodey, C.F. (1996). The psychopolitics of learning and disability in 17th century thought. In D. Wright & A. Digby (Eds.), *From idiocy to mental deficiency: Historical perspectives on people with learning disabilities* (pp. 93-117). London: Routledge.

Gooding, C. (1996). *Blackstone's guide to the Disability Discrimination Act 1995.* London: Blackstone Press Limited.

Gordan, J. C. (1885). Deaf-mutes and the public schools from 1815 to the present day. *American Annals of the Deaf, 30,* 121-143.

Gorwitz, K. (1974). Census enumeration of the mentally ill and the mentally retarded in the 19th century. *Health Services Reports, 89,* 180-187.

Gosney, E. S., & Popenoe, P. (1929). *Sterilization for human betterment.* New York: Macmillan.

Gould, S. J. (1981). *The mismeasure of man.* New York: Norton.

Gowman, A. G. (1957). *The war blind in American social structure.* New York: American Foundation of the Blind.

Griffin, J. D., & Greenland, C. (1981). Institutional care of the mentally disordered in Canada: A 17th-century record. *Canadian Journal of Psychiatry, 26,* 274-278.

Grimes, J. M. (1964). *Institutional care of mental patients in the United States.* Chicago: Author.

Grob, G. N. (1966). *The state and the mentally ill: A history of Worcester State Hospital in Massachusetts, 1830-1920.* Chapel Hill: University of North Carolina Press.

Grob, G. N. (1973). *Mental institutions in America: Social policy to 1875.* New York: Free Press.

Grob, G. N. (1983). *Mental illness and American society, 1875-1940.* Princeton, NJ: Princeton University Press.

Grob, G. N. (1990). Marxian analysis and mental illness. *History of Psychiatry, 1,* 223-232.

Grob, G. N. (1994). *The mad among us.* New York: Free Press.

Gussow, Z. (1989). *Leprosy, racism, and public health.* Boulder, CO: Westview.

Hahn, H. (1985). Disability policy and the problem of discrimination. *American Behavioral Scientist, 28,* 293-318.

Haines, T. H. (1925). Mental defect and poverty. *Proceedings and addresses of the American Association for the Study of the Feebleminded, 30,* 136-145.

Haller, B. (1993). The little papers: Newspapers at 19th-century schools for deaf persons. *Journalism History, 19,* 43-50.

Hamilton, S. W. (1944). *One hundred years of American psychiatry.* New York: Columbia University Press.

Harms, E. (1955). The origin and early history of electrotherapy and electroshock. *American Journal of Psychiatry, 111,* 933-934.

Harris, C. C. (1971). The treatment of mental deficiency in colonial Virginia. *Virginia Cavalcade, 17,* 34-41.

Hayden, M. F. (1997). Class-action, civil rights litigation for institutionalized persons with mental retardation and other developmental disabilities. *Mental and Physical Disability Law Reporter, 21,* 411-423.

Hayden, M. F., & Senese, D. (1996). *Self-advocacy groups: 1996 directory for North America.* Minneapolis: University of Minnesota.

Hecht, I. W. D., & Hecht, F. (1973). Mara and Benomi Buck: Familial mental retardation in colonial Jamestown. *Journal of the History of*

Medicine and Allied Sciences, 28, 171-176.

Hirsch, K. (1995). Culture and disability: The role of oral history. *Oral History Review, 22*, 1-27.

Hoakley, Z. P. (1922). Extra-institutional care for the feebleminded. *Journal of Psycho-Asthenics, 27,* 117-137.

Hodgson, K. W. (1953). The deaf and their problems. *New York Philosophical Library, 66.*

Hoffman, A., & Field, S. (1995). Promoting self-determination through effective curriculum development. *Intervention in School and Clinic, 30,* 147-156.

Holstein, M., & Cole, T. (1995). The evolution of long-term care in America. In L. B. McCullough & N.L. Wilson (Eds.), *Long-term care decisions: Ethical and conceptual dimensions* (pp. 19-47). Baltimore: Johns Hopkins Press.

Howard, J. (1789). *An account of the principal lazarettos in Europe.* London: Warrington.

Howe, S. G. (1848). *Report made to the Legislature of Massachusetts upon idiocy.* Boston: Coolidge & Wiley.

Howe, S. G. (1851). On training and educating idiots: Second annual report to the Massachusetts legislature. *American Journal of Insanity, 8,* 97-118.

Hughes, S. L. (1986). *Long-term care: Options in an expanding market.* Homewood, IL: Dow Jones-Irwin.

Humphrey, J. C. (2000). Researching disability politics, or, some problems with the social model in practice. *Disability & Society, 15*(1), 63-85.

Hurd, H. M. (1910). *A history of institutional care of the insane in the United States and Canada.* American Medico-Psychological Association.

Innes, B., Enders, A., Seekins, T., Merritt, D.J., Kirshenbaum, A., & Arnold, N. (2000). Assessing the geographic distribution of Centers for Independent Living across urban and rural areas: Toward a policy of universal access. *Journal of Disability Policy Studies, 10*(2), 207-224.

Itard, J.M. (1802). *The wild boy of Aveyron.* Richard Phillips.

Itard, J. M. (1821a). *Traite des maladies de l'oreille et de l'audition: I.* Paris: Chez Mequignon-Marvis.

Itard, J. M. (1821b). *Traite des maladies de l'oreille et de l'audition: II.* Paris: Chez Mequignon-Marvis.

Jackson, M. (1998). "It begins with the goose and ends with the goose": Medical, legal, and lay understandings of imbecility in Ingram v. Wyatt, 1824-1832, *Social History of Medicine, 11*, 361-380.

Jackson, S. W. (1988). Introduction. In W. Pargeter, *Observations on maniacal disorders.* London: Routledge.

Jacobson, J. W., Burchard, S. N., & Carling, P. J. (1992). *Community living for people with developmental and psychiatric disabilities.* Baltimore: Johns Hopkins University Press.

Jankauskas, R., & Urbanavicius, A. (1998). Diseases in European historical populations and their effects on individuals and society. *Collegium Antropologicum, 22*, 465-476.

Janicki, M., & Ansello, E. (2000). Supports for community living: Evaluation of an aging with lifelong disabilities movement. In M. Janicki & E. Ansello (Eds.), *Community supports for aging adults with lifelong disabilities* (pp. 519-537). Baltimore: Brookes.

Johnson, A. (1896). Permanent custodial care. *Proceedings of the National Conference of Social Work,* 207-219.

Johnson, A. (1899). The self-supporting imbecile. *Journal of Psycho-Asthenics, 4,* 91-99.

Jones, L. A. (1987). *Doing justice: A history of the Association of Retarded Citizens of Washington.* Olympia, WA: The Arc of Washington.

Jørgensen, S. (1982). Independent living for handicapped persons in Denmark. In D. G. Tate & L. M. Chadderdon (Eds.), *Independent living: An overview of efforts in five countries* (pp. 11-29). East Lansing: University Center for International Rehabilitation, Michigan State University.

Kanner, L. (1964). *A history of the care and study of the mentally retarded.* Springfield, IL: Charles C. Thomas.

Keith, K., & Schalock, R. (2000). *Cross-cultural perspectives on quality of life.* Washington, DC: American Association on Mental Retardation.

Kennedy, J. F. (1961). Statement by the President regarding the need for a national plan in mental retardation. In the President's Panel on Mental Retardation (Ed.), *National action to combat mental retardation* (pp. 196-201). Washington, DC: U.S. Government Printing Office.

Kerlin, I. N. (1877). The organization of establishments for the idiotic and imbecile classes. *Proceedings of the Association of Medical Officers of American Institutions for Idiotic and Feebleminded Persons, 3*, 19-24.

Kerlin, I. N. (1887). Moral imbecility. *Proceedings of the Association of Medical Officers of American Institutions for Idiotic and Feebleminded Persons, 12*, 32-37.

Kevles, D. J. (1985). *In the name of eugenics: Genetics and the uses of human heredity.* New York: Alfred A. Knopf.

Kipp, R. S. (1994). The evangelical uses of leprosy. *Social Science & Medicine, 39*, 165-178.

Kirchner, C., Peterson, R., & Suhr, C. (1988). Trends in school enrollment and reading methods among legally blind school children, 1963-1978. In C. Kirchner (Ed.), *Data on blindness and visual impairment in the U.S.: A resource manual on social demographic characteristics, education, employment, and income, and Service Delivery* (2nd ed.). New York: American Foundation for the Blind.

Kirkbride, T. (1845). A sketch of the history, buildings, and organization of the Pennsylvania Hospital for the Insane. *American Journal of Insanity, 2*, 97-114.

Kirkbride, T. (1973). *On the construction, organization, and general arrangements of hospitals for the insane.* New York: Arno Press. (Original work published 1880)

Knight, G. H. (1891). Colony care for adult idiots. *Proceedings of the National Conference of Social Work*, 107-108.

Knight, G. H. (1895). The feebleminded. *Proceedings of the Association of Medical Officers of American Institutions for Idiotic and Feebleminded Persons*, 559-563.

Koegel, L. K., Koegel, R. L., & Dunlap, G. (1996). *Positive behavioral support: Including people with difficult behavior in the community.* Baltimore: Brookes.

Koestler, F. A. (1976). *The unseen minority.* New York: David McKay.

Koven, S. (1994). Remembering and dismemberment: Crippled children, wounded soldiers, and the great war in Great Britain. *American Historical Review, 99*, 1167-1202.

Kroll, J. (1973). A reappraisal of psychiatry in the middle ages. *Archives of General Psychiatry, 29*, 276-283.

Kuhlmann, F. (1940). One hundred years of special care and training. *American Journal of Mental Deficiency, 45*, 18-24.

Lakin, K. C. (1979). *Demographic studies of residential facilities for the mentally retarded: An historical review of methodologies and findings.* Minneapolis: University of Minnesota.

Lane, H. (1989). *When the mind hears: A history of the deaf.* New York: Vintage Books.

Lazar, I., & Darlington, R. B. (1982). Lasting effects of early education. *Monographs of the society for research in child development, 47* (2-3, Serial No. 195).

Lefley, H. (1996). *Family caregiving in mental illness.* Thousand Oaks, CA: Sage.

Lende, H. (1941). *What of the blind?* New York: American Foundation for the Blind.

Levy, R. M., & Rubenstein, L. S. (1996). *The rights of people with mental disabilities: The authoritative ACLU guide to the rights of people with mental illness and mental retardation.* Carbondale & Edwardsville: Southern Illinois University.

Linton, S. (1998). *Claiming disability: Knowledge and identity.* New York: New York University Press.

Locke, J. (1690). *An essay concerning human understanding.* London: Basset.

Longhurst, N. A. (1994) *The self-advocacy movement: A demographic study and directory.* Washington, DC: American Association on Mental Retardation.

Lupton, D. (2000). The social construction of the body. In G. L. Albrecht, R. Fitzpatrick, & S. C. Scrimshaw (Eds.), *The handbook of social studies in health and medicine* (pp. 250-263). London: Sage Publications.

Lutterman, T., Hirad, A., & Poindexter, B. (1999). *Funding sources and expenditures of state mental health agencies: Fiscal year 1997.* Alexandria, VA: National Association of State Mental Health Program Directors Research Institute.

Lysack, C., & Kaufert, J. (1994). Comparing the origins and ideologies of the independent living movement and community-based rehabilitation. *International Journal of Rehabilitation Research, 17*, 231-240.

MacAndrew, C., & Edgerton, R. (1964). The everyday life of institutionalized "idiots." *Human Organization, 23*, 312-318.

MacArthur, W. (1953). Mediaeval "leprosy" in the British Isles. *Leprosy Review, 24*, 10-11.

MacDonald, M. (1981). *Mystical Bedlam: Madness, anxiety, and healing in 17th-century England.* Cambridge: Cambridge University Press.

Mackelprang, R. W., & Salsgiver, R. O. (1996). People with disabilities and social work: Historical and contemporary issues. *Social Work, 41*, 7-14.

MadNation. (1999). *Movement history of the consumer/survivor/ex-patient/user community.* Available at: http://madnation.org/csxuhistory.htm

Maher, W. B. & Maher, B. (1982). The ship of fools: Stultifera navis or ignis fatuus? *American Psychologist, 37,* 756-761.

Marcus, J. (1999). A note on Markan optics. *New Testament Studies, 45*, 250-256.

Martin, E. W., Martin, R., & Terman, D. L. (1996). The legislative and litigation history of special education. *Special Education for Students with Disabilities, 6*, 25-38.

Martin, F. (1924). Artifical limbs: Appliances for the disabled. Studies and reports, Series E (Disabled Men) No. 5. *International Labour Office.* Liége, Belgium: Georges Thone.

Mastin, J. T. (1916). The new colony plan for the feebleminded. *Journal of Psycho-Asthenics, 21*, 25-35.

Matson, F. (1990). *Walking alone and marching together: A history of the organized blind movement in the United States, 1940-1990.* Baltimore: National Federation of the Blind.

Matthews, M. A. (1921). One hundred institutionally trained male defectives in the community under supervision. *Journal of Psycho-Asthenics, 26*, 60-70.

Metts, R. L. (2000). *Disability issues, trends, and recommendations for the World Bank.* Washington, DC: The World Bank.

Miles, M. (2000). Signing in the Seraglio: Mutes, dwarfs and jestures at the Ottoman Court 1500-1700. *Disability & Society, 15*(1), 115-134.

Minski, L. (1957). *Deafness, mutism, and mental deficiency in children.* New York: Philosophical Library.

Mitchell, D. (2000). *Narrative prosthesis: Disability and the dependencies of discourse.* Ann Arbor: University of Michigan Press.

Mora, G. (1992). The history of psychiatry in the United States: Historiographic and theoretical considerations. *History of Psychiatry, 3*, 187-201.

The moral treatment of insanity. (1847). *American Journal of Insanity, 4*, 1-15.

Moreno, J. (1999). *Undue risk: Secret state experiments on humans.* New York: W.H. Freeman.

Morton, T. G. (1897). *The history of Pennsylvania Hospital 1751-1895.* Philadelphia: Times Printing House.

Nagi, S. Z. (1970). *Disability and rehabilitation: legal, clinical, and self-concepts and measurements.* Columbus: Ohio State University Press.

National Association of State Mental Health Program Directors Research Institute. (1996). *FY'96 SMHA Profiling System.* Alexandria, VA: Author. Available at: http://www.nasmhpd.org/nri/CLI_T1.HTM

National Council on Disability. (1997, July 26). *Equality of opportunity: The making of the Americans with Disabilities Act.* Washington, DC: Author.

Navon, L. (1998). Beggars, metaphors, and stigma: A missing link in the social history of leprosy. *Social History of Medicine, 11*, 89-105.

Neaman, J. (1978). *Suggestion of the devil:*

Insanity in the Middle Ages and the 20th century. New York: Octagon Books.

Neugebauer, R. (1978). Treatment of the mentally ill in medieval and early modern England: A reappraisal. *Journal of the History of the Behavioral Sciences, 14*, 158-169.

Neugebauer, R. (1979). Medieval and early modern theories of mental illness. *Archives of General Psychiatry, 36*, 477-483.

Neugebauer, R. (1987). Exploitation of the insane in the New World: Benoni Buck, the first reported case of mental retardation in the American Colonies. *Archives of General Psychiatry, 44*, 481-483.

Neugebauer, R. (1996). Mental handicap in medieval and early modern England: Criteria, measurement, and care. In D. Wright & A. Digby (Eds.), *From idiocy to mental deficiency: Historical perspectives on people with learning disabilities* (pp. 22-43). London: Routledge.

Nirje, B. (1976). The normalization principle and its human management implications. In R. B. Kugel & A. Shearer (Eds.), *Changing patterns in residential services for the mentally retarded* (pp. 231-240). Washington, DC: President's Committee on Mental Retardation.

Noll, S. (1996). *The feebleminded in our midst: Institutions for the mentally retarded in the south, 1900-1940*. Chapel Hill: University of North Carolina Press.

Obermann, C. E. (1968). *A history of vocational rehabilitation in America* (5th ed.). Minneapolis: T.S. Dennison.

Oliver, M. (1983). *Social work with disabled people*. Basingstoke, England: Macmillan.

Oliver, M. (1990). *The politics of disablement*. Basingstoke, England: Macmillan.

Oliver, M. (1992). Changing the social relations of research production. *Disability, Handicap, & Society, 7*(2), 101-114.

Oliver, M., & Barnes, C. (1999). *Disabled people and social policy: From exclusion to inclusion*. London: Longman.

Packard, E. P. W. (1868). *The prisoner's hidden life, or, insane asylums unveiled: As demonstrated by the Report of the Investigating Committee of the Legislature of Illinois*. Chicago: J.N. Clarke.

Pargeter, W. (1988). *Observations on maniacal disorders*. London: Routledge. (Originally published 1792)

Park, E., & Daston, L. (1981). Unnatural conceptions: The study of monsters in 16th- and 17th-century France and England. *Past & Present, 92*, 20-54.

Parry, J. (1995). *Mental disability law: A primer* (5th ed.). Washington, DC: American Bar Association.

Parry-Jones, W. L. (1972). *The trade in lunacy: A study of private madhouses in England in the 18th and 19th centuries*. London: Routledge.

Pennsylvania Ass'n., Retarded Child. v. Commonwealth of PA. 334 F.Supp.1257 (1971).

Percy, S. (1989). *Disability, civil rights, and public policy: The politics of implementation*. Tuscaloosa: University of Alabama Press.

Pernick, M. S. (1996). *The black stork: Eugenics and the death of "defective" babies in American medicine and motion pictures since 1915*. New York: Oxford University Press.

Peterson, D. (1982). *A mad people's history of madness*. Pittsburgh: University of Pittsburgh Press.

Pinel, P. (1977). *Treatise on insanity*. (H. Maudsley, Trans.). Washington, DC: University Publications of America. (Original work published 1801)

Pinel, P. (1809). *Traité médico-philosophique sur l'aliénation mentale* (2nd ed.). Paris: J.A. Brosson.

Plann, S. (1997). *A silent minority: Deaf education in Spain, 1550-1835*. Berkeley: University of California Press.

Pollock, H. M. (1945). A brief history of family care of mental patients in America. *American Journal of Psychiatry, 102*, 351-361.

Popenoe, P. (1927). Success on parole after sterilization, *Proceedings and addresses of the American Association for the Study of Feeblemindedness, 32*, 86-109.

Porter, R. (1987). *Mind forg'd manacles: A history of madness in England from the restoration to the regency*. London: Athlone Press.

Porter, R. (1987). *A social history of madness: The world through the eyes of the insane.* New York: Weidenfeld & Nicolson.

Porter, S. (1894). The suppression of signs by force. *American Annals of the Deaf, 39*, 169-178.

Public Law 100-407. (1988). Technology Related Assistance for Individuals with Disabilities Act of 1988.

Public Law 105-394. (1998). Assistive Technology Act of 1998.

Quartararo, A. T. (1995). The perils of assimilation in modern France: The deaf community, social status, and educational opportunity, 1815-1870, *Journal of Social History, 29*, 5-23.

Radford, J. P. (1994). Eugenics and the asylum. *Journal of Historical Sociology, 7*, 462-473.

Rafter, N. H. (1988). *White trash: The eugenic family studies, 1877-1919*. Boston: Northeastern University Press.

Ramirez-Moreno, S. (1937). History of psychiatry and mental hospitals in Mexico. *The Journal of Nervous and Mental Disease, 86*(5), 513-524.

Ramirez-Moreno, S. (1942). History of the first psychopathic institution on the American Continent. *American Journal of Psychiatry, 99*(2), 194-195.

Ramsey, G. V. (1952). A short history of psychosurgery. *American Journal of Psychiatry, 108*, 813-816.

Reilly, P. R. (1991). *The surgical solution: A history of involuntary sterilization in the United States*. Baltimore: Johns Hopkins University Press.

Roberts, E. V. (1989). A history of the Independent Living Movement: A founder's perspective. In B. W. Heller, L. M. Flohr, & L. S. Zegans (Eds.), *Psychosocial interventions with physically disabled persons* (pp.231-244). New Brunswick, NJ: Rutgers University Press.

Roberts, F. K. (1986). Education of the visually handicapped: A social and educational history. In

G. T. Scholl (Ed.), *Foundations of education for blind and visually handicapped children and youth: Theory and practice*. New York: American Foundation for the Blind.

Roberts, J. A. F. (1952). The genetics of mental deficiency. *Eugenics Review, 44*, 71-83.

Rochefort, D. A. (1981). Three centuries of care of the mentally disabled in Rhode Island and the nation, 1650-1950. *Rhode Island History, 40*, 111-132.

Rockey, D. (1980). *Speech disorder in 19th century Britain*. London: Croom Helm.

Roosens, E. (1979). *Mental patients in town life: Gheel-Europe's first therapeutic community*. Beverly Hills, CA: Sage.

Rosen, G. (1968). *Madness in society: Chapters in the historical sociology of mental illness*. Chicago: University of Chicago Press.

Rosenfeld, S. (1997). Deaf men on trial: Language and deviancy in late 18th-century France. *Eighteenth Century Life, 21*, 157-175.

Rothfels, N. (1996). Aztecs, aborigines, and ape-people: Science and freaks in Germany, 1850-1900. In R.G. Thomson (Ed.), *Freakery: Cultural spectacles of the extraordinary body* (pp. 158-172). New York: New York University Press.

Rothman, D. J. (1990). *The discovery of the asylum: Social order and disorder in the New Republic* (Rev. ed.). Boston: Little, Brown.

Rothman, D. J., & Rothman, S. M. (1984). *The Willowbrook wars*. New York: Harper & Row.

Rouse v. Cameron, 373 F.2d 451, 452 (D.C. Cir. 1966).

Rousseau, J. J. (1991). *The social contract*. Norwalk, CT: Easton Press. (Original work published 1762)

Rumbaut, R. D. (1972). The first psychiatric hospital of the Western world. *American Journal of Psychiatry, 128*(10), 1305-1309.

Rush, B. (1812). *Medical inquiries and observations, upon the diseases of the mind*. Philadelphia: Kimber & Richardson.

Rushton, P. (1988). Lunatics and idiots: Mental disability, the community, and the Poor Law in northeast England, 1600-1800. *Medical History,*

32, 34-50.

Rushton, P. (1996). Idiocy, the family, and the community in early modern northeast England. In D. Wright & A. Digby (Eds.), *From idiocy to mental deficiency: Historical perspectives on people with learning disabilities* (pp. 44-64). London: Routledge.

Russell, J. B. (1972). *Witchcraft in the Middle Ages.* Ithaca, NY: Cornell University Press.

Russell, J. B. (1980). *A history of witchcraft: Sorcerers, heretics, and pagans.* New York: Thames & Hudson.

Sacks, O. (1989). *Seeing voices: A journey into the world of the deaf.* Berkeley: University of California Press.

Sarason, S. B., & Gladwin, T. (1958). Psychological and cultural problems in mental subnormality, Part II. In R.L. Masland, S.B. Sarason, & T. Gladwin, *Mental subnormality: Biological, psychological, and cultural factors.* New York: Basic Books.

Schafer, R. J. (1980). *A guide to historical method* (3rd ed.). Chicago: Dorsey Press.

Scheerenberger, R.C. (1983). *A history of mental retardation.* Baltimore: Brookes.

Scotch, R. (1984). *From goodwill to civil rights: Transforming federal disability policy.* Philadelphia: Temple University Press.

Scotch, R. K. (1989). Politics and policy in the history of the disability rights movement. *The Milbank Quarterly, 67* (Suppl. 2, Pt. 2), 380-400.

Scotch, R. K., & Berkowitz, E. (1990). One comprehensive system? A historical perspective on federal disability policy. *Journal of Disability Policy Studies, 1,* 1-19.

Scott, R. (1968). *The making of blind men: A study of adult socialization.* New Brunswick, NJ: Transaction Books.

Scull, A. (1979). *Museums of madness: The social organization of insanity in 19th century England.* London: Allen Lane.

Scull, A. (1991). Psychiatry and social control in the 19th and 20th centuries. *History of Psychiatry, 2,* 149-169.

Seguin, E. (1846). *Traitement moral hygiene et education des idiots et des autres enfants erroires.* Paris: Bailliere.

Seguin, E. (1870). *New facts and remarks concerning idiocy, being a lecture before the New York Medical Journal Association, October 15, 1869.* New York: William Wood.

Semi-deaf lady. (1908). The sign language and the human right to expression. *American Annals of the Deaf, 53,* 141-148.

Semonin, P. (1996) . Monsters in the marketplace: The exhibition of human oddities in early modern England. In R.G. Thomson (Ed.), *Freakery: Cultural spectacles of the extraordinary body* (pp. 69-81). New York: New York University Press.

Shapiro, J. P. (1993). *No pity: People with disabilities forging new civil rights movement.* New York: Times Books.

Sheldon, E. W. (1921). Historical review. In H. Townsend, B. Winthrop, & R. H. Gallatin (Eds.), *A psychiatric milestone: Bloomingdale Hospital Centenary: 1821-1921* (pp. 7-16). New York: Society of the New York Hospital.

Silverstein, R. (2000). *Disability policy framework: A guidepost for analyzing public policy.* Washington, DC: Center for the Study and Advancement of Disability Policy and the Arc of the United States.

Simpson, M. K. (1999). The moral government of idiots: Moral treatment in the work of Seguin. *History of Psychiatry, 10,* 227-243.

Skeels, H. M., & Harms, I. (1948). Children with inferior social histories: Their mental development in adoptive homes. *Journal of Genetic Psychology, 72,* 283-294.

Skeels, H. M., Updegraff, R., Wellman, B. L., & Williams, H. M. (1938). A study of environmental stimulation, an orphanage preschool project. *University of Iowa Studies in Child Welfare, 15*(4).

A sketch of the history, buildings, and organization of the Pennsylvania Hospital for the Insane, extracted principally from the reports of Thomas S. Kirkbride, M.D., Physician to the institution. (1845). *American Journal of Insanity, 2,* 97-114.

Sloan, W., & Stevens, H. A. (1976). *A century of concern: A history of the American Association on Mental Deficiency, 1876-1976*. Washington, DC: American Association on Mental Deficiency.

Smith, S., Wilkinson, M. W., & Wagoner, L. C. (1914). A summary of the laws of the several states governing I. Marriage and divorce of the feebleminded, the epileptic, and the insane. II. Asexualization. III. Institutional commitment and discharge of the feebleminded and epileptic. *The Bulletin of the University of Washington, 82*, Bailey and Babette Gatzert Foundation for Child Welfare.

Social Security Board. (1946). *Recommendations of the Children's Bureau Advisory Committee on Services to Crippled Children: December 1935 to April 1946*. Washington, DC: Department of Health and Human Services Archives.

Solecki, R. (1971). *Shanidar: The first flower people*. New York: Knopf.

Speer, G.S. (1940). The intelligence of foster children. *Journal of Genetic Psychology, 57*, 49-55.

Spierenburg, P. (1984). The sociogenesis of confinement and its development in early modern Europe. In P. Spierenburg (Ed.), *The emergence of carceral institutions: Prisons, galleys and lunatic asylums, 1550-1900*. Rotterdam: Erasmus Universiteit, Centrum voor Maatschappij Geschiedenenis.

Statistics of speech training in American schools. (1920). *Volta Review, 22*, 361-375.

Stevens, H. (1858). Insane colony of Gheel. *The Asylum Journal of Mental Science, 4*, 426-436.

Stewart, J., Harris, J., & Sapey, B. (1999). Disability and dependency: Origins and futures of 'special needs' housing for disabled people. *Disability & Society, 14*, 5-20.

Stewart, J. Q. A. (1882). The industrial department of the Kentucky Institution for the Education and Training of Feebleminded Children. *Proceedings of the Association of Medical Officers of American Institutions for Idiotic and Feebleminded Persons*, 236-239.

Stewart, T. D. (1958). Report of committee on

research: Anthropology. *Yearbook of the American Philosophical Society*, 274-278.

Stiker, H. (1997). *A history of disability*. (W. Sayers, Trans.). Ann Arbor: University of Michigan Press.

Straus, W. L., & Cave, A. J. E. (1957). Pathology and the posture of Neanderthal man. *Quarterly Review of Biology, 32*, 348-363.

Strype, J. (1720). Description of Bethlem Hospital commonly called Bedlam. In R. Hunter & I. Macalpine (1982) *Three hundred years of psychiatry 1535-1860: A history presented in selected English texts* (pp. 192-197). Hartsdale, NY: Carlisle.

Survey and Research Corporation. (1965, July). *Mental retardation program statistics of U.S.: Report to the Department of Health, Education, and Welfare pursuant to contract PH-86-64-99*. Washington, DC: U.S. Department of Health, Education, and Welfare.

Suzuki, A. (1991). Lunacy in 17th- and 18th-century England: Analysis of Quarter Sessions records: Part I. *History of Psychiatry, 2*, 437-456.

Suzuki, A. (1998). The household and the care of lunatics in 18th-century London. In P. Horden & R. Smith (Eds.), *The locus of care: Families, communities, institutions, and the provision of welfare since antiquity* (pp. 153-175). London: Routledge.

Swain, B. (1932). *Fools and folly during the Middle Ages and the Renaissance*. New York: Columbia University Press.

Swayze, V. W. (1995). Frontal leukotomy and related psychosurgical procedures in the era before antipsychotics (1935-1954): A historical overview. *American Journal of Psychiatry, 152*, 505-515.

Swinburne, H. (1590). *A brief treatise of testaments and last willes*. London: John Windet.

Switzky, H. N., Dudzinski, M., Van Acker, R., & Gambro, J. (1988). Historical foundations of out-of-home residential alternatives for mentally retarded persons. In L. W. Heal, J. I. Haney, & A. R. Novak Amado (Eds.), *Integration of developmentally disabled individuals into the community* (2nd ed., pp. 19-35). Baltimore: Brookes.

Symonds, B. (1995). The origins of insane asylums in England during the 19th century: A brief sociological review. *Journal of Advanced Nursing, 22,* 94-100.

Szasz, T. (1970). *The manufacture of madness: A comparative study of the inquisition and the mental health movement.* Syracuse, NY: Syracuse University Press.

Szasz, T. (1973). *The age of madness: The history of involuntary mental hospitalization.* New York: Jason Aronson.

Talbot, M. (1967). Edouard Seguin. *American Journal of Mental Deficiency, 72,* 184-189.

Thiher, A. (1999). *Revels in madness: Insanity in medicine and literature.* Ann Arbor: University of Michigan Press.

Thompson, T., & Grabowski, J. (Eds.) (1977). *Behavior modification of the mentally retarded* (2nd ed.). New York: Oxford University Press.

Thomson, R. G. (1996). *Freakery: Cultural spectacles of the extraordinary body.* New York: New York University Press.

Thomson, R. G. (1997). *Extraordinary bodies: Figuring physical disability in American culture and literature.* New York: Columbia University Press.

Trent, J. W. (1995). *Inventing the feeble mind: A history of mental retardation in the United States.* Berkeley: University of California Press.

Trombley, S. (1988). *The right to reproduce: A history of coercive sterilization.* London: Winfield & Nicolson.

Tuke, D. H. (1878). *Insanity in ancient and modern life.* London: Macmillan.

Tuke, D. H. (1968). *Chapters in the history of the insane in the British Isles.* Amsterdam, Holland: E.J. Bonset. (Original work published 1882)

Tuke, S. (1815). *A letter on pauper lunatic asylums.* New York: Samuel Wood & Sons.

Tyor, P. L. (1972). *Segregation or surgery: The mentally retarded in America, 1850-1920.* Unpublished doctoral dissertation, Northwestern University, Chicago.

Tyor, P. L., & Bell, L. V. (1984). *Caring for the retarded in America: A history.* Westport, CT: Greenwood Press.

United Nations. (1971). General Assembly Resolution 2856 (XXVI), *On the Declaration on the Rights of Mentally Retarded Persons.* New York: Author.

United Nations. (1975). General Assembly Resolution 3447 (XXX), *On the Declaration on the Rights of Disabled Persons.* New York: Author.

United Nations. (1982). *World program of action concerning people with disabilities.* New York: Author.

United Nations. (1994). *The standard rules on the equalization of opportunities for persons with disabilities.* New York: Author.

U.S. Bureau of the Census. (1914). *Insane and feeble-minded in institutions, 1910.* Washington, DC: Author.

U.S. Bureau of the Census. (1939). *Patients in mental institutions.* Washington, DC: Author.

U.S. Bureau of the Census. (1940). *Patients in mental institutions.* Washington, DC: Author.

U.S. Bureau of the Census. (1997). *International data base.* Washington, DC: Bureau of the Census, International Programs Center, Information Resources Branch.

U.S. Department of Education. (1998). *Twentieth annual report to Congress on the implementation of the Individuals With Disabilities Education Act.* Washington, DC: Author.

U.S. Department of Health, Education, and Welfare. (1972, September). *Mental retardation sourcebook of the DHEW.* Washington, DC: Author, Office of the Secretary, Office of Mental Retardation Coordination.

U.S. Holocaust Memorial Museum. (nodate). *The mentally and physically handicapped victims of the Nazi era.* Washington, DC: Author.

U.S. Office of Management and Budget. (1999). *Budget of the United States Government, Fiscal Year 1999: Budget information for states.* Washington, DC: U.S. Government Printing Office.

Valenstein, E. S. (1986). *Great and desperate cures: The rise and decline of psychosurgery and other radical treatments for mental illness.* New York: Basic Books.

Vaux, C. L. (1935). Family care of mental defectives. *The Journal of Psycho-Asthenics, 40,* 168-189.

Walker, T. (1950). *Rise up and walk.* New York: E.P. Dutton.

Wallace, G. L. (1929). Are the feebleminded criminals? *Mental Hygiene, 13,* 93-98.

Ward, M. J. (1946). *The snake pit.* New York: Random House.

Ward, N., & Schoultz, B. (1996). People First of Nebraska: Eight years of accomplishment. In G. Dybwad & H. Bersani (Eds.), *New voices: Self-advocacy by people with disabilities* (pp. 216-236). Cambridge, MA: Brookline Books.

Warkany, J. (1959). Congenital malformations in the past. *Journal of Chronic Disabilities, 10,* 84-96.

Watkins, H. M. (1930). Selective sterilization. *Proceedings and addresses of the American Association for the Study of the Feeble-minded,* 51-67.

Welsford, E. (1966). *The fool: His social and literary history.* Gloucester, MA: Peter Smith. (Original work published 1935)

Weymouth, A. (1938). *Through the leper-squint: A study of leprosy from pre-Christian times to the present day.* London: Selwyn & Blount.

Whitney, E. A. (1949). The historical approach to the subject of mental retardation. *American Journal of Mental Deficiency, 53,* 419-424.

Wilbur, C. T. (1888). Institutions for the feeble-minded. *Proceedings of the 15th National Conference of Charities and Correction, 17,* 106-113.

Willeford, W. (1969). *The fool and his sceptre: A study in clowns and jesters and their audience.* London: Edward Arnold.

Winship, M. P. (1994). Prodigies, puritanism, and the perils of natural philosophy: The example of Cotton Mather. *The William and Mary Quarterly, 51,* 92-105.

Winspear, C. W. (1895). The protection and training of feebleminded women. *Proceedings of the Association of Medical Officers of American Institutions for Idiotic and Feebleminded Persons, 20,* 160-163.

Winzer, M. A. (1986). Early developments in special education: Some aspects of Enlightenment thought. *Remedial & Special Education (RASE), 7,* 42-49.

Winzer, M. A. (1993). *The history of special education: From isolation to integration.* Washington, DC: Gallaudet University Press.

Witchcraft and insanity. (1849). *American Journal of Insanity, 5,* 246-261.

Wolfensberger, W. (1972). *The principle of normalization in human services.* Toronto: National Institute on Mental Retardation.

Wolfensberger, W. (1976). On the origin of our institutional models. In R. Kugel & A. Shearer (Eds.), *Changing patterns in residential services for the mentally retarded* (Rev. ed., pp. 35-82). Washington, DC: President's Committee on Mental Retardation.

Wolfensberger, W. (1981). The extermination of handicapped people in World War II Germany. *Mental Retardation, 19,* 1-7.

Wood, G. B. (1853). History of the Pennsylvania Hospital for the Insane, *American Journal of Insanity, 9,* 209-213.

Woodill, G., & Velche, D. (1995). From charity and exclusion to emerging independence: An introduction to the history of disabilities. *Journal on Developmental Disabilities, 4,* 1-11.

Woodside, M. (1950). *Sterilization in North Carolina: A sociological and psychological study.* Chapel Hill: University of North Carolina Press.

Woodward, S. (1845). *Annual report of the Worcester State Hospital.* Worcester, MA: Worcester State Hospital.

Woolfson, R. C. (1984). Historical perspective on mental retardation. *American Journal of Mental Deficiency, 89,* 231-235.

World Health Organization. (1980). *International classification of impairments, disabilities, and handicaps.* Geneva: Author.

Wright, D. (1969). *Deafness.* New York: Stein & Day.

Wright, D., & Digby, A. (1996). *From idiocy to*

mental deficiency: Historical perspectives on people with learning disabilities. London: Routledge.

Wright, H. (1920). *Survey of cripples in New York City.* New York: New York Committee on After Care of Infantile Paralysis.

Wright, L., & Hamburger, A. M. (1918). *Education and occupation of cripples juvenile and adult: A survey of all the cripples of Cleveland, Ohio in 1916.* New York: Red Cross Institute for Crippled and Disabled Men.

Wyatt v. Stickney, 325 F. Supp. 781 (M.D. Ala. 1971), enforced in 334 F. Supp. 1341 (1971); 344 F. Supp. 387 (1972); Wyatt v. Aderholt, 503 F. 2d. 1305 (5th Cir. 1974).

Zola, I. K. (1979). Helping one another: Speculative history of the self-help movement. *Archives of Physical Medicine, 60*(10), 452-456.

PART I
Cross Disability Perspectives
CHAPTER 2

Public Financial Support for Disability at the Dawn of the 21st Century

David Braddock

This chapter describes a study which is an exploratory effort to quantitatively assess the level of public sector financial commitments for disability programs in the United States. The study integrates the methodological approaches of Berkowitz and Greene's (1989) study assessing disability expenditures by the federal government with the longitudinal studies of public spending for developmental disabilities services in the states (Braddock, Hemp, Parish, & Westrich, 1998; Braddock, Hemp, Parish, & Rizzolo, 2000), and the National Association of State Mental Health Program Directors' studies of mental health spending in the states (Lutterman, Hirad, & Poindexter, 1999). The specific purpose of the present study was to determine the approximate level of federal, state, and local cross-disability governmental expenditures in each state and nationally (i.e., spending for services and income maintenance to persons with mental retardation, mental illness, and physical disabilities). A monograph provides an historical overview of public financial commitments for disability programs in the United States dating to colonial times (Braddock, 2001). This chapter is an extended version of an article appearing in the *American Journal on Mental Retardation* (Braddock, in press).

The analysis of budgetary decisions using states as the primary unit of analysis permits comparisons to be made on disability spending across the states so that "leaders and laggards" can be identified. Such state-by-state analyses are useful for state planning. They are particularly useful to state and national disability advocacy constituencies because, for many consumers with disabilities and their families, the budgetary and programmatic decisions made in state legislatures, and in rehabilitation, mental disability, public health, education, and public welfare agencies in the states, are frequently more important for determining who receives which services and supports than are the general budgetary and programmatic decisions on disability programs made in Washington, DC. For example, the varied patterns in the states in the utilization of federal Medicaid Home and Community Based Services (HCBS) Waiver funding in developmental disabilities illustrate the great latitude state governments have in deploying financial resources for institutional versus home and community services objectives (Braddock et al., 2000).

METHOD

This study is believed to be the first to quantify cross-disability public spending commitments for disability programs nationally and in each of the American states. The study was guided by three research questions: First, how much public sector spending was allocated for disability programs in the United States in 1997 and how many recipients with disabilities received support? Second, to what degree were expenditures in long-term care for persons with disabilities allocated for institutional versus community services objectives? Third, what is the level of fiscal effort (Bahl, 1982) commitment in the states for long-term care?

The principal "disability-related programs" incorporated into the assessment of spending levels in this study included seven income maintenance programs, three major general (acute) health care programs, long-term care, and special education services. The income maintenance programs included six federal programs: Supplemental Security Income (SSI); Social Security Disability Insurance (DI); the Social Security Adult Disabled Child (ADC) program; Food Stamps; Housing and Urban Development (HUD) rental subsidies and vouchers; and the Department of Veterans Affairs (DVA) Veterans' Compensation. The seventh income maintenance program was state government supplementation of SSI.

General health care included the state-federal Medicaid Program, Medicare, and DVA Medical Care. Long-term care included public spending for persons with mental and physical disabilities residing in institutional settings operated by public and private providers (including nursing homes), and community residential, rehabilitation, housing, and social services operated by public and private providers in the states. Special education programs included local school district, state government, and federal Individuals with Disabilities Education Act financial assistance for the education of children with disabilities in local school systems and in state-operated special schools for students who are deaf, blind, or have a mental disability.

Research and training spending in federal agencies such as the National Institutes of Health and the National Institute on Disability and Rehabilitation Research was excluded from the analysis. The intent of the study was to focus on services and income support programs. Many federal, state, and local disability programs, most with comparatively modest budgets, were also excluded to simplify the task of data collection by restricting the focus of the study to the largest and most important disability programs.

The data sources utilized for gathering financial and recipient data in the study were necessarily many and varied. The major data sources for income maintenance programs included the Social Security Administration's Statistical Supplements (Social Security Administration, 1998, 1999), U.S. Department of Agriculture publications (1998), and agency records and websites for HUD (2000a, 2000b). General health care disability spending data were primarily obtained from the Centers for Medicare and Medicaid Services (formerly Health Care Financing Administration, HCFA), from DVA agency records, and from the Medicare and Medicaid Statistical Supplement (HCFA, 1998).

State-by-state long-term care data for mental retardation/developmental disabilities and mental health were obtained from two nationwide financial and programmatic data bases on these topics, respectively: the State of the States in Developmental Disabilities Project at the University of Illinois at Chicago (Braddock et al., 2000) and the National Association of State Mental Health Program Directors (Lutterman et al., 1999). Nursing home data for people with developmental, mental, and physical disabilities were developed from data obtained from the Centers for Medicare and Medicaid Ser-

vices (HCFA, 2000a, 2000b) and from Harrington, Carillo, Thollaug, Summers, & Wellin (2000). State and local special education data were estimated based on data published by the Center for Special Education Finance (Chambers, Parrish, Lieberman, & Wolman, 1998), Congressional reports by the U.S. Department of Education (1992, 1998), and the *Budget of the United States Government for Fiscal Year 1999* (U.S. Office of Management and Budget, 1999). Additional information on sources of data is presented in a monograph available from the author (Braddock, 2001).

The financial data presented in this chapter reflect the vast majority of expenditures for income maintenance and service programs provided by the public sector for persons with mental, physical, and developmental disabilities in the United States. Disability spending data were collected for a single year: fiscal year 1997. This was the most current fiscal year for which comprehensive mental health expenditure data were available on a state-by-state basis.

RESULTS

Public Sector Spending for Disability Programs in the United States

Public spending for disability-related programs in the United States totaled $293.9 billion in FY 1997. Sixty-four percent of these funds ($188.6 billion) was allocated by the federal government, 31% ($92.1 bil-

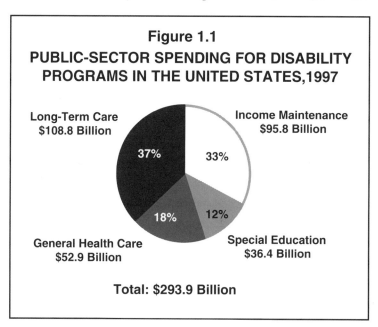

Figure 1.1
PUBLIC-SECTOR SPENDING FOR DISABILITY PROGRAMS IN THE UNITED STATES, 1997

Long-Term Care $108.8 Billion
Income Maintenance $95.8 Billion
General Health Care $52.9 Billion
Special Education $36.4 Billion

37% 33% 18% 12%

Total: $293.9 Billion

lion) by the states and 5% of the funding ($13.2 billion) emanated from local units of government, primarily local school districts. The majority of federal funding (54%) stemmed from income maintenance programs including DI, SSI, ADC, Veterans Compensation and HUD rental payments. State government expenditures stemmed primarily from Medicaid matching funds, long-term care spending commitments for state funded mental disability services, and state funds allocated for special education services to local school districts. Ninety-three percent of local government's commitment to disability services was associated with special education programs; 7% was expended by local mental retardation and developmental disabilities and mental health authorities, including municipalities, county governments, and special districts. Total public spending for disability programs is illustrated in *Figure 1.1* by category of expenditure.

The number of recipients with disabilities assisted by the $293.9 billion in public sector financial commitments was 41.511 million persons. This duplicated count included the following components of recipients: income maintenance, 18.989 million; general health care, 11.912 million; long-term care, 4.873 million; special education, 5.737. Further research is required to determine an unduplicated count.

Income Maintenance

The income maintenance component of total disability spending constituted 33% of such funds in 1997. Social Security Disability Insurance (DI), authorized by Title II of the Social Security Act as Amended,

comprised almost one half of total payments, Supplemental Security Income (SSI) constituted one quarter of the payments, and the remaining 29% of payments was distributed among the Adult Disabled Child Program, Veteran's Compensation, HUD payments/subsidies, and the Food Stamps program (*Figure 1.2*). *Figure 1.2* includes $1.6 billion appropriated by state legislatures as supplementation to federal SSI payments. One state—California—provided 54% of state supplement payments for persons with disabilities across the nation.

General Health Care

General health care had three disability expenditure components: (a) Medicare, which supports Hospital Insurance and Supplemental Medical Insurance including home health care, hospital care, and time-limited skilled nursing facility care; (b) Medicaid, which provides general health care services to persons with disabilities; and, (c) Veteran's Medical Care. The general health care expenditure in 1997 was $52.9 billion. This figure included $22.3 billion for Medicare; $21.8 billion for Medicaid; and $8.8 billion for Veteran's Medical Care.

Long-Term Care

The long-term care spending component included three institutional program elements: nursing homes, institutions for people with mental retardation/developmental disabilities, and institutions for people with mental illness. An institution was defined in the study to refer to a 24-hour facility providing residential services and related program support for 16 or more persons in a public or private setting. Fifty-two percent of the $108.8 billion in total long-term care spending in the United States in 1997 was associated with institutional settings.

Five program elements provided resources for community residential settings — defined as settings for 15 or fewer persons and related community services and supports. The programs included mental retardation/developmental disabilities community programs (primarily Medicaid HCBS Waiver and ICF/MR funded), and mental health community spending

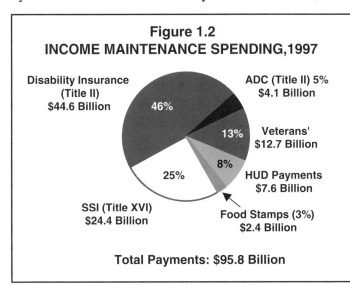

Figure 1.2
INCOME MAINTENANCE SPENDING, 1997

Disability Insurance (Title II) $44.6 Billion — 46%

ADC (Title II) 5% $4.1 Billion

Veterans' $12.7 Billion — 13%

8%

HUD Payments $7.6 Billion

Food Stamps (3%) $2.4 Billion

25%

SSI (Title XVI) $24.4 Billion

Total Payments: $95.8 Billion

(including state and local government "own-source" spending for mental health and developmental disabilities community services); physical disability community Medicaid (including personal care, home health, targeted case management and HCBS Waiver funding); rehabilitation programs financed by the federal-state vocational rehabilitation and independent living programs; and HUD construction loans for community-based housing for persons with disabilities.

Community spending for long-term care was $51.8 billion in 1997. This represented 48% of total expenditures for long-term care. Vocational Rehabilitation spending and HUD construction funds were included in the community long-term care category because these programs supported employment integration and housing for persons with disabilities, both significant components of community living. *Figure 1.3* illustrates long-term care spending for institutional and community services objectives in the United States.

Special Education

Total special education spending totaled $36.39 billion in 1997. This represented 12% of total disability financial commitments; 33.7% of the special education funding was derived from local school district sources, 58.0% from state governments, and 8.3% represented the federal component. The federal share was derived primarily from the formula grant program authorized by the Individuals with Disabilities Education Act.

Institutional Versus Community Services Spending

One of the primary purposes of this study was to assess state-by-state commitments for community services versus institutional long term care. Analysis of the data revealed that the typical state budgeted 48% of the federal-state long-term care resources under its management for community services and 52% for institutional pur-

poses. Thirty-one states devoted 50% or less of their long-term care financial resources for community services; 46 states spent 60% or less of their total long-term care funding allocations for community services in 1997; and only one state, Alaska, committed more than 70% of its resources for community services activities (see *Table 1*).

Seventy-one percent of total public expenditures for persons with physical disabilities in United States long-term care settings was associated with institutions, including nursing homes. The institutional proportion was 40% and 32% for mental illness and mental retardation/developmental disabilities, respectively. The state-by-state long-term care data on expenditures for physical disability, mental illness, and mental retardation/developmental disabilities are presented in a monograph available from the author (Braddock, 2001).

Medicaid Long-Term Care Spending

Medicaid is by far the largest long-term care financial assistance program. State-federal spending was $57.9 billion for the program in 1997, representing 53% of total spending for long-term care services in the United States Fifty-nine percent of total Medicaid resources was budgeted by federal and state governments to pay for institutional services and only 41%

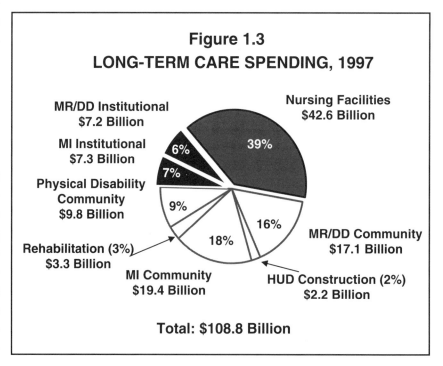

Figure 1.3
LONG-TERM CARE SPENDING, 1997

MR/DD Institutional
$7.2 Billion

MI Institutional
$7.3 Billion

Physical Disability
Community
$9.8 Billion

Rehabilitation (3%)
$3.3 Billion

MI Community
$19.4 Billion

Nursing Facilities
$42.6 Billion

MR/DD Community
$17.1 Billion

HUD Construction (2%)
$2.2 Billion

6%   7%   9%   18%   16%   39%

Total: $108.8 Billion

Table 1.1
PERCENTAGE OF PUBLIC SPENDING FOR LONG-TERM CARE ALLOCATED
TO COMMUNITY CARE SERVICES IN THE STATES, 1997

	State	All Disabilities	MR/DD	Mental Illness	Physical Disabilities
1	Alaska	73%	86%	82%	48%
2	Vermont	66%	97%	82%	33%
3	Arizona	65%	93%	86%	35%
4	New Mexico	65%	86%	80%	36%
5	Nevada	65%	59%	84%	35%
6	California	60%	77%	77%	24%
7	Michigan	58%	91%	67%	32%
8	Montana	58%	73%	71%	38%
9	Oregon	58%	63%	73%	45%
10	Rhode Island	58%	96%	60%	31%
11	Washington	56%	61%	74%	38%
12	Dist Col	55%	97%	56%	24%
13	New Hampshire	55%	97%	64%	27%
14	Minnesota	54%	82%	63%	31%
15	Colorado	54%	85%	67%	29%
16	New York	54%	81%	46%	44%
17	Hawaii	53%	74%	75%	23%
18	Maine	52%	82%	64%	28%
19	South Carolina	52%	61%	68%	33%
20	Utah	51%	57%	71%	27%
21	West Virginia	50%	84%	38%	43%
22	Wyoming	49%	72%	44%	28%
23	Idaho	49%	72%	62%	30%
24	Texas	48%	59%	63%	32%
25	North Carolina	47%	65%	56%	34%
26	Massachusetts	46%	67%	51%	32%
27	Ohio	46%	64%	57%	28%
28	Maryland	44%	77%	51%	24%
29	Wisconsin	44%	61%	65%	26%
30	Connecticut	44%	70%	58%	20%
31	North Dakota	43%	71%	56%	17%
32	Kansas	43%	69%	54%	22%
33	Alabama	42%	58%	56%	26%
34	Iowa	42%	54%	70%	18%
35	South Dakota	42%	74%	53%	17%
36	Kentucky	42%	43%	65%	29%
37	Oklahoma	42%	62%	61%	19%
38	Arkansas	42%	43%	54%	35%
39	Georgia	41%	51%	51%	27%
40	Missouri	40%	60%	51%	24%
41	New Jersey	40%	47%	57%	26%
42	Louisiana	39%	55%	47%	21%
43	Pennsylvania	38%	65%	56%	16%
44	Virginia	38%	55%	45%	24%
45	Illinois	37%	53%	48%	21%
46	Florida	35%	58%	60%	17%
47	Delaware	35%	51%	49%	19%
48	Indiana	35%	58%	55%	13%
49	Mississippi	34%	23%	50%	26%
50	Nebraska	33%	66%	35%	18%
51	Tennessee	31%	46%	40%	22%
	UNITED STATES	**48%**	**68%**	**60%**	**29%**

Source: Braddock, D. (2001). *Public financial support for disabilty programs at the close of the 20th century.*

supported community settings for 15 or fewer persons. The Medicaid programs supporting long-term care for people with disabilities are displayed in *Figure 1.4*.

Thirty-nine states committed the majority of their federal-state Medicaid funding to public and private institutional operations. Twelve states—Oregon, Vermont, Arizona, Michigan, New Mexico, DC, Colorado, Washington, Maine, New York, New Hampshire, and Rhode Island—committed more than one half of their Medicaid resources for community services objectives in 1997; only Oregon, Vermont, Arizona, and Michigan allocated 60% or more of their Medicaid resources for community services. More de-

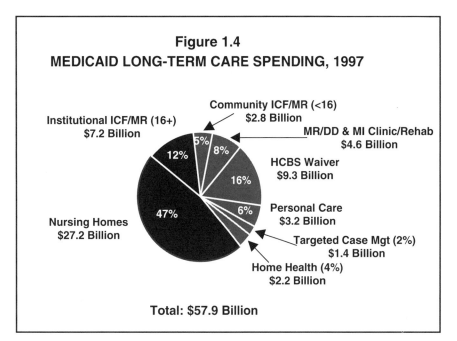

Figure 1.4
MEDICAID LONG-TERM CARE SPENDING, 1997

Institutional ICF/MR (16+) $7.2 Billion

Community ICF/MR (<16) $2.8 Billion

MR/DD & MI Clinic/Rehab $4.6 Billion

HCBS Waiver $9.3 Billion

Personal Care $3.2 Billion

Targeted Case Mgt (2%) $1.4 Billion

Home Health (4%) $2.2 Billion

Nursing Homes $27.2 Billion

12% 5% 8% 16% 6% 47%

Total: $57.9 Billion

tailed state-by-state expenditure data are presented in a monograph available from the author (Braddock, 2001).

Assessing Fiscal Effort in the States

Financial commitments for community long-term care services in the individual states varied greatly in terms of the funds budgeted for such programs per $1,000 of aggregate state personal income (fiscal effort). In fact, there was a 295% difference between the leading and lagging states on this fiscal effort measure, which raised a key question as to what factors accounted for such great differences in state commitments for community services (see *Table 1.2*).

Investigators have theorized that, due to the greater availability of "slack resources," heavily populated and wealthy states are more likely to commit proportionally greater resources to any given programmatic area than are the less wealthy and populous states (Dye & Robey, 1980; Fabricant, 1952; Hofferbert, 1972; Savage, 1978; Walker, 1969). However, research on public spending variations in the states has soundly rejected this theory with respect to community services for persons with mental retardation/developmental disabilities (Braddock & Fujiura, 1991; Braddock et al., 2000). Two factors that do predict community services spending levels in the states for mental retardation/developmental disabilities, however, are degree of state participation in the HCBS Waiver Program and a state political culture historically supportive of civil rights for minorities generally, i.e., early adoption of state civil rights statutes promoting nondiscrimination in public accommodations, public housing, and employment. Under the federal Medicaid statute, states are required to allocate funding for matching purposes in order to receive federal Waiver reimbursement. Much of the variation across the states in community services fiscal effort for developmental disabilities programs was associated with state leadership in utilizing the HCBS Waiver.

As noted in the introduction to this chapter, one explicit purpose of the study included focusing analysis on identifying variables accounting for differences across the states in fiscal effort commitments for community services objectives in long-term care. A hierarchical regression analysis was completed using the Statistical Package for the Social Sciences (SPSS) 11.0 software to explore the relationship between community services fiscal effort for long-term care disability services program commitments in the states in 1997 (the dependent variable) and the four independent variables noted above: state size (population), state wealth, the presence of a progressive civil rights po-

Table 1.2

**PUBLIC SPENDING FOR COMMUNITY LONG-TERM CARE SERVICES FOR PERSONS
WITH DISABILITIES IN THE STATES PER $1,000 OF PERSONAL INCOME, 1997**

Rank	State	Spending per $1,000 of Personal Income
1	District of Columbia	$15.72
2	New York	$15.27
3	Vermont	$14.82
4	Rhode Island	$13.66
5	Maine	$12.91
6	Montana	$12.54
7	Minnesota	$12.00
8	Alaska	$10.55
9	North Dakota	$10.39
10	Massachusetts	$10.02
11	New Hampshire	$10.01
12	Oregon	$9.97
13	Connecticut	$9.78
14	Ohio	$9.63
15	Michigan	$9.62
16	South Carolina	$9.36
17	New Mexico	$9.32
18	West Virginia	$9.20
19	Washington	$9.13
20	Arizona	$9.08
21	Wisconsin	$8.74
22	North Carolina	$8.72
23	South Dakota	$8.62
24	Iowa	$8.61
25	Wyoming	$8.48
26	Arkansas	$7.77
27	Kansas	$7.52
28	Pennsylvania	$7.44
29	Missouri	$7.26
30	Kentucky	$7.18
31	Louisiana	$7.08
32	California	$6.86
33	Oklahoma	$6.74
34	Idaho	$6.60
35	Colorado	$6.45
36	New Jersey	$6.02
37	Maryland	$6.02
38	Utah	$6.01
39	Hawaii	$5.97
40	Texas	$5.92
41	Mississippi	$5.91
42	Indiana	$5.86
43	Alabama	$5.82
44	Delaware	$5.40
45	Nebraska	$5.32
46	Nevada	$4.91
47	Illinois	$4.85
48	Tennessee	$4.79
49	Georgia	$4.56
50	Florida	$4.37
51	Virginia	$3.98
	UNITED STATES	$7.84

Source: Braddock, D. (2001). *Public financial support for disability programs at the close of the 20th century.*

litical culture in the state historically, and state leadership to expand HCBS Waiver funding. State size was measured by general state population in 1997; state wealth by aggregate statewide personal income in 1997; the civil rights variable was indexed according to the states' ranking in how soon they adopted state statutes in public accommodations, public housing, and employment for racial minorities (Gray, 1973); and the HCBS Waiver variable was expressed as per capita (per member of the general population) state government Waiver expenditure.

Sixty-three percent of the variance in state fiscal effort for community services for persons with disabilities was accounted for in the overall regression. The equation, with all variables entered, was statistically significant at the $p < .001$ level, $F(4,43) = 20.721$. As in the aforementioned mental retardation/developmental disabilities analysis, neither state population nor state wealth was a statistically significant predictor. The entry of the civil rights and HCBS Waiver variables made the overall regression equation statistically significant. Over two thirds of the variance in the states was attributable to the degree of HCBS Waiver participation in the states. The civil rights variable correlated with state HCBS Waiver spending per capita at a significance level of .01 ($r = .54$) and with state wealth at a significance level of .01 ($r = .61$). Waiver funding also correlated with state wealth at a significance level of .05 ($r = .34$).

DISCUSSION AND CONCLUSION

On a nationwide basis, public spending of $293.9 billion for disability programs in 1997 constituted 12.2% of total federal-state expenditures of $2.404 trillion that year. This percentage of total expenditure is similar to the figure we computed for a 1986 data set developed by revising Berkowitz and Greene's (1989) earlier data set. We excluded noncomparable private insurance spending and included our 1986 state and local government data sets for mental health (Lutterman et al., 1999), developmental disabilities (Braddock et al., 2000), and special education spending in the states (Chambers et al., 1998). We calculated that 11.9% of total federal and state expenditures was being expended

for publicly financed disability programs in 1986.

Total public disability expenditure in 1986 was estimated to be $177 billion in constant 2002 dollar terms. For fiscal year 2002, total disability expenditure in the United States was projected to be $426 billion in current (2002) dollar terms. This projection was based on the rate of growth in disability spending between 1986-97.

A second major finding of this study is that the majority of public resources being allocated for long-term care services for persons with disabilities in the United States supports placements in institutions and nursing homes. It is especially noteworthy that an extremely large percentage of the nation's resources for long-term care for persons with physical disabilities (71%) is being allocated for institutional care in nursing homes. In 1997, $9.7 billion was allocated for community long-term care services for persons with physical disabilities, compared to $35.3 billion for institutional care in nursing facilities. No state allocated a majority of its long-term care funding base for community services and supports for this group of persons with disabilities. In contrast, approximately two thirds of total public funding for long-term care services for persons with mental disabilities is allocated for community services and supports.

The analysis of state variations in community long-term care services fiscal effort indicated that variations were tied to the extent of state participation in the Medicaid Waiver and Personal Assistance programs and to the states' histories in the adoption of civil rights legislation promoting racial equality. However, the civil rights variable was statistically significant only in the case of the mental retardation/developmental disabilities group and, due to its strength in this category, in the combined analysis for all three disability groups. This suggests that long-term care for persons with mental retardation/developmental disabilities has become more fully manifest as a civil rights issue in the states than it has for persons with physical disabilities and mental illness. In fact, more than 70 MR/DD class action right-to-habilitation lawsuits in 38 states were litigated between 1970 and 1996 (Hayden, 1997). Currently, 31 additional lawsuits are being litigated in 25 states on access to community Medicaid services and implementation of the community services mandates of the *Olmstead* (1999) Supreme Court decision (Smith, 2002).

In this paper, a methodology has been presented comparing the states in terms of the degree to which they are committed to financing community long-term care services for persons with disabilities and their families. However, differentiating meaningfully among the states on their levels of financial commitments to community long-term care services requires that the state rankings presented in this paper be interpreted generally; i.e., according to their quintile or decile positions in groups of 5 to 10 states rather than in the seemingly precise numerical rankings presented in the Tables.

There is considerable value in comparing public sector disability spending in the states over time. State governments should be held accountable for the policy and budgetary decisions they make that tend to segregate people with disabilities in institutional settings versus supporting them in home, community, and family settings. In the present study "community services" was operationally defined in terms of residential settings for "15 or fewer persons." This was an extremely generous interpretation of the concept of community services today. It would have been preferable to use a six person or fewer metric to define community services commitments in the states; however, working with the many existing data sets across the spectrum of disability programs required a "lowest common denominator" approach to be inclusive of the major programs. Had community services been restricted in the study to refer only to residential settings for six or fewer persons, a slightly smaller percentage of financial resource commitments in most states would have been identified as being allocated for community services activities, and a correspondingly larger proportion of the states' resources would have been identified with financing disability services in institutional settings.

A critically important underlying reason for the great variability in state-to-state commitments for disability programs stems from the semi-autonomous role constitutionally granted to state governments in our federal system. The United States Government has only been active in disability policymaking for a few decades, and, unlike many European nations, the United States government lacks fully comprehensive and nationally uniform entitlement policies in health care, employment, and social welfare. However, a new legal framework on disability support has begun to emerge in the United States based on self-determination, community and family support, independent living, inclusive education, and broad civil rights protections. The new framework is embodied in statutes such as the Individuals with Disabilities Education Act, the Americans with Disabilities Act, the Developmental Disabilities Act, the Medicaid HCBS Waiver program, the Fair Housing Act, the Rehabilitation Act, and in numerous federal and state court rulings on the rights of persons with disabilities (Silverstein, 2000).

It is clear that the United States has made enormous strides in the implementation of disability programs over the past 30 years. However, the incentives embedded in many disability financial assistance programs administered by the federal government and in the states today, particularly those programs financing long-term care, have not kept pace with innovations in community and family support and independent living. This is especially true for persons with physical disabilities but also for persons with mental illness, where there is an almost complete absence of public sector community long-term care support in the states' Medicaid programs (Braddock, 1992; Hatfield, 1987; Koyanagi, 1990). In 1997, for example, only Colorado and Vermont utilized Medicaid HCBS Waiver or Personal Assistance funding to support individuals with severe and persistent mental illness in community settings.

In the future, greater emphasis should be placed on extending the availability and improving the quality of HCBS Waiver and Personal Assistance services to all persons with disabilities in the states who require such services, while reducing reliance on institutions and nursing homes. Replication of the present study every few years could be useful in promoting the diffusion of home and community long-term care services to persons with disabilities in the states, including persons with physical disabilities and mental illness, and in contributing to the national dialogue on disability policy reform. Perhaps most importantly, it could assist in the assessment of progress in the states and by the federal government in the implementation of the United States Supreme Court's *Olmstead* (1999) decision.

REFERENCES

Bahl, R. (1982). Fiscal health of state and local governments: 1982 and beyond. *Public Budgeting and Finance, 2*, 5-21.

Berkowitz, M., & Greene, C. (1989, Spring). Disability expenditures. *American Rehabilitation*, pp. 7-15.

Braddock, D. (1992). Community mental health and mental retardation services in the American states: A comparative study of resource allocation. *American Journal of Psychiatry, 149*, 175-183.

Braddock, D. (2001). Public financial support for disability programs at the close of the 20th century. Boulder: Coleman Institute for Cognitive Disabilities, University of Colorado.

Braddock, D. (in press). Public financial support for disability programs at the close of the 20th century. *American Journal on Mental Retardation.*

Braddock, D., & Fujiura, G. (1991). Politics, public policy, and the development of community mental retardation services in the United States. *American Journal on Mental Retardation, 95*(4), 369-387.

Braddock, D., Hemp, R., Parish, S., & Rizzolo, M. C. (2000). *The state of the states in developmental disabilities: 2000 study summary.* Chicago, IL: Department of Disability and Human Development, University of Illinois at Chicago.

Braddock, D., Hemp, R., Parish, S., & Westrich, J. (1998). The state of the states in developmental disabilities (5th ed.). Washington, DC: American Association on Mental Retardation.

Chambers, J. G., Parrish, T. B., Lieberman, J. C., & Wolman, J. M. (1998, February). What are we spending on special education in the U.S.? *CSEF Brief No. 8.* (Center for Special Finance; Palo Alto, CA).

Dye, T., & Robey, J. S. (1980). Politics versus economics: Development of the literature on policy determination. In T. R. Dye & V. Gray (Eds.), *The determinants of public policy* (pp. 3-18). Lexington, MA: D.C. Heath.

Fabricant, S. (1952). *The trend of government activity in the United States since 1900.* New York: National Bureau of Economic Research.

Gray, V. (1973). Innovation in the states: A diffusion study. *The American Political Science Review, 67*, 1174-1185.

Harrington, C., Carillo, H., Thollaug, S. C., Summers, P.R., & Wellin, V. (2000, January). *Nursing facilities, staffing, residents, and facility deficiencies, 1992 - 1998.* San Francisco: University of California – San Francisco, Department of Social and Behavioral Sciences.

Hatfield, A. B. (1987). Consumer issues in mental illness. In *Families of the mentally ill: Meeting the challenges.* San Francisco: Jossey-Bass.

Health Care Financing Administration. (1998, December). *Health Care Financing Review Medicare and Medicaid statistical supplement.* Baltimore: Author.

Health Care Financing Administration. (2000a). *Online data based on HCFA 64 forms.* Baltimore: Author. Available at: http://hcfa.gov/medicaid/MCD97T10.htm.

Health Care Financing Administration. (2000b). *Online data based on HCFA 2082 data system: Table 32-Medicaid long-term care recipients and days of care by state: Fiscal year 1997.* Baltimore: Author. Available at: http://www.hcfa.gov/medicaid/msis/MCD97T32.htm

Hofferbert, R. I. (1972). State and community policy studies: A review of comparative input-output analyses. In J. A. Robinson (Ed.), *Political science annual: An international review* (Vol. 3). Indianapolis: Bobbs-Merrill Company.

Koyanagi, C. (1990). The missed opportunities of Medicaid. *Hospital & Community Psychiatry, 41,* 135-138.

Lutterman, T., Hirad, A., & Poindexter, B. (1999). *Funding sources and expenditures of state mental health agencies: Fiscal year 1997.* Alexandria, VA: National Association of State Mental Health Program Directors Research Institute.

Olmstead v. L. C., 119 S. Ct. 2176 (1999).

Savage, R. L. (1978). Policy innovativeness as a trait of American states. *Journal of Politics, 40,* 212-224.

Silverstein, R. (2000). *Disability policy frame-*

work: A guidepost for analyzing public policy. Washington, DC: Center for the Study and Advancement of Disability Policy and the Arc of the United States.

Smith, G. A. (2002, March). *Status report: Litigation concerning Medicaid services for persons with developmental disabilities.* Tulatin, OR: Human Services Research Institute.

Social Security Administration. (1998, November). *Annual statistical supplement, 1998, to the Social Security Bulletin.* Washington, DC: Author.

Social Security Administration. (1999, November). *Annual statistical supplement, 1999, to the Social Security Bulletin.* Washington, DC: Author.

U.S. Department of Agriculture. (1998, August). *Reaching those in need: How effective is the Food Stamp program?* Washington, DC: Author.

U.S. Department of Education. (1992). *Fourteenth annual report to Congress on the implementation of the Individuals with Disabilities Education Act.* Washington, DC: Author.

U.S. Department of Education. (1998). *Twentieth annual report to Congress on the implementation of the Individuals with Disabilities Education Act.* Washington, DC: Author.

U.S. Department of Housing and Urban Development. (2000a). *Homes and communities.* Washington, DC: Author. Available at: http://www.hud.gov

U.S. Department of Housing and Urban Development. (2000b). *A picture of subsidized households: Project, agency, and state summaries: Fiscal year 1997.* Washington, DC: Author. Available at: http://www.huduser.org/datasets/assthsg/statedata97/allst.html

U.S. Office of Management and Budget. (1999). *Budget of the United States Government, fiscal year 1999: Budget information for states.* Washington, DC: U.S. Government Printing Office.

Walker, J. L. (1969). The diffusion of innovation among the American states. *American Political Science Review, 63,* 880-899.

APPENDICES:
Public Financial Support for Disability

Appendix 1

PUBLIC FINANCIAL SUPPORT FOR DISABILITY SERVICES IN THE UNITED STATES, 1997

Rank[1]	State	Health Care	Long-Term Care	Special Education	Disability Services Total	Disability Services Fiscal Effort[2]	Income Maintenance	Services & Income Maintenance
1	Alabama	$1,206,401,403	$1,213,647,421	$327,019,433	$2,747,068,257	$31.08	$2,075,802,617	$4,822,870,874
2	Alaska	$90,693,993	$215,711,256	$222,841,751	$529,247,000	$35.40	$164,577,713	$693,824,713
3	Arizona	$675,037,689	$1,339,661,455	$370,269,117	$2,384,968,261	$24.67	$1,415,945,471	$3,800,913,732
4	Arkansas	$737,154,059	$897,434,337	$130,556,343	$1,765,144,739	$36.50	$1,336,243,254	$3,101,387,993
5	California	$5,878,639,120	$9,348,648,510	$3,594,182,824	$18,821,470,455	$22.90	$10,976,337,711	$29,797,808,166
6	Colorado	$544,095,185	$1,206,209,044	$268,922,025	$2,019,226,254	$19.92	$1,159,331,577	$3,178,557,831
7	Connecticut	$611,637,691	$2,560,056,634	$747,670,609	$3,919,364,933	$34.34	$1,016,560,845	$4,935,925,778
8	Delaware	$140,252,453	$310,199,299	$95,178,344	$545,630,096	$26.87	$235,549,230	$781,179,326
9	District of Columbia	$396,121,707	$527,421,394	$122,183,242	$1,045,726,344	$56.24	$241,237,233	$1,286,963,577
10	Florida	$1,792,120,936	$4,366,340,418	$1,713,361,700	$7,871,823,054	$22.24	$5,327,471,023	$13,199,294,077
11	Georgia	$1,769,221,971	$1,933,087,516	$858,326,453	$4,560,635,941	$26.21	$2,749,020,173	$7,309,656,114
12	Hawaii	$233,665,705	$335,728,653	$161,146,166	$730,540,524	$24.32	$310,283,326	$1,040,823,850
13	Idaho	$179,199,017	$325,231,136	$100,811,324	$605,241,477	$25.18	$342,216,280	$947,457,757
14	Illinois	$2,305,879,290	$4,222,755,189	$2,399,701,515	$8,928,335,994	$27.58	$3,804,288,927	$12,732,624,921
15	Indiana	$907,534,865	$2,216,648,804	$400,112,907	$3,524,296,575	$26.50	$1,810,928,613	$5,335,225,188
16	Iowa	$443,937,113	$1,315,349,273	$304,752,425	$2,064,038,811	$31.97	$772,817,833	$2,836,856,643
17	Kansas	$456,578,800	$1,050,993,492	$398,820,936	$1,906,393,228	$31.49	$708,880,746	$2,615,273,974
18	Kentucky	$1,166,584,109	$1,331,452,272	$334,639,831	$2,832,676,212	$36.23	$2,231,764,541	$5,064,440,753
19	Louisiana	$1,293,161,323	$1,573,134,266	$395,519,988	$3,261,815,577	$37.45	$2,003,414,070	$5,265,229,647
20	Maine	$285,029,461	$657,828,772	$164,532,226	$1,107,390,460	$41.54	$567,004,728	$1,674,395,187
21	Maryland	$848,372,498	$1,931,168,924	$893,046,152	$3,672,587,573	$25.84	$1,427,541,559	$5,100,129,132
22	Massachusetts	$1,579,608,864	$4,022,630,611	$1,223,667,176	$6,825,906,650	$36.78	$2,619,760,982	$9,445,667,632
23	Michigan	$1,943,923,034	$3,990,199,337	$1,436,216,399	$7,371,437,769	$30.53	$3,472,995,240	$10,844,433,009
24	Minnesota	$687,302,863	$2,655,428,177	$797,901,989	$4,140,633,030	$34.41	$1,217,248,501	$5,357,881,531
25	Mississippi	$980,819,011	$834,003,453	$173,728,497	$1,988,550,961	$41.17	$1,502,720,183	$3,491,271,144
26	Missouri	$1,117,333,072	$2,241,253,894	$487,719,289	$3,846,306,255	$30.79	$1,980,991,020	$5,827,297,275
27	Montana	$138,921,090	$365,566,161	$61,624,784	$566,112,035	$33.41	$317,252,828	$883,364,863
28	Nebraska	$267,344,406	$627,603,933	$125,112,756	$1,020,061,095	$26.45	$434,574,246	$1,454,635,341
29	Nevada	$244,760,864	$326,403,942	$265,816,799	$838,981,605	$19.43	$488,953,167	$1,327,934,772
30	New Hampshire	$144,588,805	$575,262,320	$201,640,217	$921,491,343	$29.17	$375,868,520	$1,297,359,863
31	New Jersey	$1,359,743,389	$3,851,062,434	$780,606,876	$5,991,412,699	$23.63	$2,482,758,092	$8,474,170,791
32	New Mexico	$348,575,785	$465,502,747	$284,048,565	$1,098,127,097	$33.72	$630,364,684	$1,728,491,781
33	New York	$4,620,740,884	$15,086,148,303	$7,276,832,948	$26,983,722,136	$50.61	$8,162,469,825	$35,146,191,960
34	North Carolina	$1,683,223,941	$3,085,719,219	$429,773,077	$5,198,716,237	$31.10	$3,046,923,442	$8,245,639,679
35	North Dakota	$87,387,320	$310,242,967	$61,440,490	$459,070,776	$35.43	$158,337,673	$617,408,449
36	Ohio	$2,043,213,446	$5,517,440,787	$1,814,397,603	$9,375,051,836	$35.47	$4,194,405,570	$13,569,457,406
37	Oklahoma	$617,046,643	$1,053,868,477	$437,455,011	$2,108,370,131	$32.09	$1,319,051,435	$3,427,421,566
38	Oregon	$488,251,405	$1,301,083,948	$392,042,007	$2,181,377,360	$28.83	$1,009,490,837	$3,190,868,197
39	Pennsylvania	$2,223,311,243	$5,877,803,431	$1,067,583,691	$9,168,698,366	$30.31	$4,270,894,934	$13,439,593,299
40	Rhode Island	$275,113,263	$582,554,845	$168,169,937	$1,025,838,045	$41.52	$448,741,289	$1,474,579,334
41	South Carolina	$907,739,895	$1,363,171,259	$266,312,928	$2,537,224,083	$33.54	$1,621,270,550	$4,158,494,632
42	South Dakota	$155,462,442	$314,681,380	$65,808,526	$535,952,348	$34.83	$216,375,464	$752,327,812
43	Tennessee	$1,777,540,912	$1,832,440,663	$285,965,637	$3,895,947,213	$32.73	$2,446,590,083	$6,342,537,296
44	Texas	$3,282,974,768	$5,522,419,570	$1,637,393,416	$10,442,787,754	$23.32	$5,179,955,740	$15,622,743,493
45	Utah	$210,958,014	$471,467,080	$143,184,655	$825,609,749	$20.47	$396,163,647	$1,221,773,396
46	Vermont	$128,542,379	$297,032,716	$99,223,594	$524,798,689	$39.51	$222,243,695	$747,042,385
47	Virginia	$1,166,229,842	$1,802,889,630	$733,721,476	$3,702,840,948	$21.60	$2,261,322,651	$5,964,163,599
48	Washington	$851,931,946	$2,335,504,288	$607,737,651	$3,795,173,885	$26.49	$1,786,097,276	$5,581,271,162
49	West Virginia	$630,274,957	$612,947,613	$166,626,191	$1,410,296,149	$42.01	$1,126,750,111	$2,537,046,260
50	Wisconsin	$890,274,957	$2,423,571,949	$802,913,228	$4,116,760,134	$33.68	$1,609,857,862	$5,726,617,996
51	Wyoming	$82,043,534	$182,375,159	$88,824,408	$353,243,101	$33.27	$134,603,574	$487,846,675
	UNITED STATES	$52,898,948,750	$108,808,087,359	$36,387,085,132	$198,094,121,242	$30.02	$95,812,250,590	$293,906,371,832

[1] States are ranked on Disability Services fiscal effort.

[2] Fiscal effort is defined as a state's spending for disability services per $1,000 of total state personal income.

Source: Braddock. D. (2001). *Public financial support for disability programs at the close of the 20th century.*

Appendix 2

PUBLIC SPENDING FOR MEDICAID LONG-TERM CARE SERVICES FOR PEOPLE WITH DISABILITIES, 1997

State	Institutional Medicaid Long-Term Care	Community Medicaid Long-Term Care	Total Medicaid Long-Term Care	Percent Community
1 Oregon	$218,718,645	$420,029,581	$638,748,226	66%
2 Vermont	$58,932,902	$111,245,991	$170,178,894	65%
3 Arizona	$244,293,181	$440,799,126	$685,092,307	64%
4 Michigan	$726,432,637	$1,183,956,921	$1,910,389,558	62%
5 New Mexico	$120,016,089	$154,011,190	$274,027,279	56%
6 District of Columbia	$139,458,654	$155,636,647	$295,095,301	53%
7 Colorado	$293,191,234	$324,686,568	$617,877,802	53%
8 Washington	$580,100,391	$618,995,198	$1,199,095,589	52%
9 Maine	$188,147,425	$200,294,213	$388,441,637	52%
10 New York	$5,796,205,482	$5,949,552,272	$11,745,757,754	51%
11 New Hampshire	$171,461,767	$175,218,111	$346,679,878	51%
12 Rhode Island	$184,868,181	$188,233,123	$373,101,304	50%
13 Minnesota	$812,695,313	$810,476,261	$1,623,171,574	50%
14 Montana	$96,079,241	$94,606,414	$190,685,655	50%
15 West Virginia	$207,712,534	$189,829,778	$397,542,312	48%
16 South Carolina	$350,117,808	$310,564,574	$660,682,382	47%
17 Alaska	$40,515,751	$32,965,356	$73,481,107	45%
18 North Carolina	$866,548,951	$691,416,802	$1,557,965,753	44%
19 Idaho	$98,826,765	$78,148,671	$176,975,436	44%
20 Nevada	$72,737,859	$57,037,479	$129,775,338	44%
21 Kansas	$266,432,538	$206,076,235	$472,508,773	44%
22 Maryland	$414,199,068	$313,629,443	$727,828,511	43%
23 California	$2,230,411,791	$1,665,798,053	$3,896,209,844	43%
24 Texas	$1,568,000,840	$1,143,012,326	$2,711,013,167	42%
25 Wyoming	$57,442,989	$41,004,489	$98,447,478	42%
26 Massachusetts	$1,332,525,200	$803,655,785	$2,136,180,985	38%
27 Virginia	$467,674,139	$273,045,405	$740,719,545	37%
28 South Dakota	$98,468,608	$57,111,520	$155,580,128	37%
29 North Dakota	$111,035,306	$64,182,626	$175,217,932	37%
30 Ohio	$1,888,667,481	$1,066,608,967	$2,955,276,447	36%
31 Connecticut	$823,562,113	$463,553,881	$1,287,115,994	36%
32 Missouri	$646,048,525	$362,517,156	$1,008,565,681	36%
33 Utah	$119,385,147	$65,284,669	$184,669,816	35%
34 Arkansas	$346,872,047	$179,319,822	$526,191,869	34%
35 New Jersey	$1,208,578,926	$623,601,559	$1,832,180,485	34%
36 Wisconsin	$844,264,551	$401,324,021	$1,245,588,572	32%
37 Oklahoma	$334,857,974	$149,331,265	$484,189,239	31%
38 Kentucky	$456,008,770	$202,652,639	$658,661,409	31%
39 Louisiana	$542,079,764	$240,460,642	$782,540,405	31%
40 Nebraska	$224,492,373	$93,390,395	$317,882,768	29%
41 Iowa	$377,554,694	$155,573,127	$533,127,821	29%
42 Delaware	$93,783,934	$38,171,625	$131,955,558	29%
43 Alabama	$497,490,038	$193,997,296	$691,487,334	28%
44 Georgia	$661,610,595	$241,089,238	$902,699,833	27%
45 Indiana	$734,740,961	$264,482,113	$999,223,074	26%
46 Tennessee	$729,442,954	$261,547,318	$990,990,272	26%
47 Florida	$1,237,355,820	$440,465,022	$1,677,820,842	26%
48 Illinois	$1,564,311,830	$541,840,196	$2,106,152,026	26%
49 Pennsylvania	$2,728,086,156	$732,502,166	$3,460,588,322	21%
50 Mississippi	$356,871,826	$93,406,503	$450,278,328	21%
51 Hawaii	$122,512,501	$31,521,897	$154,034,398	20%
UNITED STATES	$34,351,830,268	$23,597,861,675	$57,949,691,943	41%

Source: Braddock, D. (2001). *Public financial support for disability at the close of the 20th century.*

Appendix 3

RECIPIENTS OF DISABILITY SERVICES, PAYMENTS, AND BENEFITS IN THE UNITED STATES, 1997

PROGRAM	RECIPIENTS
Income Maintenance	**18,989,032**
Supplemental Security Income (SSI)	5,101,400
Supplemental Security Disability Insurance (SSDI)	4,598,020
Adult Disabled Child (ADC)	691,610
Veterans' Compensation	2,226,053
Food Stamps	2,012,000
Housing and Urban Development (HUD) Payments	2,600,925
SSI State Supplement	1,759,024
Health Care	**11,911,793**
Medicare	4,876,755
Medicaid	6,222,529
Veterans' Medical Care	812,509
Long-Term Care	**4,872,605**
Institutional LTC	**1,516,175**
Nursing Facilities	1,332,177
MR/DD	93,542
Mental Illness	90,456
Community LTC	**3,356,430**
MR/DD Residential & Day Programs	488,899
Mental Illness Services	682,535
Vocational Rehabilitation (VR)	220,936
VR Independent Living	99,323
Veterans' Rehabilitation	53,138
Home and Community Based Waiver	578,089
Medicaid Home Health Care	766,000
Medicaid Personal Care	467,510
Special Education	**5,737,420**
TOTAL RECIPIENTS (DUPLICATED COUNT)	**41,510,850**

Source: Braddock, D. (2001). *Public financial support for disability programs at the close of the 20th century.*

Appendix 4
LONG-TERM CARE SPENDING AND PARTICIPANTS, 1997

PHYSICAL DISABILITY

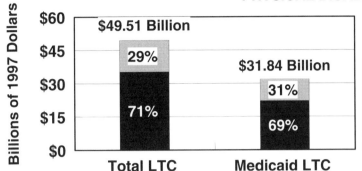

Participants Served		
	Total LTC	Medicaid LTC
Inst & Comm	2,951,815	2,687,904
Community	1,854,968	1,591,057
Institution	1,096,847	1,096,847

MENTAL ILLNESS

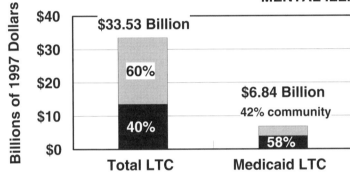

Participants Served		
	Total LTC	Medicaid LTC
Inst & Comm	1,030,910	139,148
Community	742,741	626
Institution	288,169	138,522

MENTAL RETARDATION/DEVELOPMENTAL DISABILITIES

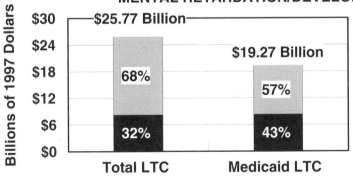

Participants Served		
	Total LTC	Medicaid LTC
Inst & Comm	889,880	386,194
Community	758,721	264,675
Institution	131,159	121,519

☐ **Community** ■ **Institution**

Source: Braddock, D. (2001). *Public financial support for disability programs at the close of the 20th century.*

PART II

The State of the States
in Developmental Disabilities

The State of the States in Developmental Disabilities: Study Summary

David Braddock, Richard Hemp, Mary C. Rizzolo, Susan Parish, & Amy Pomeranz

This chapter presents the results of the seventh State of the States in Developmental Disabilities study of financing and programming trends in the United States. The first study was initiated in 1982 to monitor the growth and development of services and funding for persons with developmental disabilities across the states (Braddock, Hemp, & Howes, 1984). Six subsequent editions of the study have been completed (Braddock et al., 1986, 1987, 1990, 1995, 1998, 2000). The current update extends the longitudinal analysis of financial and programmatic trends in the states through fiscal year 2000 and pays particular attention to trends in services from 1996 through 2000. During this four-year period, the nation experienced ongoing economic growth. Data were analyzed to determine whether this growth was paralleled in the states' mental retardation and developmental disability (MR/DD) service systems.

Data were collected from each state's principal MR/DD agency to assess trends in the structure and financing of developmental disabilities services. State health and social services agencies that administered programs for individuals with developmental disabilities, such as the Medicaid program and the Social Ser-

vices Block Grant, were also surveyed, as necessary. This summary focuses on describing the structure of residential and community services in the states; and identifying trends in the financing of institutional and community services, and individual and family support which consists of family support, supported living, personal assistance, and supported employment. The chapter concludes with a discussion of issues that will have an impact on the future of provisions for MR/DD services in the states, including aging caregivers and their increased need for support, waiting lists for services, class-action litigation and the potential impact of a declining economy on developmental disabilities services.

INTRODUCTION

Since the 1970s, many states have vigorously reduced their reliance on institutional facilities and developed community residential settings including group homes, foster care, and supported living options. During the 1996-2000 period, the number of individuals served in all types of residential settings in the United States advanced 11%, from 390,586 to

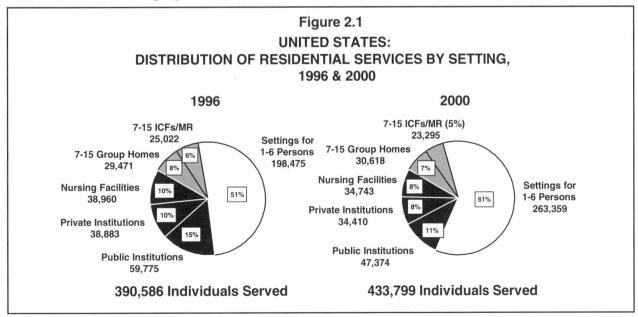

Figure 2.1
UNITED STATES:
DISTRIBUTION OF RESIDENTIAL SERVICES BY SETTING,
1996 & 2000

1996

7-15 ICFs/MR 25,022
7-15 Group Homes 29,471
Nursing Facilities 38,960
Private Institutions 38,883
Public Institutions 59,775
Settings for 1-6 Persons 198,475

6% 8% 10% 10% 15% 51%

390,586 Individuals Served

2000

7-15 ICFs/MR (5%) 23,295
7-15 Group Homes 30,618
Nursing Facilities 34,743
Private Institutions 34,410
Public Institutions 47,374
Settings for 1-6 Persons 263,359

7% 8% 8% 11% 61%

433,799 Individuals Served

Table 2.1
INDIVIDUALS SERVED BY RESIDENTIAL SETTING, FY 2000

Rank[1]	State	1-6 Residents[2] Number	%	7-15 Residents Number	%	16+ Residents Number	%	Total	Placements Per 100K[3]
44	Alabama	1,918	43%	979	22%	1,544	35%	4,441	100
1	Alaska	864	97%	25	3%	6	1%	895	141
4	Arizona	3,298	92%	42	1%	258	7%	3,598	75
51	Arkansas	1,232	26%	893	19%	2,631	55%	4,756	184
18	California	37,647	77%	2,548	5%	8,524	17%	48,719	148
9	Colorado	6,229	87%	522	7%	417	6%	7,168	174
22	Connecticut	4,678	71%	463	7%	1,416	22%	6,557	200
29	Delaware	585	63%	0	0%	350	37%	935	123
28	District of Columbia	786	63%	383	31%	84	7%	1,253	240
38	Florida	6,303	50%	2,937	23%	3,378	27%	12,618	83
33	Georgia	3,863	54%	0	0%	3,299	46%	7,162	91
6	Hawaii	1,177	91%	7	1%	105	8%	1,289	106
26	Idaho	2,076	65%	672	21%	464	14%	3,212	247
47	Illinois	8,124	40%	3,208	16%	9,073	44%	20,405	169
42	Indiana	4,958	44%	2,754	24%	3,550	32%	11,262	188
34	Iowa	5,562	54%	1,405	14%	3,293	32%	10,260	356
12	Kansas	3,942	82%	223	5%	614	13%	4,779	180
41	Kentucky	1,661	45%	276	8%	1,736	47%	3,673	92
45	Louisiana	3,455	43%	795	10%	3,861	48%	8,111	184
8	Maine	2,795	87%	217	7%	192	6%	3,204	255
7	Maryland	5,538	89%	0	0%	709	11%	6,247	120
23	Massachusetts	9,238	71%	1,000	8%	2,792	21%	13,030	211
5	Michigan	11,664	91%	0	0%	1,088	9%	12,752	131
15	Minnesota	11,568	81%	1,241	9%	1,403	10%	14,212	296
50	Mississippi	1,867	34%	617	11%	2,943	54%	5,427	194
39	Missouri	4,062	47%	1,724	20%	2,798	33%	8,584	156
30	Montana	1,049	59%	437	25%	292	16%	1,778	194
21	Nebraska	2,690	72%	300	8%	754	20%	3,744	222
13	Nevada	900	82%	15	1%	181	17%	1,096	60
3	New Hampshire	1,744	95%	8	0%	88	5%	1,840	152
36	New Jersey	5,768	52%	674	6%	4,757	42%	11,199	137
11	New Mexico	1,987	86%	217	9%	110	5%	2,314	129
49	New York	16,716	39%	18,168	42%	8,340	19%	43,224	238
19	North Carolina	11,135	76%	596	4%	2,937	20%	14,668	190
32	North Dakota	1,199	56%	506	24%	445	21%	2,150	332
40	Ohio	9,396	47%	2,772	14%	7,925	39%	20,093	178
46	Oklahoma	2,385	42%	231	4%	3,082	54%	5,698	169
17	Oregon	3,581	78%	597	13%	384	8%	4,562	136
25	Pennsylvania	14,883	68%	689	3%	6,376	29%	21,948	181
14	Rhode Island	1,614	81%	180	9%	187	9%	1,981	199
37	South Carolina	2,394	50%	1,073	23%	1,280	27%	4,747	123
31	South Dakota	1,366	57%	643	27%	373	16%	2,382	315
43	Tennessee	2,486	44%	1,237	22%	1,939	34%	5,662	102
48	Texas[4]	7,313	39%	550	3%	10,721	58%	18,584	92
27	Utah	1,713	63%	44	2%	945	35%	2,702	125
2	Vermont	1,063	96%	0	0%	42	4%	1,105	183
35	Virginia	3,646	51%	360	5%	3,148	44%	7,154	103
16	Washington	9,669	79%	409	3%	2,089	17%	12,167	210
10	West Virginia	3,213	87%	390	11%	99	3%	3,702	203
24	Wisconsin	9,638	70%	819	6%	3,342	24%	13,799	261
20	Wyoming	721	76%	67	7%	163	17%	951	189
	United States	263,359	61%	53,913	12%	116,527	27%	433,799	159

[1] States' ranking in terms of percentage in 1-6 person settings

[2] Settings for 6 or fewer persons included 98,300 supported living/personal assistance participants.

[3] Per 100,000 citizens of the general population.

[4] Texas officials reported numbers of persons served and associated expenditures in the categories of 8 or fewer persons and 9-14 persons, slightly different than the project's categories of 6 or fewer persons and 7-15 persons.

15%. In 1996, 51% of the total number of individuals receiving residential services lived in settings for 1 to 6 persons, and 35% resided in settings for 16 or more persons. In 2000, the proportion of persons living in settings for 1 to 6 increased to 61%, while institutional placements dropped to 27% (*Figure 2.1*). However, there was great state-by-state variation in the use of residential settings of different sizes. For example, in 2000, 61% of out-of-home residential placements in the United States were in settings for six or fewer persons, yet the range across the states was from 26% in Arkansas to 97% in Alaska. *Table 2.1* illustrates this variability and presents state-by-state data on the proportion of persons living in settings for 16 or more persons (including nursing facilities), for 7 to15 persons, and for 6 or fewer persons. In 2000, 24 states provided 70% or more of their residential services in settings for six or fewer persons. However, in 10 states, Arkansas, Georgia, Illinois, Kentucky, Louisiana, Mississippi, New Jersey, Oklahoma, Texas, and Virginia, 40% or more of all persons living in out-of-home residential placements lived in public and private institutional facilities for 16 or more persons.

433,799 (*Figure 2.1*). The number of people living in settings for six or fewer people grew by 33%. In contrast, residents in the nation's public and private institutional facilities for 16 or more persons declined by

Table 2.1 also presents out-of-home residential placement rates per 100,000 of the state general population. In 2000, placements per 100,000 ranged from 60 in Nevada to 356 in Iowa. The average for the United States was 159. As evident in *Table 2.1*, a state may serve a large proportion of all persons in family-scale settings for six or fewer persons, but still have a relatively small total out-of-home residential service system. In Nevada and Arizona, for example, 82% and 92%, respectively, of total placements were in settings for six or fewer persons, well above the 61% national average. However, these two states had the nation's lowest placement rates per 100,000.

COMMUNITY RESIDENTIAL SERVICES

Community residential services for 15 or fewer persons include public and private ICFs/MR, group homes, foster care, apartments, and supported living. Supported living was defined for purposes of this study to include housing in which individuals choose where and with whom they live, ownership is by someone other than the support provider, and the individual has a personalized support plan that changes as her or his needs and abilities change. Nationwide, placements in settings for 7 to 15 people declined slightly (less than 1%) between 1996 and 2000. The number of individuals served in ICFs/MR for 7 to 15 persons declined 7% during the same period.

Between 1996 and 2000, placements in community residences for 1 to 15 persons per capita (per 100,000 of state general population) advanced 21% while institutional placements per capita declined 17%. Nationwide, there were 116 community placements per 100,000 in 2000 (*Table 2.2*). Placements per capita ranged from 39 in Texas to 267 in Minnesota. Change during 1996-2000 in the number of community residential placements per capita ranged from a decline of 27% in Wyoming to expansion of 150% in North Carolina. North Carolina's percentage gain was partially attributable to improved tracking of personal assistance recipients during fiscal year 2000.

Supported living and personal assistance placements in the United States expanded from a 23% share of all community residential placements nationwide in 1996 to 31% in 2000.

Table 2.2
COMMUNITY RESIDENCES FOR 1 TO 15 Persons: GROWTH IN PER CAPITA PLACEMENTS, FY 2000

State	FY 2000 Community Placements per 100K[1]	FY 2000 Ranking: Community Placements per 100K[1]	% Change in Community Placements: 1996-2000
Alabama	65	45	71%
Alaska	140	23	78%
Arizona	70	43	32%
Arkansas	82	38	-9%
California	122	28	1%
Colorado	164	16	52%
Connecticut	157	19	10%
Delaware	77	42	14%
District of Columbia	224	6	9%
Florida	61	46	17%
Georgia	49	49	98%
Hawaii	97	33	-21%
Idaho	211	7	13%
Illinois	94	35	23%
Indiana	129	25	25%
Iowa	242	4	72%
Kansas	157	20	63%
Kentucky	49	50	47%
Louisiana	97	34	-19%
Maine	240	5	32%
Maryland	106	31	31%
Massachusetts	165	15	31%
Michigan	120	29	35%
Minnesota	267	1	27%
Mississippi	89	37	71%
Missouri	105	32	29%
Montana	162	17	6%
Nebraska	177	12	25%
Nevada	50	48	46%
New Hampshire	144	22	9%
New Jersey	79	40	22%
New Mexico	122	27	41%
New York	192	10	14%
North Carolina	152	21	150%
North Dakota	263	3	1%
Ohio	108	30	24%
Oklahoma	78	41	20%
Oregon	124	26	15%
Pennsylvania	129	24	32%
Rhode Island	180	11	33%
South Carolina	90	36	2%
South Dakota	266	2	17%
Tennessee	67	44	28%
Texas[2]	39	51	8%
Utah	81	39	18%
Vermont	176	13	25%
Virginia	58	47	7%
Washington	174	14	18%
West Virginia	198	9	7%
Wisconsin	198	8	22%
Wyoming	157	18	-27%
United States	**116**		**21%**

[1]Community placements for 15 or fewer persons per 100,000 citizens of the general population.

[2]Texas officials reported numbers of persons served in settings for 14 or fewer persons.

Cost by Setting

Table 2.3 presents annual costs of care in three types of community residential programs: private ICFs/MR for 15 or fewer persons, public ICFs/MR for 15 or fewer persons, and supported living/personal assistance. The annual nationwide cost per resident for the reporting states ranged from $16,868 in supported living to $86,074 in publicly operated ICFs/MR. The annual cost per resident in the 34 states funding private ICFs/MR ranged from below $40,000 in Alabama, Colorado, and Illinois to more than $100,000 in Connecticut, Florida, Maine, Tennessee, and Vermont.

Between 1992 and 2000, Alaska, Delaware, Massachusetts, Michigan, Montana, Nebraska, New Hampshire, Oregon, Rhode Island, and Wisconsin terminated their utilization of all private ICFs/MR, and converted them to Home and Community Based Services (HCBS) Waiver programs. Arizona, Georgia, Kentucky, Maryland, Mississippi, New Jersey, and Wyoming have never funded private ICFs/MR for 15 or fewer persons.

Publicly operated ICFs/MR for fewer than 15 persons were provided by 12 states (*Table 2.3*). The annual public ICF/MR cost per person ranged from $37,381 in Louisiana to over $100,000 in Connecticut, Kentucky, Nevada, New York, and Rhode Island. The national average cost was $86,074. New York's high annual cost of care in 2000 was largely due to the transfer of the majority of the state's public ICF/MR residents to the HCBS Waiver. During 1995-2000, New York's public ICF/MR population dropped from 3,277 to 76 persons. Public ICF/MR costs were also high in Connecticut and Kentucky due to small numbers of persons served: 16 and 24 persons, respectively.

The final column in *Table 2.3* presents the combined annual costs for supported living and personal assistance services. All states but Hawaii provided supported living or personal assistance services in 2000. Spending per participant in supported living and personal assistance ranged from below $2,000 in Mississippi and West Virginia to over $60,000 in Maine, Michigan, and Oklahoma. The majority of Oklahoma's 1,379 supported living and personal assistance participants were class mem-

Table 2.3
ANNUAL COST OF CARE
PER AVERAGE DAILY RESIDENT, FY 2000

State	Private ICFs/MR for 15 or fewer persons	Public ICFs/MR for 15 or fewer persons	Supported Living/Personal Assistance
Alabama	$37,646		n/a
Alaska			$40,259
Arizona		$69,142	$18,229
Arkansas	$46,582		$24,702
California	$42,585		$9,438
Colorado	$29,847		$11,565
Connecticut	$130,158	$193,619	$26,477
Delaware			$22,304
District of Columbia	$92,355		n/a
Florida	$101,916		$5,742
Georgia			$26,821
Hawaii	$64,660		
Idaho	$72,524		n/a
Illinois	$38,101		$8,205
Indiana	$54,092		$12,216
Iowa	$70,020		$18,755
Kansas	$69,193		n/a
Kentucky		$199,329	$6,867
Louisiana	$46,744	$37,381	$31,959
Maine	$109,156	$55,890	$72,557
Maryland			$20,737
Massachusetts			$10,118
Michigan			$62,493
Minnesota	$57,808	$92,973	$16,683
Mississippi		$70,710	$1,386
Missouri	$43,857		$34,393
Montana			$9,590
Nebraska			$7,968
Nevada	$63,135	$109,500	$17,884
New Hampshire			$2,880
New Jersey			$19,000
New Mexico	$60,957		$42,669
New York	$76,021	$438,065	$2,681
North Carolina	$74,407		$10,784
North Dakota	$62,928		$19,666
Ohio	$59,771		$33,304
Oklahoma	$57,121		$73,309
Oregon			$9,877
Pennsylvania	$80,285		$4,090
Rhode Island		$146,041	$53,591
South Carolina	$65,060	$70,818	$6,952
South Dakota*	$55,768		$5,543
Tennessee	$104,215		$47,819
Texas	$51,498	$53,532	$6,692
Utah	$59,641		$9,682
Vermont	$131,082		n/a
Virginia	$72,454		$7,741
Washington	$55,738		$21,602
West Virginia	$88,846		$1,354
Wisconsin			$9,364
Wyoming			$10,714
United States	**$57,877**	**$86,074**	**$16,868**

All cost data were determined by dividing total annual spending by average daily residents; day program costs are not included. A blank space indicates the state did not provide the service and "n/a" indicates that data were not available.

bers in the federal lawsuit *Homeward Bound v. Hissom Memorial Center* (1990).

Community Staff Wage Initiatives

Direct support staff in community residential settings work for lower compensation and fewer benefits compared to institutional personnel (Association of Developmental Disabilities Providers, 1999; Larson, Lakin, & Bruininks, 1998; Mitchell & Braddock, 1993; Rubin, Park, & Braddock, 1998). Community residential service providers must also cope with difficulties in direct service staff recruitment, training, and retention (Larson, Hewitt, & Lakin, 1994; Larson et al., 1998). Several states are launching initiatives to address low direct service staff wages. In 1999, Arizona appropriated $5 million for a 43 cents per hour increase in community services staff wages. Maine's legislature unanimously approved a 1999 appropriation of $2.6 million for an increase in entry wages of direct service workers to $7.99 per hour. The Michigan legislature increased direct service personnel wages by 50 cents per hour in 1999 and by 75 cents per hour in 2000. Illinois appropriated $23 million for direct service staff wage increases in 1999 (Arc of Illinois, 1999; "1998 Summary of State Legislation," 1999). In 2001, funds were appropriated for $1 per hour increases for direct service staff working in privately operated facilities.

In January 2000, New Hampshire authorized wage increases of $1.13 per hour for direct service workers, which brought the average hourly wage in the state to $8.67. Missouri appropriated funds to provide direct service staff working in privately operated facilities with a $1 per hour wage increase in 2001.

In Pennsylvania, the Legislative Budget and Finance Committee on Wages, Turnover, and Quality reported that direct service staff hourly wages of $8.13 were below the federal poverty guideline for a family of four ("Correlation Between Wages," 1999). Direct service wages in Illinois ($6.53 in 1997), in Minnesota ($7.07 in 2000), and in Massachusetts in 1996 ($8.06) were also below the poverty level (Association of Developmental Disabilities Providers, 1999; Larson et al., 1998; Rubin et al., 1998).

In 2001, Maryland passed legislation that required an increase in reimbursement rates for community service providers. This increase, to be phased in over five years, will address the inequities in the pay and benefits of direct service workers in community settings. Providers are expected to use the funds to bring their direct service workers into parity with the wages and benefits of institutional workers (National Association of State DD Directors, 2001b).

PUBLIC AND PRIVATE INSTITUTIONS

The consolidated data in *Figure 2.2* depict the nation's progress in the last decade in downsizing all public and private residential settings serving 16 or more people. During 1990-2000, the number of residents of public and private institutions for 16 or more

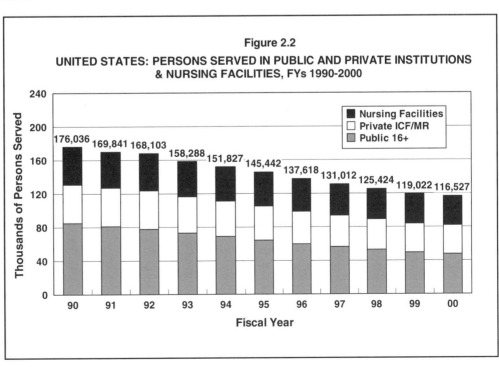

Figure 2.2

UNITED STATES: PERSONS SERVED IN PUBLIC AND PRIVATE INSTITUTIONS & NURSING FACILITIES, FYs 1990-2000

Table 2.4
PUBLIC INSTITUTION CENSUS, FYs 1977, 1996, & 2000

State	1977	1996	2000	% Change 1977-2000	% Change 1996-2000	Placements per 100K[1]: 2000
Alabama	1,643	826	614	-63%	-26%	14
Alaska	100	28	0	-100%	-100%	0
Arizona	959	243	166	-83%	-32%	3
Arkansas	1,380	1,263	1,241	-10%	-2%	48
California	9,764	4,823	3,795	-61%	-21%	12
Colorado	1,580	194	147	-91%	-24%	4
Connecticut	3,058	1,218	970	-68%	-20%	30
Delaware	534	292	253	-53%	-13%	33
District of Columbia	1,100	0	0	-100%		0
Florida	4,414	1,605	1,534	-65%	-4%	10
Georgia	2,909	1,961	1,489	-49%	-24%	19
Hawaii	570	60	0	-100%	-100%	0
Idaho	454	131	110	-76%	-16%	8
Illinois	6,580	3,645	3,221	-51%	-12%	27
Indiana	2,477	1,261	782	-68%	-38%	13
Iowa	1,397	687	679	-51%	-1%	24
Kansas	1,456	696	386	-73%	-45%	15
Kentucky	839	746	735	-12%	-1%	18
Louisiana	3,245	2,030	1,717	-47%	-15%	39
Maine	522	76	11	-98%	-86%	1
Maryland	2,725	720	548	-80%	-24%	10
Massachusetts	5,229	1,884	1,293	-75%	-31%	21
Michigan	6,047	362	250	-96%	-31%	3
Minnesota	3,085	442	59	-98%	-87%	1
Mississippi	1,720	1,442	1,382	-20%	-4%	49
Missouri	2,305	1,494	1,509	-35%	1%	27
Montana	299	157	130	-57%	-17%	14
Nebraska	1,008	404	399	-60%	-1%	24
Nevada	118	150	141	19%	-6%	8
New Hampshire	684	0	0	-100%		0
New Jersey	7,603	4,338	3,556	-53%	-18%	44
New Mexico	584	177	0	-100%	-100%	0
New York	18,799	3,589	2,009	-89%	-44%	11
North Carolina	3,848	2,229	1,933	-50%	-13%	25
North Dakota	1,139	148	152	-87%	3%	23
Ohio	6,838	2,087	1,990	-71%	-5%	18
Oklahoma	2,158	548	407	-81%	-26%	12
Oregon	1,873	435	105	-94%	-76%	3
Pennsylvania	9,189	3,272	1,969	-79%	-40%	16
Rhode Island	736	0	0	-100%		0
South Carolina	3,440	1,574	1,115	-68%	-29%	29
South Dakota	843	323	196	-77%	-39%	26
Tennessee	2,071	1,513	903	-56%	-40%	16
Texas	10,843	5,517	5,338	-51%	-3%	27
Utah	841	303	236	-72%	-22%	11
Vermont	443	0	0	-100%		0
Virginia	3,836	2,148	1,744	-55%	-19%	25
Washington	2,504	1,295	1,138	-55%	-12%	20
West Virginia	1,165	80	0	-100%	-100%	0
Wisconsin	2,405	1,214	899	-63%	-26%	17
Wyoming	533	145	123	-77%	-15%	24
United States	149,892	59,775	47,374	-68%	-21%	17

[1] Per 100,000 citizens of the general population.

persons, including nursing facilities, declined 34%, from 176,036 to 116,527. Public institutions alone declined 44%, from 84,818 to 47,374. The number of private institutional residents in facilities for 16 or more persons declined 26%, and the number of nursing facility residents declined 23%.

Public Institutions

State-operated institutions include publicly operated institutions, developmental centers, training centers, state schools, and designated MR/DD units in state psychiatric hospitals. Since 1977, total spending for the nation's public institutions has declined 13% in inflation-adjusted terms. Average daily costs per person have advanced dramatically, however, from $45 in 1977 to $321 in 2000. Improved staffing levels accounted for some of the cost increases. Total inflation-adjusted spending for state-operated institutions declined 11% between 1996 and 2000.

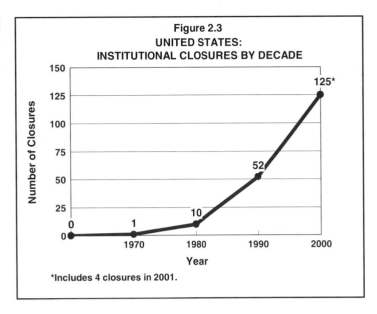

Figure 2.3
UNITED STATES:
INSTITUTIONAL CLOSURES BY DECADE

*Includes 4 closures in 2001.

Census Trends

The number of state-operated institutional residents continued to decline during 1996-2000. During this period, the population residing in these facilities dropped by 21%, from 59,775 in 1996 to 47,374 in 2000 (*Table 2.4*). The census in state-operated institutions peaked at 194,650 in 1967 and diminished by an average of 4% per year through 1992. The rate of annual decline accelerated to 6% during 1993-99 and then declined by 4% from 1999-2000 . All states except Missouri and North Dakota reduced their public institutional populations during 1996-2000. Excluding states that closed all public institutions, the states with the greatest percentage reduction in their public institutional censuses during the 1996-2000 period were Kansas, Maine, Minnesota, New York, Oregon, and Tennessee. These six states reduced their public institutional censuses by 40-86%.

Public institutional placements per 100,000 of state general population ranged from 0 in the states that have closed all public institutional facilities to more than 40 per 100,000 in Arkansas, Mississippi, and New Jersey. *Table 2.4* presents state-by-state insti-

tutional census data (average daily residents for fiscal years 1977, 1996, and 2000); the percentage change in the institutional census from 1977-2000 and from 1996-2000; and 2000 institutional placement rates per 100,000 of the state general population.

Public Institutional Closures

Institutional closures were defined as completed or in-progress terminations of state-operated institutions for people with mental retardation/developmental disabilities (MR/DD) or closures of psychiatric facilities that included designated MR/DD units. An in-progress closure implied that the MR/DD state agency was implementing a legislatively sanctioned phase-out of the facility. Institutional closures typically could be verified by examining published state budget documentation. The trend toward closing institutions gained momentum during the recession of the early 1980s and has continued. In a national survey, Braddock and Heller (1985) identified 24 closures in 12 states between 1970-1984. The 1988 national study of public spending (Braddock et al., 1990) identified a total of 44 closures in 20 states. The present study has identified 125 closures, or planned closures by 2000, in 37 states (*Table 2.5*). The number of institutional closures by decade in the United States is illustrated in *Figure 2.3*.

In 1991, New Hampshire closed the Laconia State School and became the nation's first state to completely terminate its public institutional system. The District of Columbia, Vermont, Rhode Island, Alaska, New Mexico, West Virginia, Hawaii, and Minnesota followed suit between 1991-2001. The six states of Alabama, Alaska, Hawaii, Maine, South Dakota, and Tennessee, which had not previously closed a state facility, did so for the first time between 1996-2000. The 14 states that have not closed at least one public institution are: Arkansas, Delaware, Idaho, Iowa, Louisiana, Mississippi, Montana, Nebraska, Nevada, North Carolina, Utah, Virginia, Wisconsin, and Wyoming. Arkansas, Louisiana, Mississippi, North Carolina, and Virginia continue to support an extensive network of public institutions.

New York, which in 1992 announced the closure of all its public institutions by 2001, has since rescinded its closure plans for several facilities. Alabama had announced plans to close the Wallace Center in September 1999, but Governor-elect Don Siegelman subsequently rescinded this plan. Public facility closures in each state are summarized in *Table 2.5*, which is current as of September 2001.

As the institutional census continues to fall and average daily costs increase, there will be continued pressure on states to close additional institutions. The United States public institutional census decline of 21% between 1996-2000 represented a reduction of 3,100 persons per year. Although the national public institution census has declined every year since 1967, a number of states reduced their public institutional population by less than 15% between 1996-2000. These states were Arkansas, Delaware, Florida, Illinois, Iowa, Kentucky, Mississippi, Missouri, Nebraska, Nevada, North Carolina, North Dakota, Ohio, Texas, and Washington.

Average Costs of Care

Average daily costs of care in public institutions increased 165% in inflation-adjusted terms from 1977-2000. The rate of growth in institutional average daily costs substantially exceeded the rate of inflation, as illustrated in *Figure 2.4*, which depicts the inflation-adjusted advance in daily public institutional costs across the study's 24-year span.

The states varied greatly in terms of average daily costs of public institutions in 2000. Rates ranged from under $230 per day in Arkansas, Indiana, Nebraska, and Texas, to over $500 per day in Connecticut, Idaho, Minnesota, New York, Oregon, and Tennessee (*Table 2.6*).

Inflation-adjusted growth rates of 30% or more during 1996-2000 occurred in Arizona, California, Connecticut, Minnesota, Mississippi, New York, Oregon, Pennsylvania, and Tennessee. The daily cost advance in Minnesota is attributable to the closure of the remaining public institution, Fergus Falls, in 2000. Among the states that still operate public institutions, inflation-adjusted costs of care were reduced during 1996-2000 in Indiana,

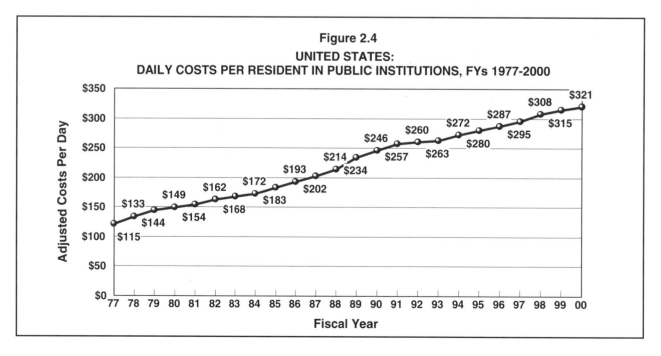

Figure 2.4
UNITED STATES:
DAILY COSTS PER RESIDENT IN PUBLIC INSTITUTIONS, FYs 1977-2000

Table 2.5
COMPLETED AND IN-PROGRESS CLOSURES OF PUBLIC INSTITUTIONS

State	Institution	Year Built/ Became MR	Original Use	# Residents, Closure Announcement	Year of Closure	Alternate Use
Alabama	Glenn Ireland	1986	MR Facility	20	1996	To be sold
Alaska	Harborview	1964	MR Facility	45	1997	Undetermined
Arizona	Phoenix	1974	MR Facility	46	1988	Pending Sale: Commercial
	Tucson	1972	MR Facility	13	1997	Outreach Offices
California	Camarillo	1935	MR Facility	497	1998	University
	DeWitt	1942/1947	Army Hospital	819	1972	Placer County Recreation
	Modesto Unit	1943/1948	Army Hospital	1,394	1969	Modesto Co. Comm. College
	Napa	1875/1967	Asylum for MR/MI	30	1988	MI Use Only
	Stockton	1852	Asylum for MI	414	1996	University
Colorado	Pueblo	1935	MI/MR Facility	163	1989	Pueblo Regional Center
Connecticut	John Dempsey Center	1964			1998	Undetermined
	Mansfield	1906/1917	Epileptic Colony	146	1993	Corrections/U. of Connecticut
	New Haven	1964	MR Facility	56	1994	Job Corps
	Seaside	1961			1996	Administrative Offices
	Waterbury	1963/1972	Convent	40	1989	Administrative Offices
D.C.	Forest Haven	1925	MR Facility	1,000	1991	Private Rehab/PH Infirmary
Florida	Orlando	1929/1959	TB Hospital	1,000	1984	Unoccupied: asbestos
	Tallahassee	1928/1967	TB Hospital	350	1983	Unoccupied: asbestos
Georgia	Brook Run	1969	MR Facility	364	1997	Undetermined
	Rivers' Crossing	1969	MR Facility	37	1994	Undetermined
Hawaii	Kula Hospital (privatized)	1984			1999	
	Waimano	1921	MR Facility	96	1999	Undetermined
Illinois	Adler	1967	MI/MR Facility	16	1982	Water Survey Offices
	Bowen	1965	MR Facility	105	1982	Corrections
	Dixon	1918	MR Facility	820	1987	Corrections/New MR Facility
	Galesburg	1950/1969	Army Hospital	350	1985	Head Start/Community Programs
	Meyer	1966/1970	MI Facility	53	1993	Women's Prison
Indiana	Central State	1848	MI/MR Facility	83	1994	Undetermined
	New Castle	1907	Epileptic Village	200	1998	Corrections
	Northern Indiana	1943	MR Facility	53	1998	Undetermined
Kansas	Norton	1926/1963	TB Hospital	60	1988	Corrections
	Winfield	1888	MR Facility	250	1998	Undetermined
Kentucky	Frankfort	1860	MR Facility	650	1972	Demolition
	Outwood	1922/1962	TB Hospital	80	1983	Demolition/New Campus
Maine	Levinson	1971			1999	
	Pineland	1908	MR Facility	265	1996	Undetermined
Maryland	Victor Cullen	1908/1974	TB Hospital	79	1991	Private Juvenile Facility
	Great Oaks	1970	MR Regional Center	273	1997	Private Senior Retire. Community
	Henryton	1928/1962	TB Hospital	312	1985	Undetermined
	Highland Health	1870/1972	General Hospital	88	1989	Sold to Johns Hopkins University
Massachusetts	Belchertown	1922	MR Facility	297	1992	Vacant
	John T. Berry	1900/1963	TB Sanitarium	101	1995	Undetermined
	Paul A. Dever	1940/1946	P.O.W. Camp	294	2001	Undetermined
Michigan	Alpine	1937/1959	TB Hospital	200	1981	Notsego County Offices
	Caro	1914			1998	
	Coldwater	1874/1939	Orphanage	113	1987	Corrections
	Fort Custer	1942/1956	Army Hospital	1,000	1972	Back to U.S. Dept. of Defense
	Hillcrest	1905/1961	TB Hospital	350	1982	Demolition
	Macomb-Oakland	1967/1970	CDA	100	1989	Reverted to Community Dev.
	Muskegon	1969	MR Facility	157	1992	Vacant
	Newberry	1896/1941	MI Facility	39	1992	Vacant
	Northville	1952/1972	MI/MR Facility	180	1983	Revert to MI Use
	Oakdale	1895	MR Facility	100	1991	Vacant/County Negotiating
	Plymouth	1960	MR Facility	837	1984	County/State Offices
	Southgate	1977		55	2001	
Minnesota	Brainerd	1958			1999	
	Faribault	1879	MR Facility	501	1998	Portion Used by Corrections
	Fergus Falls	1969			2000	
	Moose Lake	1938/1970	Psychiatric Hosp	34	1993	Corrections
	Owatonna	1895/1947	Orphanage	250	1970	Abuse
	Rochester	1879/1972	MI Facility	150	1982	Federal Corrections
	St. Peter	1968			1996	
	Willmar	1973			1996	

Table 2.5 continued

State	Institution	Year Built/ Became MR	Original Use	# Residents, Closure Announcement	Year of Closure	Alternate Use
Missouri	Albany	1967	MR Facility	4	1991	Administrative Offices
	Hannibal	1967	MR Facility	3	1989	Administrative Offices
	Joplin	1967	MR Facility	5	1992	Administrative Offices
	Kansas City	1970	MR Facility	12	1993	Administrative Offices
	Kirksville	1968	MR Facility	4	1988	Administrative Offices
	Poplar Bluff	1968	MR Facility	50	1993	Administrative Offices
	Rolla	1968	MR Facility	2	1984	Administrative Offices
	Sikeston	1969	MR Facility	40	1993	Administrative Offices
	Springfield	1967	MR Facility	12	1990	Administrative Offices
New Hampshire	Laconia	1903	MR Facility	4	1991	Corrections
New Jersey	Edison	1975/1981	Corrections	70	1988	Sold at Public Auction
	Johnstone	1955	MR Facility	239	1992	Corrections
	North Princeton	1898/1975	Epileptic Colony	512	1998	Undetermined
New Mexico	Fort Stanton	1964	Army Apache Outpos	145	1995	Skilled Nursing/Respite
	Los Lunas	1929	MR Facility	252	1997	Undetermined - State Use
	Villa Solano	1964/1967	Missile Base	82	1982	Housing
New York	J.N. Adam	1912/1967	TB Hospital	180	1993	Undetermined
	Bronx	1977	MR Facility	217	1992	Plans Not Final
	Craig	1896/1935	Epilepsy Hospital	120	1988	Corrections
	Gouverneur	1962	MR Facility	N/A	1978	Leased site
	Letchworth	1911	MR Facility	704	1996	Undetermined
	Long Island	1965	MR Facility	682	1993	Undetermined
	Manhattan	1919/1972	Warehouse	197	1991	OMRDD Office
	Newark	1878	Custodial Asylum	325	1991	Community College
	Rome	1825/1894	County Poorhouse	638	1989	Corrections
	Sampson	1860/1961	Naval Base	695	1971	Office of Mental Health
	Staten Island	1942/1952	Army Hospital	692	1987	OMRDD & Community College
	Syracuse	1851/1972	MR Facility	409	1997	Undetermined
	Valatie	1971	MR Facility	N/A	1974	Private Holdings and ICFs/MR
	Westchester	1932/1979	MI Facility	195	1988	Office of MH
	Wilton	1960	MR Facility	370	1995	Sold to Private Industry
North Dakota	San Haven	1922/1973	TB Hospital	86	1987	Vacant
Ohio	Broadview	1930/1967	TB Hospital	178	1992	City Administration Building/Retirement
	Cleveland	1855/1963	MI Facility	149	1988	Vacant/Negot. with City of Cleveland
	Orient	1898	MR Facility	800	1984	Corrections
Oklahoma	Hissom	1967	MR Facility	451	1994	Corrections/Educational
Oregon	Columbia Park	1929/1963	TB Hospital	304	1977	College
	Eastern Oregon	1929/1963	TB Hospital	240	1984	Corrections/Opened New MR Facility
	Fairview	1907	MR Facility	327	2000	Undetermined
Pennsylvania	Cresson	1912/1964	TB Hospital	155	1982	Corrections
	Embreeville	1880/1972	County Poorhouse	152	1998	Undetermined
	Hollidaysburg	1974	MR Facility	60	1976	Revert to MI Use
	Laurelton	1920	MR Facility	192	1998	Undetermined
	Marcy Center	1915/1974	TB Hospital	152	1982	Vacant
	Pennhurst Center	1908	MR Facility	179	1988	Veterans' Medical Center
	Philadelphia	1983	MI/MR Facility	60	1989	Vacant
	Western	1962		133	1999	
	Woodhaven	1974	MR Facility	N/A	1985	Became Private Institution
Rhode Island	Dix Building	1945/1982	WPA	80	1989	Corrections
	Ladd Center	1907	MR Facility	292	1994	Undetermined
South Carolina	Clyde Street	1973	mothers	20	1995	Administrative Offices
	Live Oak	1987	Nursing home	50	1999	To Be Sold
South Dakota	Custer	1964	TB Hospital	76	1996	Boot Camp for Delinquent Boys
Tennessee	Winston	1979			1998	
Texas	Forth Worth	1976	MR Facility	339	1995	Undetermined
	Travis	1934	MR Facility	585	1997	Undetermined
Vermont	Brandon	1915	MR Facility	26	1993	For Sale, Local Realty
Washington	Interlake School	1946/1967	Geriatric MI	123	1995	Other State Agency
West Virginia	Colin Anderson	1920s	MR Facility	85	1998	Possible Juvenile Corrections
	Greenbrier	1801/1974	Women's College	56	1994	Community College
	Spencer	1893	MI/MR Facility	150	1989	Vacant/Possible Corrections
	Weston	1864/1985	MI/MR Facility	99	1988	Revert to MI Use

Table 2.6
STATE INSTITUTION DAILY COSTS, 1996 & 2000

State	1996	2000	% Real Change 1996-2000
Alabama	$229.59	$303.88	20%
Alaska	$743.58	$0.00	
Arizona	$167.32	$249.84	35%
Arkansas	$165.26	$205.54	13%
California	$296.98	$428.67	31%
Colorado	$287.36	$358.92	13%
Connecticut	$384.48	$552.23	30%
Delaware	$286.52	$369.94	17%
District of Columbia	$0.00	$0.00	
Florida	$210.65	$264.58	14%
Georgia	$230.27	$263.91	4%
Hawaii	$394.10	$0.00	
Idaho	$404.73	$502.03	12%
Illinois	$238.49	$279.94	6%
Indiana	$239.85	$207.80	-22%
Iowa	$267.31	$308.13	4%
Kansas	$272.07	$308.63	3%
Kentucky	$190.20	$243.92	16%
Louisiana	$187.02	$262.32	27%
Maine	$443.94	$258.45	-47%
Maryland	$285.57	$315.60	0%
Massachusetts	$448.55	$438.95	-11%
Michigan	$401.57	$494.49	11%
Minnesota	$364.43	$546.69	36%
Mississippi	$157.91	$234.77	35%
Missouri	$265.14	$289.33	-1%
Montana	$267.29	$340.63	15%
Nebraska	$171.96	$220.87	16%
Nevada	$276.99	$342.14	12%
New Hampshire	$0.00	$0.00	
New Jersey	$240.98	$286.26	7%
New Mexico	$363.21	$0.00	
New York	$360.20	$563.46	42%
North Carolina	$253.28	$336.14	20%
North Dakota	$369.49	$313.03	-23%
Ohio	$276.52	$309.36	1%
Oklahoma	$286.22	$386.25	22%
Oregon	$491.62	$822.66	51%
Pennsylvania	$260.83	$389.72	35%
Rhode Island	$0.00	$0.00	
South Carolina	$213.37	$253.95	8%
South Dakota	$221.57	$230.11	-6%
Tennessee	$262.47	$519.49	79%
Texas	$181.05	$204.82	2%
Utah	$252.38	$356.87	28%
Vermont	$0.00	$0.00	
Virginia	$199.88	$272.75	23%
Washington	$295.78	$336.91	3%
West Virginia	$448.48	$0.00	
Wisconsin	$274.57	$359.88	19%
Wyoming	$316.04	$409.60	17%
United States	**$259.81**	**$320.66**	**12%**

Maine, Maryland, Massachusetts, Missouri, North Dakota and South Dakota. Among these states, daily costs in Indiana, Maine, and South Dakota were substantially below the national average of $321 in 2000.

Privately Operated Institutions and Nursing Facilities

Private institutional facilities provided 24-hour care for 16 or more persons in the same location, and included state-funded facilities, whether or not the facilities were certified as ICFs/MR. The total population of these facilities (excluding nursing facilities) declined 12% between 1996-2000, from 38,883 to 34,410 persons. There was a 9% decline in the number of persons residing in private ICFs/MR for 16 or more persons (decrease of 2,670 persons) and an 18% decline (decrease of 1,803 persons) in private settings not certified as ICFs/MR. Public financial support for all private institutions declined by 2% in inflation-adjusted terms during 1996-2000. In 2000, no public funds were used to support private institutions in the 10 states of Alabama, Alaska, Colorado, Massachusetts, Michigan, Montana, Nevada, South Dakota, Vermont, and Wyoming.

Nursing Facility Utilization

An additional objective of the study included the collection of data on the number of persons with MR/DD residing in nursing facilities. In previous studies, data were based on figures the states reported to the Health Care Financing Administration in accordance with their reporting requirements under Pub. L. 100-203 (OBRA-1987). Although the OBRA-87 statutory reporting requirements have since been modified, in the present study data were collected according to the original provisions of this federal legislation defining persons with "mental retardation and related conditions."

Between 1996-2000, the number of people with MR/DD reported to be residing in nursing facilities in the United States declined by 11%, from 38,960 to 34,743 residents (*Table 2.7*). There was marked state variation in the utilization of nursing facilities. Population declines were reported by 37 states. Leading states in the rate of facility census decline were Alaska (81%), West Virginia (76%), Nebraska and Idaho (75%),

Table 2.7
NURSING FACILITY RESIDENTS WITH
DEVELOPMENTAL DISABILITIES, FYs 1996 & 2000

State	1996	2000	% Change 1996-2000	Placements per 100K[1]: 2000
Alabama	791	930	18%	21
Alaska	31	6	-81%	1
Arizona	67	57	-15%	1
Arkansas	1,000	867	-13%	33
California	1,232	1,409	14%	4
Colorado	295	270	-8%	7
Connecticut	422	378	-10%	12
Delaware	75	34	-55%	4
District of Columbia	37	36	-3%	7
Florida	232	191	-18%	1
Georgia	1,897	1,700	-10%	22
Hawaii	45	97	116%	8
Idaho	110	28	-75%	2
Illinois	1,971	1,267	-36%	10
Indiana	2,057	1,933	-6%	32
Iowa	520	536	3%	19
Kansas	n/a	13		0
Kentucky	1,100	744	-32%	19
Louisiana	1,267	1,109	-12%	25
Maine	207	145	-30%	12
Maryland	462	121	-74%	2
Massachusetts	1,777	1,499	-16%	24
Michigan	869	838	-4%	9
Minnesota	1,074	491	-54%	10
Mississippi	1,046	900	-14%	32
Missouri	1,657	830	-50%	15
Montana	169	162	-4%	18
Nebraska	454	115	-75%	7
Nevada	104	40	-62%	2
New Hampshire	107	64	-40%	5
New Jersey	847	593	-30%	7
New Mexico	148	94	-36%	5
New York	3,055	3,497	14%	19
North Carolina	385	397	3%	5
North Dakota	191	184	-4%	28
Ohio	2,173	2,430	12%	22
Oklahoma	912	1,210	33%	36
Oregon	260	180	-31%	5
Pennsylvania	2,353	2,350	0%	19
Rhode Island	184	162	-12%	16
South Carolina	104	121	16%	3
South Dakota	169	177	5%	23
Tennessee	1,351	892	-34%	16
Texas	2,864	2,919	2%	15
Utah	218	203	-7%	9
Vermont	68	42	-38%	7
Virginia	1,086	1,272	17%	18
Washington	646	659	2%	11
West Virginia	164	40	-76%	2
Wisconsin	664	471	-29%	9
Wyoming	43	40	-7%	8
United States	**38,960**	**34,743**	**-11%**	**13**

[1]Per 100,000 citizens of the general population.

and Maryland (74%). During 2000, only six persons with developmental disabilities received support in nursing facilities in Alaska. With plans underway to provide these individuals with personal assistance services, Alaska could become the first state in the nation with no nursing facility placement of persons with MR/DD. Kansas supported 13 persons with MR/DD in nursing facilities.

Thirteen states increased the number of nursing facility residents with developmental disabilities by a total of 1,620 people between 1996-2000. The census of nursing facility residents with developmental disabilities increased by more than 100 people in six states: Alabama, California, New York, Ohio, Oklahoma, and Virginia. The lowest per capita utilization rates of nursing facilities, at less than 3 per 100,000 of state population, were reported by Alaska, Arizona, Florida, Idaho, Kansas, Maryland, Nevada, South Carolina, and West Virginia. The highest utilization rates, 32-36 per 100,000, were reported by Arkansas, Indiana, Mississippi, and Oklahoma. The national average utilization of nursing facilities for persons with developmental disabilities was 13 per 100,000 of state population.

GENERAL TRENDS IN SYSTEM FINANCING

Total public spending for MR/DD services in the United States expanded from $3.5 billion in 1977 to $29.3 billion in 2000, an inflation-adjusted increase of 215%. Inflation-adjusted spending for community services, including individual and family support, advanced an average 10% per year during 1977-2000. The increase in total spending was largely attributable to the expansion of funds allocated to community services activities. In contrast to the vigorous growth of community spending, inflation-adjusted spending for public and private institutions posted average annual growth rates of less than 1% during the 24-year period. Institutional spending grew 2% per year between 1977-91, and declined 3% per year during 1992-2000.

Spending for community services first surpassed institutional spending in 1989 (*Figure 2.5*). Total MR/DD spending increased 18% in inflation-adjusted terms during 1996-2000.

The nation's gross domestic product (GDP) rose an inflation-adjusted 18% from 1996-2000, more than 4% annually (Bureau of Economic Analysis, 2002). Most state economies also fared well during this period. Gross state product (GSP) is the state-level equivalent to the GDP. During the 1996-99 period, gross state product percentage change rates ranged from a 4% decline in Alaska to a 23% increase in Colorado (Bureau of Economic Analysis, 2001). Fiscal year 1999 was the latest year for which GSP data were available.

Total MR/DD spending declined in the District of Columbia and advanced at least 40% in three states (Idaho, Oregon, and Tennessee) during the 1996-99 period. *Table 2.8* identifies the change in each state's GSP and in total MR/DD spending during 1996-99.

In 28 states, total MR/DD spending outpaced advances in GSP from 1996 to 1999. There was tremendous growth in MR/DD spending, over 30% during the period, in Tennessee, Idaho, Oregon, Utah, Maine, Nebraska, Mississippi, and Alaska. The 32% growth in Alaska is especially noteworthy -- Alaska was the only state in which GSP declined from 1996 to 1999.

Conversely, 23 states with expanding GSPs did not make increased appropriations for MR/DD services. In the District of Columbia, Indiana, and Wyoming, MR/DD spending declined even though GSP advanced. Nationwide, the aggregate MR/DD spending advance of 14% exceeded the GSP advance of 13%.

States vary markedly in the level of total MR/DD spending, and also in the allocation of funding to community versus institutional services. Changes in community services spending during 1996-2000 ranged from a decline of 17% in the District of Columbia to a growth of 119% in Oregon. Twenty-eight states posted advances to their total public and private institutional spending between 1996-2000, ranging from 1% to 40%. Twenty-two states decreased spending during 1996-2000 for public and private institutional facilities for 16 or more people, and Vermont spent no funds on institutional care during the period. States that increased their institutional spending included: Arizona, Arkansas, California, Connecticut, Delaware, the District of Columbia, Florida, Idaho, Illinois, Iowa, Kentucky, Louisiana, Mississippi, Montana, Nebraska, Nevada, North Carolina, North Dakota, Ohio, Oklahoma, Pennsylvania, Rhode Island, Tennessee, Texas, Utah, Virginia, Wisconsin, and Wyoming. The District

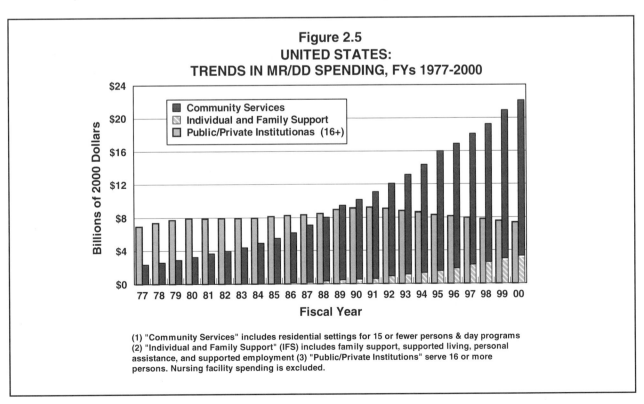

Figure 2.5
UNITED STATES:
TRENDS IN MR/DD SPENDING, FYs 1977-2000

(1) "Community Services" includes residential settings for 15 or fewer persons & day programs
(2) "Individual and Family Support" (IFS) includes family support, supported living, personal assistance, and supported employment (3) "Public/Private Institutions" serve 16 or more persons. Nursing facility spending is excluded.

Table 2.8
INFLATION-ADJUSTED CHANGE IN GSP & TOTAL MR/DD SPENDING, 1996-1999

State	MR/DD Spending	Gross State Product
MR/DD Spending Advanced More Rapidly than GSP		
Tennessee	44%	12%
Idaho	41%	14%
Oregon	40%	12%
Utah	37%	14%
Maine	35%	11%
Nebraska	34%	6%
Mississippi	32%	7%
Alaska	32%	-4%
North Carolina	29%	19%
Texas	27%	17%
Arizona	26%	20%
Colorado	26%	23%
Oklahoma	25%	8%
Kentucky	24%	12%
Kansas	21%	11%
Wisconsin	21%	11%
South Carolina	21%	12%
Arkansas	19%	7%
West Virginia	19%	3%
Alabama	16%	9%
Pennsylvania	15%	9%
Ohio	15%	11%
Missouri	15%	9%
North Dakota	12%	1%
Montana	8%	7%
Iowa	7%	4%
Louisiana	7%	4%
Hawaii	4%	2%
GSP Advanced More Rapidly than MR/DD Spending		
Washington	17%	21%
Nevada	17%	20%
California	14%	19%
Massachusetts	14%	17%
Rhode Island	13%	15%
Minnesota	12%	15%
Virginia	11%	14%
Delaware	11%	12%
New York	11%	12%
Connecticut	8%	15%
Michigan	8%	9%
Vermont	7%	10%
New Mexico	7%	9%
Florida	7%	14%
New Hampshire	5%	18%
Georgia	5%	18%
New Jersey	4%	9%
Illinois	3%	11%
Maryland	1%	13%
South Dakota	0%	5%
Wyoming	-2%	3%
Indiana	-4%	10%
District of Columbia	-14%	8%
United States	**14%**	**13%**

of Columbia did not operate any institutional facilities within its own jurisdiction, but did expend funds to serve individuals with developmental disabilities in out-of-state institutional placements. Rhode Island opened a private ICF/MR facility for 25 persons in 1997.

For more than two decades, the rate of expansion of resources for community services in the United States has been extremely strong. Across the 1977-2000 period, inflation-adjusted community spending increased 845%. Concurrently, public and private institutional spending rose 6% between 1977-2000, but there was a steady decline in public and private institutional spending after the peak in 1991 (*Figure 2.5*). From 1996-2000, community services spending, including individual and family support, has grown from $15.3 billion to $22.1 billion, an inflation-adjusted increase of 31%.

Spending for public and private facilities serving 16 or more persons constituted 25% of total MR/DD system-wide spending in 2000. Of the $7.2 billion total in institutional spending, 78%, or $5.6 billion, was allocated for the 47,374 residents of publicly operated state institutions. The remaining $1.6 billion was spent for the 34,410 persons residing in private institutional facilities.

Spending for community services in 2000 totalled $22.1 billion, or 75% of total MR/DD spending in the nation. Of this, $3.3 billion, or 15%, was spent on individual and family supports including family support, supported living/personal assistance, and supported employment.

Impact of Economic Recession in the States

During the second Clinton administration, the nation experienced ongoing economic growth, part of the strongest record of economic expansion in the nation's history. All states but Alaska had real growth in GSP between 1996 and 1999; in 31 states, there was 10%-23% growth (*Table 2.8*).

However, the record-setting pace of economic growth during the 1990s has faltered. State budgets began slowing in the fall of 2000 (Eckl & Perez, 2001), and the September 11 attacks exacerbated the economic problems the states were beginning to experience (National Association of State Budget Officers, 2001a). Unemployment rates have climbed, and state and local tax revenues have declined to their lowest rates since the 1950s (Zandi, 2001). Many states are bearing the extra costs of heightened security measures. As of October 31, 2001, state budget shortfalls were estimated to exceed $15 billion for fiscal year 2002, and most states had cut, or were planning to cut, their budgets (National Association of State Budget Officers, 2001b).

During 1996-99, a period of nearly unparalleled economic expansion, 6 states cut their adjusted MR/DD funding, and 12 others increased inflation-adjusted spending by less than 5%. The prospect of at least some period of continued slow down in the economic momentum in the United States means that advocates of expanded MR/DD services in the states must intensify their efforts to forestall likely cutbacks in the rates of growth in funding for these services.

COMMUNITY SERVICES TRENDS

Sources of Revenue

All states but the District of Columbia increased their inflation-adjusted community spending from 1996 to 2000. The enactment of the Home and Community Based Services (HCBS) Waiver in 1981 enabled states to expand federal Medicaid support for community services. The growing contribution of federal funds in the financing of community services across the nation is evident in *Figure 2.6*. In 1977, federal funds represented 23% of total allocations for community services. By 2000, that proportion had increased to 48% of total community services spending. Between 1990-2000, federal spending as a proportion of total community services spending advanced from 27%-48%.

State government general revenues, including state augmentation of federal Supplemental Security Income (SSI) payments, comprised 49% of total community services revenues in 2000. Federal funds, primarily Medicaid, constituted 48% of community services spending, while local funds made up the 4% balance (*Figure 2.7*). As a portion of total community spending, state funds declined from 56% in 1996 to 48% in 2000, due primarily to the rapid expansion of federal Medicaid HCBS Waiver funding accessed by the states. State funds comprised 63% of all community services spending in 1981, before HCBS Waiver funds were available to the states. However, in 2000, federal HCBS Waiver funds and federal income maintenance payments (SSI/ADC) for Waiver participants represented 69% of federal funding for community services, and roughly 33% of all funding allocated for community services in 2000 (*Figure 2.7*).

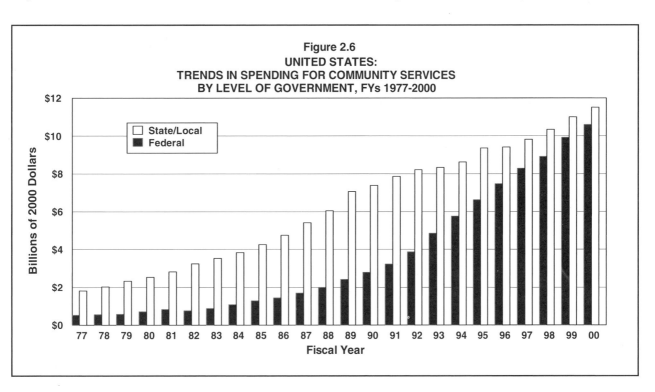

Figure 2.6
UNITED STATES:
TRENDS IN SPENDING FOR COMMUNITY SERVICES
BY LEVEL OF GOVERNMENT, FYs 1977-2000

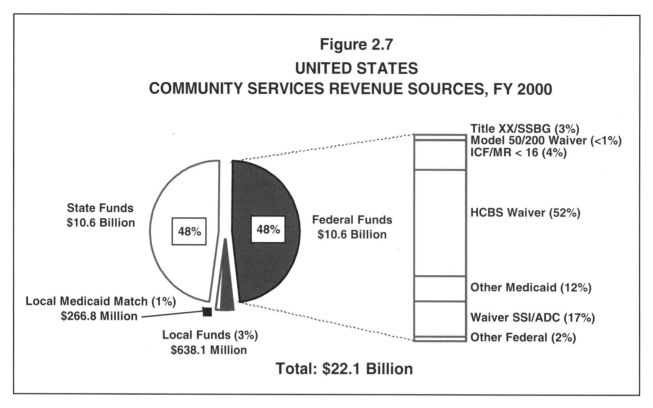

Figure 2.7
UNITED STATES
COMMUNITY SERVICES REVENUE SOURCES, FY 2000

State Funds
$10.6 Billion

48%   48%   Federal Funds
$10.6 Billion

Local Medicaid Match (1%)
$266.8 Million

Local Funds (3%)
$638.1 Million

Title XX/SSBG (3%)
Model 50/200 Waiver (<1%)
ICF/MR < 16 (4%)

HCBS Waiver (52%)

Other Medicaid (12%)

Waiver SSI/ADC (17%)
Other Federal (2%)

Total: $22.1 Billion

The remaining federal funds supporting community services were composed of funding for public and private ICFs/MR for 15 or fewer persons, constituting 14% of all community services federal funds; Medicaid funding for targeted case management, clinic/rehabilitative services, and personal care constituted 12%; the Social Services Block Grant constituted 3%; and the remaining 2% of federal funding consisted of various other federal project funds including vocational rehabilitation and education.

The Social Services Block Grant (SSBG), authorized under Title XX of the Social Security Act, has represented a declining portion of revenue for developmental disability services in the states since enactment of the HCBS Waiver and the implementation of disability services funding cuts in 1981 (Braddock, 1986, 1987). The Social Services Block Grant was authorized by Pub. L. 97-35, the Omnibus Budget Reconciliation Act of 1981 (OBRA 81). That legislation represented the Reagan Administration's efforts, with block grants, the Medicaid Home and Community Based Services (HCBS) Waiver, and other budgetary provisions, to devolve authority to the states and to cut federal health and welfare spending. Prior to passage of OBRA 81, Title XX of the Social Security Act was a social services formula grant program authorized in 1962 to help prevent welfare dependence.

Title XX was instrumental in a number of states' early efforts in the 1960s and 1970s to establish community residential and day programs, notably in Nebraska. In 1977, 10 states (Arkansas, Florida, Georgia, Mississippi, Montana, New Hampshire, New Mexico, South Dakota, Washington, and Wyoming) underwrote more than 50% of their community MR/DD spending with federal Title XX funding, and Title XX funding constituted 18% of community MR/DD spending nationwide that year.

With OBRA 81, nationwide Title XX/SSBG spending for persons with MR/DD declined 31% in inflation-adjusted terms between 1981 and 1982, and nearly every state experienced revenue declines as well. Moreover, there was a 10% adjusted decline nationwide between 1981 and 1982 in the combined federal funding that derived from both the SSBG and Medicaid (the Waiver and ICFs/MR for 15 or fewer persons) (Braddock & Hemp, 1996). The Social Services Block Grant funding for community MR/DD services in the United States declined by 3%-4% per year from 1982 through 2000. Between 1999 and 2000 Congress cut the SSBG program by $605 million, a 25% reduction ("Status of the Arc's Legislative Goals," 1999). In 2000, nationwide SSBG funding for MR/DD services totaled $267 million. Inflation-adjusted SSBG funds for MR/DD declined from 1996 to 2000 by 12%.

Inflation-adjusted spending for ICFs/MR supporting 15 or fewer persons declined 9% during 1996-2000. Alaska, Delaware, Michigan, Montana, Nebraska, and New Hampshire converted all their community ICFs/MR to HCBS Waiver group homes during the 1996-2000 period. Rhode Island, South Dakota, and Vermont have also substantially reduced their reliance on smaller ICFs/MR during 1996-2000. Michigan, Minnesota, and New York had the greatest absolute reductions in community-based ICF/MR placements for 15 or fewer persons. Forty- seven percent of the nation's reduction in community ICF/MR placements was attributable to Michigan alone. Conversely, 16 states expanded their community ICF/MR programs, creating 3,335 new ICF/MR placements. Forty-five percent of the new placements (1,499) were in California alone. In 2000, 42,432 persons were supported in public and private ICFs/MR in the community, at a federal reimbursement level of $1.5 billion.

The HCBS Waiver

First authorized by Congress in 1981, HCBS Waiver spending grew from $1.2 million in federal reimbursements in 1982 to $2.7 billion in 1996. In 2000, federal HCBS Waiver reimbursement totaled $5.5 billion and supported 293,713 participants. The types of services financed by the Waiver include case management, assistive technology, homemaker assistance, home health aides, personal care, residential habilitation, day habilitation, respite care, transportation, supported employment, adapted equipment, home modification, and occupational, speech, physical, and behavioral therapy. No state financed all of these options, and there was considerable variability in the services that states opted to fund via the Waiver.

Connecticut, Maine, Rhode Island, Vermont, and Wyoming had the largest Waiver programs in 2000 on the basis of federal spending per person of the state general population. In terms of the absolute number of participants served, large HCBS Waiver programs in 2000 were, predictably, in the populous states of California, Florida, New York, and Pennsylvania. In terms of total expenditure, the largest HCBS Waiver programs were in California, Massachusetts, Michigan, Minnesota, New York, and Pennsylvania.

Table 2.9 presents data on each state's per capita spending rank (rank of federal Waiver spending per citizen of the state's general population), number of HCBS Waiver participants, years the Waiver has been in effect, per capita spending amount, and total federal-state Waiver spending as a percentage of total MR/DD spending. The HCBS Waiver has been an essential part of community services expansion, including the development of supported living and personal assistance, family support, and supported employment.

The HCBS Waiver was established in every state by 2000, although the District of Columbia in 2000 had not yet drawn down federal Waiver dollars (see "years in effect" column in *Table 2.9*). Federal Waiver revenues increased by an average of 15% per year in inflation-adjusted terms during 1996-2000. The overall inflation-adjusted growth between 1996 and 2000 was 77%. This rapid growth in the HCBS Waiver, contrasted with the decline in federal ICF/MR funding, is illustrated in *Figure 2.8*. In the figure, Other Medicaid consists of federal Medicaid spending for clinic and rehabilitative services, targeted case management, personal care, and Medicaid financing of community services administration in some states.

The role played by the HCBS Waiver seems likely to grow even larger in the years ahead due to the increasing flexibility of the Centers for Medicare and Medicaid Services (CMS) in permitting innovation in the states, and due to state's efforts to utilize currently unmatched state and local funds to draw down additional federal HCBS Waiver revenue (Hemp, Braddock, Parish, & Smith, 2001). For example, Hemp et al. (2001) concluded that unmatched funding levels exceeded 30% in the states of California, Georgia, Missouri, and Ohio. In addition, the Supreme Court's recent landmark ruling in the *Olmstead* case (*Olmstead v. L.C.*, 1999) is likely to stimulate increased utilization of the Waiver to finance community long-term care supports. Judge Ruth Bader Ginsburg, writing for the 6-3 Court majority, described the essence of the Court's ruling: "We confront the question of whether the proscription of discrimination may require placement of persons with mental disabilities in community settings rather than in institutions. The answer, we hold, is a qualified yes" (*Olmstead v. L.C.*, 1999).

Table 2.9
FEDERAL HCBS WAIVER EXPENDITURES, FY 2000

Rank[1]	State	Participants	Years in Effect	Federal $s Per Capita[2]	Federal-State Waiver Spending as % of Total Spending
1	Rhode Island	2,471	17	$78.83	68%
2	Maine	1,840	17	$67.50	59%
3	Vermont	1,719	18	$65.44	80%
4	Wyoming	1,226	10	$56.35	60%
5	Connecticut	4,783	13	$53.19	44%
6	New York	38,696	9	$46.67	40%
7	Minnesota	7,689	16	$46.59	53%
8	South Dakota	1,988	18	$45.53	57%
9	New Mexico	2,160	16	$44.88	70%
10	North Dakota	1,923	17	$42.90	36%
11	New Hampshire	2,638	17	$41.13	76%
12	Kansas	5,500	17	$38.21	54%
13	Massachusetts	11,360	16	$37.65	43%
14	West Virginia	1,910	17	$34.87	53%
15	Oregon	5,858	19	$33.84	53%
16	Oklahoma	3,276	15	$32.62	43%
17	Wisconsin	8,865	17	$32.56	42%
18	Arizona	10,816	12	$31.22	62%
19	Nebraska	2,320	13	$30.51	49%
20	Pennsylvania	15,943	17	$29.39	42%
21	Alaska	681	7	$29.24	50%
22	Michigan	8,300	13	$26.54	47%
23	Montana	1,276	19	$26.43	41%
24	Colorado	5,799	17	$24.83	64%
25	Utah	3,147	13	$24.35	44%
26	Tennessee	4,318	14	$21.31	40%
27	Delaware	489	16	$20.70	36%
28	South Carolina	4,489	9	$20.42	28%
29	Missouri	7,775	12	$20.30	35%
30	Iowa	4,591	8	$18.35	21%
31	Maryland	4,982	17	$18.19	44%
32	New Jersey	6,894	17	$18.15	31%
33	Washington	10,530	17	$16.97	35%
34	Louisiana	3,450	14	$15.26	19%
35	Alabama	4,337	18	$15.09	48%
36	North Carolina	5,735	17	$14.76	21%
37	Virginia	4,698	10	$10.76	31%
38	Kentucky	1,200	17	$10.71	32%
39	Hawaii	1,089	17	$9.54	50%
40	Ohio	5,593	10	$9.45	12%
41	Arkansas	2,012	11	$9.10	13%
42	Florida	20,442	17	$8.88	33%
43	California	28,233	16	$8.66	18%
44	Idaho	653	17	$8.03	11%
45	Indiana	2,069	11	$7.98	17%
46	Georgia	3,612	11	$7.72	26%
47	Texas	5,140	15	$7.24	16%
48	Illinois	7,400	17	$6.15	13%
49	Nevada	950	18	$3.57	22%
50	Mississippi	848	5	$1.22	2%
51	District of Columbia	0	4	$0.00	0%
	United States	293,713	19	$19.99	33%

[1]States are ranked by federal waiver spending per capita.

[2]Per citizen of the general population.

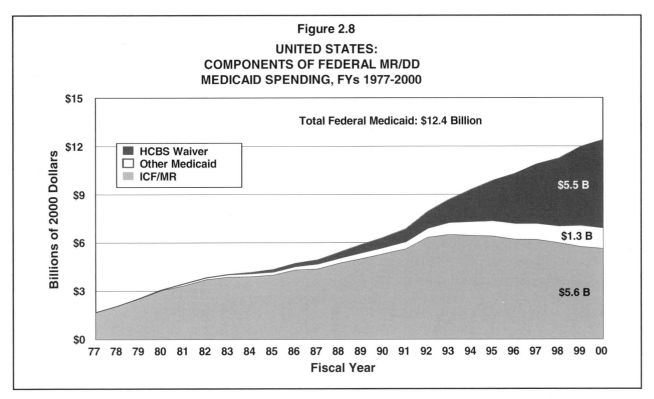

Figure 2.8
UNITED STATES:
COMPONENTS OF FEDERAL MR/DD
MEDICAID SPENDING, FYs 1977-2000

Leveraging Federal Funds

Table 2.10 presents the estimated amounts of "unmatched" state-by-state funding potentially available to draw down increased federal financial participation under the Medicaid HCBS Waiver or the ICF/MR program. Fifteen states had higher percentages of unmatched state funds than the 18% national average. The reasons for the levels of unmatched state funds are multiple and complex, including Medicaid-eligibility issues and the reluctance of many states to "Medicaid" family support services.

Currently, there are a number of initiatives in the states to leverage unmatched state funds. Ohio and Pennsylvania have plans to substantially expand their HCBS Waivers. Colorado and Montana are capturing additional Waiver funding for supported employment services, and Wyoming has extended its HCBS Waiver to include individuals previously funded only through state contracts ("Ohio Requests Expansion of Waiver Resources," 2000). States with relatively high volumes of unmatched state funds should engage stakeholders in the identification of barriers to the expansion of Medicaid reimbursement. Using unmatched state funds to match additional Medicaid HCBS re-

sources is one way many states may be able to expand the capacity of their community services and family support programs, even as the economies of these states may be slowing down and restricting tax revenues. It is also a means by which states can be responsive to the Supreme Court's *Olmstead* (1999) decision and to growing waiting lists.

Local Funding

Local government resources allocated for community MR/DD services are derived from county, township, or municipal entities, and grew from $691.4 million in 1996 to $904.9 million in 2000, an inflation-adjusted advance of 18%. Twenty-nine percent of these resources was used as part of the required state matching funds for the Medicaid HCBS Waiver or ICF/MR programs. The remaining funds supported county government-operated group homes, day programs, or other community supports.

Local resources constituted major revenue components in several states, most notably in Ohio, Iowa, and Wisconsin, where county funding comprised 45%, 26%, and 20%, respectively, of each state's total community spending. In Minnesota, Missouri, Texas, and Virginia, local governments contributed between 5%

Table 2.10
STATE FUNDS POTENTIALLY AVAILABLE TO
MATCH ADDITIONAL FEDERAL MEDICAID FUNDING, FY 2000

State	Total MR/DD Spending	Unmatched State Funds	Unmatched % of Total Spending
California	$3,018,455,649	$1,216,962,846	40%
Georgia	$387,482,752	$136,610,417	35%
Maryland	$429,010,818	$147,851,855	34%
Ohio	$1,496,733,246	$470,277,392	31%
Alaska	$62,199,891	$18,229,964	29%
Missouri	$529,327,689	$137,435,106	26%
New Jersey	$964,924,023	$246,382,759	26%
North Carolina	$884,387,390	$224,020,030	25%
District of Columbia	$100,976,671	$24,937,848	25%
Virginia	$459,640,282	$113,421,535	25%
Illinois	$1,189,482,024	$290,729,774	24%
Massachusetts	$1,082,548,662	$254,247,030	23%
Texas	$1,471,066,279	$334,797,016	23%
Connecticut	$792,010,671	$179,266,642	23%
Iowa	$404,383,045	$84,159,786	21%
Montana	$82,437,039	$15,066,687	18%
Nevada	$59,510,674	$10,524,257	18%
Pennsylvania	$1,586,326,786	$268,962,117	17%
Mississippi	$219,714,390	$36,702,792	17%
Delaware	$86,438,507	$14,328,507	17%
Colorado	$317,147,739	$51,773,707	16%
Oklahoma	$363,373,002	$58,764,002	16%
Oregon	$354,737,292	$57,069,014	16%
Wisconsin	$696,730,140	$103,215,532	15%
Kentucky	$191,045,772	$27,946,645	15%
Nebraska	$170,534,352	$24,595,132	14%
Arizona	$367,652,283	$48,818,486	13%
Hawaii	$45,613,825	$6,014,554	13%
South Carolina	$407,416,390	$51,198,771	13%
New Mexico	$157,100,948	$16,568,847	11%
Indiana	$453,434,400	$47,602,153	10%
Minnesota	$825,368,640	$80,048,461	10%
Florida	$726,115,999	$67,084,539	9%
Washington	$547,319,612	$49,920,385	9%
Wyoming	$74,070,492	$6,524,150	9%
Louisiana	$492,170,115	$41,029,028	8%
West Virginia	$160,356,604	$12,508,159	8%
Rhode Island	$212,729,515	$14,901,558	7%
Tennessee	$468,475,727	$31,347,200	7%
South Dakota	$87,910,751	$5,570,268	6%
Michigan	$993,355,629	$55,134,520	6%
North Dakota	$108,829,336	$5,874,809	5%
Kansas	$313,046,654	$15,982,059	5%
New Hampshire	$130,818,027	$6,186,873	5%
Maine	$216,804,537	$9,541,051	4%
Utah	$166,999,686	$7,209,213	4%
Vermont	$79,935,565	$2,874,688	4%
Arkansas	$243,299,093	$8,740,014	4%
Alabama	$201,072,041	$6,461,760	3%
Idaho	$137,459,137	$0	0%
New York	$4,292,345,285	$0	0%
United States	$29,310,325,076	$5,145,419,938	18%

and 15% of total community services revenues in 2000. Fifty-two percent of all local funding supporting community services in the United States in 2000 was attributable to a single state, Ohio.

Variations in State Commitments for MR/DD Services

National data inevitably obscure state variability in the financing of institutional and community services, as is revealed by inspecting the state-by-state graphics in *Figure 2.9*. Data for 1977-2000 are presented for all 50 states, the District of Columbia, and the United States. Public and private institutional spending, defined in terms of facilities for 16 or more persons, is indicated in each state's graphic by the light gray bar. The black bar represents community services spending for individuals served in settings for 15 or fewer people and community day, sheltered work, and other non-residential services. The white sub-component of the black community bar represents combined spending for supported living, personal assistance, supported employment, and family support.

Inspection of the state-by-state data in *Figure 2.9* reveals two broad trends: community services funding has grown steadily in virtually every state for more than a decade and institutional spending has declined in most states during this same period. Five empirical characteristics of states' patterns of financing institutional and community services can be used to gauge resource allocation trends in the states over the past two decades:

Figure 2.9
PUBLIC SPENDING FOR DEVELOPMENTAL DISABILITIES BY STATE, FYs 1977-2000

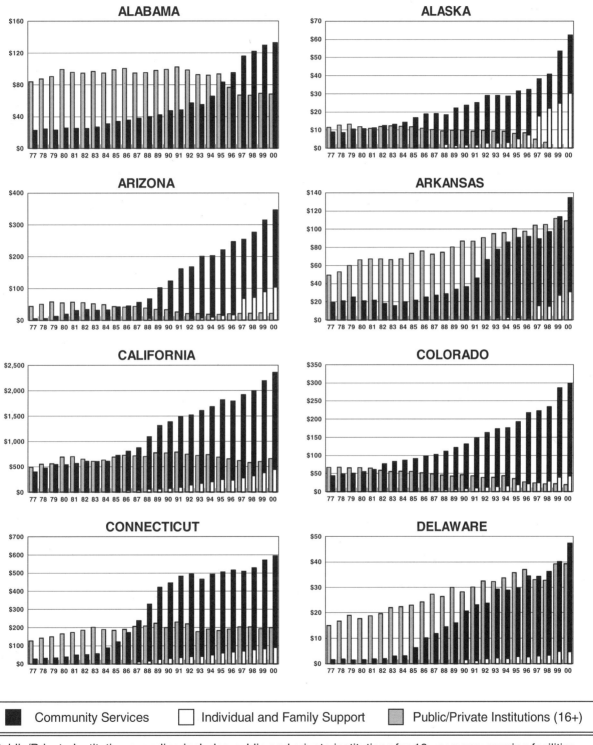

Community Services   Individual and Family Support   Public/Private Institutions (16+)

Public/Private Institution spending includes public and private institutions for 16+ persons; nursing facilities are not included. Community spending includes residential programs for 15 or fewer persons and non-residential community services. Individual and Family Support consists of spending for family support, supported employment, and supported living/personal assistance. The spending amounts for each state are in millions of constant 2000 dollars and, for the United States, in billions of constant 2000 dollars.

Figure 2.9 continued

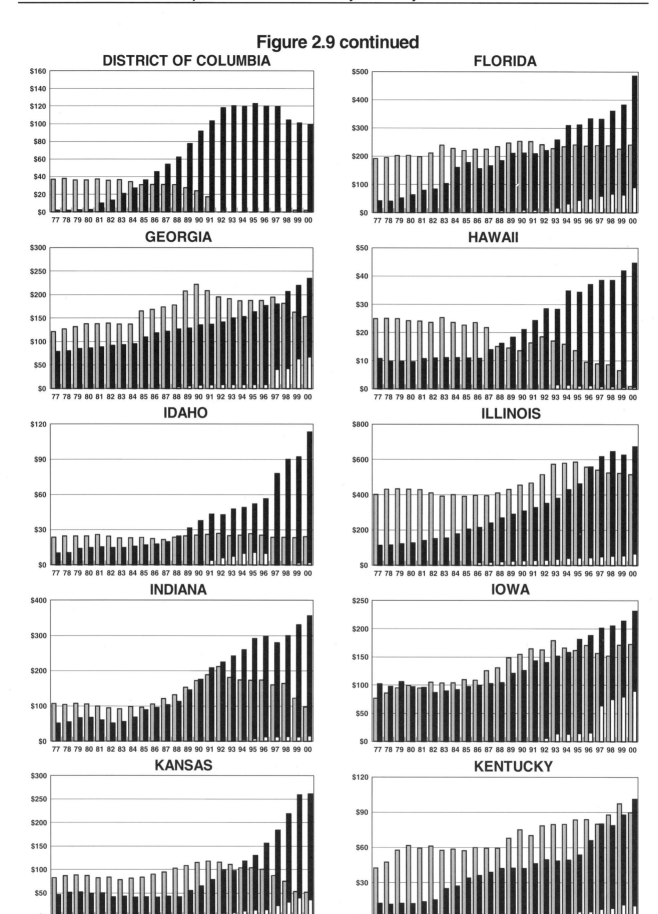

Figure 2.9 continued

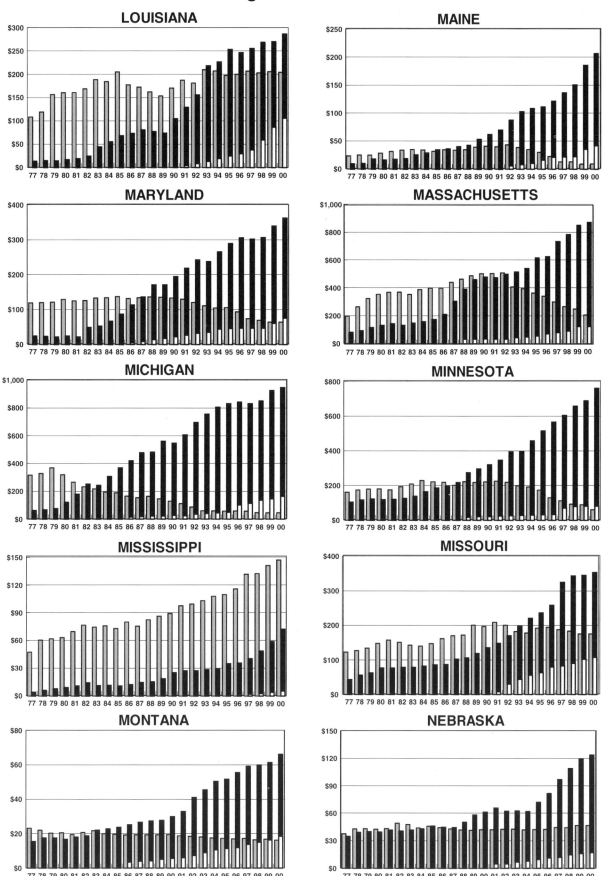

Figure 2.9 continued

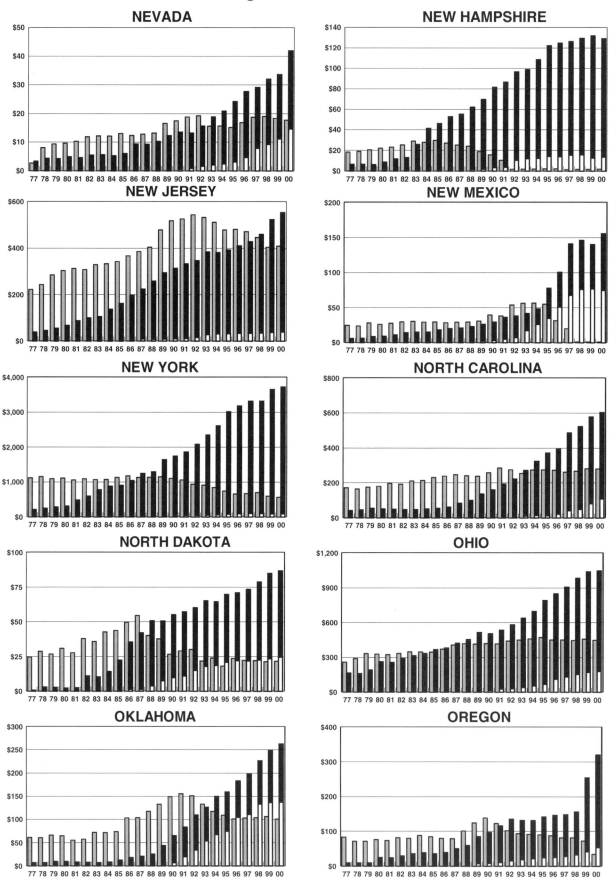

Figure 2.9 continued

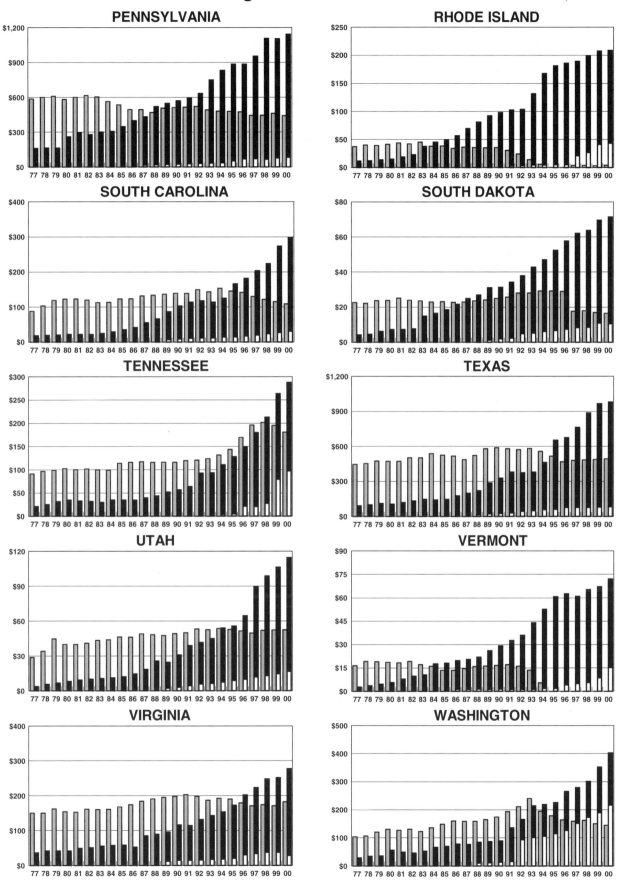

Figure 2.9 continued

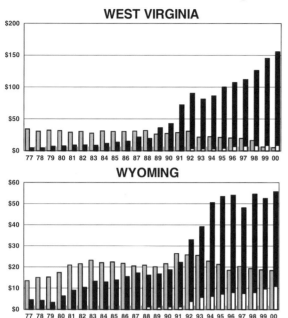

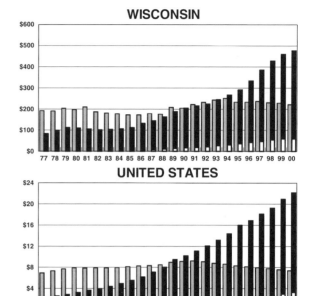

(a) the year in which community spending first exceeded institutional spending; (b) the rate at which community services resources have grown over time; (c) the rate at which institutional spending has declined; (d) the proportion of total MR/DD resources in 2000 committed to community services versus institutional services; and e) the extent of resource commitments in the states to individual and family support activities.

Public spending for community services in the United States first exceeded institutional spending in 1989. In 2000, all states but Mississippi were spending more for community services than for institutional services. Alaska, in 1981, and Colorado and Michigan, in 1982, were the first three states to allocate a majority of their total MR/DD funding base to community services, followed between 1983-84 by Montana, New Hampshire, Rhode Island, and Vermont. An additional 15 states and the District of Columbia began committing the majority of their MR/DD resources to community services activities during 1985-89. Twenty states reached this benchmark of community spending during 1990-96. Community services spending first surpassed institutional allocations in 1997-98 in Delaware, Georgia, Illinois, New Jersey, and Tennessee. Arkansas reached parity in 1999, followed by Kentucky in 2000.

During 1996-2000, inflation-adjusted community spending in the United States advanced 31%. In this period, community services spending growth ranged from 3% in Wyoming to 119% in Oregon. Other leaders in the expansion of community services resources during 1996-2000 were Mississippi (102%), Idaho (101%), Alaska (93%), and Tennessee (93%). The District of Columbia was the only jurisdiction to reduce community spending during this period. The District's inflation-adjusted community funding declined by 17% from 1996 to 2000.

Another mechanism for gauging trends in the states is the rate of decline in state financing of institutional care. Across the nation during 1977-1991, the public and private institutional care sector grew every year in inflation-adjusted terms. After the peak in spending in 1991, institutional spending declined each year from 1991 to 2000. During 1996-2000, inflation-adjusted institutional spending in the United States declined 10%. Among the states that have not completely closed their public institutions, Indiana, Kansas, Maine, Massachusetts, Oregon, and South Dakota reduced their inflation-adjusted institutional spending by more than 39% during 1996-2000. During 1996-2000, 18 states expanded their inflation-adjusted institutional spending by 1%-27%. These states included Arizona, Arkansas, California, Connecticut, Delaware, Florida, Iowa, Kentucky, Louisiana, Mississippi, Nebraska, Nevada, North Carolina, Rhode Island, Tennessee, Texas, Utah, and Virginia. In all of these states except Arkansas, Iowa, Rhode Island, and Texas, advances in institutional spending were accompanied by reductions in the number of public and private institutional residents. Rhode Island's increase in spending is attributable to the opening of a private ICF/MR facility for 25 persons in 1997.

The proportion of total MR/DD resources dedicated to community services activities in 2000 was another significant aspect of state MR/DD financing. Nationally, 75% of total MR/DD resources was dedicated to community services and supports in 2000 (*Table 2.11*). Alaska and Vermont devoted 100% of their MR/DD resources to community services. Twelve states dedicated at least 90% of their total resources to community services in 2000: Arizona, Colorado, the District of Columbia, Hawaii, Maine, Michigan, Minnesota, New Hampshire, New Mexico, Oregon, Rhode Island, and West Virginia. At the other end of the spectrum of the proportion of community spending, Mississippi allocated 33% of total MR/DD resources for community services.

A final dimension by which to evaluate current trends in the states is the continued expansion of resources for individual and family support, consisting of family support, supported employment, supported living, and personal assistance. Combined spending for family support, personal assistance, supported employment, and supported living constituted 11% of total community services allocations in 1996, and 15% in 2000. However, great variability existed among the states. Individual and family support spending ranged from 1% of total MR/DD spending in Hawaii, to 40% or more in Alaska, New Mexico, and Washington State. Supported living/personal assistance spending of $1.7 billion for 98,300 persons represented 6% of the nation's total MR/DD spending. Family support spending of $1.0 billion represented 4% and supported employment spending of $618 million represented 2% of total MR/DD spending in 2000. The next section addresses the growth of individual and family sup-

Table 2.11

PERCENTAGE OF TOTAL MR/DD SPENDING ALLOCATED FOR COMMUNITY SERVICES, FY 2000

State	Community Services Spending %	Rank
Alaska	100%	1
Vermont	100%	1
New Mexico	99%	3
New Hampshire	99%	4
Rhode Island	98%	5
District of Columbia	98%	6
Hawaii	98%	7
West Virginia	97%	8
Maine	96%	9
Michigan	95%	10
Arizona	94%	11
Colorado	94%	12
Minnesota	93%	13
Oregon	90%	14
New York	87%	15
Maryland	85%	16
Kansas	83%	17
Idaho	82%	18
South Dakota	81%	19
Massachusetts	81%	20
Montana	80%	21
North Dakota	80%	22
Indiana	79%	23
California	78%	24
Wyoming	75%	25
Connecticut	75%	26
Washington	74%	27
South Carolina	73%	28
Nebraska	73%	29
Oklahoma	72%	30
Pennsylvania	72%	31
Nevada	70%	32
Ohio	70%	33
Utah	69%	34
North Carolina	68%	35
Wisconsin	68%	36
Missouri	67%	37
Florida	67%	38
Texas	67%	39
Alabama	66%	40
Tennessee	61%	41
Georgia	61%	42
Virginia	60%	43
Louisiana	58%	44
New Jersey	58%	45
Iowa	57%	46
Illinois	57%	47
Arkansas	55%	48
Delaware	55%	49
Kentucky	53%	50
Mississippi	33%	51
United States	**75%**	

port activities and funding in the states.

Individual and Family Support

Combined individual and family support spending of $3.3 billion constituted 11% of the $29.3 billion in total MR/DD spending across the United States in 2000. Fifty percent of the nationwide funding for individual and family support was allocated for supported living and personal assistance, 31% for family support, and the remaining 19% funded supported employment activities. Aggregate spending for the three components of individual and family support increased 80% in inflation-adjusted terms between 1996 and 2000, compared to a 31% increase in total community services spending, and a 9% decline in institutional spending. Individual and family support represented the fastest-growing portion of most states' MR/DD budgets during 1996-2000.

The expansion of community residences for six or fewer persons and individual and family support in the states has largely been underwritten by the HCBS Waiver. States varied in their utilization of Waiver funds for family support, supported living/personal assistance and supported employment. For the reporting states, federal/state Waiver funds constituted 48% of family support spending (40 of 50 participating states reporting); 63% of supported living spending (39 of 46 participating states reporting); 59% of personal assistance services (16 of 20 participating states reporting) and 29% of supported employment spending (45 of 51 participating states reporting).

The percentage of supported employment spending funded by the Waiver is likely to increase substantially as more states take full advantage of the provisions of the Balanced Budget Act of 1997 (Pub. L. 105-33). The Act expanded supported employment opportunities for HCBS Waiver participants. Previously, only those Waiver participants who had resided in nursing facilities or ICFs/MR were eligible for prevocational, education, or supported employment services funded through the Waiver. The Arc (1997) estimated that an additional 150,000 Waiver participants would be eligible for Waiver reimbursed supported employment services under the auspices of the new law.

A national initiative with potential impact on individual and family support was the Self-Determination for Persons with Developmental Disabilities project financed in 1997 by the Robert Wood Johnson Foundation. Nineteen states received from $100,000 to $400,000 to initiate projects consistent with principles of consumer freedom, authority, support, and responsibility ("Declaration of Self-Determination," 1998). A major impetus for the Robert Wood Johnson Self-Determination project came from a small project in southwestern New Hampshire that tested whether gradual and responsible reduction of professional control over basic life choices might enhance quality and other positive outcomes, but not increase public costs. This initial demonstration, with support provided to 45 participants over a 20-month period, reduced public costs by 12%-15% per individual, while substantially improving participants' assessment of areas including self-determination, number of friends, quality of the home, vocational options, and challenging behavior (Nerney, 1999).

Thirty-six states responded to the Robert Wood Johnson request for proposals, and 19 grants were initially awarded. The 18 states, in addition to New Hampshire, were Arizona, Connecticut, Florida, Hawaii, Iowa, Kansas, Maryland, Massachusetts, Michigan, Minnesota, Ohio, Oregon, Pennsylvania, Texas, Utah, Vermont, Washington, and Wisconsin ("Declaration of Self-Determination," 1998). A number of states, including Utah, have established their own self-determination and person-centered planning initiatives. These states are Alaska, Louisiana, North Carolina, and South Carolina ("Paving the Road," 1997; "Louisiana Maps," 1998; "North Carolina Division," 1999; "New Person-Centered System," 1998; "Utah Plans," 1997).

Family Support Services

Family support consisted of any community-based service administered or financed by the state MR/DD agency providing for vouchers, direct cash payments to families, reimbursement, or direct payments to service providers which the state agency identified as family support. Examples of family support programs included cash subsidy payments, respite care, family counseling, architectural adaptation of the home, in-home training, sibling support programs, education and behavior management services and the purchase of specialized equipment. Family support emerged as a significant priority for MR/DD state agencies in the early 1980s (Agosta & Bradley, 1985; Fujiura, Garza, & Braddock, 1990). Michigan's establishment of a cash subsidy program was a particularly notable early development (Fujiura et al., 1990; Herman, 1991; Meyers & Marcenko, 1989).

Family support data were collected in the present study in two categories: cash subsidy payments, and all other family support services. Inflation-adjusted total family support expenditures advanced from $569 million for 279,266 families in 1996 to $1.0 billion for 385,414 families in 2000. Family support spending constituted 3.6% of total MR/DD resources in 2000, up from 2.3% in 1996. The 85% family support spending advance between 1996 and 2000 was more than two times the 31% increase in overall community spending over the same period. The number of families receiving some form of assistance increased by 38% during the same period, as many states increased per-family allocations rather than the number of participating families. All 50 states reported a family support initiative in either cash subsidy or other family support activity. The District of Columbia did not fund family support services in 2000. *Figure 2.10* depicts the advances in the number of families served, and in the inflation-adjusted resources allocated for family support services across the nation during 1990-2000.

In 2000, 19 states reported cash subsidy payments, down from 20 states in 1996. Total cash payments to families increased, however, from $42.8 million in 1996 to $69.0 million in 2000, and the number of families receiving subsidies grew from 17,495 to 25,802 during 1996-2000. The average annual subsidy payment to a family in the United States in the year 2000 was $2,674 and ranged from $351 in North Carolina to $8,524 in Illinois. The combined cash subsidy programs in Illinois, Michigan, and Texas accounted for 62% of all subsidy payments in the United States during 2000. Spending for family support in 2000 averaged $383,376 per 100,000 citizens across the nation, and ranged from a low of $5,668 in Arkansas to over $1,000,000 in Arizona, Kansas, Louisiana, and Vermont. While 17 states spent more than $500,000 per 100,000 of the general population on family support services, 18 spent less than $100,000, and the District of Columbia did not offer any support, reflecting the tremendous differences among the states in their levels of commitment to supporting families.

The total annual allocation per family (cash subsidy and other family support) was another metric by which to assess states' family support services. In 2000, the average spending per family in the United States was $2,722 (*Table 2.12*). Annual per-family spending ranged from $234 in Alabama to $13,614 in North Carolina. Twelve states spent more than $5,000 per family in 2000, while seven spent less than $1,000. During 1996-2000, inflation-adjusted family support spending growth exceeded 300% in Arizona, Delaware, Louisiana, North Carolina, and South Dakota.

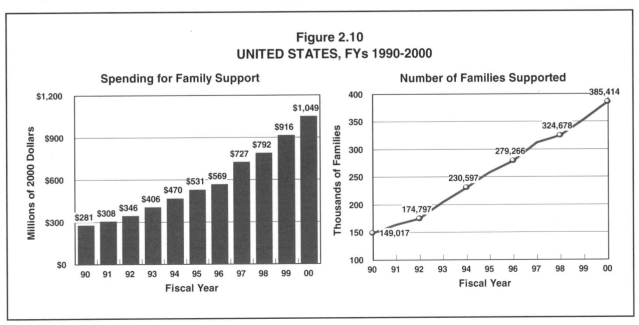

Figure 2.10
UNITED STATES, FYs 1990-2000

Spending for Family Support

Number of Families Supported

Table 2.12
FAMILY SUPPORT PROGRAMS, FY 2000

State	Cash Subsidy Expenditures	Families	Other Family Support Expenditures	Families	Total Family Support Expenditures	Families	Average Spending Per Family	Families Served Per 100K[1]
Alabama	$0	0	$654,916	2,800	$654,916	2,800	$234	63
Alaska	$0	0	$4,367,936	1,361	$4,367,936	1,361	$3,209	214
Arizona	$886,136	151	$82,821,203	13,037	$83,707,339	13,188	$6,347	275
Arkansas	$0	0	$146,876	49	$146,876	49	$2,997	2
California	$0	0	$233,701,772	101,194	$233,701,772	101,194	$2,309	308
Colorado	$0	0	$4,465,314	4,014	$4,465,314	4,014	$1,112	98
Connecticut	$988,067	911	$6,209,898	3,108	$7,197,965	4,019	$1,791	122
Delaware	$0	0	$1,362,779	1,218	$1,362,779	1,218	$1,119	160
D.C.	$0	0	$0	0	$0	0	$0	0
Florida	$1,000,598	636	$63,355,404	12,021	$64,356,002	12,021	$5,354	79
Georgia	$0	0	$1,817,307	5,648	$1,817,307	5,648	$322	72
Hawaii	$0	0	$265,210	632	$265,210	632	$420	52
Idaho	$0	0	$471,747	988	$471,747	988	$477	76
Illinois	$16,545,171	1,941	$21,428,298	14,493	$37,973,469	16,434	$2,311	136
Indiana	$0	0	$875,000	2,400	$875,000	2,400	$365	40
Iowa	$1,520,000	379	$55,000	38	$1,575,000	417	$3,777	14
Kansas	$2,623,200	1,093	$30,054,600	1,937	$32,677,800	3,030	$10,785	114
Kentucky	$0	0	$3,902,000	1,950	$3,902,000	1,950	$2,001	49
Louisiana	$4,405,038	1,574	$53,542,251	4,055	$57,947,289	5,629	$10,294	128
Maine	$0	0	$532,687	500	$532,687	500	$1,065	40
Maryland	$0	0	$23,237,173	5,383	$23,237,173	5,383	$4,317	103
Massachusetts	$0	0	$39,575,391	15,010	$39,575,391	15,010	$2,637	243
Michigan	$13,720,845	5,264	$15,919,109	7,943	$29,639,954	13,207	$2,244	136
Minnesota	$2,099,000	1,118	$17,812,454	1,428	$19,911,454	2,546	$7,821	53
Mississippi	$0	0	$3,028,128	640	$3,028,128	640	$4,731	23
Missouri	$1,042,666	901	$5,748,555	4,117	$6,791,221	5,018	$1,353	91
Montana	$0	0	$9,088,814	2,762	$9,088,814	2,762	$3,291	301
Nebraska	$0	0	$2,974,715	753	$2,974,715	753	$3,950	45
Nevada	$752,975	278	$625,825	1,018	$1,378,800	1,296	$1,064	70
New Hampshire	$0	0	$7,269,655	4,917	$7,269,655	4,917	$1,478	406
New Jersey	$3,361,930	1,852	$17,303,012	4,590	$20,664,942	4,590	$4,502	56
New Mexico	$0	0	$9,327,667	1,737	$9,327,667	1,737	$5,370	97
New York	$0	0	$46,845,000	63,343	$46,845,000	63,343	$740	348
North Carolina	$351,069	1,001	$57,481,242	3,247	$57,832,311	4,248	$13,614	55
North Dakota	$589,417	387	$3,505,284	508	$4,094,701	895	$4,575	138
Ohio	$0	0	$12,543,967	12,110	$12,543,967	12,110	$1,036	107
Oklahoma	$2,690,100	997	$20,826,303	993	$23,516,403	1,990	$11,817	59
Oregon	$0	0	$6,902,210	999	$6,902,210	999	$6,909	30
Pennsylvania	$0	0	$24,957,407	21,500	$24,957,407	21,500	$1,161	178
Rhode Island	$184,448	54	$9,120,125	911	$9,304,573	965	$9,642	97
South Carolina	$2,600,000	544	$18,700,000	6,459	$21,300,000	6,749	$3,156	174
South Dakota	$0	0	$1,601,572	1,613	$1,601,572	1,613	$993	214
Tennessee	$0	0	$4,411,532	3,048	$4,411,532	3,048	$1,447	55
Texas	$12,707,989	5,148	$37,174,744	5,247	$49,882,733	10,395	$4,799	52
Utah	$932,100	1,573	$5,313,300	1,528	$6,245,400	2,366	$2,640	109
Vermont	$0	0	$12,284,420	1,003	$12,284,420	1,003	$12,248	166
Virginia	$0	0	$2,324,080	2,164	$2,334,080	2,164	$1,079	31
Washington	$0	0	$32,751,199	7,095	$32,751,199	7,095	$4,616	122
West Virginia	$0	0	$5,397,195	2,031	$5,397,195	2,031	$2,657	111
Wisconsin	$0	0	$11,237,793	6,908	$11,237,793	6,908	$1,627	131
Wyoming	$0	0	$4,841,131	641	$4,841,131	641	$7,552	128
United States	$69,000,749	25,802	$980,159,200	363,089	$1,049,169,949	385,414	$2,722	141

[1]Per 100,000 citizens of the general population.

114

Mississippi first began funding family support in 1997. Conversely, Arkansas, Hawaii, and Maine, which had relatively small programs in 2000, cut their family support funding between 1996 and 2000. Other states with small relative commitments for family support services in 2000 included Alabama, Idaho, and Indiana. *Table 2.12* provides state-by-state data regarding the allocation of family support resources for cash subsidy and other family support. The final two columns of *Table 2.12* detail the average spending per family and families served per 100,000 of the state general population.

In 1998, a federal Family Support Program administered by the Department of Health and Human Services' Administration on Developmental Disabilities (ADD) was designed to stimulate the development of innovative family support services (Parish, Pomeranz, Hemp, Rizzolo, & Braddock, 2001). ADD has provided family support grants to the states for training and technical assistance, integration and coordination of services, outreach, and policy development. Grants have also been awarded to promote culturally competent services and self- or family-directed supports.

Supported Employment

In the early 1980s, state MR/DD agencies began providing long-term support for workers with developmental disabilities. These services supplemented the employment options that were available through states' vocational rehabilitation (VR) agencies. Research since that time, along with advances in employment services and legislative mandates such as the Americans with Disabilities Act of 1990 (Pub. L. 101-336), have reinforced the need for supported employment (Blanck, 1998; Wehman, West, & Kane-Johnston, 1997), even though most states have maintained their commitments to sheltered work settings (McGaughey, Kiernan, McNally, & Gilmore, 1995). Longitudinal studies of people moving from sheltered to supported employment have also pointed to benefits for both consumers and taxpayers (Helms, Moore, & McSewyn, 1991; Hill & Wehman, 1983; Kregel, Wehman, & Banks, 1989; Lagomarcino, 1986; Thompson, Powers, & Houchard, 1992; Vogelsberg, Ashe, & Williams, 1985).

Supported employment was defined in the present study to include MR/DD state agency-financed programs for the long-term support of individuals in integrated work settings, work stations in industry, enclaves, or work crews, where developing independent work skills and earning competitive wages were the goals. Activities sponsored by the state's vocational rehabilitation agency, with the exception of Arizona and California's transfer of MR/DD sheltered workshop/day activity programs to their states' VR agencies, were not identified in data collected for this study. Supported employment spending grew from $420 million in 1996 to $617 million in 2000, a 33% inflation-adjusted increase. The number of supported workers increased by 22%, from 88,662 to 108,004, during 1996-2000.

In 2000, 23% of all vocational and day program participants in the United States worked in supported or competitive employment, while the remaining 77% of participants received services in sheltered employment, day activity, or day habilitation programs (*Table 2.13*). The proportion of total day-work participants who worked in supported or competitive employment services in 2000 ranged from less than 10% in Alabama, Arkansas, Hawaii, and West Virginia, to 40% or more in Connecticut, Maryland, Massachusetts, Oklahoma, Utah, and Washington. In 2000, supported employment spending per 100,000 of the state general population ranged from $11,585 in Arkansas to over $1,000,000 in Connecticut and Massachusetts; the national average was $225,670. *Table 2.13* provides state-by-state data regarding supported employment programs in the states, including total program spending and workers supported, spending and workers adjusted per 100,000 of the general population, and the percentage of all participants in supported employment.

The most recent legislation aimed at improving work opportunities for people with disabilities was the Ticket to Work and Work Incentives Improvement Act, enacted December 17, 1999. This legislation was designed to address the barriers to work that people with disabilities confront as a result of the potential loss of publicly funded health care services when they become employed. The Act (Pub. L. 106-170) provided $150 million in grants to the states so that workers with disabilities who return to work could continue

Table 2.13
SUPPORTED EMPLOYMENT, FY 2000

State	Participants	Spending	Participants Per 100K[1]	Spending Per 100K[1]	% in Supported Employment[2]
Alabama	348	n/a	8	n/a	8%
Alaska	125	$989,955	20	$155,592	35%
Arizona	1,133	$10,478,354	24	$218,839	19%
Arkansas	150	$300,180	6	$11,585	4%
California	8,974	$79,566,000	27	$242,335	18%
Colorado	2,253	n/a	55	n/a	39%
Connecticut	3,552	$47,423,112	108	$1,444,499	49%
Delaware	345	$2,587,824	45	$340,159	31%
D.C.	0	$0	0	$0	
Florida	3,734	$9,210,330	25	$60,706	28%
Georgia	2,566	$8,813,497	33	$112,537	23%
Hawaii	53	$366,866	4	$30,040	5%
Idaho	n/a	$1,747,859	n/a	$134,518	n/a
Illinois	2,455	$11,819,696	20	$97,767	10%
Indiana	1,824	$5,991,266	30	$99,955	17%
Iowa	2,379	$6,400,909	82	$221,891	31%
Kansas	471	$3,686,207	18	$138,526	13%
Kentucky	633	$2,126,512	16	$53,458	29%
Louisiana	1,208	$6,597,236	27	$149,988	34%
Maine	688	$3,280,391	55	$261,173	20%
Maryland	3,390	$32,455,582	65	$621,360	41%
Massachusetts	5,100	$65,187,598	82	$1,053,608	41%
Michigan	5,648	$27,673,589	58	$284,556	37%
Minnesota	4,831	$24,118,966	101	$502,190	n/a
Mississippi	300	$1,310,894	11	$46,947	13%
Missouri	480	$1,654,936	9	$30,067	10%
Montana	249	$1,857,808	27	$202,731	15%
Nebraska	890	$4,440,912	53	$263,475	27%
Nevada	450	$540,000	24	$29,346	34%
New Hampshire	483	$5,181,673	40	$427,331	26%
New Jersey	1,623	$10,185,335	20	$124,809	19%
New Mexico	1,122	$6,363,632	62	$353,550	33%
New York	10,420	$35,442,000	57	$194,908	12%
North Carolina	2,148	$13,218,570	28	$171,361	24%
North Dakota	326	$1,863,883	50	$287,710	19%
Ohio	8,538	$29,443,769	76	$260,845	23%
Oklahoma	1,630	$12,955,420	48	$384,945	46%
Oregon	1,500	$15,884,054	45	$473,222	34%
Pennsylvania	6,803	$27,515,147	56	$227,435	30%
Rhode Island	497	$2,996,597	50	$301,344	19%
South Carolina	1,187	$5,190,000	31	$134,044	18%
South Dakota	745	$4,856,723	99	$643,218	37%
Tennessee	801	$1,898,370	14	$34,080	14%
Texas	3,971	$16,792,498	20	$83,570	31%
Utah	860	$5,292,000	40	$244,049	41%
Vermont	698	$4,580,753	115	$756,686	35%
Virginia	2,312	$14,699,870	33	$211,968	28%
Washington	3,247	$17,505,588	56	$301,447	52%
West Virginia	390	$1,078,107	21	$59,108	9%
Wisconsin	4,157	$21,240,405	79	$401,655	24%
Wyoming	317	$2,202,627	63	$438,507	33%
United States	**108,004**	**$617,013,500**	**39**	**$225,465**	**23%**

[1] Per 100,000 citizens of the general population.

[2] % in Supported Employment includes competitive employment.

to receive Medicaid. The law was scheduled to be phased in over a three-year period, with 30% of states participating beginning in January 2001. The 13 states in which the new law is being piloted are Arizona, Colorado, Delaware, Florida, Illinois, Iowa, Massachusetts, New York, Oklahoma, Oregon, South Carolina, Vermont, and Wisconsin.

Supported Living and Personal Assistance

Supported living was first initiated in Colorado, Florida, Missouri, North Dakota, Ohio, Oregon, and Wisconsin in the mid-1980s (Bauer & Smith, 1993; Pittsley, 1990; Smith, 1990). The increased funding to emphasize individual choice, control over housing, and individualized, person-centered planning reflected in part the growing strength of self-advocacy organizations (Dybwad & Bersani, 1996; Hayden & Senese, 1996; Longhurst, 1994). Self-advocates articulated where they wished to live and the types of support they preferred (e.g., Kennedy, 1990; Nelis, 1995; Nelis & Ward, 1995).

Supported living was defined for purposes of this study to include housing in which individuals choose where and with whom they live, in which ownership is by someone other than the support provider (i.e., by the individual, the family, a landlord, or a housing cooperative), and in which the individual has a personalized support plan that changes as her or his needs and abilities change (Karan, Granfield, & Furey, 1992; Racino & Taylor, 1993; Smith, 1990; Smull, 1989). According to this definition, 46 states reported providing supported living services to 79,474 individuals in 2000 at a cost of $1.5 billion (*Table 2.14*). From 1996-2000, inflation-adjusted growth in supported living funding advanced 110%.

Personal assistance services were defined as support provided to people living in their own homes financed by either state funds or federal/state Medicaid funds and defined by the state as "personal assistance." In 2000, initiatives in personal assistance were identified in 20 states. From 1996 to 2000, inflation adjusted growth in personal assistance funding advanced 88%. Funding for supported living and personal assistance combined totaled $1.7 billion in 2000, and constituted 2% of total MR/DD spending. During

1996-2000, supported living and personal assistance spending advanced 108% in inflation-adjusted terms. The number of participants increased from 56,392 to 98,300 persons between 1996 and 2000.

In 2000, substantial efforts to finance supported living and personal assistance were evident in Alaska, Maine, New Mexico, Oklahoma, and Rhode Island. These states spent $3,000,000 or more per 100,000 members of the state general population for supported living and personal assistance; the United States average was $605,896. Supported living spending per participant varied greatly across the states from $1,020 in Mississippi to $101,735 in Oklahoma; the national average was $18,406. Personal assistance cost per participant in the 19 states reporting spending data ranged from West Virginia's $844 to Oklahoma's $40,960; the national average was $10,373.

These cost extremes highlight state service systems that vary from those financing comprehensive supported living and personal assistance services as an integral part of deinstitutionalization plans (e.g., Oklahoma, Maine, and Washington), to more limited support intended for individuals with fewer needs (e.g., Mississippi and West Virginia). *Table 2.14* provides state-by-state data regarding the number of supported living and personal assistance participants and associated spending, and combined supported living/personal assistance participants and spending per 100,000 of the general population. Personal assistance data for individuals participating in Medicaid, social service, or VR agency programs, or those receiving personal assistance funding while living in out-of-home residential settings, are excluded.

There was considerable growth during 1996-2000 in supported living and personal assistance programs in Alaska, Arkansas, Colorado, Iowa, North Carolina, and Tennessee. Inflation-adjusted spending advanced at least four-fold in these states between 1996-2000. As a result of this funding expansion, Alaska, Iowa, and Tennessee were ranked in the top 10 for supported living and personal assistance spending per 100,000 of state population in 2000. There were inflation-adjusted declines of 4%-40% in spending for supported living and personal assistance in Indiana, New Hampshire, New York, and Virginia. Alabama, the District of Columbia, and Idaho each offered supported living/personal assistance services,

Table 2.14
SUPPORTED LIVING AND PERSONAL ASSISTANCE, FY 2000

State	Supported Living		Personal Assistance		Spending Per 100K[1]	Participants Per 100K[2]
	Spending	Participants	Spending	Participants		
Alabama	n/a	225	n/a	60	n/a	6
Alaska	$24,540,721	578	$339,408	40	$3,910,433	97
Arizona	$10,044,147	551	$0	0	$209,770	12
Arkansas	$30,433,176	1,232	$0	0	$1,174,488	48
California	$130,351,725	13,812	$0	0	$397,014	42
Colorado	$38,788,187	3,354	$0	0	$943,277	82
Connecticut	$35,320,231	1,334	$0	0	$1,075,847	41
Delaware	$713,738	32	$0	0	$93,818	4
District of Columbia	n/a	12	$0	0	n/a	2
Florida	$16,320,109	2,839	$5,618	4	$107,603	19
Georgia	$57,344,078	2,138	$0	0	$732,212	27
Hawaii	$0	0	$0	0	$0	0
Idaho	n/a	931	$0	0	n/a	72
Illinois	$16,041,014	1,955	$0	0	$132,683	16
Indiana	$502,945	60	$7,974,985	634	$141,441	12
Iowa	$81,905,145	4,354	$298,219	29	$2,849,627	152
Kansas	$0	0	$0	0	$0	0
Kentucky	$4,779,498	696	$0	0	$120,151	17
Louisiana	$42,058,437	1,316	$0	0	$956,196	30
Maine	$38,527,933	531	$0	0	$3,067,462	42
Maryland	$20,882,137	1,007	$0	0	$399,787	19
Massachusetts	$22,481,712	2,222	$0	0	$363,365	36
Michigan	$106,987,507	1,712	$0	0	$1,100,107	18
Minnesota	$0	0	$38,538,341	2,310	$802,422	48
Mississippi	$471,281	462	$559,910	282	$36,930	27
Missouri	$94,866,472	2,393	$5,216,552	517	$1,818,313	53
Montana	$7,662,803	799	$0	0	$836,195	87
Nebraska	$9,896,736	1,242	$0	0	$587,164	74
Nevada	$12,643,788	707	$0	0	$687,115	38
New Hampshire	$982,176	341	$0	0	$81,000	28
New Jersey	$8,986,780	473	$0	0	$110,123	6
New Mexico	$59,182,164	1,387	$0	0	$3,288,040	77
New York	$6,594,740	1,463	$3,175,274	2,181	$53,729	20
North Carolina	$14,582,583	594	$23,580,328	2,945	$494,729	46
North Dakota	$18,263,136	897	$655,461	65	$2,920,289	148
Ohio	$139,044,718	4,175	$0	0	$1,231,811	37
Oklahoma	$74,673,486	734	$26,418,962	645	$3,003,767	41
Oregon	$13,597,250	2,013	$17,782,514	1,164	$934,874	95
Pennsylvania	$31,916,031	7,803	$0	0	$263,812	64
Rhode Island	$30,921,875	577	$0	0	$3,109,572	58
South Carolina	$0	0	$4,449,000	640	$114,906	17
South Dakota	$3,952,012	713	$0	0	$523,399	94
Tennessee	$83,858,421	1,724	$6,806,656	172	$1,627,661	34
Texas	$16,449,384	2,458	$0	0	$81,862	12
Utah	$4,252,000	441	$957,000	97	$240,221	25
Vermont	n/a	n/a	$0	0	n/a	n/a
Virginia	$4,141,653	1,212	$7,578,185	302	$168,997	22
Washington	$125,480,390	3,713	$40,552,541	3,973	$2,859,097	132
West Virginia	$1,238,300	350	$1,263,573	1,498	$137,167	101
Wisconsin	$17,166,801	1,541	$9,137,883	1,268	$497,420	53
Wyoming	$3,975,000	371	$0	0	$791,358	74
United States	$1,462,822,420	79,474	$195,290,410	18,826	$605,896	36

[1] Spending for supported living and personal assistance per 100,000 citizens of the general population.

[2] Participants in supported living and personal assistance per 100,000 citizens of the general population.

but were unable to provide spending data on these initiatives.

The implementation of supported living programs requires a major public commitment to reallocate existing financial and human resources and to identify new funds. Federal, state, and local governments have been instrumental in structuring and extending resources for supported living and personal assistance. In Ohio, for example, collaborative efforts by counties and the state's MR/DD agency established support policies and identified available funding. In 1991, Ohio increased its supported living spending from $2 million to $10 million, including a reallocation of $6 million from the department's group homes budget. In 2000, Ohio budgeted $139 million for supported living. This was the highest funding level in the nation, followed by the $130 million committed by California, $125 million by Washington State and $107 million by Michigan.

In recent years, the federal government has encouraged supported living by increasing flexibility in the HCBS Waiver program (Smith, 1998; Smith & Gettings, 1997). The Medicaid Community Supported Living Arrangement (CSLA) legislation enacted in 1990 (Pub. L. 101-508) also endorsed supported living principles and provided funding for eight states from 1991-95. Five of the eight CSLA states —Florida, Illinois, Maryland, Michigan, and Rhode Island—used CSLA funds to establish statewide supported living initiatives. In 1996, Colorado, Wisconsin, and Florida established new HCBS Waiver programs as a continuation of their CSLA initiatives. Michigan revised its Mental Health Code in 1996 to incorporate provisions for person-centered planning ("Michigan's Revised Mental Health Code," 1996) and to provide a framework for state-wide expansion of supported living. Michigan's supported living spending more than tripled between 1996-2000, from $29.8 million to $107 million.

SIGNIFICANCE OF MEDICAID

It is clear that Medicaid is the essential financial underpinning for MR/DD services in the United States Combined federal and state Medicaid spending in 2000 constituted 75% of all MR/DD spending of $29.3 billion. States rely on Medicaid's stability, especially when undergoing major service system reform efforts including institutional downsizing and closure.

Medicaid funding is attractive to states, because state spending is matched by federal reimbursement of between 50%-79%, depending on the level of state per capita personal income. Medicaid therefore represents an unsurpassed opportunity for states to expand their services beyond what the allocation of their own resources would otherwise allow. The proportion of states' community services budgets that are made up of federal Medicaid funds and state/local matches has increased substantially in recent years, from 35% in 1990 to 94% in 2000. Much of this expansion, of course, can be attributed to growth of the HCBS Waiver program.

Based on the 1993-2000 trend, HCBS Waiver spending will surpass combined institutional and community-based ICF/MR spending in 2001. Continued expansion of family-scale homes and individual and family support initiatives hinges on continued efforts by the states to redirect institutional ICF/MR funding to community alternatives. During the past decade the vast majority of states have demonstrated that individualized supports are effectively financed by the Waiver and by other non-institutional Medicaid programs including personal assistance, targeted case management, and clinic/rehabilitative services.

Comprehensive reform of Medicaid in order to reduce expenditures was seriously considered by the Congress in 1995-96. The major target was poor people and welfare programs, but people with developmental disabilities and their families became targets as well, due to significant levels of Medicaid spending on their behalf (Braddock & Hemp, 1996). But for the president's veto, the 104th Congress' Contract with America would have converted Medicaid to a block grant and limited Medicaid optional services essential to persons with developmental disabilities and their families (e.g., ICF/MR, clinic/rehab services, the HCBS Waiver, personal assistance, targeted case management). If this Medicaid reform had been enacted, an estimated 55,000 persons with developmental disabilities might have become ineligible for Medicaid long-term care services in 2002, the target year for the 7-year "Medigrant" plan (Braddock & Hemp, 1996).

However, Medicaid growth slowed during the mid-1990s, thus reducing political support for Medicaid budget cuts. Subsequently, the Balanced Budget Act of 1997 and the 2001 United States budget did not fundamentally alter the program. The essential source of funding for the majority of services received by people with developmental disabilities was unchanged. Moderate Medicaid spending growth in the late 1990s was due primarily to the strong economy, which reduced the need for access to publicly funded health care, and to the impact of managed care, which controlled costs (Starr, 1999). The recent downturn in the economy could redirect the attention of elected officials to containing Medicaid spending.

ASSESSING FISCAL EFFORT IN THE STATES

Fiscal effort is a ratio that can be utilized to rank states according to the proportion of their total statewide personal income devoted to the financing of developmental disabilities services (Braddock & Fujiura, 1987). It is tied theoretically to the competitive resource allocation struggle described by Key (1949) and Wildavsky (1974) as the essence of politics. Some states are financing developmental disabilities services more vigorously than others. Comparative state fiscal effort analysis enables distinctions to be made between those states making a strong effort and those that are not (Bahl, 1982). According to Caiden (1978), this knowledge is useful in providing objective standards of comparison among the states in policy making and in the enforcement of accountability.

Fiscal effort was defined as a state's spending for MR/DD services per $1,000 of total state personal income. *Figure 2.11* illustrates changes in fiscal effort across the United States during the 1977-2000 period. In 1977, $2.26 per $1,000 of aggregate United States personal income was expended for MR/DD services across the nation. In 1990, fiscal effort had increased by 42% to $3.21, and in 2000 the figure was $3.65 per $1,000. The composition of this robust 24-year trend consists of two major sub-components: the dynamic and continuing growth of community services resources and the slow but steady decline in states' spending for institutions, that has accelerated since 1991.

Community services fiscal effort has grown nearly five-fold from $.57 per $1,000 of personal income in 1977 to $2.75 per $1,000 in 2000. In contrast, institutional fiscal effort peaked in 1980 at $1.73 per $1,000 and declined each year to $0.90 per $1,000 in 2000.

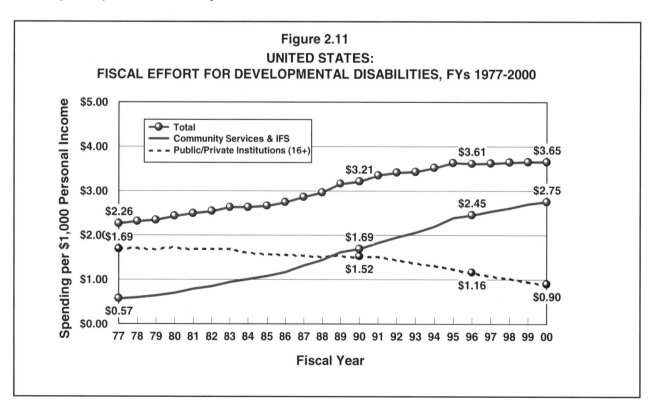

Figure 2.11
UNITED STATES:
FISCAL EFFORT FOR DEVELOPMENTAL DISABILITIES, FYs 1977-2000

State Spending Patterns

There were wide variations in fiscal effort among the states in 2000 and several notable developments in the performance of individual states over the preceding four year period. North Dakota led the nation in 2000 in total fiscal effort, spending $7.16 per $1,000 of state personal income on MR/DD services. Other states with the most substantial financial commitments to MR/DD services in 2000 included Maine, New York, and Rhode Island. At the other end of the spectrum, Nevada committed $1.02 per $1,000 of state wealth to MR/DD services, the lowest level in the nation. Other states that allocated less than $2.00 per $1,000 included Alabama, Florida, Georgia, Hawaii, Kentucky, and Virginia.

Community services fiscal effort exhibited the same variability as total spending fiscal effort in 2000. Community fiscal effort ranged from $0.72 per $1,000 in Nevada to Rhode Island's $6.95 per $1,000. The nation's average was $2.75 in 2000. *Table 2.15* presents state-by-state fiscal effort data for community, institutional, and total MR/DD spending in 1977, 1996, and 2000.

Between 1996-2000, total MR/DD fiscal effort increased in 34 states and by 42% in Idaho. Increases of 25%-35% were posted in Alaska, Maine, Mississippi, Oregon, and Tennessee. Total fiscal effort declined by 1%-21% during 1996-2000 in the District of Columbia, Georgia, Hawaii, Illinois, Indiana, Iowa, Louisiana, Maryland, Massachusetts, Michigan, Minnesota, Nevada, New Hampshire, New Jersey, Rhode Island, South Dakota, and Wyoming. Declines in total fiscal effort exceeded 10% in D.C., Georgia, Indiana, New Hampshire, South Dakota, and Wyoming.

Changes in community services fiscal effort during the 1996-2000 period were more uniform. Advances in community services fiscal effort were posted by 46 states, with the most significant increases, those exceeding 60%, in Alaska, Idaho, Mississippi, Oregon, and Tennessee. Community services fiscal effort during 1996-2000 was flat in Michigan, and it declined by between 2%-22% in the District of Columbia, New Hampshire, Rhode Island, and Wyoming.

The most significant changes in total MR/DD fiscal effort rankings between 1996-2000 in the states occurred in Alaska, Idaho, Mississippi, and Oregon which advanced 9-16 positions in the rankings (*Table 2.16*). Idaho's ranking increased from 32nd to 16th, and Oregon advanced from 34th to 26th. Mississippi advanced from 36th to 27th between 1996-2000, and Alaska moved forward in the rankings from 42nd to 32nd.

In each state, the basis of the increase in total resources was attributable to expanded spending for community services. Declines in total fiscal effort rankings occurred in 21 states between 1996-2000. The greatest declines were by 12 positions in Indiana, and 10 in New Hampshire. Fiscal effort rankings for community services in the states showed unusually strong advances during 1996-2000 in Oregon (+19 positions) and Alaska (+16 positions); Idaho advanced 14 positions. There were major declines in community fiscal effort rankings in New Hampshire (-11 positions) and Michigan (-10 positions).

In the public and private institutional care sector, the most dramatic declines in fiscal effort rankings occurred in South Dakota (-19 positions); Kansas (-14); Massachusetts, New Mexico, and Oregon (-13); Indiana (-11); and South Carolina (-10). Institutional downsizing and closures were influential in these rankings. Major enhancements of institutional fiscal effort rankings occurred in Kentucky (+9 positions); Connecticut (+8); and Montana, Nebraska, Texas, and Virginia (+7). Mississippi led the nation in institutional fiscal effort ranking in 2000, followed by Iowa. *Table 2.16* provides fiscal effort rankings for the states for 1977, 1996, and 2000.

CONCLUSION

Aging Caregivers and the Growing Demand for Services

The aging of our society, the increasing longevity of persons with developmental disabilities, growing waiting lists in the states, waiting list and access-to-Medicaid services litigation, and the future of funding for MR/DD services in the midst of our current recession are the focal points of this concluding section. These demographic, budgetary, litigation, and economic factors impact state service delivery systems and challenge their capacities to meet current and projected demands for residential, vocational, and family

Table 2.15
FISCAL EFFORT, FYs 2000, 1996, & 1977

State	Community Spending			Institutional Spending			Total Spending		
	2000	1996	1977	2000	1996	1977	2000	1996	1977
Alabama	$1.28	$1.02	$0.40	$0.66	$0.83	$1.49	$1.95	$1.85	$1.88
Alaska	$3.42	$2.00	$0.69	$0.00	$0.52	$0.90	$3.42	$2.53	$1.59
Arizona	$2.76	$2.48	$0.12	$0.17	$0.20	$1.10	$2.93	$2.69	$1.22
Arkansas	$2.31	$1.81	$0.61	$1.88	$1.93	$1.58	$4.19	$3.75	$2.19
California	$2.27	$2.09	$0.83	$0.64	$0.77	$1.02	$2.91	$2.86	$1.85
Colorado	$2.22	$2.09	$0.86	$0.14	$0.26	$1.32	$2.36	$2.34	$2.18
Connecticut	$4.47	$4.33	$0.39	$1.50	$1.61	$1.86	$5.96	$5.94	$2.25
Delaware	$1.99	$1.64	$0.13	$1.65	$1.76	$1.25	$3.64	$3.40	$1.38
D.C.	$4.61	$5.92	$0.11	$0.09	$0.00	$2.12	$4.71	$5.92	$2.22
Florida	$1.13	$0.91	$0.26	$0.56	$0.64	$1.23	$1.69	$1.55	$1.50
Georgia	$1.06	$0.99	$0.96	$0.69	$1.05	$1.48	$1.75	$2.04	$2.43
Hawaii	$1.34	$1.13	$0.57	$0.03	$0.29	$1.32	$1.37	$1.42	$1.89
Idaho	$3.81	$2.24	$0.70	$0.81	$1.01	$1.63	$4.62	$3.25	$2.34
Illinois	$1.74	$1.65	$0.46	$1.33	$1.65	$1.65	$3.07	$3.30	$2.11
Indiana	$2.24	$2.13	$0.51	$0.61	$1.24	$1.09	$2.85	$3.37	$1.61
Iowa	$3.07	$2.82	$1.91	$2.29	$2.57	$1.44	$5.37	$5.39	$3.34
Kansas	$3.57	$2.49	$1.09	$0.71	$1.60	$1.93	$4.28	$4.09	$3.02
Kentucky	$1.07	$0.81	$0.23	$0.95	$1.03	$0.78	$2.02	$1.85	$1.00
Louisiana	$2.82	$2.69	$0.22	$2.01	$2.17	$1.74	$4.83	$4.86	$1.96
Maine	$6.53	$4.38	$0.56	$0.30	$0.81	$1.34	$6.83	$5.20	$1.89
Maryland	$2.11	$2.07	$0.29	$0.37	$0.63	$1.39	$2.48	$2.70	$1.68
Massachusetts	$3.81	$3.25	$0.73	$0.91	$1.77	$1.75	$4.72	$5.02	$2.48
Michigan	$3.29	$3.30	$0.33	$0.16	$0.23	$1.67	$3.44	$3.53	$2.00
Minnesota	$5.03	$4.54	$1.40	$0.40	$1.04	$2.14	$5.43	$5.59	$3.53
Mississippi	$1.24	$0.71	$0.12	$2.51	$2.29	$1.47	$3.75	$3.00	$1.59
Missouri	$2.39	$1.98	$0.51	$1.18	$1.49	$1.43	$3.57	$3.48	$1.94
Montana	$3.32	$3.10	$1.21	$0.81	$0.95	$1.82	$4.14	$4.05	$3.03
Nebraska	$2.67	$2.06	$1.26	$1.01	$1.07	$1.37	$3.68	$3.13	$2.63
Nevada	$0.72	$0.64	$0.23	$0.30	$0.39	$0.19	$1.02	$1.02	$0.42
New Hampshire	$3.30	$3.78	$0.42	$0.04	$0.06	$1.20	$3.34	$3.85	$1.63
New Jersey	$1.86	$1.55	$0.24	$1.37	$1.81	$1.40	$3.24	$3.35	$1.64
New Mexico	$3.98	$2.93	$0.32	$0.03	$0.92	$1.35	$4.02	$3.85	$1.67
New York	$5.99	$5.69	$0.57	$0.90	$1.18	$3.06	$6.89	$6.86	$3.63
North Carolina	$2.94	$2.29	$0.48	$1.36	$1.58	$1.98	$4.30	$3.88	$2.47
North Dakota	$5.72	$5.26	$0.08	$1.44	$1.76	$2.42	$7.16	$7.02	$2.51
Ohio	$3.35	$3.05	$0.82	$1.44	$1.62	$1.28	$4.78	$4.67	$2.11
Oklahoma	$3.33	$2.67	$0.15	$1.28	$1.47	$1.31	$4.61	$4.14	$1.46
Oregon	$3.44	$1.88	$0.19	$0.37	$1.13	$1.81	$3.81	$3.00	$2.01
Pennsylvania	$3.25	$2.79	$0.71	$1.26	$1.50	$2.60	$4.51	$4.28	$3.32
Rhode Island	$6.95	$7.12	$0.67	$0.14	$0.00	$2.17	$7.09	$7.12	$2.84
South Carolina	$3.16	$2.30	$0.42	$1.16	$1.80	$2.07	$4.31	$4.09	$2.48
South Dakota	$3.76	$3.63	$0.40	$0.87	$1.82	$2.17	$4.62	$5.45	$2.57
Tennessee	$1.99	$1.20	$0.31	$1.25	$1.36	$1.35	$3.24	$2.55	$1.67
Texas	$1.73	$1.47	$0.38	$0.87	$1.02	$1.88	$2.60	$2.48	$2.26
Utah	$2.23	$1.56	$0.19	$1.02	$1.25	$1.42	$3.25	$2.80	$1.61
Vermont	$5.03	$4.96	$0.38	$0.00	$0.00	$2.12	$5.03	$4.96	$2.50
Virginia	$1.31	$1.13	$0.39	$0.86	$1.00	$1.62	$2.17	$2.13	$2.01
Washington	$2.22	$1.81	$0.39	$0.80	$1.12	$1.40	$3.01	$2.92	$1.79
West Virginia	$4.01	$3.00	$0.15	$0.13	$0.57	$1.18	$4.14	$3.56	$1.32
Wisconsin	$3.22	$2.61	$0.97	$1.50	$1.83	$2.26	$4.72	$4.44	$3.23
Wyoming	$4.25	$4.84	$0.57	$1.41	$1.66	$1.69	$5.66	$6.51	$2.26
United States	$2.75	$2.45	$0.57	$0.90	$1.16	$1.69	$3.65	$3.61	$2.26

Table 2.16
Fiscal Effort Rankings: FYs 2000, 1996, & 1977

State	Community			Institutional			Total Spending		
	2000	1996	1977	2000	1996	1977	2000	1996	1977
Alabama	46	46	28	32	36	25	47	47	33
Alaska	17	33	14	50	42	49	32	42	43
Arizona	29	24	49	41	47	46	39	40	49
Arkansas	32	36	16	4	4	24	22	24	22
California	33	29	9	33	38	48	40	37	34
Colorado	36	30	8	43	45	39	44	44	23
Connecticut	8	9	30	7	15	14	5	5	20
Delaware	40	39	47	5	10	42	29	28	47
District of Columbia	7	2	50	46	49	9	14	6	21
Florida	48	48	38	35	39	43	49	49	45
Georgia	50	47	7	31	28	26	48	46	16
Hawaii	44	44	18	49	44	38	50	50	32
Idaho	13	27	13	28	32	22	16	32	17
Illinois	42	38	24	13	13	21	37	31	24
Indiana	34	28	21	34	23	47	41	29	42
Iowa	26	18	1	2	1	28	8	9	3
Kansas	15	23	5	30	16	12	21	19	7
Kentucky	49	49	41	21	30	50	46	48	50
Louisiana	28	20	42	3	3	18	10	13	29
Maine	2	8	20	40	37	37	4	10	31
Maryland	38	31	37	37	40	33	43	39	36
Massachusetts	12	13	11	22	9	17	12	11	14
Michigan	22	12	34	42	46	20	31	26	28
Minnesota	6	7	2	36	29	7	7	7	2
Mississippi	47	50	48	1	2	27	27	35	44
Missouri	31	34	22	17	19	29	30	27	30
Montana	20	14	4	27	34	15	24	20	6
Nebraska	30	32	3	20	27	34	28	33	9
Nevada	51	51	40	39	43	51	51	51	51
New Hampshire	21	10	25	47	48	44	33	23	40
New Jersey	41	41	39	11	7	32	36	30	39
New Mexico	11	17	35	48	35	36	25	22	37
New York	3	3	17	23	24	1	3	3	1
North Carolina	27	26	23	12	17	11	20	21	15
North Dakota	4	4	51	9	11	3	1	2	11
Ohio	18	15	10	8	14	41	11	14	25
Oklahoma	19	21	45	14	20	40	17	17	46
Oregon	16	35	43	38	25	16	26	34	27
Pennsylvania	23	19	12	15	18	2	18	16	4
Rhode Island	1	1	15	44	50	5	2	1	8
South Carolina	25	25	26	18	8	10	19	18	13
South Dakota	14	11	27	25	6	6	15	8	10
Tennessee	39	43	36	16	21	35	35	41	38
Texas	43	42	33	24	31	13	42	43	19
Utah	35	40	44	19	22	30	34	38	41
Vermont	5	5	32	51	51	8	9	12	12
Virginia	45	45	29	26	33	23	45	45	26
Washington	37	37	31	29	26	31	38	36	35
West Virginia	10	16	46	45	41	45	23	25	48
Wisconsin	24	22	6	6	5	4	13	15	5
Wyoming	9	6	19	10	12	19	6	4	18

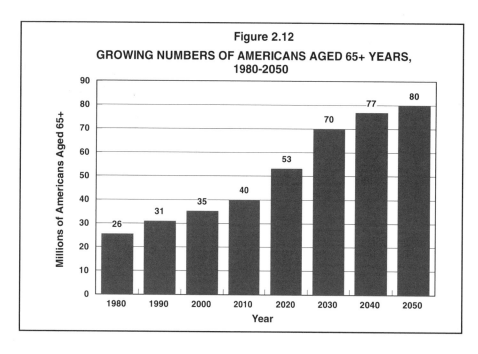

Figure 2.12
GROWING NUMBERS OF AMERICANS AGED 65+ YEARS,
1980-2050

of the system of residential care was modest, in light of an inflation-adjusted spending increase of 5% per year over the 24-year period.

The aging of our society directly influences demand for developmental disabilities services. This occurs because the majority of people with developmental disabilities in the United States currently reside with family caregivers. As these caregivers age beyond their caregiving capacities, formal living arrangements must be established to support their relatives with disabilities (Braddock, 1999).

support services for individuals with developmental disabilities.

Formal out-of-home residential services were being provided to 433,799 persons in the states in 2000. The vast majority of these settings are operated by private, non-profit service providers. The structure of the residential care system has changed markedly over the past 20 years as state-operated residential institutions have increasingly been supplanted by community residential services. The nation's overall residential system capacity grew by 24% between 1977 and 2000, an average annual rate of 2% per year, while the United States general population increased by 1% annually. The 2% annual growth in the capacity

The aging of our society is the product of several forces, primary among them the size of the baby boom generation, consisting of persons born during 1946-64, declining fertility rates, and increased longevity. Baby boomers will begin to reach age 65 in 2010. The number of persons in our society aged 65+ years is projected by the U.S. Bureau of the Census (1996) to reach 35 million in 2000 and 80 million in 2050 (*Figure 2.12*). Currently, 13% of the United States general population is aged 65+ years. Census Bureau demographers anticipate that this percentage will grow steadily for the next three decades, finally leveling off at 22% of the United States population in 2030. Problems loom even larger in countries such as Japan and Germany, where the 65+ cohort is projected to constitute approximately one third of their general populations by the year 2040 (U.S. Bureau of the Census, 1997).

Estimating the impact of aging on the increased demand for developmental disabilities services in the states requires data on the prevalence of developmental disabilities in our society. Based on the 1994/95 data from the National Health Interview Survey--Disability Supplement

Figure 2.13
UNITED STATES:
DISTRIBUTION OF INDIVIDUALS WITH MR/DD BY LIVING
ARRANGEMENT, FY 2000

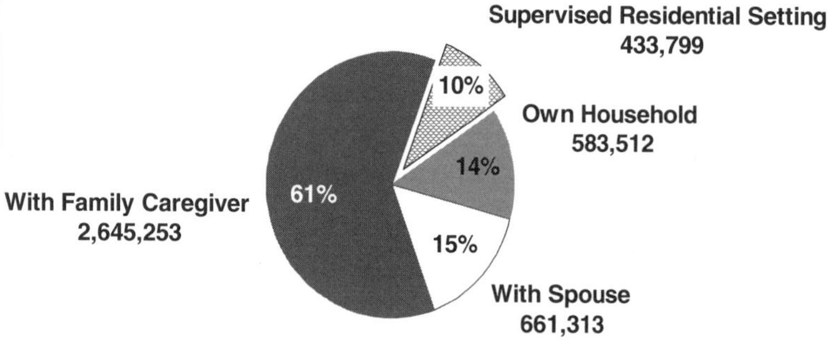

Supervised Residential Setting
433,799

Own Household
583,512

10%

14%

61%

15%

With Family Caregiver
2,645,253

With Spouse
661,313

Total Estimated Population: 4,323,877

(NHIS-D), Larson et al. (2001) recommended using a rate of 1.58% to estimate prevalence for persons with mental retardation, cerebral palsy, autism, epilepsy, and other childhood disabilities originating prior to 22 years of age. Fujiura (1998) determined that, in 1991, 60% of persons with developmental disabilities in the United States resided with family caregivers, and 40% lived on their own or within the formal out-of-home residential care system in the states.

We updated Fujiura's 1991 analysis using data pertaining to the 2000 out-of-home residential system, and the United States general population in 2000. The results are presented in *Figure 2.13*, which indicates that 2.65 million of the 4.32 million persons with developmental disabilities in the United States population in 2000 were receiving residential care from family caregivers. This "informal" system of residential care served about six times the number of persons served by the formal out-of-home residential care system (433,799 persons).

Fujiura (1998) determined that 25% of individuals with developmental disabilities in the United States lived with family caregivers aged 60+ years, and an additional 35% were in "households of middle-aged caretakers for whom transition issues are near-term considerations" (p. 232). In *Figure 2.14*, we reconfigured *Figure 2.13* to draw specific attention to the size of the aging family caregiver cohort (672,994 persons) in 2000.

How large is the aging caregiver cohort in each of the states? State-by-state estimates can be generated by taking into account differences in states' utilization of out-of-home placements and the number of the states' caregivers who are over age 60. For example, 8% of persons with developmental disabilities in Michigan live in out-of-home settings while the figure is 21% in North Dakota. The percentage of older individuals in the general population in the "oldest" state, Florida (18.3%), is three times the percentage of older individuals in the youngest state, Alaska (5.5%) (U.S.

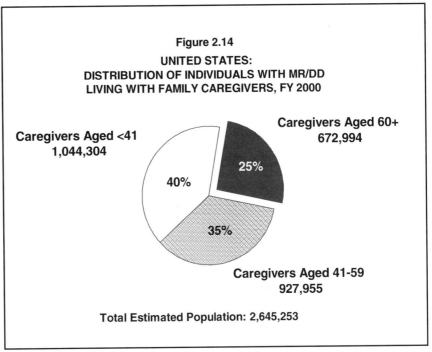

Figure 2.14

**UNITED STATES:
DISTRIBUTION OF INDIVIDUALS WITH MR/DD
LIVING WITH FAMILY CAREGIVERS, FY 2000**

Caregivers Aged <41
1,044,304

Caregivers Aged 60+
672,994

40%

25%

35%

Caregivers Aged 41-59
927,955

Total Estimated Population: 2,645,253

Census Bureau, 2000). State-by-state estimates of the number of individuals with developmental disabilities living with older caregivers appear in *Table 2.17*.

Increased Longevity of Persons with Developmental Disabilities

A second factor impinging on the growing demand for MR/DD services has to do with increases in the lifespan of individuals with developmental disabilities. The mean age at death for persons with mental retardation was 66 years in 1993—up from 19 years in the 1930s and 59 years in the 1970s. The mean age at death for the general population in 1993 was 70 years (Janicki, 1996). Janicki observed that with continued improvement in their health status, individuals with mental retardation—particularly those without severe impairments—could be expected to have a lifespan equal to that of the general population. Longevity has also increased dramatically for persons with Down syndrome. Average age at death for persons with Down syndrome in the 1920s was 9 years; it rose to 31 years in the 1960s and to 56 years in 1993 (Janicki, Dalton, Henderson, & Davidson 1999).

As persons with developmental disabilities live longer, they require services and support for longer periods of time. This directly impacts the finite capacities of state service delivery systems. The increased life expectancy of persons with developmental disabili-

Table 2.17
INDIVIDUALS WITH DEVELOPMENTAL DISABILITIES LIVING IN HOUSEHOLDS WITH CAREGIVERS AGED 60+ YEARS, 2000

State	Estimated Individuals/Households
Alabama	11,872
Alaska	727
Arizona	13,048
Arkansas	7,056
California	69,401
Colorado	7,810
Connecticut	8,710
Delaware	2,007
D.C.	1,189
Florida	55,674
Georgia	15,589
Hawaii	3,336
Idaho	2,726
Illinois	28,755
Indiana	14,412
Iowa	7,330
Kansas	6,904
Kentucky	10,304
Louisiana	9,918
Maine	3,338
Maryland	12,007
Massachusetts	15,932
Michigan	24,141
Minnesota	10,394
Mississippi	6,521
Missouri	14,739
Montana	2,371
Nebraska	4,336
Nevada	4,287
New Hampshire	2,895
New Jersey	21,648
New Mexico	4,258
New York	43,858
North Carolina	17,920
North Dakota	1,656
Ohio	29,318
Oklahoma	8,729
Oregon	8,642
Pennsylvania	36,766
Rhode Island	2,773
South Carolina	9,511
South Dakota	1,902
Tennessee	14,223
Texas	41,218
Utah	3,736
Vermont	1,497
Virginia	15,978
Washington	12,416
West Virginia	5,353
Wisconsin	12,728
Wyoming	1,138
United States	**672,994**

Note: State-by-state aging caregiver data for 2000 was estimated using a prevalence rate of 1.58% for persons with developmental disabilities (Larson et al., 2001). Data for 1998, presented in the 2000 Study Summary (Braddock et al., 2000), utilized a prevalence rate of 1.2% based on earlier work by Fujiura (1998).

ties since 1970 accounts for a significant percentage of the increased demand for residential services in the states today. The likelihood of older persons with developmental disabilities living into their own retirement and outliving their family caregivers has increased substantially in recent years. This has stimulated a growing demand for additional services and supports. The need to provide these services is frequently unanticipated by federal, state, and local agencies, often resulting in a crisis situation for families. It is an unfortunate reality that many family caregivers must die before the disabled relative for whom they are caring can receive services from the publicly financed system (Braddock, 1999).

Waiting Lists in the States

Prouty, Smith, and Lakin (2001) reported that, in 2000, an estimated nationwide total of 71,922 persons with developmental disabilities were on formal state waiting lists for residential services. A survey conducted by the Arc/United States (Davis, 1997) confirmed the magnitude of waiting lists in the states. Demographic trends clearly suggest that as baby boomers age, waiting lists will accelerate markedly in the states, unless a concerted state-federal effort is mounted to address this issue.

Some states maintain detailed waiting lists of service needs for persons with developmental disabilities. Some do not officially collect data on the number of persons waiting for services, although state officials informally acknowledge that significant demand for services exists. The Prouty et al. (2001) survey found an 18% increase in persons requesting residential services compared to a survey conducted eight years earlier (Hayden & DePaepe, 1994). Eight states did not furnish waiting list data in the 2000 survey (Arizona, the District of Columbia, Illinois, Indiana, Iowa, Michigan, Mississippi, and Washington) and six additional states indicated that their waiting lists were zero (California, Hawaii, Idaho, North Dakota, Rhode Island, and Wyoming). We need more accurate waiting list data from the states, which should conduct rigorous needs assessments and develop plans to serve the burgeoning number of families awaiting services.

Lakin (1998) has noted that waiting list initiatives in the states have generally involved expanding family support to prevent or delay the need for placement, and obtaining new or reallocated resources from the following sources: institutions, ICF/MR conversion to HCBS Waiver programs, capping reimbursement for existing programs, or seeking additional Medicaid funding.

Several states have, in fact, begun to address the need for services. New Jersey appropriated $30 million in fiscal year 1999 to reduce its waiting list for community residential services. An additional $72 million was proposed for fiscal year 2001 to expand services ("New Jersey Continues," 2000). Between 1986-96, the New Jersey waiting list increased from 767 to 4,600 persons. The "urgent" category in 1996 consisted of 2,286 persons. New Jersey's Division of Developmental Disabilities projected the need for a 10-year waiting list reduction initiative with appropriations of $30 million per year through 2008 (New Jersey Department of Human Services, 1998).

New Hampshire enacted a special appropriation to address its waiting list and required an annual status report to the governor regarding progress in addressing the waiting list ("Wait List Costs," 1997). Connecticut and Massachusetts have also commenced waiting list initiatives ("Connecticut Budget," 1999; "Massachusetts to Cut Waiting List," 1998). For fiscal year 2001, Connecticut's governor proposed new spending to support 212 persons in community settings ("State Budget Highlights," 2000).

Civil Rights and Advocacy

States vary dramatically in the vigor with which they are financing community services. Analysis by Braddock and Fujiura (1987) revealed that MR/DD spending was not a simple function of state size and wealth (reviewed in Braddock & Fujiura, 1991; and in Braddock et al., 1998, 2000). Spending for MR/DD community long-term care services was associated with a history of innovativeness on civil rights issues promoting racial equality in the states, a strong advocacy group presence, and state utilization of the HCBS Waiver.

In a recent study by Braddock (in press, see Part II), the relationship between community services fiscal effort (the dependent variable) and state wealth, state population, civil rights innovativeness and utilization of Medicaid HCBS Waiver and personal assistance funding (the independent variables) was assessed for individuals with mental retardation, individuals with mental illness, and individuals with physical disabilities. The state variations in community long-term care

services fiscal effort were in part attributable to the extent of state participation in the Medicaid Waiver and Personal Assistance programs and to the states' histories in the adoption of civil rights legislation promoting racial equality. However, the civil rights variable was statistically significant only in the case of the mental retardation/developmental disabilities group.

The importance of a civil rights history and a strong advocacy presence is suggested by the extent of MR/DD class action litigation in the nation after 1971. For example, there were more than 70 pending and completed class action right-to-habilitation suits in 38 states between 1970 and 1996 (Hayden, 1997). Significantly, most of the cases filed or reformulated after 1974 resulted in court orders or consent agreements requiring the states to develop community-based alternatives to institutions (Herr, 1983, 1992). This stimulated many defendant state governments to request substantial additional funds from their legislatures to implement new community services initiatives.

The link between interest group activity and spending is often direct; for example, developmental disabilities advocacy organizations were frequently the moving parties or plaintiff intervenors in key litigation (*Table 2.18*), and most state Arc organizations (formerly Associations for Retarded Citizens) operated active governmental affairs programs. Theoretically, the state governments most responsive from a fiscal standpoint to community services development (i.e., the 10 top ranking states in community services fiscal effort) were significantly influenced by the efforts of these highly motivated special interest groups.

Numerous state Protection and Advocacy agencies operated under the rubric of the Federal Developmental Disabilities Act have played key roles in many of these cases, including New Mexico (counsel) and Wyoming (counsel). Protection and Advocacy agencies also participated in major cases stimulating community services development in California (counsel, *Coffelt v. Department of Developmental Srvs.*, 1994), Georgia (amicus, *Olmstead v. L.C.*, 1999), Iowa (plaintiff, *Conner v. Branstad*, 1986), and Oregon (plaintiff intervenor, *United States v. Oregon*, 1987). Nationwide, Protection and Advocacy agencies are currently involved in more than 30 cases related to community integration, rights violations in facilities, and access to housing in the community for

Table 2.18
FISCAL EFFORT FOR PEOPLE WITH DEVELOPMENTAL DISABILITIES
AND RIGHT TO HABILITATION CLASS-ACTION LITIGATION

Rank[1]	State	Class Action Litigation Filed	State ARC Involvement
1	Rhode Island	*Iasimone v. Garrahy* 1977	Court Monitor
2	Maine	*Wouri et al. v. Zitnay* 1975	No Official Role
3	New York	*New York State ARC v. Rockefeller* 1972	Plaintiff
4	North Dakota	*ARC of North Dakota v. Olson* 1980	Plaintiff
5	Vermont	*In re Brace* (Judicial Review) 1978	No Official Role
6	Minnesota	*Welsch v. Likins* 1972	Plaintiff
7	District of Columbia	*Evans v. Washington* 1976	Court Monitor
8	Connecticut	*Connecticut ARC v. Thorne* 1978	Plaintiff NARC was Amicus Curiae
9	Wyoming	*Weston v. Wyoming* 1990	ARC participated in the consent decree, monitoring
10	West Virginia	*Medley v. Ginsberg* 1980	Plaintiff

[1]State community services fiscal effort rank in 2000 (Table 2.16).

persons with developmental disabilities (National Association of Protection and Advocacy Systems, 2000).

Litigation in the States

During the 1970s and 1980s, federal class-action lawsuits were used by advocates to improve conditions in public institutions in many states. Judge Frank Johnson issued a landmark decision in the *Wyatt v. Stickney* case, filed in 1970, establishing minimum standards for treatment and habilitation in state facilities for people with mental illness and/or mental retardation. After 30 years, a settlement agreement has been signed which will implement a three-year plan to downsize state facilities and expand community services in Alabama. Clearly, litigation continues to influence the delivery of MR/DD services in the states.

In the late 1990s, three types of class-action litigation emerged in the states: Lawsuits filed to force states to expand services to people on waiting lists; lawsuits filed to force states to meet the requirements of the *Olmstead* decision; and lawsuits filed on behalf of individuals who had been found eligible for Medicaid services, but did not receive them. As of March 2002, 22 waiting list lawsuits, 9 *Olmstead* lawsuits, and eight Medicaid access lawsuits have been filed

(Smith, 2002).

The most significant waiting list lawsuit to date was decided by a federal district court in Florida. In *Doe v. Bush*, the state was directed to develop a plan to serve 600 children and adults with developmental disabilities on the state's ICF/MR waiting list. In *Doe v. Bush,* the state was found to have a responsibility to provide services to Medicaid recipients with developmental disabilities with "reasonable promptness," which the court stipulated must occur within 90 days. The defendants in *Doe v. Bush* lost both in federal district court, and on appeal in the 11th Circuit ("Waiting List Suit," 1999).

Advocates in other states, inspired by *Doe v. Bush,* have filed their own suits, and have frequently borrowed the language of the Florida court in seeking remedies. As of March 2002, waiting list lawsuits have been filed in Alabama, Alaska, Colorado, Connecticut, Florida, Hawaii, Illinois, Kentucky, Maine, Massachusetts, Montana, New Hampshire, New Mexico, Ohio, Oregon, Pennsylvania, Tennessee, (2 cases), Virginia, Washington, and West Virginia (*Table 2.19*).

Decisions or settlements in waiting list lawsuits have been reached in Massachusetts, Oregon, Virginia, Florida, West Virginia, Washington, and Hawaii

(Smith, 2002). Generally, these settlements stipulate how the needs of the class will be met, and have called for the phased-in expansion of services in the states. For instance, a settlement in *Makin et al. v. State of Hawaii* was obtained in August 2000. The settlement called for a near two-fold expansion of HCBS Waiver participants from 1,087 in 2000 to nearly 2000 by July 1, 2003. The settlement reached in the Massachusetts waiting list lawsuit compels the Commonwealth to provide services to all wait-listed individuals, an estimated 2,800 persons, by fiscal year 2006 (National Association of State DD Directors, 2001a). This would entail a more than 20% increase in the Commonwealth's out-of-home residential service system. In Oregon, a settlement reached in October 2000 requires the State to provide community services or supports to over 5,000 people over six years (National Association of State DD Directors, 2000). This would represent more than two-times the capacity of the Oregon out-of-home residential system in 2000 (4,562 persons).

Olmstead lawsuits have been filed in the eight states of California, Florida, Indiana, Kentucky, Louisiana, Massachusetts, Michigan (2 cases), and New Hampshire. Lawsuits seeking Medicaid services for individuals previously determined to be eligible have been filed in the states of Arizona, California, Florida, Louisiana, Maine, Pennsylvania, Texas, and West Virginia. Settlement agreements had not been reached in any

Table 2.19
COMMUNITY SERVICES LITIGATION

State	Lawsuit	Issue
Alabama	*Susan J. et al. v. Siegelman et al.*	waiting list
Alaska	*Carpenter et al. v. Alaska Department of Health and Social Services*	waiting list
Arizona	*Ball et al v. Biedess et al.*	access to Medicaid benefits
California	*Sanchez et al. v. Johnson et al.*	access to Medicaid benefits
	Capitol People First et al. v. California Department of Developmental Disabilities et al.	Olmstead
Colorado	*Mandy R. et al. v. Owens et al.*	waiting list
Connecticut	*ARC/Connecticut v. O'Meara and Wilson-Coker*	waiting list
Florida	*John/Jane Doe v. Bush et al.*	waiting list
	Wolf Prado-Steiman et al. v. Bush et al.	waiting list access to Medicaid benefits
	Brown et al. v. Bush et al.	Olmstead
Hawaii	*Makin et al. v. State of Hawaii*	waiting list
Illinois	*Boudreau et al. v. Ryan et al.*	waiting list
Indiana	*Inch et. al. v. Humphrey and Griffin*	Olmstead
Kentucky	*Doe v. Kentucky Cabinet for Human Services*	Olmstead
	Michelle P. et al. v. Morgan et al.	waiting list
Louisiana	*Barthelemy et al. v. Louisiana Department of Health and Hospitals*	Olmstead
	Malen v. Hood	access to Medicaid benefits
Maine	*Rancourt et al. v. Maine Department of Human Services et al.*	waiting list
	Risinger et al. v. Concannon et al.	access to Medicaid benefits
Massachusetts	*Boulet et al. v. Cellucci et al.*	waiting list
	Rolland et al. v. Cellucci et al.	Olmstead
Michigan	*Olesky et al. v. Haveman et al.*	Olmstead
	Eager et al. v. Engler and Haveman	Olmstead
Montana	*Travis D. et al. v. Eastmont Human Services Center*	waiting list
New Hampshire	*Bryson Shepardson et al. v. Shumway and Fox*	Olmstead
	Harris et al. v. Shaheen et al.	waiting list
New Mexico	*Lewis et al. v. New Mexico Department of Health et al.*	waiting list
Ohio	*Martin et al. v. Taft et al.*	waiting list
Oregon	*Staley et al. v Kitzhaber et al.*	waiting list
Pennsylvania	*Gross et al. v. Houston*	waiting list
	Network for Quality Mental Retardation Services in Pennsylvania v. Department of Public Welfare Access to Medicaid Services	waiting list
Tennessee	*Brown et al. v. The Tennessee Department of Mental Health and Developmental Disabilities and Rukeyser*	waiting list
	People First of Tennessee v. Neal et al.	waiting list
Texas	*Private Povider Association of Texas v. Texas Health Human Services Commission et al.*	access to Medicaid benefits
Virginia	*Quibuyen v. Allen and Smith*	waiting list
Washington	*The Arc of Washington State et al. v. Lyle Quasim et al.*	waiting list
West Virginia	*Benjamin H. et al. v. Ohl*	waiting list access to Medicaid benefits

Source: Smith, G. A. (2002, March). *Status report: Litigation concerning Medicaid services for persons with developmental disabilities*. Tualatin, OR: Human Services Research Institute.

these cases as we went to press.

Settlement agreements have been reached in Louisiana, which compels the state to provide personal care and other services for Medicaid-eligible adults who would otherwise go into nursing homes. In addition, the settlement stipulated that people waiting for services could not wait longer than 90 days after being found eligible (*Barthelemy et al. v. Louisiana Department of Health and Hospitals,* 2001).

Since the *Olmstead* decision, however, some states have challenged the constitutionality of the Americans with Disabilities Act itself, and this battleground could have significant implications for people with developmental disabilities and the services that states fund for them. The Supreme Court ruled in February 2001 that suits attempting to recover monetary damages from states are barred by the Eleventh Amendment *(Board of Trustees of the University of Alabama et al. v. Garrett et al.,* 2001). While this case did not directly address individuals with developmental disabilities, it was a direct challenge to the constitutionality of the ADA, and was widely perceived by advocates to be a setback. The United States Supreme Court heard oral arguments in November 2001 on new ADA cases. If the Court takes measures to limit the ADA, states may feel less obliged to address the Act's integration mandate.

Class-action litigation was a powerful force in compelling many states to improve the quality of MR/DD services in the states. It will be critical to evaluate the impact of these waiting list cases and related Medicaid services cases as they develop in the months ahead.

REFERENCES

1998 summary of state legislation. (1999). *Community Services Reporter, 6*(2), 9.

Agosta, J. M., & Bradley, V. J. (Eds.). (1985). *Family care for persons with developmental disabilities: A growing commitment.* Cambridge, MA: Human Services Research Institute.

The Arc of Illinois. (1999, June 11). Wages & waiting lists. *The Arc of Illinois-Today,* p. 1. Springfield, IL: Author.

The Arc of the United States. (1997). *Budget reconciliation.* (Memorandum to state chapters of July 31st). Washington, DC: Author.

Association of Developmental Disabilities Providers. (1999). *The crisis in care for people with disabilities: A system of care at the breaking point.* A position paper of the Association. Waltham, MA: Author.

Bahl, R. (1982). Fiscal health of state and local governments: 1982 and beyond. *Public Budgeting and Finance, 2,* 5-21.

Barthelemy et al. v. Louisiana Department of Health and Hospitals, 2001

Bauer, L., & Smith, G. (1993). Community living for the developmentally disabled. *State Legislative Report* (An information service of the National Conference of State Legislatures), *18*(12), 1-6.

Blanck, P. (1998). *The emerging workforce: Employment integration, economic opportunity, and the Americans with Disabilities Act; Empirical study from 1990-1996.* Washington, DC: American Association on Mental Retardation.

Board of Trustees of the University of Alabama et al. v. Garrett et al., 2001

Braddock, D. (1986). Federal assistance for mental retardation and developmental disabilities: II. The modern era. *Mental Retardation, 24,* 175-182.

Braddock, D. (1987). *Federal policy toward mental retardation and developmental disabilities.* Baltimore: Brookes.

Braddock, D. (1999). Aging and developmental disabilities: Demographic and policy issues affecting American families. *Mental Retardation, 37,* 155-161.

Braddock, D. (in press). Public financial support for disability at the dawn of the 21st century. *American Journal on Mental Retardation.*

Braddock, D., & Fujiura, G. (1987). State government financial effort in mental retardation. *American Journal of Mental Deficiency, 91*(5), 450-459.

Braddock, D., & Fujiura, G. (1991). Politics, public policy, and the development of community mental retardation services in the United States. *American Journal on Mental Retardation, 95*(4), 369-387.

Braddock, D., & Heller, T. (1985). The closure of mental retardation institutions: I. Trends in the United States. *Mental Retardation, 23,* 168-176.

Braddock, D., & Hemp, R. (1996). Medicaid spending reductions and developmental disabilities. *Journal of Disability Policy Studies, 7*(1), 1-32.

Braddock, D., Hemp, R., Bachelder, L., & Fujiura, G. T. (1995). *The state of the states in developmental disabilities* (4th ed.). Washington: American Association on Mental Retardation.

Braddock, D., Hemp, R., & Fujiura, G. T. (1986). *Public expenditures for mental retardation and developmental disabilities in the United States: State profiles* (2nd ed.). Chicago: University of Illinois at Chicago, Institute for the Study of Developmental Disabilities.

Braddock, D., Hemp, R., & Fujiura, G. T. (1987). National study of public spending for mental retardation and developmental disabilities. *American Journal of Mental Deficiency, 92,* 121-133.

Braddock, D., Hemp, R., Fujiura, G. T., Bachelder, L., & Mitchell, D. (1990). *The state of the states in developmental disabilities.* Baltimore: Brookes.

Braddock, D., Hemp, R., & Howes, R. (1984). *Public expenditures for mental retardation and developmental disabilities in the United States: State profiles* (1st ed.). Chicago: University of Illinois at Chicago, Institute for the Study of Developmental Disabilities.

Braddock, D., Hemp, R., Parish, S., & Westrich, J. (1998). *The state of the states in developmental disabilities* (5th ed.). Washington, DC: American Association on Mental Retardation.

Braddock, D., Hemp, R. Parish, S., & Rizzolo, M. C. (2000). *The state of the states in developmental disabilities: 2000 study summary.* Chicago: University of Illinois at Chicago, Department of Disability and Human Development.

Bureau of Economic Analyisis. (2001, June 4). *Regional accounts data, Gross State Product Data, 1977-00.* Washington, DC: Author. Available at: http://www.bea.doc.gov/regional/gsp/action.cfm

Bureau of Economic Analysis. (2002). *National accounts data: Current-dollar and "real" GDP, 1929-00.* Washington, DC: Author.

Caiden, N. (1978) *Collection of data on public expenditures for care of the mentally disabled.* (Memorandum prepared for Commission on the Mentally Disabled). Washington, DC: American Bar Association, Division of Public Service Activities.

Coffelt v. Department of Developmental Servs., No. 91-6401 (Cal. Super. Ct. Jan.19, 1994), 18 MPDLR 185.

Connecticut budget focuses on waiting lists and young adults. (1999). *Community Services Reporter, 6*(4), 2.

Conner v. Branstad, No. 4-86-CV-30871 (S.D. Iowa, 1993), 839 F. Supp. 1346 (S.D. Iowa, 1993).

Correlation between wages, turnover and quality examined in PA. (1999). *Community Services Reporter, 6*(4), 6-7.

Davis, S. (1997, November). *A status report to the nation on people with mental retardation waiting for community services.* Arlington, TX: The Arc of the United States.

Declaration of self-determination. (1998). *Common Sense, 1*(1), 4 (publication of the National Program Office on Self-Determination).

District of Columbia Auditor. (2000, December 18). *Cost of care for the District's mentally retarded and developmentally disabled exceeded $300 million over a three-year period.* Washington, DC: Author. Available at: http://www.dcwatch.com/auditor/audit030.htm

Doe v. Bush (U.S. 11th Cir., 2001).

Dybwad, G., & Bersani, H. (Eds.). (1996). *New voices: Self-advocacy by people with disabilities.* Cambridge, MA: Brookline Books.

Eckl, C., & Perez, A. (2001, August). *State budget & tax actions 2001. Preliminary report: Executive summary.* Denver, CO: National Conference of State Legislatures. Available at: http://www.ncsl.org/programs/fiscal/presbta01.htm

Fujiura, G. T. (1998). Demography of family households. *American Journal on Mental Retardation, 103,* 225-235.

Fujiura, G. T., Garza, J., & Braddock, D. (1990). *National survey of family support services in developmental disabilities.* Chicago: University of Illinois at Chicago, University Affiliated Program in Developmental Disabilities.

Harrington, C., Carrillo, H., Thollaug, S. C., Summers, P.R., & Wellin, V. (2000, October). *Nursing facilities, staffing, residents, and facility deficiencies, 1993 through 1999.* San Francisco: University of California – San Francisco, Department of Social and Behavioral Sciences.

Hayden, M. F. (1997, May-June). Class-action, civil rights litigation for institutionalized persons with mental retardation and other developmental disabilities: A review. *Mental and Physical Disabilities Law Reporter,* pp. 411-423.

Hayden, M. F., & DePaepe, P. (1994). Waiting for community services: The impact on persons with mental retardation and other developmental disabilities. In M. F. Hayden & B. H. Abery (Eds.), *Challenges for a service system in transition: Ensuring quality community experiences for persons with developmental disabilities* (pp. 173-206). Baltimore:Brookes.

Hayden, M. F., & Senese, D. (1996). *Self-advocacy groups: 1996 directory for North America.* Minneapolis: University of Minnesota, Research and Training Center on Community Living, Institute on Community Integration.

Helms, B. J., Moore, S. C., & McSewyn, C. A. (1991). Supported employment in Connecticut: An examination of integration and wage outcomes. *Career Development of Exceptional Individuals, 14,* 159-166.

Hemp, R., Braddock, D., Parish, S., & Smith, G. A. (2001). Leveraging federal funding in the states to address *Olmstead* and growing waiting lists. *Mental Retardation, 39*, 241-243.

Herman, S. E. (1991). Use and impact of a cash subsidy program. *Mental Retardation, 29*, 253-258.

Herr, S. S. (1983). *Rights and advocacy for retarded people*. Lexington, MA: D.C. Heath.

Herr, S. S. (1992). Beyond benevolence: Legal protection for persons with special needs. In L. Rowitz (Ed.), *Mental retardation in the year 2000* (pp. 279-298). New York: Springer-Verlag.

Hill, M., & Wehman, P. (1983). Cost benefit analysis of placing moderately and severely handicapped individuals into competitive employment. *Journal of the Association for Persons with Severe Handicaps, 8*, 30-38.

Homeward Bound v. Hissom Mem'l Ctr., No. 85-C-437-E (N.D. Okla. Jan. 12, 1990), 14 MPDLR 133.

Janicki, M. P. (1996, Fall). Longevity increasing among older adults with an intellectual disability. *Aging, Health, & Society, 2, 2.*

Janicki, M. P., Dalton, A. J., Henderson, C. M., & Davidson, P. W. (1999). Mortality and morbidity among older adults with intellectual disability: Health service considerations. *Disability & Rehabilitation, 21*(5/6), 284-294

Karan, O. C., Granfield, J. M., & Furey, E. M. (1992). Supported living: Rethinking the rules of residential services. *AAMR News and Notes, 5*(1), 5.

Kennedy, M. J. (1990). What quality assurance means to me: Expectations of consumers. In V.J. Bradley & H.A. Bersani (Eds.), *Quality assurance for individuals with developmental disabilities: It's everybody's business* (pp. 35-45). Baltimore: Brookes.

Key, V. O., Jr. (1949) *Southern politics in state and nation*. New York: Knopf.

Kregel, J., Wehman, P., & Banks, P. D. (1989). The effects of consumer characteristics and type of employment model on individual outcomes in supported employment. *Journal of Applied Behavior Analysis, 22*, 407-415.

Lagomarcino, T. R. (1986). Community services: Using the supported work model with an adult service agency. In F. R. Rusch (Ed.), *Competitive employment: Issues and strategies*. Baltimore: Brookes.

Lakin, K. C. (1998). Perspectives. On the outside looking in: Attending to waiting lists in systems of services for people with developmental disabilities. *Mental Retardation, 36*, 157-162.

Larson, S. A., Hewitt, A., & Lakin, K .C. (1994). Residential services personnel: Recruitment, training, and retention. In M. F. Hayden & B. Abery (Eds.), *Community living for persons with mental retardation and related conditions* (pp. 313-341). Baltimore: Brookes.

Larson, S. A., Lakin, K. C., Anderson, L., Kwak, N., Lee, J., & Anderson, D. (2001). Prevalence of mental retardation and developmental disabilities: Estimates from the 1994/1995 National Health Interview Survey Disability Supplements. *American Journal of Mental Retardation, 106*(3), 231-252.

Larson, S. A., Lakin, K. C., & Bruininks, R. H. (1998). *Staff recruitment and retention: Study results and intervention strategies*. Washington, DC: American Association on Mental Retardation.

Longhurst, N. (1994). *The self-advocacy movement by persons with developmental disabilities: A demographic study and directory of groups in the United Sates*. Washington, DC, and Chicago: American Association on Mental Retardation, in cooperation with People First of Illinois and the Institute on Disability and Human Development (UAP).

Louisiana maps out system change strategy. (1998). *Community Services Reporter, 5*(3), 3, 7.

Makin v. Hawaii, D. Haw. 1999.

Massachusetts to cut waiting list. (1998). *Community Services Reporter, 5*(10), 2-3.

McGaughey, M. J., Kiernan, W. E., McNally, L. C., & Gilmore, D.S. (1995). A peaceful coexistence? State MR/DD agency trends in integrated employment and facility-based services. *Mental Retardation, 33*, 170-179.

Meyers, J. C., & Marcenko, M. O. (1989). Impact of a cash subsidy program for families of children with severe developmental disabilities. *Mental Retardation, 27*, 383-387.

Michigan's revised Mental Health Code makes sweeping changes. (1996). *Community Services Reporter, 3*(6), 8-9.

Mitchell, D., & Braddock, D. (1993). Compensation and turnover of direct care staff in developmental disabilities residential facilities in the United States: I. Wages and benefits. *Mental Retardation, 31*, 429-437.

National Association of Protection and Advocacy Systems. (2000, Winter). *Docket of significant protection and advocacy cases related to community integration.* Washington, DC: Author.

National Association of State Budget Officers. (2001a, September 25). *Fiscal update – State budgets, post-attacks.* Washington, DC: Author. Available at: http://www.nasbo.org

National Association of State Budget Officers. (2001b, November). *State budgets – update.* Washington, DC: Author. Available at: http://www.nasbo.org

National Association of State DD Directors. (2000, October). Oregon settles waiting list lawsuit. *Community Services Reporter, 7*(10), 1, 6.

National Association of State DD Directors. (2001a, February). Massachusetts settles waiting list lawsuit. *Community Services Reporter, 8*(2), 1, 5-6.

National Association of State DD Directors. (2001b, June). Maryland governor signs wage parity measure. *Community Services Reporter, 8*(2), 1, 5-6.

Nelis, T. (1995). The realities of institutions. *Impact, 9*(1), 1, 27. Minneapolis: University of Minnesota, Institute on Community Integration.

Nelis, T., & Ward. N. (1995). Operation Close the Doors: Working for freedom. *Impact, 9*, 12. Minneapolis: University of Minnesota, Institute on Community Integration.

Nerney, T. (1999). *Synopsis of the self-determination initiative for people with developmental disabilities.* Durham: University of New Hampshire, Institute on Disability, National Program Office on Self-Determination.

New Jersey continues ten-year plan to eliminate community waiting list. (2000, February). *Community Services Reporter, 7*(2), 6.

New Jersey Department of Human Services. (1998). *A plan to eliminate the waiting list for community residential services by 2008.* Trenton, NJ: Division of Developmental Disabilities' Waiting List Planning Work Group.

New person-centered system to expand consumer choice in SC. (1998). *Community Services Reporter, 5*(9), 6.

North Carolina Division makes commitment to self-determination pilots. (1999). *Community Services Reporter, 6*(5), 8.

Ohio requests expansion of Waiver resources to cut MR/DD waiting list. (2000, December). *Community Services Reporter, 7*(12), 5.

Olmstead v. L.C., 119 S. Ct. 2176 (1999).

Parish, S. L., Pomeranz, A., Hemp, R., Rizzolo, M. C., & Braddock, D. (2001, June). Family support for families of persons with developmental disabilities in the U.S.: Status and trends. *Policy Research Brief, 12*(2), 1-12 [University of Minnesota].

Paving the road to individual choice in Alaska. (1997). *Community Services Reporter, 4*(11), 7.

Pittsley, R. (1990). North Dakota: Individualized supported living arrangement. *DD Network News, 3*(3), 7-8.

Prouty, R. W., & Lakin, K. C. (2000, May). *Residential services for persons with developmental disabilities: Status and trends through 1999.* Minneapolis: University of Minnesota, College of Education and Human Development, Institute on Community Integration, Research and Training Center on Community Living.

Prouty, R. W., Smith G., & Lakin, K. C. (2001, June). *Residential services for persons with developmental disabilities: Status and trends through 2000.* Minneapolis: University of Minnesota, College of Education and Human Development, Institute on Community Integration, Research and Training Center on Community Living.

Pub. L. 97-35. (1981, July 31). Omnibus Budget Reconciliation Act 0f 1981.

Pub. L. 100-203. (1987, December 22). Omnibus Budget Reconciliation Act of 1987.

Pub. L. 101-336. (1990, July 26). Americans with Disabilities Act of 1990.

Pub. L. 101-508. (1990, October 27). Omnibus Budget Reconciliation Act of 1990.

Pub. L. 105-33.(1997, August 5). The Balanced Budget Act of 1997.

Pub. L. 106-170. (1999, December 17). Ticket to Work and Work Incentives Improvement Act.

Racino, J. A., & Taylor, S. J. (1993). "People first": Approaches to housing and support. In J.A. Racino, P. Walker, S. O'Connor, & S.J. Taylor (Eds.), *Housing, support, and community: Choices and strategies for adults with disabilities* (pp. 33-56). Baltimore: Brookes.

Ricci v. Okin, Civ. A. Nos. 72-0469-T, 74-2768-T, 75-3910-T, 75-5023-T and 75-5210-T (D. Mass.) 537 F. Supp. 817 (D. Mass. 1982); 97 F.R.D. 737 (1983); 576 F. Supp. 415 (D. Mass., 1983); 646 F. Supp. 378 (D. Mass., 1986); 781 F. Supp. 826 (D. Mass. 1992).

Rubin, S. S., Park, H. J., & Braddock, D. (1998). *Wages, benefits, and turnover of residential direct care staff serving individuals with developmental disabilities in Illinois.* Chicago: University of Illinois at Chicago, Department of Disability and Human Development.

Smith, G. A. (1990). *Supported living: New directions in services to people with developmental disabilities.* Alexandria, VA: National Association of State Mental Retardation Program Directors.

Smith, G. A. (1998). *Medicaid & system change: Finding the fit.* Alexandria, VA: National Association of State Directors of Developmental Disabilities Services.

Smith, G.A. (2002, March). *Status report: Litigation concerning Medicaid services for persons with developmental disabilities.* Tualatin, OR: Human Services Research Institute.

Smith, G. A., & Gettings, R. M. (1997, April). *Medicaid Home and Community-Based Waiver services and supports for people with developmental disabilities: Trends through 1997.* Alexandria, VA: National Association of State Directors of Developmental Disabilities Services.

Smith, G. A., Prouty, R., & Lakin, K. C. (2001). Medicaid long-term care services for people with developmental disabilities—That was then, this is now. *Mental Retardation, 39*, 488-491.

Smull, M. (1989). *Crisis in the community.* Baltimore: University of Maryland at Baltimore, Applied Research and Evaluation Unit, Department of Pediatrics, School of Medicine.

Starr, P. (1999, October 17). The return of health reform, *Washington Post.*

State Budget Highlights. (2000, February). *Community Services Reporter, 7*(2), 5.

Status of the Arc's legislative goals at end of first session of the 106th Congress. (1999, December 31). *Government Report, 29*(12), 1, 3-11.

Thompson, L., Powers, G., & Houchard, B. (1992). The wage effects of supported employment. *Journal of the Association for Persons with Severe Handicaps, 17*, 87-94.

U.S. Bureau of the Census. (1996, April). *Current population reports. Special studies (P23-190).* Washington, DC: U.S. Government Printing Office.

U.S. Bureau of the Census. (1997). *International data base.* Washington, DC: Bureau of the Census, International Programs Center, Information Resources Branch.

U.S. Census Bureau. (2000). *ST-98-40, Population estimates for states by age, sex, race, and Hispanic origin: July 1, 1998.* Available at: http://www.census.gov/population/estimates/state/st98elderly.txt

United States v. Oregon, 675 F. Supp. 1249 (D. Or. 1987), 12 MPDLR 253.

Utah plans person-centered reimbursement methodology. (1997). *Community Services Reporter, 4*(12), 1, 3.

Vogelsberg, R.T., Ashe, W., & Williams, W. (1985). Community based service delivery in a rural state: Issues for development and implementation. In R. Horner, L.M. Voeltz, & B. Fredericks (Eds.), *Education for learners with severe handicaps: Exemplary service strategies.* Baltimore: Brookes.

Wait list costs calculated annually in NH. (1997). *Community Services Reporter, 4*(8), 3.

Waiting list suit filed in Washington. (1999, December). *Community Services Reporter, 7*(12), 3, 6.

Wehman, P., West, M., & Kane-Johnston, K. (1997). Improving access to competitive employment for persons with disabilities as a means of reducing Social Security expenditures. *Focus on Autism and Other Developmental Disabilities, 12*(1), 23-30.

Wildavsky, A. (1974). *The politics of the budgetary process* (2nd ed.). Boston: Little, Brown.

Wyatt v. Stickney Wyatt v. Stickney 325 F. Supp 781(M.D. Ala.1971), 334 F. Supp. 1341 (M.D.Ala 1971), 344 F. Supp. 373 (M.D. Ala. 1972), sub nom Wyatt v. Aderholt, 503 F. 2d 1305 (5th Cir. 1974).

Zandi, M.M. (2001). *The outlook for state tax revenues.* West Chester, PA: Economy.com. Report commissioned by the National Governor's Association. Available at: http://www.nga.org

NOTES ON DATA SOURCES

Alabama. Data were provided by Anne Evans, Division of Mental Retardation, Department of Mental Health and Mental Retardation. Evans indicated that the numbers of nursing home residents with mental retardation and related condition reported for Alabama during FYs 1996-00 (791, 860, 930, 930, and 930), were substantially higher than the number of nursing home residents who were supported by the Department of Mental Health and Mental Retardation.

Alaska. Data were provided by Barbara Knapp, Division of Mental Health and Developmental Disabilities Central Office, Department of Health and Social Services. Data for prior years that had been based on estimates were substantially revised.

Arizona. Data were provided by Lynne Larson, Finance Manager, and by Kim Simmons, Division of Developmental Disabilities, Department of Economic Security. State officials concurred with our decision to exclude Arizona Long Term Care System (ALTCS) acute care medical services that had been reported in the category, community services' other Medicaid funding, for fiscal years 1990 through 1998.

Arkansas. Data were provided by Dennis Bonge, Fiscal Manager, and by Judy Routon, Grants Administration, Division of Developmental Disabilities, Department of Human Services.

California. Data were provided by Kathy Owen, Information Systems and Services Branch, Department of Developmental Services, and by Tom Graham, Department of Social Services. State officials confirmed the approximate 10% drop from 1998 to 2000 in federal Supplemental Security Income (SSI) State Supplement Payments for persons with developmental disabilities. This drop was primarily attributable to the California Needs Index that establishes the joint State Supplement and federal SSI monthly payment levels. During 1998 to 2000, the California Needs Index increased substantially less than did the federal SSI annual cost

of living adjustments; therefore State Supplement monthly payments declined.

Colorado. Data were provided by Lynne Struxness, Research Analyst, Program Evaluation and Information Services, Developmental Disabilities Services, Office of Health and Rehabilitation Services, Department of Human Services.

Connecticut. Data were provided by Lawrence Johnson, Management Information Group, Department of Mental Retardation.

Delaware. Data were provided by Lois Brown, Division of Mental Retardation, Department of Health and Social Services.

District of Columbia. Data were primarily obtained from information presented in the December 18, 2000, report of the District of Columbia Auditor entitled *Cost of Care for the District's Mentally Retarded and Developmentally Disabled Exceeded $300 Million Over a Three-Year Period*. Available at: http://www.dcwatch.com/auditor/audit030.htm

Florida. Data were provided by Amy Claiborne, Operations and Management Consultant, and by Susan Dickerson, Chief, Program Initiatives, Developmental Services, Department of Children and Families.

Georgia. Data were provided by Charles Hopkins, Mental Retardation Program Chief, and Sarah Hopper, Mental Retardation Program Specialist, Division of Mental Health, Mental Retardation, and Substance Abuse, Department of Human Resources.

Hawaii. Data were provided by David Kanno, Developmental Disabilities Division, Department of Health.

Idaho. Data were provided by Gary Baker, Diane Helton, and Ron Enright, Bureau of Developmental

Disabilities, Division of Family and Community Services, Department of Health and Welfare.

Illinois. Data were provided by Tom Armitage and Marie Havens, Office of Developmental Disabilities, Bureau of Disability and Behavioral Health, Department of Human Services.

Indiana. Data were provided by Ann January and Randy Krieble, Bureau of Developmental Disabilities Services Central Office, Department of Disability, Aging, and Rehabilitation Services, Family and Social Services Administration.

Iowa. Data were provided by Larry Allen, Division of Mental Health, Mental Retardation, and Developmental Disabilities, Department of Human Services.

Kansas. Data were provided by Becky Ross, Division of Health Care Policy, Department of Social and Rehabilitation Services.

Kentucky. Data were provided by Ray Anderson, Division of Mental Retardation, Department for Mental Health and Mental Retardation Services, Cabinet for Human Resources.

Louisiana. Data were provided by Christine Reeves, Josie Criscoe, Clinton Goff, Helene Robinson, and Ron Young, Director of Financial Services, Office of Citizens with Developmental Disabilities, Department of Health and Hospitals. There was a reduction in the amount of state funding previously reported for Jefferson Parish in 1997 and 1998.

Maine. Data were provided by David Goddu and Scott Pratt, Division of Mental Retardation, Department of Mental Health, Mental Retardation, and Substance Abuse Services. In 2000, the remaining institutional service in Maine, Aroostook Residential Center, served 11 individuals with mental retardation.

Maryland. Data were provided by Audrey Waters, Budget Director, Developmental Disabilities

Administration, Department of Health and Mental Hygiene.

Massachusetts. Data were provided by Ron Sanfield, Director of Evaluation, Department of Mental Retardation. There was a reduction in the number of supported living participants previously reported for 1997 and 1998.

Michigan. Data were provided by Judy Webb, Director, Division of Mental Health Quality, and Mark Hyllested, Department of Community Health.

Minnesota. Data were obtained by project staff from a variety of published documents provided by Laura Doyle, Division for Persons with Developmental Disabilities, Department of Human Services. Project staff used these published sources to complete the Minnesota data collection worksheets and to construct the Minnesota state profile of charts, tables, and a financial spreadsheet.

Mississippi. Data were provided by Glynne Kegley and Lisa Romine, Bureau of Mental Retardation, Department of Mental Health and by Bob Pilgrim and Louise Milton, Office of the Governor, Division of Medicaid.

Missouri. Data were provided by Jeff Grosvenor, Deputy Division Director of Administrative Services, by Gary Schanzmeyer, Fiscal and Administrative Manager, and by John Bright, Division of Mental Retardation and Developmental Disabilities, Department of Mental Health.

Montana. Data were provided by Janice Frisch, Developmental Disabilities Program, Department of Public Health and Human Services.

Nebraska. Data were provided by Frank Faughn, Grants and Cost Management Unit, Division of Developmental Disabilities, Department of Health and Human Services.

Nevada. Data were provided by Thomas Lee, Management Analyst, Developmental Services,

Division of Mental Hygiene and Mental Retardation, Department of Human Resources.

New Hampshire. Data were provided by Karen Kimball, Division of Developmental Disabilities, Department of Health and Human Services.

New Jersey. Data were provided by Bill Holloway, Division of Developmental Disabilities, Department of Human Services. The numbers of nursing home residents with mental retardation and related conditions receiving services from New Jersey Division of Developmental Disabilities during 1996-98 were 571, 617, and 553, respectively.

New Mexico. Data were provided by Marilyn Price, Deputy Director, Long Term Services Division, Department of Health.

New York. Data were provided by Alan Metevia and Paul Audino, Budget Office, Office of Mental Retardation and Developmental Disabilities. At the direction of the OMR/DD Commissioner's office, data were provided to project staff utilizing a "community services" definition that included residential programs serving fewer than 30 persons (i.e., 1 to 29 persons). We reconfigured their data sets to conform to our definition of community services as settings for 1 to 15 persons.

North Carolina. Data were provided by Laura Nuss and Maxine Terry, Division of Mental Health, Developmental Disabilities, and Substance Abuse Services, Department of Health and Human Services.

North Dakota. Data were provided by Mark Kolling, Director, and Vicci Pederson, Disabilities Services Division, Department of Human Services.

Ohio. Data were provided by Mary Beth Wickerham, Debbie Hoffine, and Matt Curran, Department of Mental Retardation and Developmental Disabilities.

Oklahoma. Data were provided by David Taylor, Developmental Disabilities Services Division, Department of Human Services.

Oregon. Data were provided by Keith Baker, Budget Analyst, and by Jeff Marshall, Developmental Disabilities Services, Mental Health and Developmental Disability Services Division, Department of Human Resources.

Pennsylvania. Data were provided by Mike Toth, Office of Mental Retardation, Department of Public Welfare.

Rhode Island. Data were provided by Brendan Mahoney, Joe Gould, and Camille LeTourneau, Division of Mental Retardation and Developmental Disabilities, Department of Mental Health, Retardation, and Hospitals. Spending and resident data for 1997-00 for the Tavares Facility, serving 25 persons, was reclassified from the category of public ICFs/MR for 15 or fewer persons to the category of private ICF/MR for 16 or more persons. The facility was operational prior to 1997, however data were not available.

South Carolina. Data were provided by Nancy Rumbaugh and Tom Waring, Mental Retardation Division, Department of Disabilities and Special Needs.

South Dakota. Data were provided by Edward Campbell, Management Analyst, Department of Human Services.

Tennessee. Data were provided by Lucia Beiler, Division of Mental Retardation Sevices, Department of Mental Health and Mental Retardation.

Texas. Data were provided by Mark Johnston and Ezekiel Harris, Department of Mental Health and Mental Retardation. State officials reported numbers of persons served and associated expenditures in the categories of 8 or fewer persons and 9-14 persons, slightly different than the project's categories of 6 or fewer persons and 7-15 persons. Project staff did not employ estimation to match Texas classification categories to the project's standard classification categories.

Utah. Data were provided by George Kelner and Paul Day, Division of Services for People with Disabilities and by Kent Roner, Director, Bureau of Financial Services, Division of Health Care Financing, Department of Health.

Vermont. Data were provided by June Bascom, Division of Developmental Services, Department of Developmental and Mental Health Services.

Virginia. Data were provided by Cheri Stierer, Office of Mental Retardation Services, Department of Mental Health, Mental Retardation, and Substance Abuse Services.

Washington. Data were provided by Rick Trosper, Lisa Weber, and John Stern, Division of Developmental Disabilities, Department of Social and Health Services.

West Virginia. Data were provided by Cynthia Beane, Division of Developmental Disabilities, Department of Health and Human Resources.

Wisconsin. Data were provided by Tom Swant, Department of Health and Family Services, and by Steve Stanek, Wisconsin Council on Developmental Disabilities.

Wyoming. Data were provided by Jon Fortune, Division of Developmental Disabilities, Department of Health.

NURSING FACILITY DATA

Representative nursing facility data were particularly difficult to collect from the states. Thus, a combination of sources was utilized to determine the numbers of persons with mental retardation and related developmental disabilities residing in non-specialized nursing homes in each of the states. Twenty-one states (AK, AL, AZ, GA, IN, KS, ME, MI, MO, MS, MT, NC, ND, NE, NH, NJ, NY, OH, PA, SC, and WI) reported the numbers of nursing home residents with MR/DD to State of the States in Developmental Disabilities project staff. Project staff estimated Oregon's nursing facility census on the basis of prior year's data.

Nursing facility data for 18 states (CA, CO, CT, FL, ID, IL, MD, MA, NV, OK, RI, SD, TN, TX, UT, VT, WV, and WY) were obtained from Prouty & Lakin (2000) for 1999 and from Prouty et al. (2001) for 2000. For Arkansas and Delaware, the 2000 figure was obtained from Prouty et al. (2001) and the 1999 figure was interpolated by State of the States project staff. The 2000 figure for Minnesota was available from Prouty et al. (2001) and the 1999 figure was available from Harrington et al. (2000). For seven states (HI, IA, KY, LA, NM, VA, and WA), data was obtained from Harrington et al. (2000). The 2000 figure for DC was obtained from the District of Columbia Auditor (2000). This number was used for 1999 as well.

A more detailed discussion of study methodology is available in the fifth edition of the *State of the States in Developmental Disabilities* (Braddock, Hemp, Parish, & Westrich, 1998).

State Profiles

TRENDS IN SPENDING

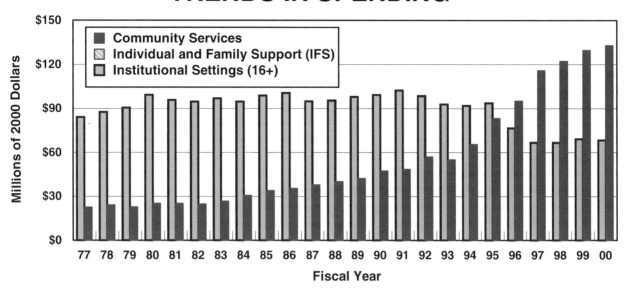

Millions of 2000 Dollars

- ■ Community Services
- ▨ Individual and Family Support (IFS)
- ▨ Institutional Settings (16+)

Fiscal Year

FISCAL EFFORT

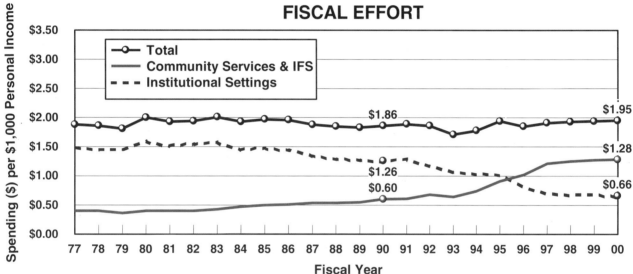

Spending ($) per $1,000 Personal Income

- —○— Total
- ——— Community Services & IFS
- - - - Institutional Settings

$1.86 $1.95

$1.26 $1.28

$0.60 $0.66

Fiscal Year

TOTAL MR/DD SPENDING AND
UNMATCHED STATE/LOCAL FUNDS

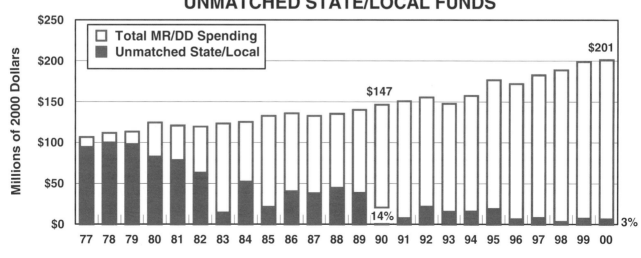

Millions of 2000 Dollars

- ☐ Total MR/DD Spending
- ■ Unmatched State/Local

$147 $201

14%   3%

Fiscal Year

Source: The Coleman Institute and Department of Psychiatry, University of Colorado, 2002.

TRENDS IN REVENUE

COMMUNITY SERVICES REVENUE IN 2000

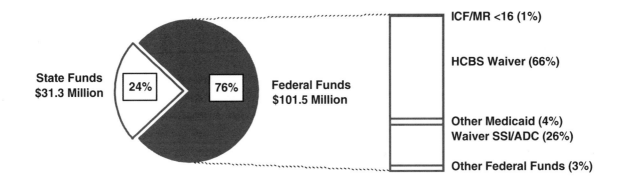

State Funds
$31.3 Million

24% **76%**

Federal Funds
$101.5 Million

ICF/MR <16 (1%)

HCBS Waiver (66%)

Other Medicaid (4%)
Waiver SSI/ADC (26%)

Other Federal Funds (3%)

Total: $132.8 Million

COMPONENTS OF FEDERAL MR/DD MEDICAID REVENUE

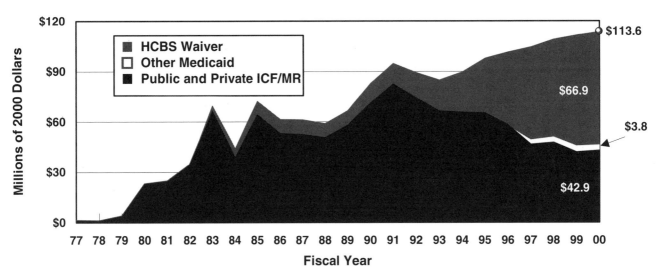

Millions of 2000 Dollars

- ■ HCBS Waiver
- □ Other Medicaid
- ■ Public and Private ICF/MR

$113.6

$66.9

$3.8

$42.9

Fiscal Year

HCBS WAIVER PARTICIPANTS

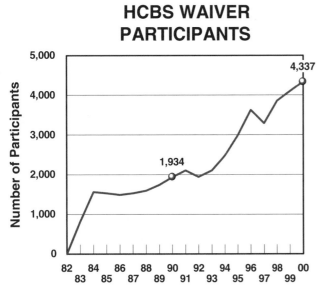

Number of Participants

4,337

1,934

WAIVER SPENDING PER PARTICIPANT

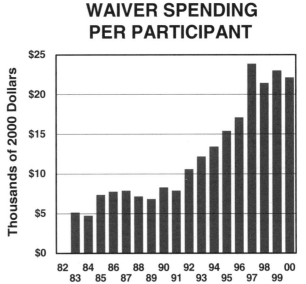

Thousands of 2000 Dollars

Source: The Coleman Institute and Department of Psychiatry, University of Colorado, 2002.

TRENDS IN RESIDENTIAL SERVICES

PERSONS SERVED BY SETTING IN 2000

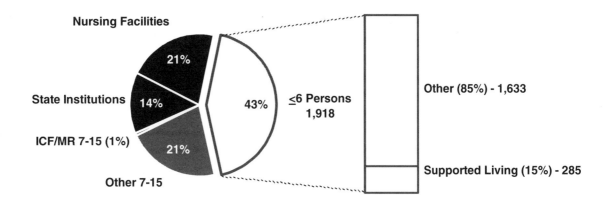

Nursing Facilities 21%

State Institutions 14%

ICF/MR 7-15 (1%)

Other 7-15 21%

≤6 Persons 1,918 43%

Other (85%) - 1,633

Supported Living (15%) - 285

Total: 4,441

PERSONS SERVED BY SETTING

	1990	1991	1992	1993	1994	1995	1996	1997	1998	1999	2000
TOTAL	3,571	3,444	3,753	3,141	3,056	3,192	3,252	3,282	3,387	3,909	4,441
16+ PERSONS	2,737	2,539	2,663	2,059	1,966	1,849	1,617	1,580	1,611	1,573	1,544
Nursing Facilities	1,429	1,321	1,401	849	838	863	791	860	930	930	930
State Institutions	1,308	1,218	1,262	1,210	1,128	986	826	720	681	643	614
Private ICF/MR	0	0	0	0	0	0	0	0	0	0	0
Other Residential	0	0	0	0	0	0	0	0	0	0	0
7-15 PERSONS	325	727	912	735	754	1,006	513	314	230	604	979
Public ICF/MR	0	0	0	0	0	0	0	0	0	0	0
Private ICF/MR	31	31	31	28	31	32	26	29	26	26	26
Other Residential	294	696	881	707	723	974	487	285	204	578	953
≤6 PERSONS	509	178	178	347	336	337	1,122	1,388	1,546	1,732	1,918
Public ICF/MR	0	0	0	0	0	0	0	0	0	0	0
Private ICF/MR	0	0	0	0	0	0	0	0	0	0	0
Other Residential	509	178	178	347	336	337	1,122	1,388	1,546	1,732	1,918

* The numbers of nursing facility residents with mental retardation and related conditions reported for Alabama during FYs 1996-98 (791, 860, and 930), are substantially higher than the number of nursing facility residents who require specialized supports and who are supported, in part, by the Department of Mental Health and Mental Retardation. FY 1998 nursing facility numbers were also used for FY 1999 and FY 2000.

PERSONS SERVED IN PUBLIC AND PRIVATE INSTITUTIONS AND NURSING FACILITIES

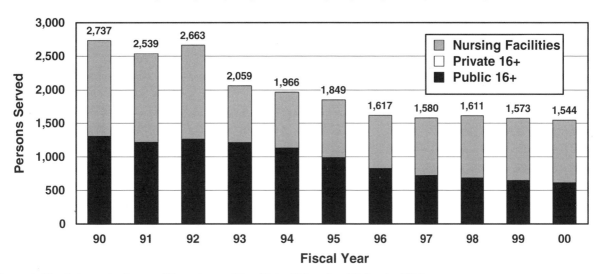

Source: The Coleman Institute and Department of Psychiatry, University of Colorado, 2002.

145

INDIVIDUAL AND FAMILY SUPPORT

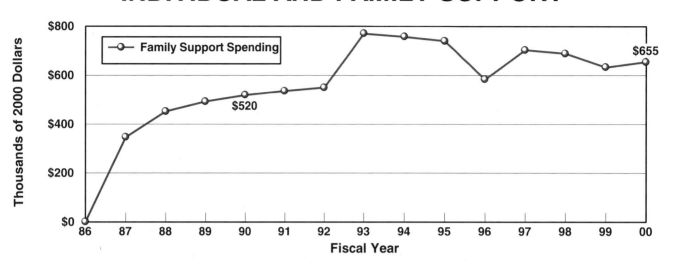

PARTICIPANTS AND SPENDING LEVELS

	1990	1991	1992	1993	1994	1995	1996	1997	1998	1999	2000
TOTAL IFS ($)	n/a	n/a	n/a	n/a	n/a	n/a	n/a	n/a	n/a	n/a	n/a
INDIVIDUAL SUPPORT ($)	n/a	n/a	n/a	n/a	n/a	n/a	n/a	n/a	n/a	n/a	n/a
Supported Employment ($)	na	na	na	na	na	na	na	na	na	na	na
# of Persons	156	183	228	322	464	570	543	229	229	286	348
Supported Living ($)	0	0	0	0	0	0	na	na	na	na	na
# of Persons	0	0	0	0	0	0	225	225	225	225	225
Personal Assistance ($)	0	0	0	na	na	na	na	na	na	na	na
# of Persons	0	0	0	34	36	39	50	63	60	60	60
FAMILY SUPPORT ($)	400,000	430,000	450,000	645,000	649,312	653,624	528,009	650,000	650,000	610,395	654,916
Total Families	3,677	3,722	3,907	3,498	3,804	3,747	2,953	2,500	2,800	2,800	2,800
Cash Subsidy/Payment ($)	0	0	0	0	0	0	0	0	0	0	0
# of Families	0	0	0	0	0	0	0	0	0	0	0
Other Family Support ($)	400,000	430,000	450,000	645,000	649,312	653,624	528,009	650,000	650,000	610,395	654,916
# of Families	3,677	3,722	3,907	3,498	3,804	3,747	2,953	2,500	2,800	2,800	2,800

PARTICIPANTS IN DAY/WORK AND SUPPORTED EMPLOYMENT

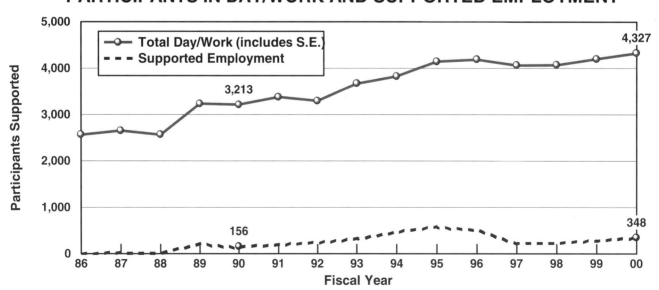

Source: The Coleman Institute and Department of Psychiatry, University of Colorado, 2002.

TRENDS IN SPENDING

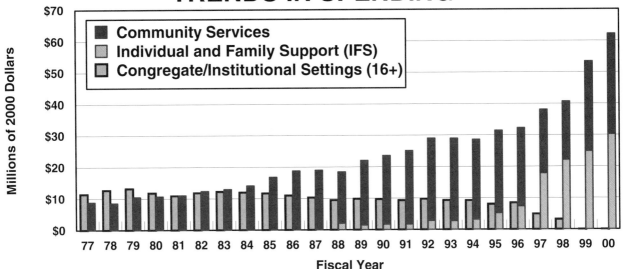

FISCAL EFFORT

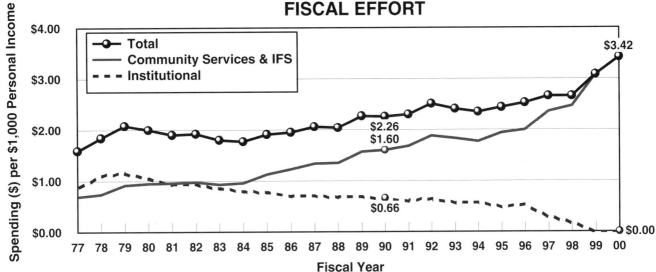

TOTAL MR/DD SPENDING AND
UNMATCHED STATE/LOCAL FUNDS

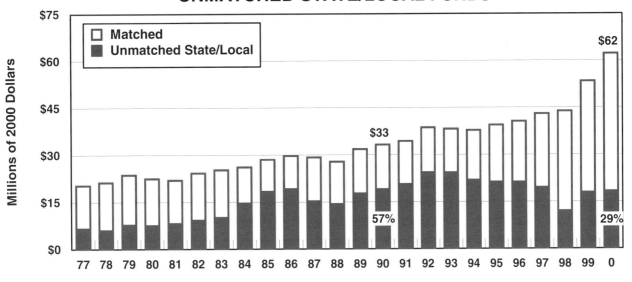

Source: The Coleman Institute and Department of Psychiatry, University of Colorado, 2002.

TRENDS IN REVENUE

COMMUNITY SERVICES REVENUE IN 2000

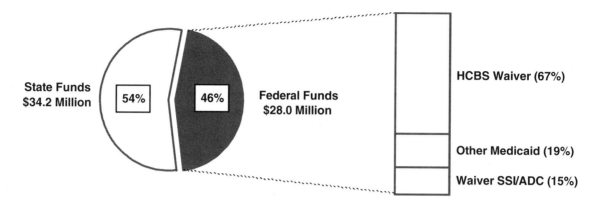

State Funds
$34.2 Million

54%

46%

Federal Funds
$28.0 Million

HCBS Waiver (67%)

Other Medicaid (19%)

Waiver SSI/ADC (15%)

Total: $62.2 Million

COMPONENTS OF FEDERAL MR/DD MEDICAID REVENUE

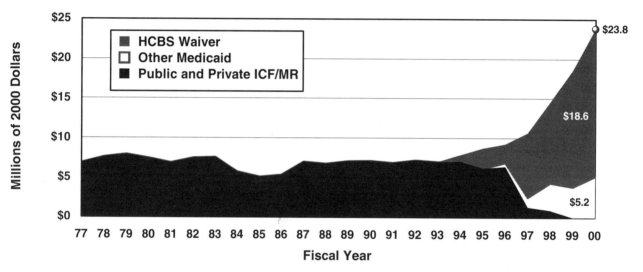

Millions of 2000 Dollars

- ■ HCBS Waiver
- □ Other Medicaid
- ■ Public and Private ICF/MR

$25

$20

$15

$10

$5

$0

$23.8

$18.6

$5.2

77 78 79 80 81 82 83 84 85 86 87 88 89 90 91 92 93 94 95 96 97 98 99 00

Fiscal Year

HCBS WAIVER PARTICIPANTS

WAIVER SPENDING PER PARTICIPANT

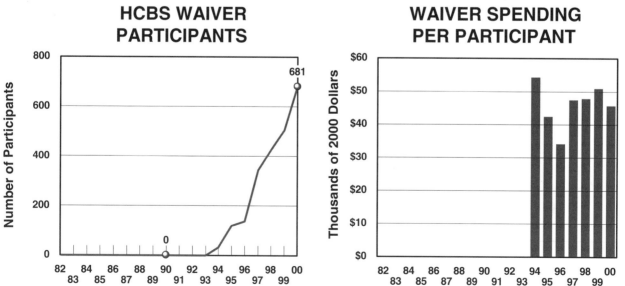

Number of Participants

800

600

400

200

0

681

0

82 84 86 88 90 92 94 96 98 00
83 85 87 89 91 93 95 97 99

Thousands of 2000 Dollars

$60

$50

$40

$30

$20

$10

$0

82 84 86 88 90 92 94 96 98 00
83 85 87 89 91 93 95 97 99

Source: The Coleman Institute and Department of Psychiatry, University of Colorado, 2002.

TRENDS IN RESIDENTIAL SERVICES

PERSONS SERVED BY SETTING IN 2000

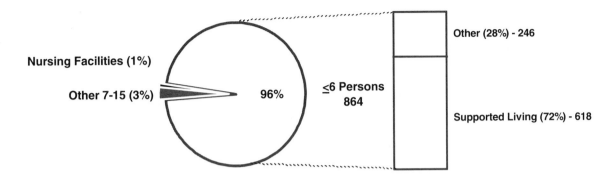

Nursing Facilities (1%)

Other 7-15 (3%)

96%

≤6 Persons
864

Other (28%) - 246

Supported Living (72%) - 618

Total: 895

PERSONS SERVED BY SETTING

	1990	1991	1992	1993	1994	1995	1996	1997	1998	1999	2000
TOTAL	n/a	n/a	446	444	454	499	533	686	768	744	895
16+ PERSONS	n/a	n/a	85	80	80	67	59	39	20	8	6
Nursing Facilities	n/a	n/a	38	35	35	35	31	19	10	8	6
State Institutions	57	53	47	45	45	32	28	20	10	0	0
Private ICF/MR	0	0	0	0	0	0	0	0	0	0	0
Other Residential	0	0	0	0	0	0	0	0	0	0	0
7-15 PERSONS	174	170	166	165	148	139	130	98	48	25	25
Public ICF/MR	54	50	46	44	37	28	19	10	0	0	0
Private ICF/MR	40	40	40	41	41	41	41	40	0	0	0
Other Residential	80	80	80	80	70	70	70	48	48	25	25
≤6 PERSONS	n/a	191	195	199	226	293	344	549	700	711	864
Public ICF/MR	0	0	0	0	0	0	0	0	0	0	0
Private ICF/MR	0	0	0	0	0	0	0	0	0	0	0
Other Residential	n/a	191	195	199	226	293	344	549	700	711	864

PERSONS SERVED IN PUBLIC AND PRIVATE INSTITUTIONS AND NURSING FACILITIES

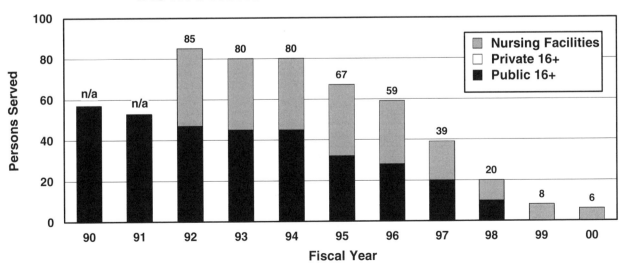

Source: The Coleman Institute and Department of Psychiatry, University of Colorado, 2002.

INDIVIDUAL AND FAMILY SUPPORT

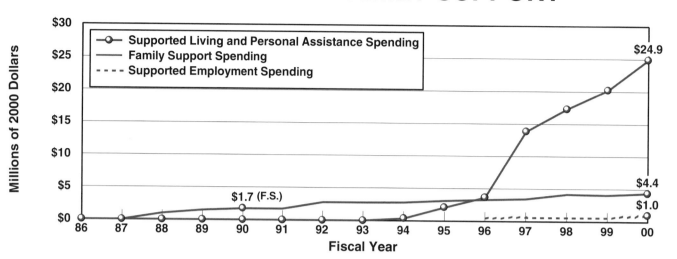

PERSONS SUPPORTED AND SPENDING LEVELS

	1990	1991	1992	1993	1994	1995	1996	1997	1998	1999	2000
TOTAL IFS ($)	1,330,944	1,403,638	2,271,542	2,310,743	2,726,998	4,574,875	6,622,121	16,491,108	20,850,927	23,971,711	30,238,020
INDIVIDUAL SUPPORT ($)	n/a	n/a	n/a	n/a	307,403	1,844,244	3,656,534	13,315,577	16,915,071	20,047,151	25,870,084
Supported Employment ($)	n/a	n/a	n/a	n/a	n/a	n/a	352,212	545,440	610,332	592,930	989,955
# of Persons	n/a	n/a	n/a	n/a	n/a	n/a	42	60	60	66	125
Supported Living ($)	0	0	0	0	307,403	1,844,244	3,230,159	12,578,505	16,038,463	19,154,086	24,540,721
# of Persons	0	0	0	0	21	83	120	306	443	442	578
Personal Assistance ($)	0	0	0	0	0	0	74,163	191,632	266,276	300,135	339,408
# of Persons	0	0	0	0	0	0	9	23	32	39	40
FAMILY SUPPORT ($)	1,330,944	1,403,638	2,271,542	2,310,743	2,419,595	2,730,631	2,965,587	3,175,531	3,935,856	3,924,560	4,367,936
Total Families	513	681	785	800	815	875	1,000	1,118	1,236	1,263	1,361
Cash Subsidy/Payment ($)	0	0	0	0	0	0	0	0	0	0	0
# of Families	0	0	0	0	0	0	0	0	0	0	0
Other Family Support ($)	1,330,944	1,403,638	2,271,542	2,310,743	2,419,595	2,730,631	2,965,587	3,175,531	3,935,856	3,924,560	4,367,936
# of Families	513	681	785	800	815	875	1,000	1,118	1,236	1,263	1,361

PARTICIPANTS IN DAY/WORK AND SUPPORTED EMPLOYMENT

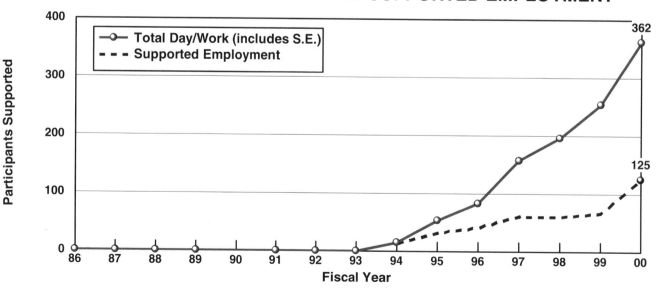

Source: The Coleman Institute and Department of Psychiatry, University of Colorado, 2002.

TRENDS IN SPENDING

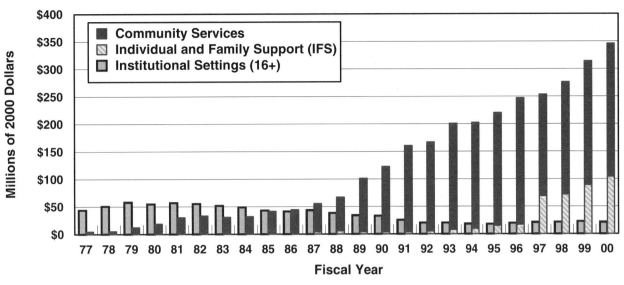

Millions of 2000 Dollars

- ■ Community Services
- ▨ Individual and Family Support (IFS)
- ▤ Institutional Settings (16+)

Fiscal Year

FISCAL EFFORT

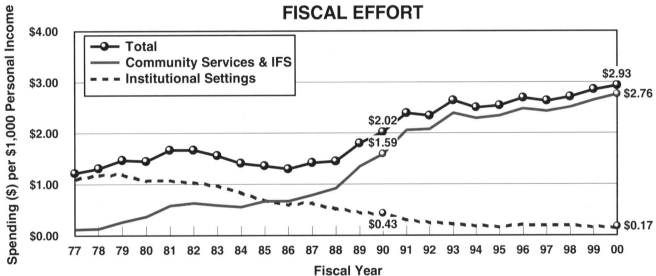

Spending ($) per $1,000 Personal Income

- —○— Total
- ——— Community Services & IFS
- - - - Institutional Settings

$2.93
$2.76
$2.02
$1.59
$0.43
$0.17

Fiscal Year

TOTAL MR/DD SPENDING AND
UNMATCHED STATE/LOCAL FUNDS

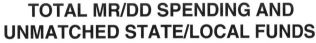

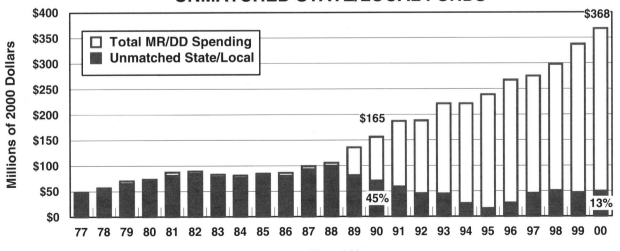

Millions of 2000 Dollars

- ☐ Total MR/DD Spending
- ■ Unmatched State/Local

$368
$165
45%
13%

Fiscal Year

Source: The Coleman Institute and Department of Psychiatry, University of Colorado, 2002.

TRENDS IN REVENUE

COMMUNITY SERVICES REVENUE IN 2000

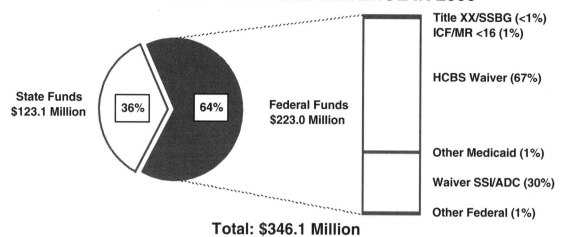

State Funds
$123.1 Million

36%

64%

Federal Funds
$223.0 Million

Title XX/SSBG (<1%)
ICF/MR <16 (1%)

HCBS Waiver (67%)

Other Medicaid (1%)

Waiver SSI/ADC (30%)

Other Federal (1%)

Total: $346.1 Million

COMPONENTS OF FEDERAL MR/DD MEDICAID REVENUE

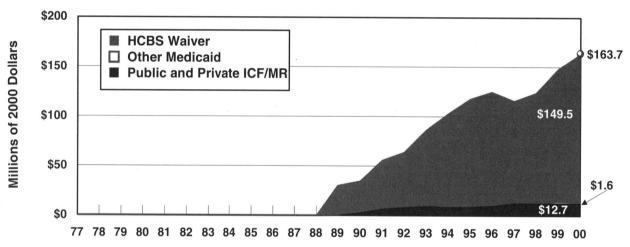

Millions of 2000 Dollars

- ■ HCBS Waiver
- □ Other Medicaid
- ■ Public and Private ICF/MR

$163.7

$149.5

$1.6

$12.7

Fiscal Year

HCBS WAIVER PARTICIPANTS

WAIVER SPENDING PER PARTICIPANT

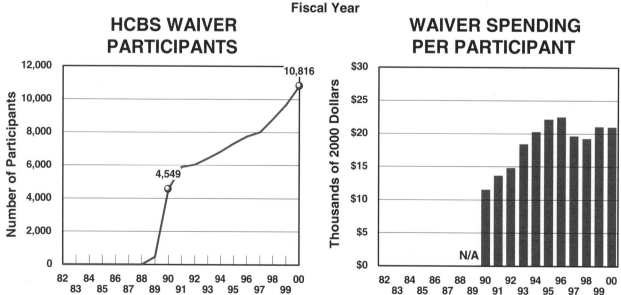

Number of Participants

10,816

4,549

Thousands of 2000 Dollars

N/A

Source: The Coleman Institute and Department of Psychiatry, University of Colorado, 2002.

TRENDS IN RESIDENTIAL SERVICES

PERSONS SERVED BY SETTING IN 2000

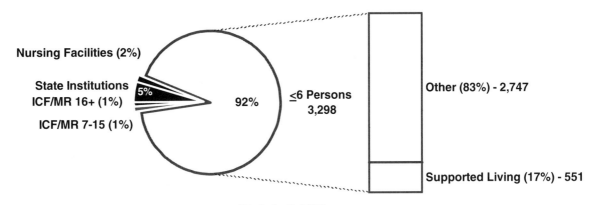

Nursing Facilities (2%)

State Institutions
ICF/MR 16+ (1%)

ICF/MR 7-15 (1%)

5%

92%

≤6 Persons
3,298

Other (83%) - 2,747

Supported Living (17%) - 551

Total: 3,598

PERSONS SERVED BY SETTING

	1990	1991	1992	1993	1994	1995	1996	1997	1998	1999	2000
TOTAL	1,938	2,154	2,170	2,444	2,574	2,694	2,668	2,936	3,193	3,537	3,598
16+ PERSONS	445	386	384	410	414	372	356	293	283	276	258
Nursing Facilities	48	47	58	85	90	76	67	50	57	62	57
State Institutions	366	310	298	287	276	248	243	196	179	174	166
Private ICF/MR	16	20	24	38	48	48	46	47	47	40	35
Other Residential	15	9	4	0	0	0	0	0	0	0	0
7-15 PERSONS	48	48	48	48	50	44	43	41	40	42	42
Public ICF/MR	48	48	48	48	50	44	43	41	40	42	42
Private ICF/MR	0	0	0	0	0	0	0	0	0	0	0
Other Residential	0	0	0	0	0	0	0	0	0	0	0
≤6 PERSONS	1,445	1,720	1,738	1,986	2,110	2,278	2,269	2,602	2,870	3,219	3,298
Public ICF/MR	0	0	0	0	0	0	0	0	0	0	0
Private ICF/MR	0	0	0	0	0	0	0	0	0	0	0
Other Residential	1,445	1,720	1,738	1,986	2,110	2,278	2,269	2,602	2,870	3,219	3,298

PERSONS SERVED IN PUBLIC AND PRIVATE INSTITUTIONS AND NURSING FACILITIES

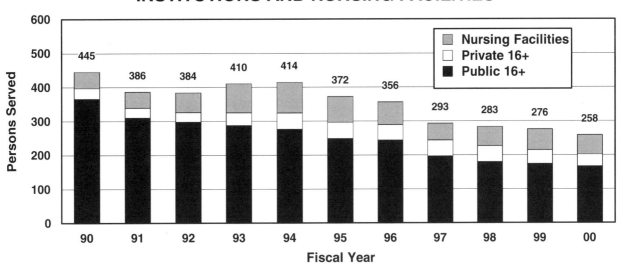

Persons Served

Nursing Facilities
Private 16+
Public 16+

445 386 384 410 414 372 356 293 283 276 258

Fiscal Year

Source: The Coleman Institute and Department of Psychiatry, University of Colorado, 2002.

INDIVIDUAL AND FAMILY SUPPORT

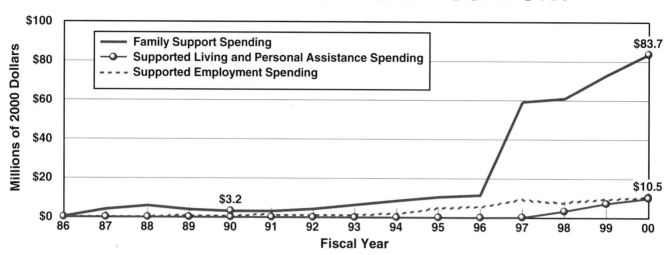

PARTICIPANTS AND SPENDING LEVELS

	1990	1991	1992	1993	1994	1995	1996	1997	1998	1999	2000
TOTAL IFS ($)	2,973,636	3,162,994	4,370,898	6,376,766	8,827,070	13,387,092	15,332,916	63,465,960	67,941,706	86,077,524	104,229,840
INDIVIDUAL SUPPORT ($)	546,259	725,781	907,698	1,092,009	1,589,176	4,144,917	4,927,507	8,729,183	10,406,816	15,836,938	20,522,501
Supported Employment ($)	546,259	725,781	907,698	1,092,009	1,589,176	4,144,917	4,927,507	8,503,183	7,181,900	8,809,690	10,478,354
# of Persons	155	205	254	304	570	1,489	1,219	1,412	1,336	1,011	1,133
Supported Living ($)	0	0	0	0	0	0	0	226,000	3,224,916	7,027,248	10,044,147
# of Persons	0	0	0	0	0	0	0	35	350	540	551
Personal Assistance ($)	0	0	0	0	0	0	0	0	0	0	0
# of Persons	0	0	0	0	0	0	0	0	0	0	0
FAMILY SUPPORT ($)	2,427,377	2,437,213	3,463,200	5,284,757	7,237,894	9,242,175	10,405,409	54,736,777	57,534,890	70,240,586	83,707,339
Total Families	2,808	3,243	3,357	3,944	5,358	5,885	6,618	9,194	10,373	13,579	13,188
Cash Subsidy/Payment ($)	413,200	463,200	463,200	549,800	603,500	578,900	761,814	615,914	591,178	635,031	886,136
# of Families	497	557	557	662	667	613	873	786	716	738	151
Other Family Support ($)	2,014,177	1,974,013	3,000,000	4,734,957	6,634,394	8,663,275	9,643,595	54,120,863	56,943,712	69,605,555	82,821,203
# of Families	2,311	2,686	2,800	3,282	4,691	5,272	5,745	8,408	9,657	12,841	13,037

PARTICIPANTS IN DAY/WORK AND SUPPORTED EMPLOYMENT

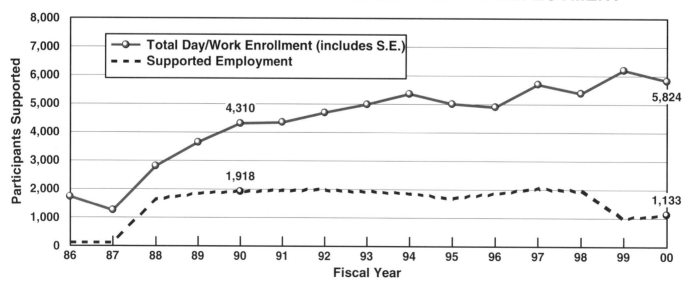

Source: The Coleman Institute and Department of Psychiatry, University of Colorado, 2002.

TRENDS IN SPENDING

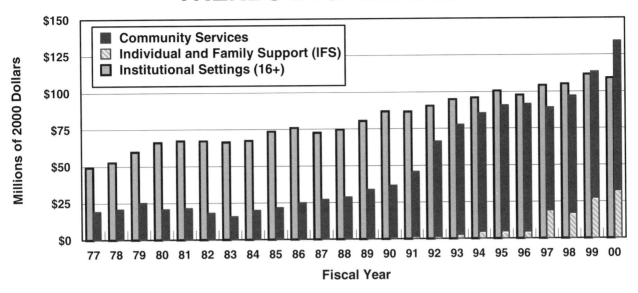

FISCAL EFFORT

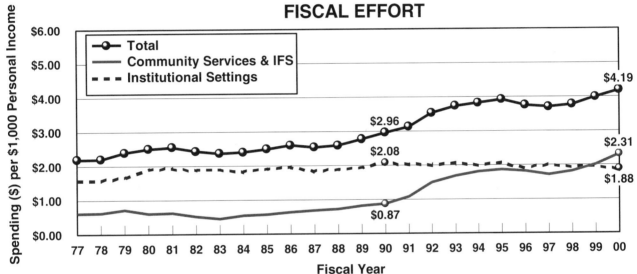

TOTAL MR/DD SPENDING AND
UNMATCHED STATE/LOCAL FUNDS

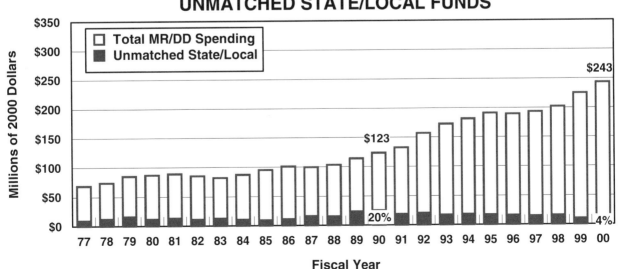

Source: The Coleman Institute and Department of Psychiatry, University of Colorado, 2002.

155

TRENDS IN REVENUE

COMMUNITY SERVICES REVENUE IN 2000

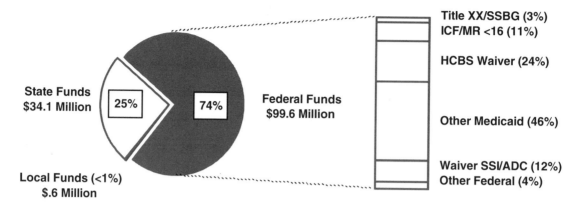

State Funds
$34.1 Million

25%

74%

Federal Funds
$99.6 Million

Local Funds (<1%)
$.6 Million

Title XX/SSBG (3%)
ICF/MR <16 (11%)

HCBS Waiver (24%)

Other Medicaid (46%)

Waiver SSI/ADC (12%)
Other Federal (4%)

Total: $134.2 Million

COMPONENTS OF FEDERAL MR/DD MEDICAID REVENUE

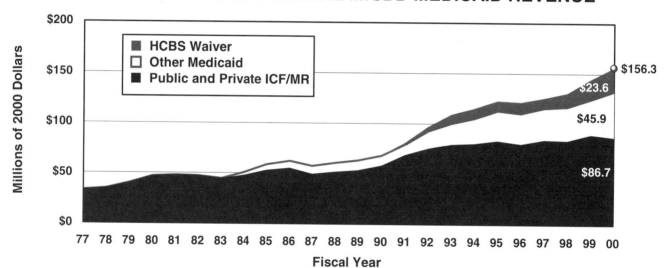

HCBS WAIVER PARTICIPANTS

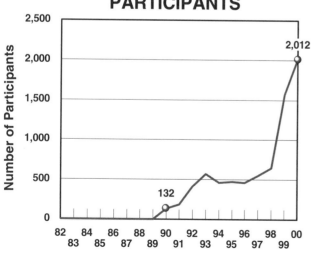

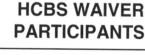

WAIVER SPENDING PER PARTICIPANT

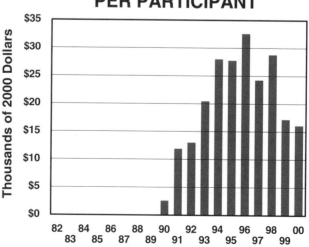

Source: The Coleman Institute and Department of Psychiatry, University of Colorado, 2002.

TRENDS IN RESIDENTIAL SERVICES

PERSONS SERVED BY SETTING IN 2000

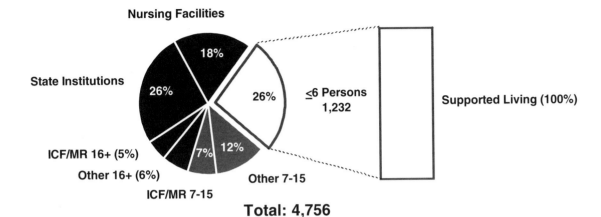

Total: 4,756

PERSONS SERVED BY SETTING

	1990	1991	1992	1993	1994	1995	1996	1997	1998	1999	2000
TOTAL	4,241	4,370	4,397	5,150	6,156	6,386	4,699	5,275	5,532	4,890	4,756
16+ PERSONS	3,109	2,874	2,370	2,601	2,427	2,452	2,445	2,766	2,745	2,701	2,631
Nursing Facilities	1,670	1,442	928	1,169	994	1,003	1,000	1,000	1,000	934	867
State Institutions	1,260	1,250	1,259	1,249	1,253	1,263	1,263	1,262	1,246	1,242	1,241
Private ICF/MR	179	182	183	183	180	186	182	204	204	230	230
Other Residential	0	0	0	0	0	0	0	300	295	295	293
7-15 PERSONS	1,132	1,496	1,107	1,031	1,080	1,170	978	1,048	1,041	894	893
Public ICF/MR	0	0	0	0	0	0	0	0	0	0	0
Private ICF/MR	25	262	300	331	322	443	314	370	377	315	320
Other Residential	1,107	1,234	807	700	758	727	664	678	664	579	573
≤6 PERSONS	0	0	920	1,518	2,649	2,764	1,276	1,461	1,746	1,295	1,232
Public ICF/MR	0	0	0	0	0	0	0	0	0	0	0
Private ICF/MR	0	0	0	0	0	0	0	0	0	0	0
Other Residential	0	0	920	1,518	2,649	2,764	1,276	1,461	1,746	1,295	1,232

PERSONS SERVED IN PUBLIC AND PRIVATE INSTITUTIONS AND NURSING FACILITIES

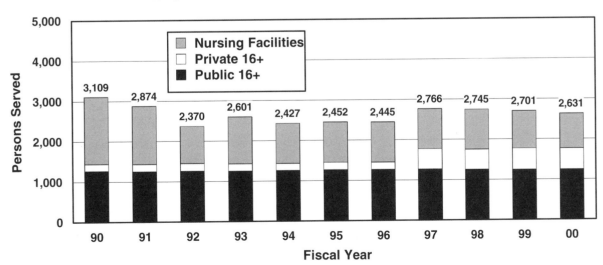

Source: The Coleman Institute and Department of Psychiatry, University of Colorado, 2002.

157

INDIVIDUAL AND FAMILY SUPPORT

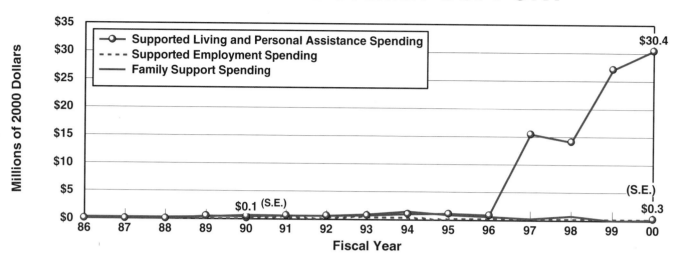

PARTICIPANTS AND SPENDING LEVELS

	1990	1991	1992	1993	1994	1995	1996	1997	1998	1999	2000
TOTAL IFS ($)	964,629	1,283,455	1,217,297	1,616,674	2,419,824	2,016,097	998,952	14,478,473	13,457,866	26,303,709	30,880,232
INDIVIDUAL SUPPORT ($)	451,164	784,008	725,934	877,979	1,174,228	1,197,668	998,952	14,478,473	13,457,866	26,303,709	30,733,356
Supported Employment ($)	90,272	271,705	196,659	260,726	292,120	216,188	194,256	215,865	176,978	208,780	300,180
# of Persons	57	133	182	219	221	223	229	304	379	150	150
Supported Living ($)	360,892	512,303	529,275	617,253	882,108	981,480	804,696	14,262,608	13,280,888	26,094,929	30,433,176
# of Persons	186	263	272	314	322	350	324	1,461	1,746	1,295	1,232
Personal Assistance ($)	0	0	0	0	0	0	0	0	0	0	0
# of Persons	0	0	0	0	0	0	0	0	0	0	0
FAMILY SUPPORT ($)	513,465	499,447	491,363	738,695	1,245,596	818,429	n/a	n/a	n/a	n/a	146,876
Total Families	544	591	847	453	1,193	981	886	625	680	n/a	49
Cash Subsidy/Payment ($)	138,337	218,451	218,451	270,750	740,198	585,318	573,190	230,145	737,151	0	0
# of Families	65	76	116	147	924	751	886	625	680	0	0
Other Family Support ($)	375,128	280,996	272,912	467,945	505,398	233,111	n/a	n/a	n/a	n/a	146,876
# of Families	479	515	731	306	269	230	n/a	n/a	n/a	n/a	49

PARTICIPANTS IN DAY/WORK AND SUPPORTED EMPLOYMENT

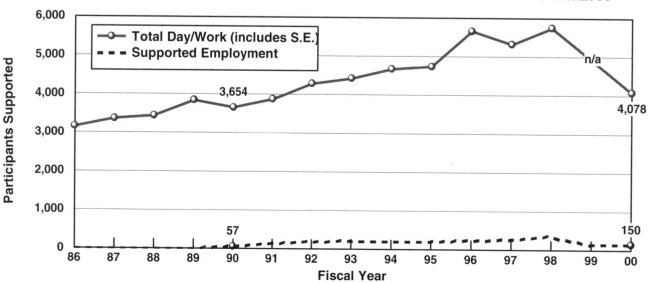

Source: The Coleman Institute and Department of Psychiatry, University of Colorado, 2002.

TRENDS IN SPENDING

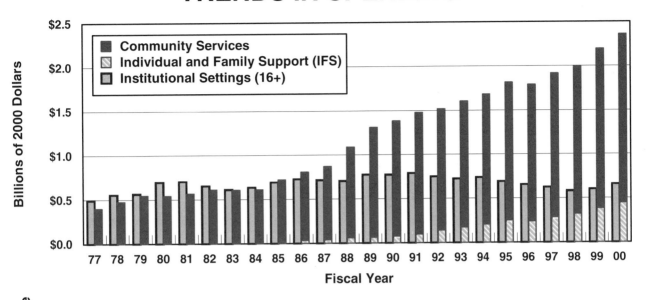

FISCAL EFFORT

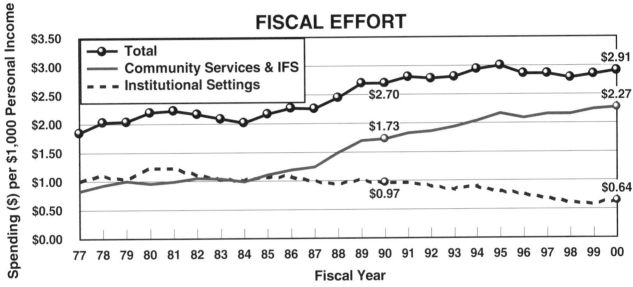

TOTAL MR/DD SPENDING AND
UNMATCHED STATE/LOCAL FUNDS

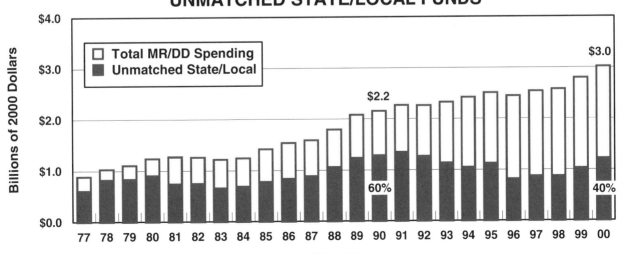

Source: The Coleman Institute and Department of Psychiatry, University of Colorado, 2002.

TRENDS IN REVENUE

COMMUNITY SERVICES REVENUE IN 2000

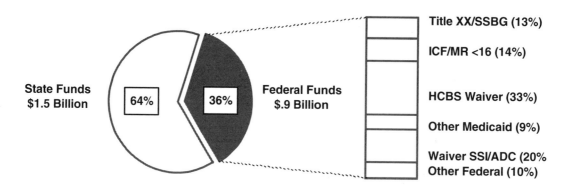

State Funds
$1.5 Billion

64%

36%

Federal Funds
$.9 Billion

Title XX/SSBG (13%)

ICF/MR <16 (14%)

HCBS Waiver (33%)

Other Medicaid (9%)

Waiver SSI/ADC (20%
Other Federal (10%)

Total: $2.4 Billion

COMPONENTS OF FEDERAL MR/DD MEDICAID REVENUE

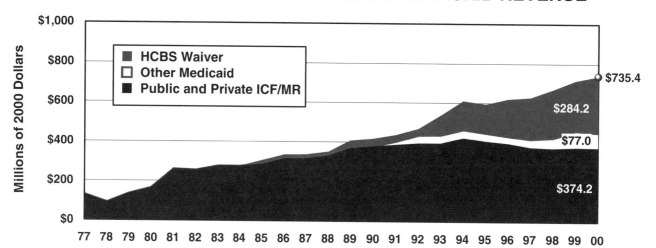

HCBS WAIVER PARTICIPANTS

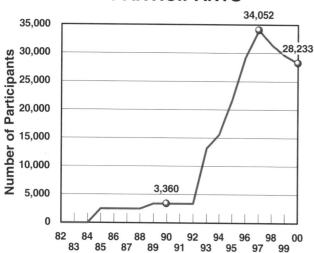

WAIVER SPENDING PER PARTICIPANT

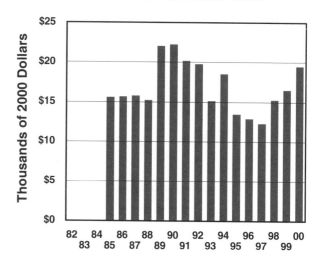

Source: The Coleman Institute and Department of Psychiatry, University of Colorado, 2002.

TRENDS IN RESIDENTIAL SERVICES

PERSONS SERVED BY SETTING IN 2000

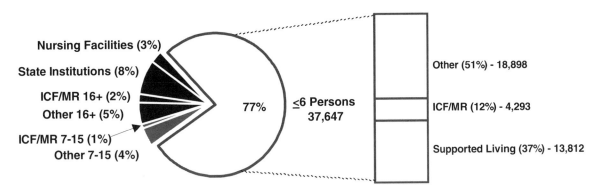

Nursing Facilities (3%)
State Institutions (8%)
ICF/MR 16+ (2%)
Other 16+ (5%)
ICF/MR 7-15 (1%)
Other 7-15 (4%)

77%

≤6 Persons
37,647

Other (51%) - 18,898

ICF/MR (12%) - 4,293

Supported Living (37%) - 13,812

Total: 48,719

PERSONS SERVED BY SETTING

	1990	1991	1992	1993	1994	1995	1996	1997	1998	1999	2000
TOTAL	32,531	33,285	42,834	44,102	46,117	48,176	48,927	46,867	48,495	47,692	48,719
16+ PERSONS	14,817	14,770	14,483	12,923	12,526	11,462	10,381	9,791	9,338	8,763	8,524
Nursing Facilities	976	1,128	1,226	997	1,058	1,064	1,232	1,342	1,365	1,416	1,409
State Institutions	6,722	6,720	6,629	6,412	6,048	5,445	4,823	4,327	4,044	3,876	3,795
Private ICF/MR	3,228	3,191	3,119	2,255	2,125	1,964	1,428	1,467	1,378	1,016	964
Other Residential	3,891	3,731	3,509	3,259	3,295	2,989	2,898	2,655	2,551	2,455	2,356
7-15 PERSONS	3,046	3,058	3,055	3,176	3,104	2,922	2,878	2,716	2,638	2,526	2,548
Public ICF/MR	0	0	0	0	0	0	0	0	0	0	0
Private ICF/MR	428	442	473	500	512	500	524	489	508	486	474
Other Residential	2,618	2,616	2,582	2,676	2,592	2,422	2,354	2,227	2,130	2,040	2,074
≤6 PERSONS	14,668	15,457	25,296	28,003	30,487	33,792	35,668	34,360	36,519	36,403	37,647
Public ICF/MR	0	0	0	0	0	0	0	0	0	0	0
Private ICF/MR	1,446	1,598	1,734	2,077	2,426	3,004	3,388	3,869	4,293	4,659	4,937
Other Residential	13,222	13,859	23,562	25,926	28,061	30,788	32,280	30,491	32,226	31,744	32,710

PERSONS SERVED IN PUBLIC AND PRIVATE
INSTITUTIONS AND NURSING FACILITIES

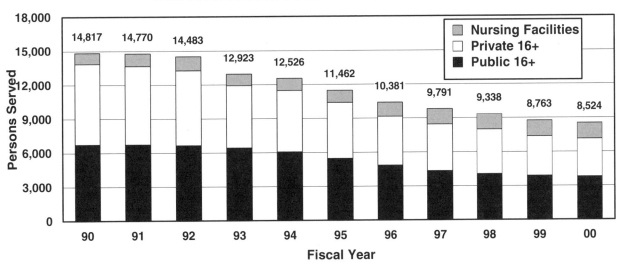

Source: The Coleman Institute and Department of Psychiatry, University of Colorado, 2002.

161

INDIVIDUAL AND FAMILY SUPPORT

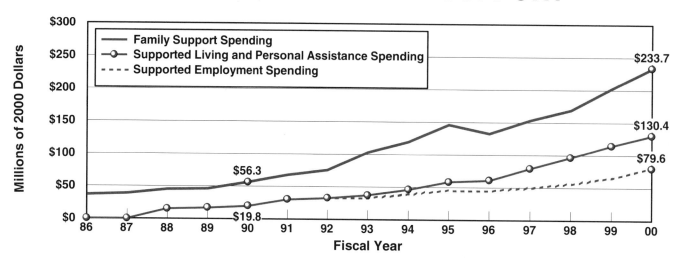

PARTICIPANTS AND SPENDING LEVELS

	1990	1991	1992	1993	1994	1995	1996	1997	1998	1999	2000
TOTAL IFS ($)	na	na	115,153,961	144,305,813	176,033,957	219,402,249	215,409,602	260,906,849	303,735,542	368,330,643	443,619,497
INDIVIDUAL SUPPORT ($)	na	na	53,358,576	57,945,963	73,378,352	90,370,801	95,271,727	118,800,684	143,964,689	173,042,821	209,917,725
Supported Employment ($)	na	na	26,700,000	26,790,000	33,689,000	38,993,000	40,216,000	45,546,072	52,988,952	62,648,105	79,566,000
# of Persons	na	na	5,023	5,362	4,438	7,213	7,115	7,601	9,091	7,312	8,974
Supported Living ($)	14,280,050	22,502,120	24,913,657	29,466,858	36,551,862	46,349,004	50,036,254	73,254,612	90,975,737	110,394,716	130,351,725
# of Persons	4,633	6,781	6,815	7,042	8,131	9,217	9,843	11,096	12,177	12,995	13,812
Personal Assistance ($)*	969,665	1,653,516	1,744,919	1,689,105	3,137,490	5,028,797	5,019,473	0	0	0	0
# of Persons*	352	531	549	734	839	958	939	0	0	0	0
FAMILY SUPPORT ($)	43,345,657	54,490,160	61,795,385	86,359,850	102,655,605	129,031,448	120,137,875	142,106,165	159,770,853	195,287,822	233,701,772
Total Families	23,881	25,773	27,507	45,486	53,855	63,015	64,517	75,591	81,809	89,636	101,194
Cash Subsidy/Payment ($)	0	0	0	0	0	0	0	0	0	0	0
# of Families	0	0	0	0	0	0	0	0	0	0	0
Other Family Support ($)	43,345,657	54,490,160	61,795,385	86,359,850	102,655,605	129,031,448	120,137,875	142,106,165	159,770,853	195,287,822	233,701,772
# of Families	23,881	25,773	27,507	45,486	53,855	63,015	64,517	75,591	81,809	89,636	101,194

*Personal Assistance spending and participants for 1997-2000 are included in the supported living category.

PARTICIPANTS IN DAY/WORK AND SUPPORTED EMPLOYMENT

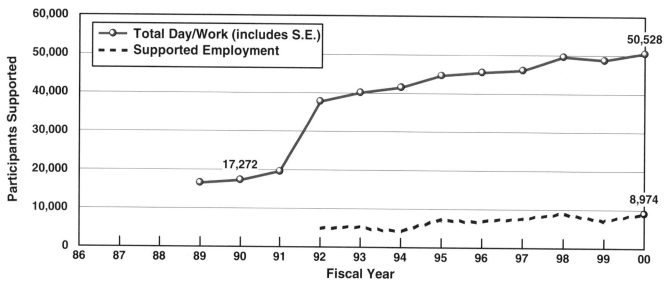

Source: The Coleman Institute and Department of Psychiatry, University of Colorado, 2002.

TRENDS IN SPENDING

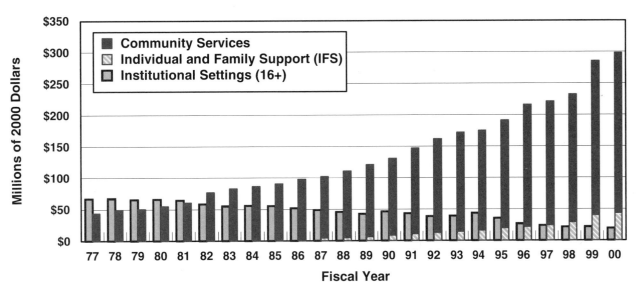

Legend:
- Community Services
- Individual and Family Support (IFS)
- Institutional Settings (16+)

Y-axis: Millions of 2000 Dollars
X-axis: Fiscal Year (77–00)

FISCAL EFFORT

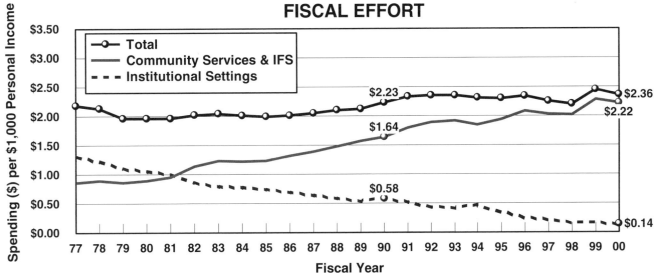

Legend:
- Total
- Community Services & IFS
- Institutional Settings

Y-axis: Spending ($) per $1,000 Personal Income
X-axis: Fiscal Year (77–00)

Data labels: $2.23, $2.36, $2.22, $1.64, $0.58, $0.14

TOTAL MR/DD SPENDING AND
UNMATCHED STATE/LOCAL FUNDS

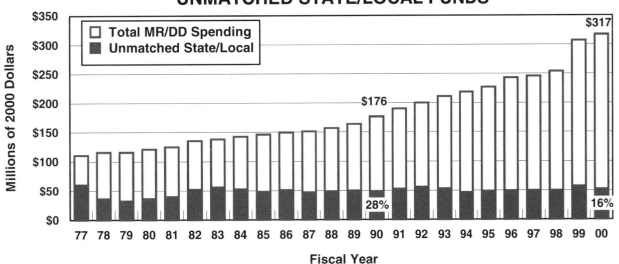

Legend:
- Total MR/DD Spending
- Unmatched State/Local

Y-axis: Millions of 2000 Dollars
X-axis: Fiscal Year (77–00)

Data labels: $317, $176, 28%, 16%

Source: The Coleman Institute and Department of Psychiatry, University of Colorado, 2002.

TRENDS IN REVENUE

COMMUNITY SERVICES REVENUE IN 2000

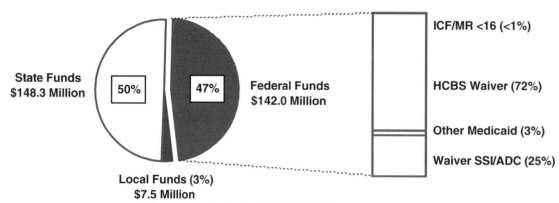

State Funds
$148.3 Million

50%

47%

Federal Funds
$142.0 Million

Local Funds (3%)
$7.5 Million

ICF/MR <16 (<1%)

HCBS Waiver (72%)

Other Medicaid (3%)

Waiver SSI/ADC (25%)

Total: $297.8 Million

COMPONENTS OF FEDERAL MR/DD MEDICAID REVENUE

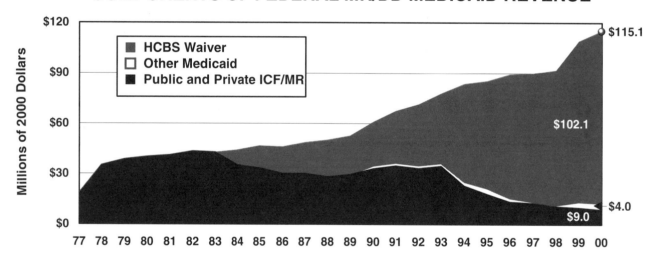

- HCBS Waiver
- Other Medicaid
- Public and Private ICF/MR

Millions of 2000 Dollars

$120

$90

$60

$30

$0

$115.1

$102.1

$4.0

$9.0

77 78 79 80 81 82 83 84 85 86 87 88 89 90 91 92 93 94 95 96 97 98 99 00

Fiscal Year

HCBS WAIVER PARTICIPANTS

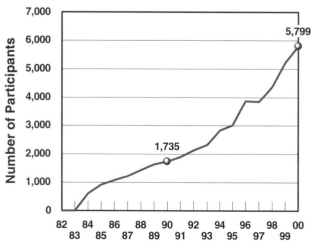

Number of Participants

7,000

6,000

5,000

4,000

3,000

2,000

1,000

0

5,799

1,735

82 83 84 85 86 87 88 89 90 91 92 93 94 95 96 97 98 99 00

WAIVER SPENDING PER PARTICIPANT

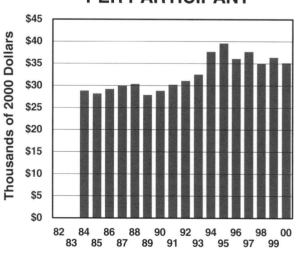

Thousands of 2000 Dollars

$45

$40

$35

$30

$25

$20

$15

$10

$5

$0

82 83 84 85 86 87 88 89 90 91 92 93 94 95 96 97 98 99 00

Source: The Coleman Institute and Department of Psychiatry, University of Colorado, 2002.

TRENDS IN RESIDENTIAL SERVICES

PERSONS SERVED BY SETTING IN 2000

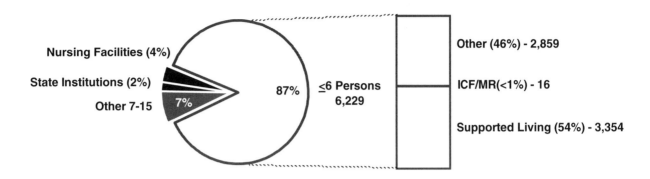

Nursing Facilities (4%)

State Institutions (2%)

Other 7-15

7%

87%

≤6 Persons
6,229

Other (46%) - 2,859

ICF/MR(<1%) - 16

Supported Living (54%) - 3,354

Total: 7,168

PERSONS SERVED BY SETTING

	1990	1991	1992	1993	1994	1995	1996	1997	1998	1999	2000
TOTAL	3,794	3,861	3,954	3,908	4,558	4,802	4,634	4,477	4,956	6,391	7,168
16+ PERSONS	1,166	1,076	949	731	693	650	549	521	460	439	417
Nursing Facilities	440	420	390	300	298	297	295	293	291	269	270
State Institutions	466	406	334	271	253	259	194	190	169	170	147
Private ICF/MR	260	250	225	160	142	94	60	38	0	0	0
Other Residential	0	0	0	0	0	0	0	0	0	0	0
7-15 PERSONS	970	723	842	273	273	261	300	534	546	524	522
Public ICF/MR	277	275	250	273	0	0	0	0	0	0	0
Private ICF/MR	0	0	0	0	0	0	0	0	0	0	0
Other Residential	693	448	592	0	273	261	300	534	546	524	522
≤6 PERSONS	1,658	2,062	2,163	2,904	3,592	3,891	3,785	3,422	3,950	5,428	6,229
Public ICF/MR	0	0	0	0	0	0	0	0	0	0	0
Private ICF/MR	0	0	0	0	0	16	16	16	16	16	16
Other Residential	1,658	2,062	2,163	2,904	3,592	3,875	3,769	3,406	3,934	5,412	6,213

PERSONS SERVED IN PUBLIC AND PRIVATE INSTITUTIONS AND NURSING FACILITIES

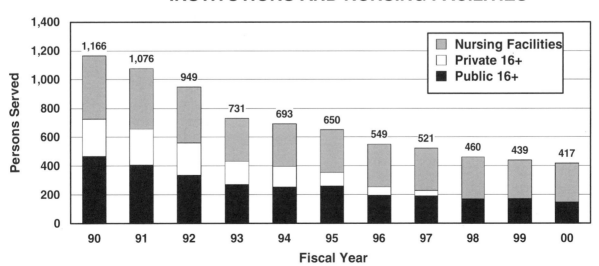

Source: The Coleman Institute and Department of Psychiatry, University of Colorado, 2002.

165

INDIVIDUAL AND FAMILY SUPPORT

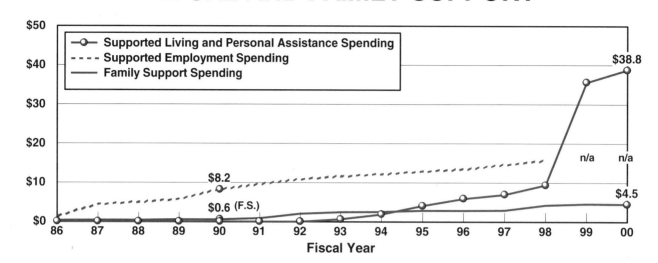

PARTICIPANTS AND SPENDING LEVELS

	1990	1991	1992	1993	1994	1995	1996	1997	1998	1999	2000
TOTAL IFS ($)	6,782,565	8,434,505	10,596,901	12,182,483	14,027,997	17,501,528	19,911,302	22,686,872	27,586,122	38,798,740	43,253,501
INDIVIDUAL SUPPORT ($)	6,316,045	7,705,340	8,904,026	10,163,482	11,888,266	14,971,988	17,367,187	19,986,134	23,578,954	34,420,948	38,788,187
Supported Employment ($)	6,316,045	7,705,340	8,904,026	9,643,226	10,272,933	11,366,585	12,000,000	13,531,575	14,716,275	n/a	n/a
# of Persons	1,426	1,673	1,880	2,006	2,101	1,945	1,986	1,927	2,105	2,256	2,253
Supported Living ($)	0	0	0	520,256	1,615,333	3,605,403	5,367,187	6,454,559	8,862,679	34,420,948	38,788,187
# of Persons	0	0	0	336	536	626	708	811	1,260	2,656	3,354
Personal Assistance ($)	0	0	0	0	0	0	0	0	0	0	0
# of Persons	0	0	0	0	0	0	0	0	0	0	0
FAMILY SUPPORT ($)	466,520	729,165	1,692,875	2,019,001	2,139,731	2,529,540	2,544,115	2,700,738	4,007,168	4,377,792	4,465,314
Total Families	115	200	733	2,137	2,603	3,134	3,498	3,500	3,587	3,897	4,014
Cash Subsidy/Payment ($)	0	0	0	0	0	0	0	0	0	0	0
# of Families	0	0	0	0	0	0	0	0	0	0	0
Other Family Support ($)	466,520	729,165	1,692,875	2,019,001	2,139,731	2,529,540	2,544,115	2,700,738	4,007,168	4,377,792	4,465,314
# of Families	115	200	733	2,137	2,603	3,134	3,498	3,500	3,587	3,897	4,014

PARTICIPANTS IN DAY/WORK AND SUPPORTED EMPLOYMENT

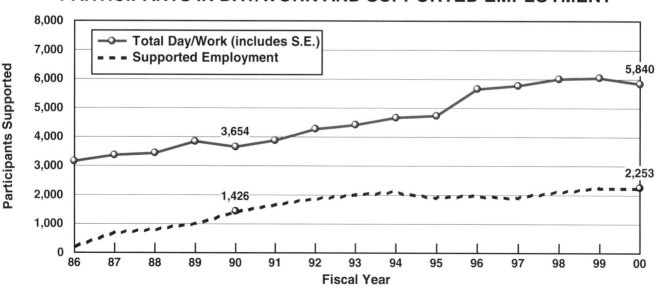

Source: The Coleman Institute and Department of Psychiatry, University of Colorado, 2002.

TRENDS IN SPENDING

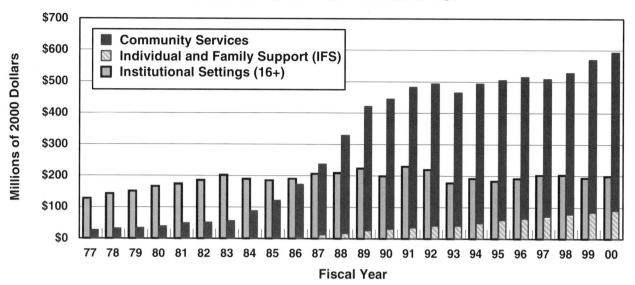

FISCAL EFFORT

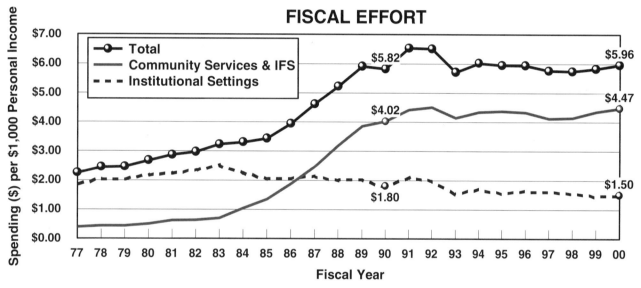

TOTAL MR/DD SPENDING AND
UNMATCHED STATE/LOCAL FUNDS

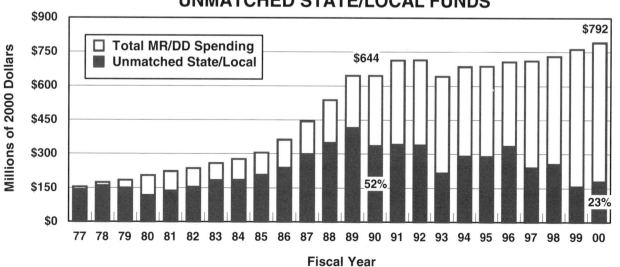

Source: The Coleman Institute and Department of Psychiatry, University of Colorado, 2002.

167

TRENDS IN REVENUE

COMMUNITY SERVICES REVENUE IN 2000

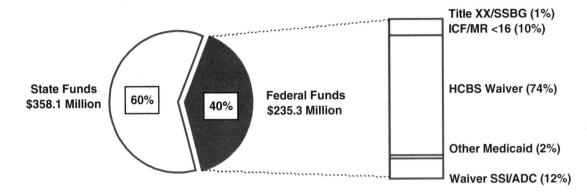

Total: $593.4 Million

COMPONENTS OF FEDERAL MR/DD MEDICAID REVENUE

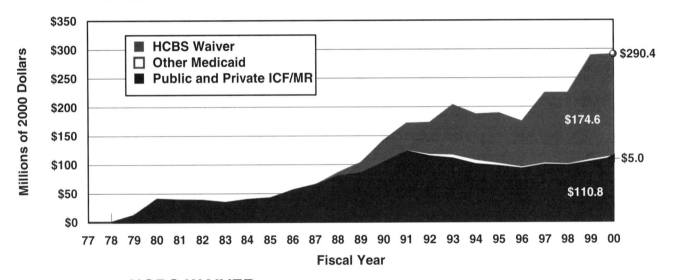

HCBS WAIVER PARTICIPANTS

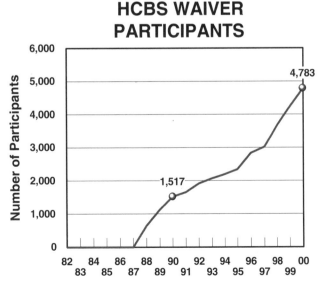

WAIVER SPENDING PER PARTICIPANT

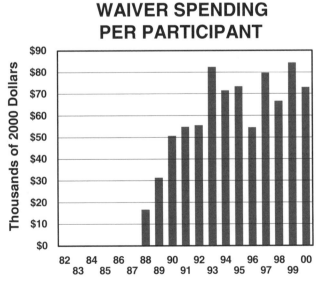

Source: The Coleman Institute and Department of Psychiatry, University of Colorado, 2002.

TRENDS IN RESIDENTIAL SERVICES

PERSONS SERVED BY SETTING IN 2000

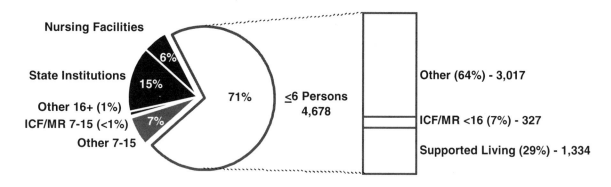

Nursing Facilities 6%
State Institutions 15%
Other 16+ (1%)
ICF/MR 7-15 (<1%)
Other 7-15 7%
71%
≤6 Persons 4,678

Other (64%) - 3,017
ICF/MR <16 (7%) - 327
Supported Living (29%) - 1,334

Total: 6,557

PERSONS SERVED BY SETTING

	1990	1991	1992	1993	1994	1995	1996	1997	1998	1999	2000
TOTAL	5,837	6,058	6,132	6,202	6,246	6,334	6,364	6,404	6,488	6,468	6,557
16+ PERSONS	2,560	2,400	2,224	2,041	1,906	1,827	1,716	1,582	1,490	1,421	1,416
Nursing Facilities	571	540	510	479	458	434	422	373	362	363	378
State Institutions	1,727	1,626	1,545	1,426	1,333	1,273	1,218	1,136	1,057	1,000	970
Private ICF/MR	20	20	20	0	0	0	0	0	0	0	0
Other Residential	242	214	149	136	115	120	76	73	71	58	68
7-15 PERSONS	3,277	636	573	632	641	569	442	460	361	432	463
Public ICF/MR	266	274	211	235	250	231	242	243	87	16	16
Private ICF/MR	269	43	54	51	72	35	32	20	10	10	10
Other Residential	2,742	319	308	346	319	303	168	197	264	406	437
≤6 PERSONS	0	3,022	3,335	3,529	3,699	3,938	4,206	4,362	4,637	4,615	4,678
Public ICF/MR	0	21	50	40	40	69	55	71	30	8	8
Private ICF/MR	0	227	206	308	302	330	327	338	325	323	319
Other Residential	0	2,774	3,079	3,181	3,357	3,539	3,824	3,953	4,282	4,284	4,351

PERSONS SERVED IN PUBLIC AND PRIVATE INSTITUTIONS AND NURSING FACILITIES

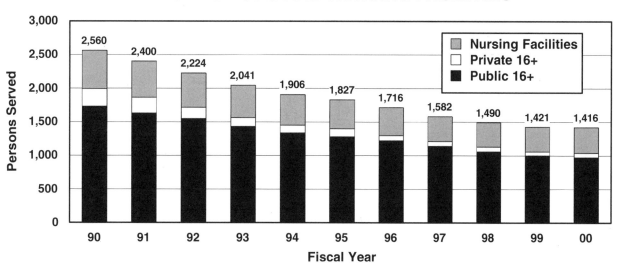

Legend:
- Nursing Facilities
- Private 16+
- Public 16+

Persons Served (y-axis): 0, 500, 1,000, 1,500, 2,000, 2,500, 3,000

Fiscal Year (x-axis): 90 (2,560), 91 (2,400), 92 (2,224), 93 (2,041), 94 (1,906), 95 (1,827), 96 (1,716), 97 (1,582), 98 (1,490), 99 (1,421), 00 (1,416)

Source: The Coleman Institute and Department of Psychiatry, University of Colorado, 2002.

INDIVIDUAL AND FAMILY SUPPORT

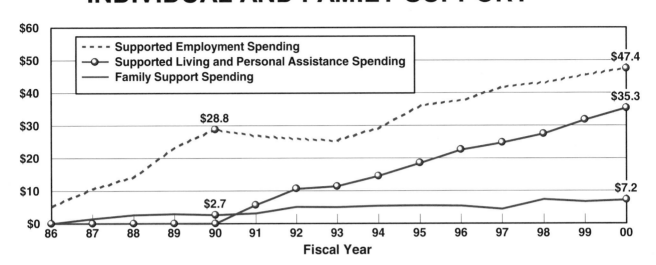

PARTICIPANTS AND SPENDING LEVELS

	1990	1991	1992	1993	1994	1995	1996	1997	1998	1999	2000
TOTAL IFS ($)	24,230,936	28,771,249	34,148,926	34,983,071	42,207,175	52,901,274	59,105,542	65,505,926	73,530,552	80,653,559	89,941,308
INDIVIDUAL SUPPORT ($)	22,191,048	26,227,794	29,929,060	30,804,090	37,523,901	48,021,202	54,200,959	61,437,493	66,582,809	74,228,429	82,743,343
Supported Employment ($)	22,191,048	21,691,280	21,241,799	21,307,191	25,083,212	31,698,422	33,783,851	38,564,216	40,694,391	43,681,180	47,423,112
# of Persons	1,576	2,060	2,206	2,372	2,562	2,817	3,006	3,147	3,245	3,439	3,552
Supported Living ($)	0	4,536,514	8,687,261	9,496,899	12,440,689	16,322,780	20,417,108	22,873,277	25,888,418	30,547,249	35,320,231
# of Persons	0	125	638	711	816	911	1,070	1,147	1,219	1,277	1,334
Personal Assistance ($)	0	0	0	0	0	0	0	0	0	0	0
# of Persons	0	0	0	0	0	0	0	0	0	0	0
FAMILY SUPPORT ($)	2,039,888	2,543,455	4,219,866	4,178,981	4,683,274	4,880,072	4,904,583	4,068,433	6,947,743	6,425,130	7,197,965
Total Families	986	1,211	1,726	2,337	2,473	2,654	2,990	3,202	3,456	3,685	4,019
Cash Subsidy/Payment ($)	50,976	280,840	589,820	966,700	967,507	968,087	966,038	968,818	996,268	968,731	988,067
# of Families	18	101	243	595	593	674	679	759	782	872	911
Other Family Support ($)	1,988,912	2,262,615	3,630,046	3,212,281	3,715,767	3,911,985	3,938,545	3,099,615	5,951,475	5,456,399	6,209,898
# of Families	968	1,110	1,483	1,742	1,880	1,980	2,311	2,443	2,674	2,813	3,108

PARTICIPANTS IN DAY/WORK AND SUPPORTED EMPLOYMENT

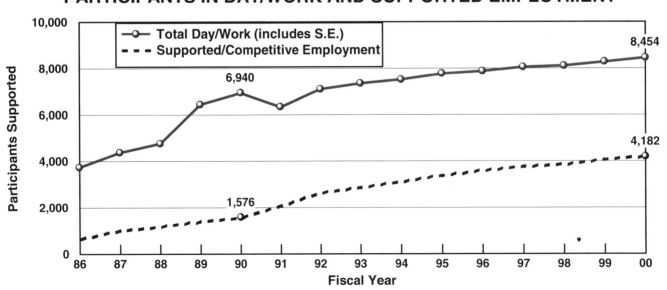

Source: The Coleman Institute and Department of Psychiatry, University of Colorado, 2002.

TRENDS IN SPENDING

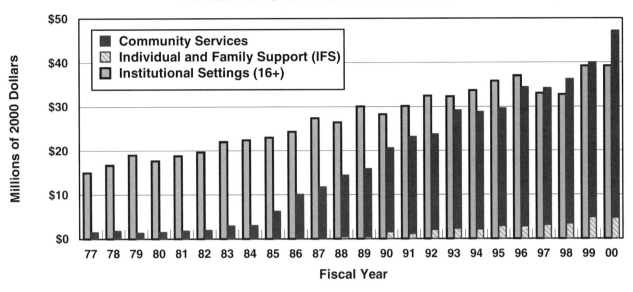

FISCAL EFFORT

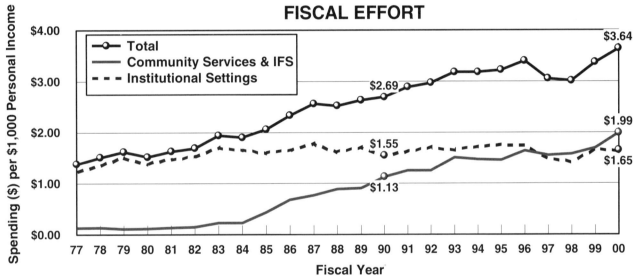

TOTAL MR/DD SPENDING AND
UNMATCHED STATE/LOCAL FUNDS

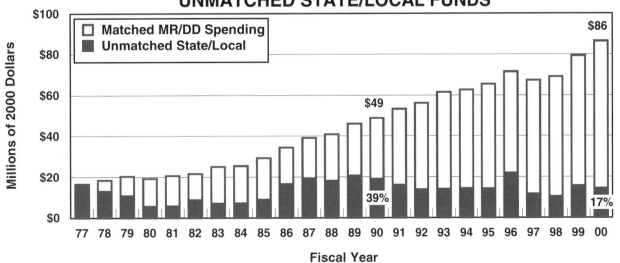

Source: The Coleman Institute and Department of Psychiatry, University sof Colorado, 2002.

DELAWARE

TRENDS IN REVENUE
COMMUNITY SERVICES REVENUE IN 2000

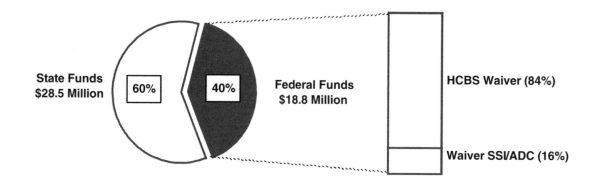

State Funds $28.5 Million — 60%

40% — Federal Funds $18.8 Million

HCBS Waiver (84%)

Waiver SSI/ADC (16%)

Total: $47.2 Million

COMPONENTS OF FEDERAL MR/DD MEDICAID REVENUE

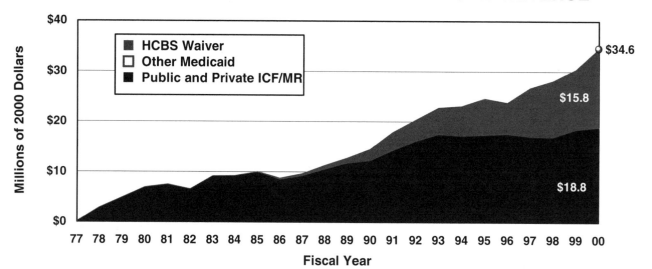

Millions of 2000 Dollars — Fiscal Year

- HCBS Waiver
- Other Medicaid
- Public and Private ICF/MR

$34.6 / $15.8 / $18.8

HCBS WAIVER PARTICIPANTS

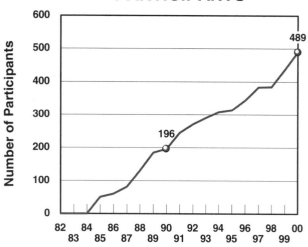

489 / 196

Number of Participants

WAIVER SPENDING PER PARTICIPANT

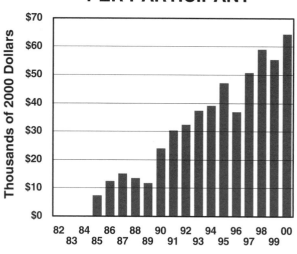

Thousands of 2000 Dollars

Source: The Coleman Institute and Department of Psychiatry, University of Colorado, 2002.

TRENDS IN RESIDENTIAL SERVICES

PERSONS SERVED BY SETTING IN 2000

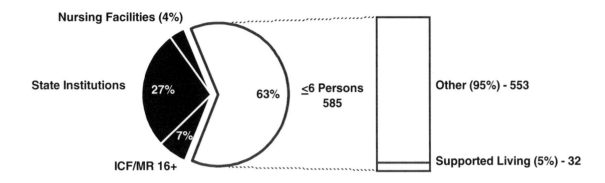

Nursing Facilities (4%)

State Institutions 27%

ICF/MR 16+ 7%

63%

≤6 Persons 585

Other (95%) - 553

Supported Living (5%) - 32

Total: 935

PERSONS SERVED BY SETTING

	1990	1991	1992	1993	1994	1995	1996	1997	1998	1999	2000
TOTAL	836	826	886	889	886	892	899	887	906	924	935
16+ PERSONS	452	427	453	445	441	430	413	377	370	355	350
Nursing Facilities	64	44	82	75	75	75	75	53	51	43	34
State Institutions	342	337	325	324	320	309	292	277	271	264	253
Private ICF/MR	46	46	46	46	46	46	46	47	48	48	63
Other Residential	0	0	0	0	0	0	0	0	0	0	0
7-15 PERSONS	384	386	71	66	36	30	21	14	15	0	0
Public ICF/MR	0	0	0	0	0	0	0	0	0	0	0
Private ICF/MR	91	90	71	66	36	30	21	14	15	0	0
Other Residential	293	296	0	0	0	0	0	0	0	0	0
≤6 PERSONS	0	13	362	378	409	432	465	496	521	569	585
Public ICF/MR	0	0	0	0	0	0	0	0	0	0	0
Private ICF/MR	0	0	6	0	0	0	0	0	0	0	0
Other Residential	0	13	356	378	409	432	465	496	521	569	585

PERSONS SERVED IN PUBLIC AND PRIVATE INSTITUTIONS AND NURSING FACILITIES

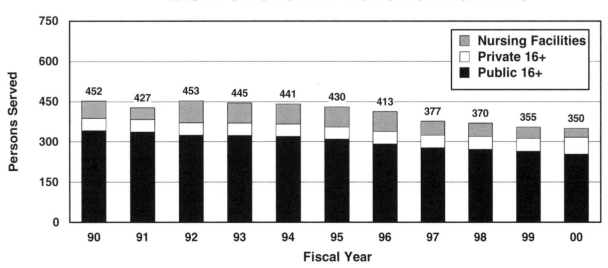

Legend:
- Nursing Facilities
- Private 16+
- Public 16+

Persons Served (y-axis): 0, 150, 300, 450, 600, 750

Fiscal Year (x-axis): 90, 91, 92, 93, 94, 95, 96, 97, 98, 99, 00

Values: 452, 427, 453, 445, 441, 430, 413, 377, 370, 355, 350

Source: The Coleman Institute and Department of Psychiatry, University of Colorado, 2002.

INDIVIDUAL AND FAMILY SUPPORT

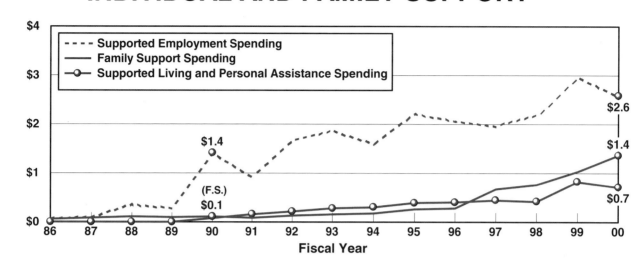

PARTICIPANTS AND SPENDING LEVELS

	1990	1991	1992	1993	1994	1995	1996	1997	1998	1999	2000
TOTAL IFS ($)	1,173,023	939,547	1,637,249	1,917,756	1,786,717	2,523,780	2,489,021	2,841,830	3,173,953	4,653,449	4,664,341
INDIVIDUAL SUPPORT ($)	1,086,679	872,355	1,532,395	1,787,523	1,632,998	2,291,847	2,231,825	2,219,285	2,450,316	3,659,452	3,301,562
Supported Employment ($)	1,086,679	744,176	1,356,163	1,554,059	1,373,721	1,947,940	1,866,978	1,807,920	2,053,440	2,864,204	2,587,824
# of Persons	113	106	147	187	192	228	243	240	279	266	345
Supported Living ($)	0	128,179	176,232	233,464	259,277	343,907	364,847	411,365	396,876	795,248	713,738
# of Persons	0	13	53	52	51	57	53	53	46	45	32
Personal Assistance ($)	0	0	0	0	0	0	0	0	0	0	0
# of Persons	0	0	0	0	0	0	0	0	0	0	0
FAMILY SUPPORT ($)	86,344	67,192	104,854	130,233	153,719	231,933	257,196	622,545	723,637	993,997	1,362,779
Total Families	318	559	621	665	732	818	772	991	1,054	1,143	1,218
Cash Subsidy/Payment ($)	0	0	0	0	0	0	0	0	0	0	0
# of Families	0	0	0	0	0	0	0	0	0	0	0
Other Family Support ($)	86,344	67,192	104,854	130,233	153,719	231,933	257,196	622,545	723,637	993,997	1,362,779
# of Families	318	559	621	665	732	818	772	991	1,054	1,143	1,218

PARTICIPANTS IN DAY/WORK AND SUPPORTED EMPLOYMENT

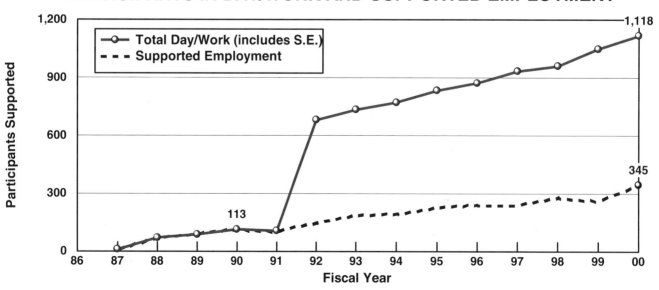

Source: The Coleman Institute and Department of Psychiatry, University of Colorado, 2002.

TRENDS IN SPENDING

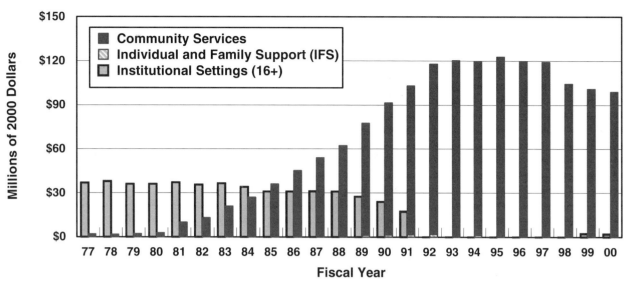

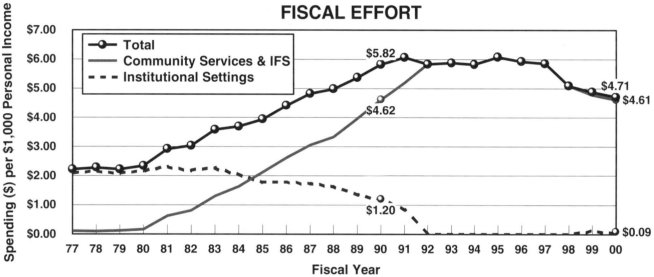

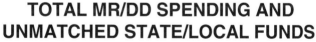

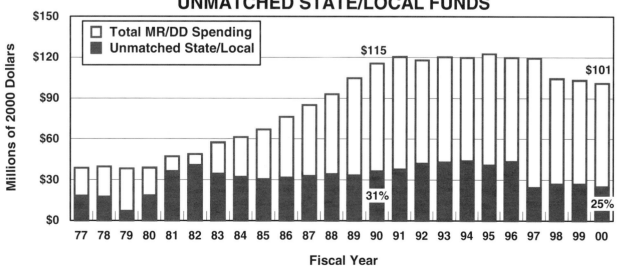

Source: The Coleman Institute and Department of Psychiatry, University of Colorado, 2002.

175

TRENDS IN REVENUE

COMMUNITY SERVICES REVENUE IN 2000

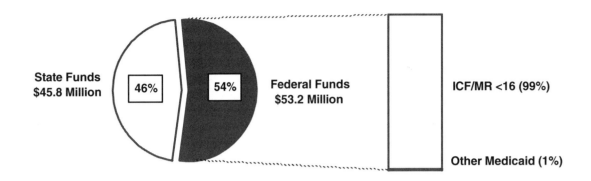

**State Funds
$45.8 Million**

46%

54%

**Federal Funds
$53.2 Million**

ICF/MR <16 (99%)

Other Medicaid (1%)

Total: $99.0 Million

COMPONENTS OF FEDERAL MR/DD MEDICAID REVENUE

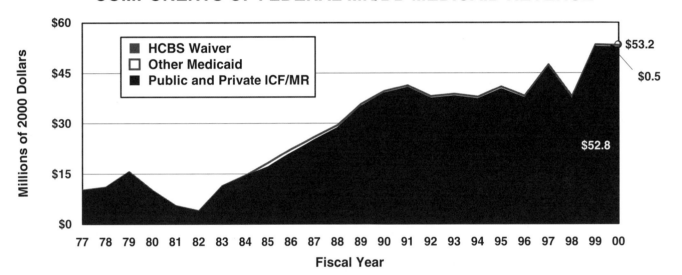

Millions of 2000 Dollars

- ■ HCBS Waiver
- □ Other Medicaid
- ■ Public and Private ICF/MR

$53.2

$0.5

$52.8

Fiscal Year

HCBS WAIVER PARTICIPANTS

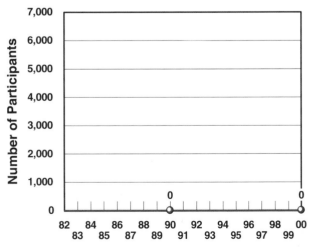

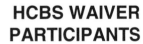

Number of Participants

WAIVER SPENDING PER PARTICIPANT

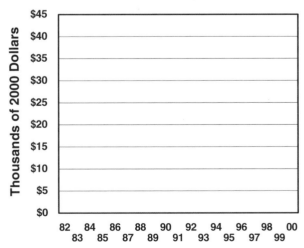

Thousands of 2000 Dollars

Source: The Coleman Institute and Department of Psychiatry, University of Colorado, 2002.

TRENDS IN RESIDENTIAL SERVICES

PERSONS SERVED BY SETTING IN 2000

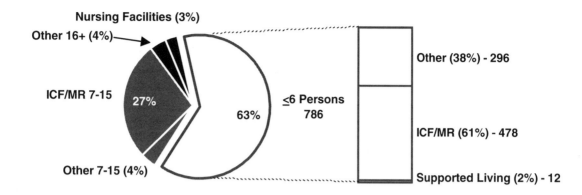

Nursing Facilities (3%)
Other 16+ (4%)
ICF/MR 7-15
27%
63%
≤6 Persons
786
Other 7-15 (4%)

Other (38%) - 296
ICF/MR (61%) - 478
Supported Living (2%) - 12

Total: 1,253

PERSONS SERVED BY SETTING

	1990	1991	1992	1993	1994	1995	1996	1997	1998	1999	2000
TOTAL	n/a	n/a	1,055	1,094	1,118	1,155	1,155	1,186	1,189	1,253	1,253
16+ PERSONS	311	189	82	55	45	37	37	28	19	84	84
Nursing Facilities	66	74	82	55	45	37	37	28	19	36	36
State Institutions	245	115	0	0	0	0	0	0	0	0	0
Private ICF/MR	0	0	0	0	0	0	0	0	0	0	0
Other Residential	0	0	0	0	0	0	0	0	0	48	48
7-15 PERSONS	720	853	649	704	744	790	790	367	399	390	383
Public ICF/MR	0	0	0	0	0	0	0	0	0	0	0
Private ICF/MR	534	604	510	560	600	642	642	301	340	338	338
Other Residential	186	249	139	144	144	148	148	66	59	52	45
≤6 PERSONS	n/a	n/a	324	335	329	328	328	791	771	779	786
Public ICF/MR	0	0	0	0	0	0	0	0	0	0	0
Private ICF/MR	0	0	164	150	135	115	115	479	471	478	478
Other Residential	n/a	n/a	160	185	194	213	213	312	300	301	308

PERSONS SERVED IN PUBLIC AND PRIVATE INSTITUTIONS AND NURSING FACILITIES

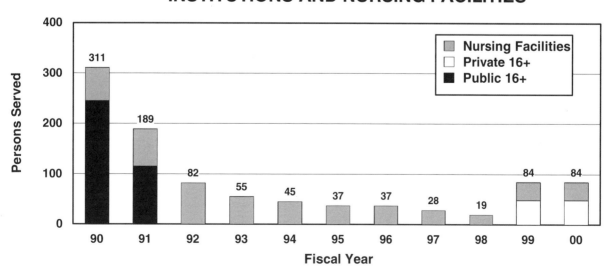

Legend:
- Nursing Facilities
- Private 16+
- Public 16+

Persons Served (y-axis): 0, 100, 200, 300, 400
Fiscal Year (x-axis): 90 (311), 91 (189), 92 (82), 93 (55), 94 (45), 95 (37), 96 (37), 97 (28), 98 (19), 99 (84), 00 (84)

Source: The Coleman Institute and Department of Psychiatry, University of Colorado, 2002.

INDIVIDUAL AND FAMILY SUPPORT

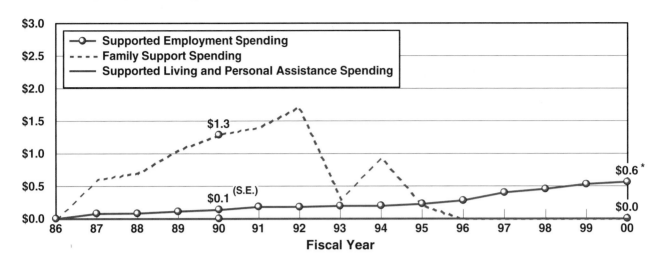

PARTICIPANTS AND SPENDING LEVELS

	1990	1991	1992	1993	1994	1995	1996	1997	1998	1999	2000
TOTAL IFS ($)	n/a	n/a	n/a	409,655	982,123	383,298	251,140	368,892	427,475	0	561,059
INDIVIDUAL SUPPORT ($)	105,965	145,294	146,359	162,467	168,966	199,801	251,140	368,892	427,475	0	561,059
Supported Employment ($)	105,965	145,294	146,359	162,467	168,966	199,801	251,140	368,892	427,475	0	0
# of Persons	36	49	49	54	59	59	72	101	112	0	0
Supported Living ($)	0	0	0	0	0	0	0	0	0	0	n/a
# of Persons	0	0	0	0	0	0	0	0	0	0	12
Personal Assistance ($)	0	0	0	0	0	0	0	0	0	0	0
# of Persons	0	0	0	0	0	0	0	0	0	0	0
FAMILY SUPPORT ($)	n/a	n/a	n/a	247,188	813,157	183,497	0	0	0	0	0
Total Families	1,110	1,268	1,492	113	99	58	0	0	0	0	0
Cash Subsidy/Payment ($)	na	na	na	0	0	0	0	0	0	0	0
# of Families	555	614	746	0	0	0	0	0	0	0	0
Other Family Support ($)	987,987	1,110,771	1,399,012	247,188	813,157	183,497	0	0	0	0	0
# of Families	555	654	746	113	99	58	0	0	0	0	0

*Supported employment figures for FY1999 and FY2000 were estimated based on 1987-1998 data.

PARTICIPANTS IN DAY/WORK AND SUPPORTED EMPLOYMENT

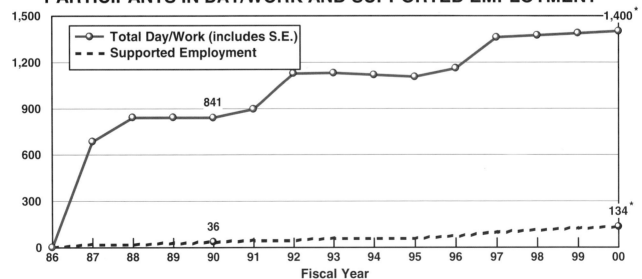

* Estimated based on 1987-1998 data.

Source: The Coleman Institute and Department of Psychiatry, University of Colorado, 2002.

TRENDS IN SPENDING

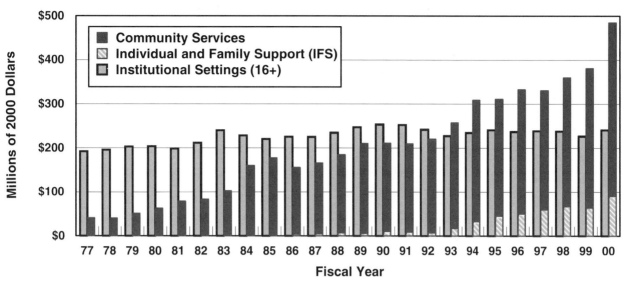

FISCAL EFFORT

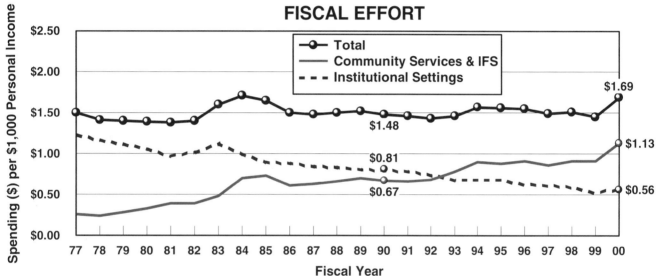

TOTAL MR/DD SPENDING AND
UNMATCHED STATE/LOCAL FUNDS

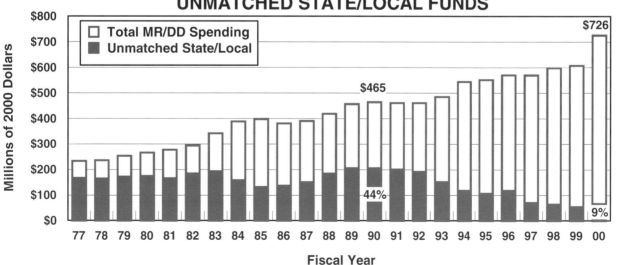

Source: The Coleman Institute and Department of Psychiatry, University of Colorado, 2002.

179

TRENDS IN REVENUE

COMMUNITY SERVICES REVENUE IN 2000

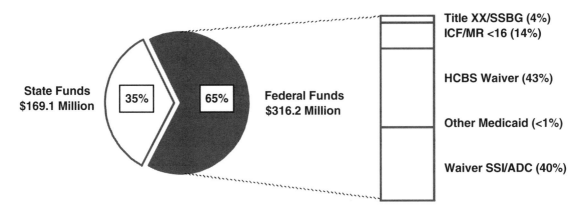

State Funds
$169.1 Million

35%

65%

Federal Funds
$316.2 Million

Title XX/SSBG (4%)
ICF/MR <16 (14%)

HCBS Waiver (43%)

Other Medicaid (<1%)

Waiver SSI/ADC (40%)

Total: $485.3 Million

COMPONENTS OF FEDERAL MR/DD MEDICAID REVENUE

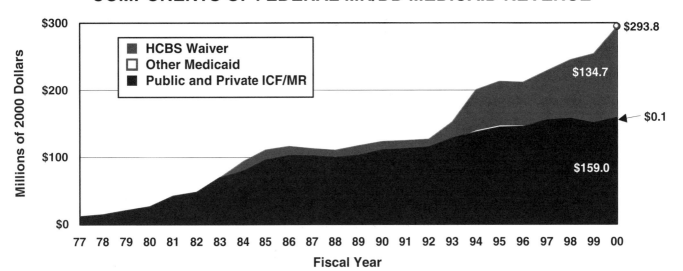

Millions of 2000 Dollars

- ■ HCBS Waiver
- □ Other Medicaid
- ■ Public and Private ICF/MR

$300 — $293.8
$134.7
$0.1
$159.0

Fiscal Year: 77 78 79 80 81 82 83 84 85 86 87 88 89 90 91 92 93 94 95 96 97 98 99 00

HCBS WAIVER PARTICIPANTS

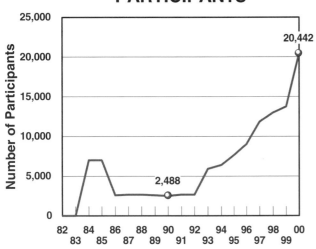

Number of Participants

20,442

2,488

82 83 84 85 86 87 88 89 90 91 92 93 94 95 96 97 98 99 00

WAIVER SPENDING PER PARTICIPANT

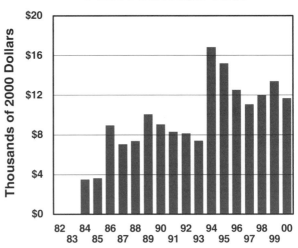

Thousands of 2000 Dollars

82 83 84 85 86 87 88 89 90 91 92 93 94 95 96 97 98 99 00

Source: The Coleman Institute and Department of Psychiatry, University of Colorado, 2002.

TRENDS IN RESIDENTIAL SERVICES

PERSONS SERVED BY SETTING IN 2000

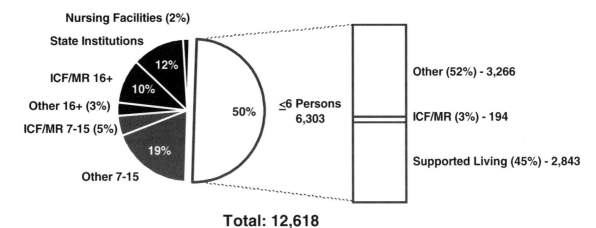

Nursing Facilities (2%)
State Institutions
ICF/MR 16+
Other 16+ (3%)
ICF/MR 7-15 (5%)
Other 7-15

12%
10%
19%
50%

≤6 Persons
6,303

Other (52%) - 3,266
ICF/MR (3%) - 194
Supported Living (45%) - 2,843

Total: 12,618

PERSONS SERVED BY SETTING

	1990	1991	1992	1993	1994	1995	1996	1997	1998	1999	2000
TOTAL	n/a	n/a	10,304	10,380	10,786	11,340	11,412	11,559	11,747	11,794	12,618
16+ PERSONS	n/a	n/a	4,319	4,081	3,980	3,961	3,968	3,533	3,476	3,295	3,378
Nursing Facilities	n/a	n/a	377	219	202	234	232	206	200	192	191
State Institutions	1,992	1,982	1,949	1,838	1,726	1,619	1,605	1,539	1,498	1,512	1,534
Private ICF/MR	1,335	1,331	1,337	1,339	1,339	1,339	1,339	1,229	1,286	1,243	1,274
Other Residential	724	707	656	685	713	769	792	559	492	348	379
7-15 PERSONS	5,252	5,323	3,782	3,385	2,988	2,849	2,701	2,588	2,495	2,872	2,937
Public ICF/MR	0	0	0	0	0	0	0	0	0	0	0
Private ICF/MR	600	600	600	600	600	600	600	559	582	558	574
Other Residential	4,652	4,723	3,182	2,785	2,388	2,249	2,101	2,029	1,913	2,314	2,363
≤6 PERSONS	n/a	n/a	2,203	2,914	3,818	4,531	4,743	5,438	5,776	5,627	6,303
Public ICF/MR	0	0	0	0	0	0	0	0	0	0	0
Private ICF/MR	0	0	0	53	107	159	173	221	229	216	194
Other Residential	n/a	n/a	2,203	2,861	3,712	4,372	4,570	5,217	5,547	5,411	6,109

PERSONS SERVED IN PUBLIC AND PRIVATE INSTITUTIONS AND NURSING FACILITIES

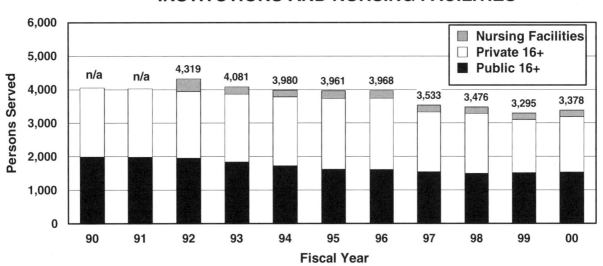

Legend:
- Nursing Facilities
- Private 16+
- Public 16+

Persons Served (y-axis: 0 to 6,000)

Fiscal Year (x-axis: 90 to 00)

Values shown: n/a, n/a, 4,319, 4,081, 3,980, 3,961, 3,968, 3,533, 3,476, 3,295, 3,378

Source: The Coleman Institute and Department of Psychiatry, University of Colorado, 2002.

INDIVIDUAL AND FAMILY SUPPORT

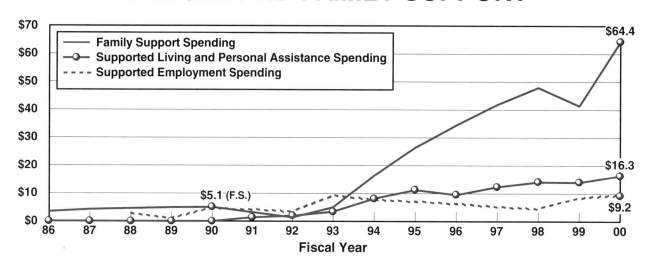

Family Support Spending
Supported Living and Personal Assistance Spending
Supported Employment Spending

$5.1 (F.S.)
$64.4
$16.3
$9.2

PARTICIPANTS AND SPENDING LEVELS

	1990	1991	1992	1993	1994	1995	1996	1997	1998	1999	2000
TOTAL IFS ($)	7,628,880	7,200,668	5,764,846	14,865,031	27,869,496	39,640,887	45,702,365	55,361,281	62,926,865	61,386,179	89,892,059
INDIVIDUAL SUPPORT ($)	3,705,780	4,617,358	4,589,944	10,677,629	13,813,903	16,340,270	14,509,018	16,577,672	17,656,577	21,429,216	25,536,057
Supported Employment ($)	3,705,780	3,517,355	2,956,407	7,812,373	6,874,525	6,396,559	5,874,173	5,158,596	4,349,714	7,960,616	9,210,330
# of Persons	1,578	2,171	2,328	2,640	2,537	2,591	2,016	2,192	2,201	3,368	3,734
Supported Living ($)	0	1,100,003	1,633,537	2,863,006	6,376,325	7,753,033	6,302,494	10,436,628	11,594,277	13,453,022	16,320,109
# of Persons	0	334	496	805	1,132	1,317	1,363	2,019	2,116	2,352	2,839
Personal Assistance ($)	0	0	0	2,250	563,053	2,190,678	2,332,351	982,448	1,712,586	15,578	5,618
# of Persons	0	0	0	2	196	537	474	156	198	6	4
FAMILY SUPPORT ($)	3,923,100	2,583,310	1,174,902	4,187,402	14,055,593	23,300,617	31,193,347	38,783,609	45,270,288	39,956,963	64,356,002
Total Families	3,981	2,386	1,640	2,458	4,716	6,729	7,604	9,697	9,798	8,166	12,021
Cash Subsidy/Payment ($)	926,757	875,974	373,777	1,007,808	913,446	825,668	780,454	485,121	457,629	650,558	1,000,598
# of Families	293	302	232	392	388	550	369	324	282	397	636
Other Family Support ($)	2,996,343	1,707,336	801,125	3,179,594	13,142,147	22,474,949	30,412,893	38,298,488	44,812,659	39,306,405	63,355,404
# of Families	3,981	2,386	1,640	2,458	4,716	6,729	7,604	9,697	9,798	8,166	12,021

PARTICIPANTS IN DAY/WORK AND SUPPORTED EMPLOYMENT

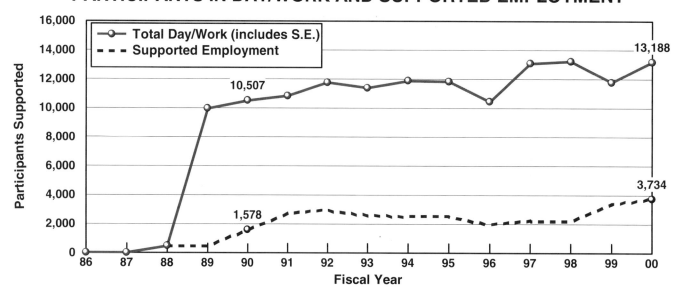

Total Day/Work (includes S.E.)
Supported Employment

10,507
1,578
13,188
3,734

Source: The Coleman Institute and Department of Psychiatry, University of Colorado, 2002.

TRENDS IN SPENDING

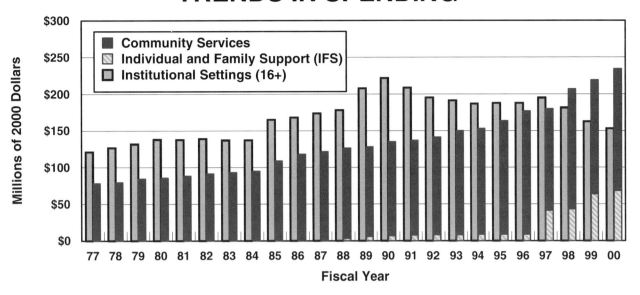

FISCAL EFFORT

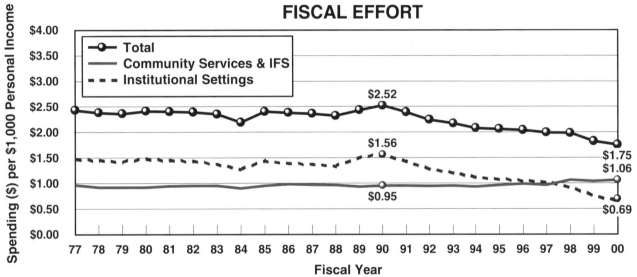

TOTAL MR/DD SPENDING AND
UNMATCHED STATE/LOCAL FUNDS

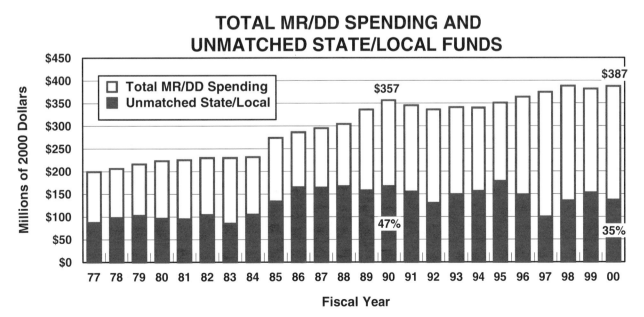

Source: The Coleman Institute and Department of Psychiatry, University of Colorado, 2002.

TRENDS IN REVENUE

COMMUNITY SERVICES REVENUE IN 2000

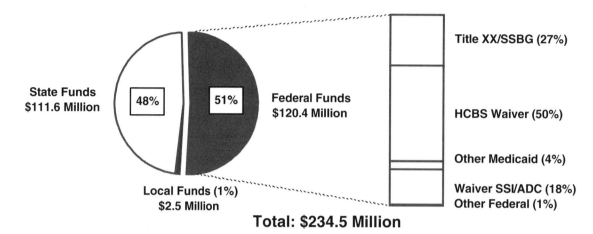

State Funds
$111.6 Million

48%

51%

Federal Funds
$120.4 Million

Local Funds (1%)
$2.5 Million

Title XX/SSBG (27%)

HCBS Waiver (50%)

Other Medicaid (4%)

Waiver SSI/ADC (18%)
Other Federal (1%)

Total: $234.5 Million

COMPONENTS OF FEDERAL MR/DD MEDICAID REVENUE

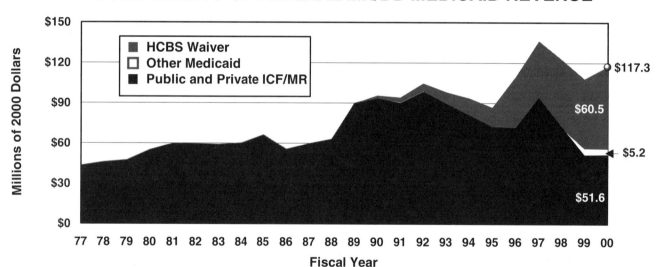

Millions of 2000 Dollars

- ■ HCBS Waiver
- □ Other Medicaid
- ■ Public and Private ICF/MR

$150
$120
$90
$60
$30
$0

$117.3
$60.5
$5.2
$51.6

77 78 79 80 81 82 83 84 85 86 87 88 89 90 91 92 93 94 95 96 97 98 99 00

Fiscal Year

HCBS WAIVER PARTICIPANTS

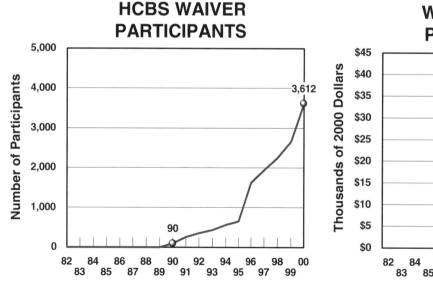

Number of Participants

5,000
4,000
3,000
2,000
1,000
0

3,612

90

82 83 84 85 86 87 88 89 90 91 92 93 94 95 96 97 98 99 00

WAIVER SPENDING PER PARTICIPANT

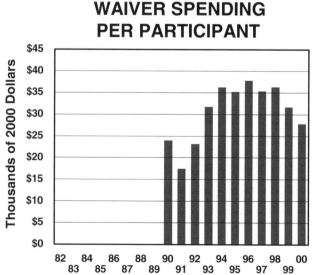

Thousands of 2000 Dollars

$45
$40
$35
$30
$25
$20
$15
$10
$5
$0

82 83 84 85 86 87 88 89 90 91 92 93 94 95 96 97 98 99 00

Source: The Coleman Institute and Department of Psychiatry, University of Colorado, 2002.

TRENDS IN RESIDENTIAL SERVICES
PERSONS SERVED BY SETTING IN 2000

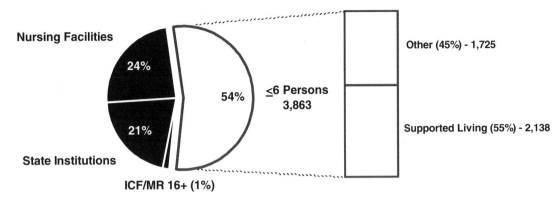

Nursing Facilities
24%
21%
State Institutions
ICF/MR 16+ (1%)
54%
≤6 Persons 3,863
Other (45%) - 1,725
Supported Living (55%) - 2,138

Total: 7,162

PERSONS SERVED BY SETTING

	1990	1991	1992	1993	1994	1995	1996	1997	1998	1999	2000
TOTAL	5,506	5,432	5,472	5,945	5,809	5,897	5,780	6,018	6,268	7,085	7,162
16+ PERSONS	3,998	3,894	3,976	4,289	4,248	4,142	3,968	3,793	3,409	3,356	3,299
Nursing Facilities	1,807	1,685	1,777	2,105	2,080	2,004	1,897	1,757	1,576	1,701	1,700
State Institutions	2,081	2,099	2,089	2,074	2,058	2,028	1,961	1,926	1,723	1,545	1,489
Private ICF/MR	110	110	110	110	110	110	110	110	110	110	110
Other Residential	0	0	0	0	0	0	0	0	0	0	0
7-15 PERSONS	0	0	7	7	7	7	7	0	0	0	0
Public ICF/MR	0	0	0	0	0	0	0	0	0	0	0
Private ICF/MR	0	0	0	0	0	0	0	0	0	0	0
Other Residential	0	0	7	7	7	7	7	0	0	0	0
≤6 PERSONS	1,508	1,538	1,489	1,649	1,554	1,748	1,805	2,225	2,859	3,729	3,863
Public ICF/MR	0	0	0	0	0	0	0	0	0	0	0
Private ICF/MR	0	0	0	0	0	0	0	0	0	0	0
Other Residential	1,508	1,538	1,489	1,649	1,554	1,748	1,805	2,225	2,859	3,729	3,863

PERSONS SERVED IN PUBLIC AND PRIVATE INSTITUTIONS AND NURSING FACILITIES

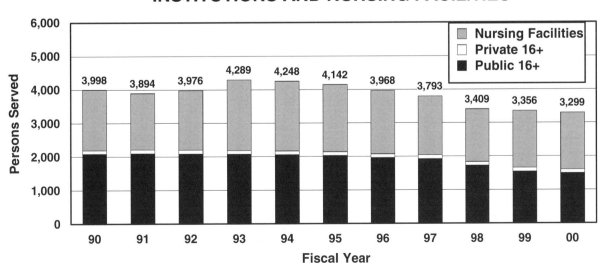

Source: The Coleman Institute and Department of Psychiatry, University of Colorado, 2002.

185

INDIVIDUAL AND FAMILY SUPPORT

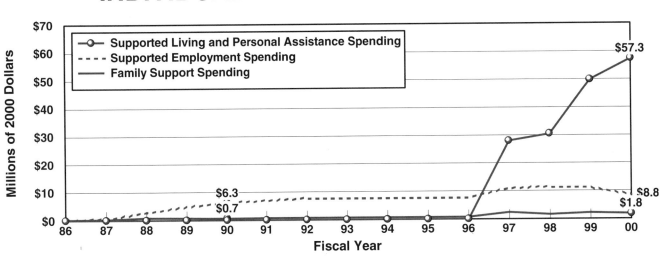

PARTICIPANTS AND SPENDING LEVELS

	1990	1991	1992	1993	1994	1995	1996	1997	1998	1999	2000
TOTAL IFS ($)	5,385,494	6,086,141	6,761,227	6,964,064	7,172,986	7,388,175	7,609,821	38,153,767	40,728,951	61,060,181	67,974,882
INDIVIDUAL SUPPORT ($)	4,830,840	5,420,544	6,117,144	6,300,658	6,489,678	6,684,368	6,884,899	35,912,302	39,239,905	58,985,239	66,157,575
Supported Employment ($)	4,830,840	5,420,544	6,117,144	6,300,658	6,489,678	6,684,368	6,884,899	10,051,239	10,514,166	10,914,642	8,813,497
# of Persons	810	891	986	1,123	1,152	1,175	1,181	2,088	2,578	2,504	2,566
Supported Living ($)	0	0	0	0	0	0	0	25,861,063	28,725,739	48,070,597	57,344,078
# of Persons	0	0	0	0	0	0	0	938	1,630	1,960	2,138
Personal Assistance ($)	0	0	0	0	0	0	0	0	0	0	0
# of Persons	0	0	0	0	0	0	0	0	0	0	0
FAMILY SUPPORT ($)	554,654	665,597	644,083	663,405	683,308	703,807	724,921	2,241,465	1,489,046	2,074,942	1,817,307
Total Families	454	545	607	1,656	2,017	2,440	2,669	7,908	7,093	7,598	5,648
Cash Subsidy/Payment ($)	0	0	0	0	0	0	0	0	0	0	0
# of Families	0	0	0	0	0	0	0	0	0	0	0
Other Family Support ($)	554,654	665,597	644,083	663,405	683,308	703,807	724,921	2,241,465	1,489,046	2,074,942	1,817,307
# of Families	454	545	607	1,656	2,017	2,440	2,669	7,908	7,093	7,598	5,648

PARTICIPANTS IN DAY/WORK AND SUPPORTED EMPLOYMENT

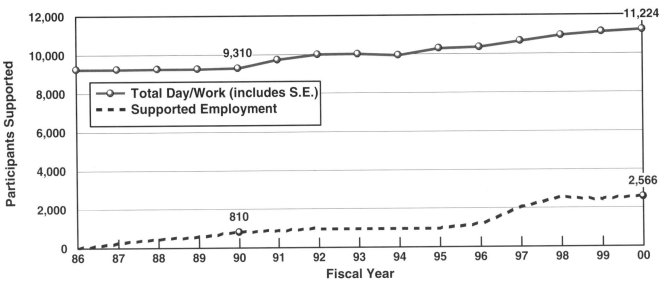

Source: The Coleman Institute and Department of Psychiatry, University of Colorado, 2002.

TRENDS IN SPENDING

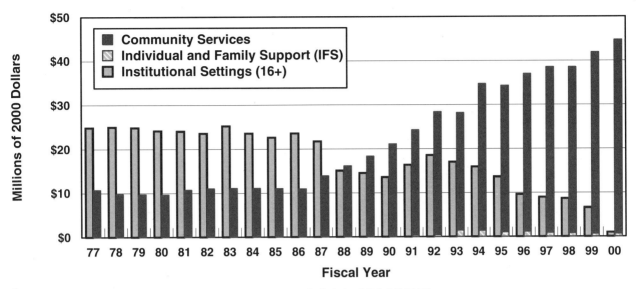

- ■ Community Services
- ▨ Individual and Family Support (IFS)
- ▨ Institutional Settings (16+)

Millions of 2000 Dollars

Fiscal Year

FISCAL EFFORT

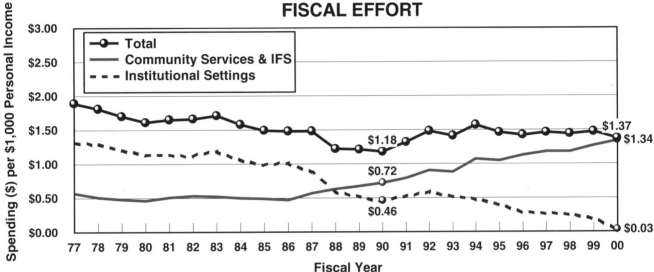

Spending ($) per $1,000 Personal Income

- —○— Total
- —— Community Services & IFS
- - - - Institutional Settings

$1.18
$0.72
$0.46
$1.37
$1.34
$0.03

Fiscal Year

TOTAL MR/DD SPENDING AND
UNMATCHED STATE/LOCAL FUNDS

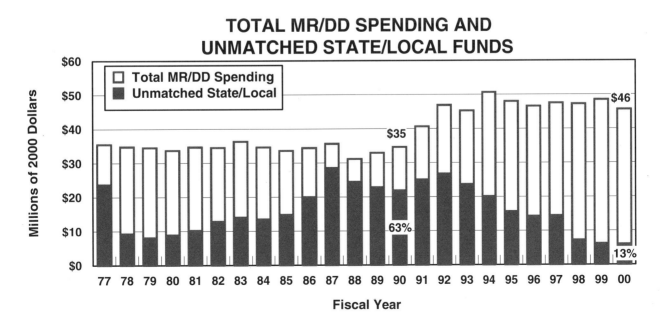

- ▢ Total MR/DD Spending
- ■ Unmatched State/Local

Millions of 2000 Dollars

$35
$46
63%
13%

Fiscal Year

Source: The Coleman Institute and Department of Psychiatry, University of Colorado, 2002.

187

TRENDS IN REVENUE

COMMUNITY SERVICES REVENUE IN 2000

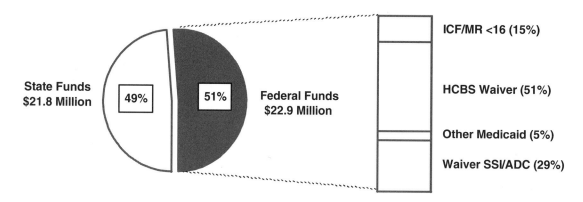

**State Funds
$21.8 Million** 49% 51% **Federal Funds
$22.9 Million**

ICF/MR <16 (15%)

HCBS Waiver (51%)

Other Medicaid (5%)

Waiver SSI/ADC (29%)

Total: $44.7 Million

COMPONENTS OF FEDERAL MR/DD MEDICAID REVENUE

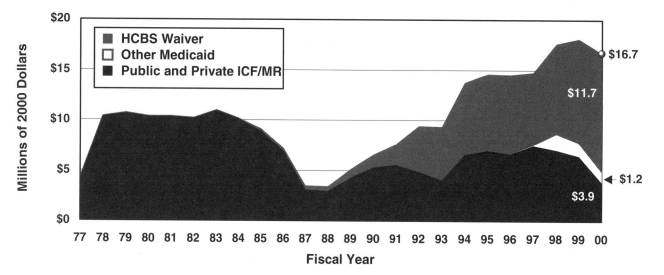

Millions of 2000 Dollars

- ■ HCBS Waiver
- □ Other Medicaid
- ■ Public and Private ICF/MR

$16.7
$11.7
$3.9
$1.2

Fiscal Year

HCBS WAIVER PARTICIPANTS

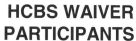
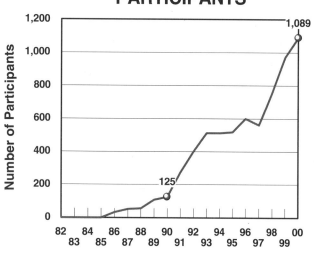

Number of Participants

1,089

125

WAIVER SPENDING PER PARTICIPANT

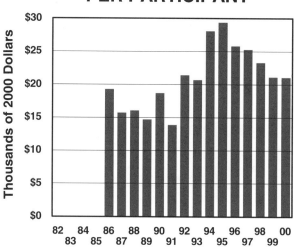

Thousands of 2000 Dollars

Source: The Coleman Institute and Department of Psychiatry, University of Colorado, 2002.

TRENDS IN RESIDENTIAL SERVICES
PERSONS SERVED BY SETTING IN 2000

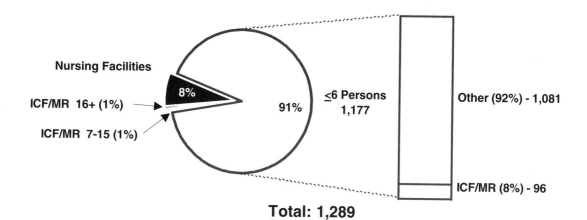

Nursing Facilities

ICF/MR 16+ (1%)

ICF/MR 7-15 (1%)

8%

91%

≤6 Persons
1,177

Other (92%) - 1,081

ICF/MR (8%) - 96

Total: 1,289

PERSONS SERVED BY SETTING

	1990	1991	1992	1993	1994	1995	1996	1997	1998	1999	2000
TOTAL	1,104	1,093	1,131	1,394	1,656	1,734	1,547	1,535	1,675	1,417	1,289
16+ PERSONS	225	187	176	155	129	129	105	127	98	109	105
Nursing Facilities	59	35	37	35	29	31	45	74	55	76	97
State Institutions	166	152	139	120	100	98	60	53	43	25	0
Private ICF/MR	0	0	0	0	0	0	0	0	0	8	8
Other Residential	0	0	0	0	0	0	0	0	0	0	0
7-15 PERSONS	102	93	6	7	7	7	7	7	7	7	7
Public ICF/MR	0	0	0	0	0	0	0	0	0	0	0
Private ICF/MR	102	93	6	7	7	7	7	7	7	7	7
Other Residential	0	0	0	0	0	0	0	0	0	0	0
≤6 PERSONS	777	813	949	1,232	1,520	1,598	1,435	1,401	1,570	1,301	1,177
Public ICF/MR	0	0	0	0	0	0	0	0	0	0	0
Private ICF/MR	na	na	36	47	41	54	75	80	89	95	96
Other Residential	777	813	913	1,185	1,479	1,544	1,360	1,321	1,481	1,206	1,081

PERSONS SERVED IN PUBLIC AND PRIVATE INSTITUTIONS AND NURSING FACILITIES

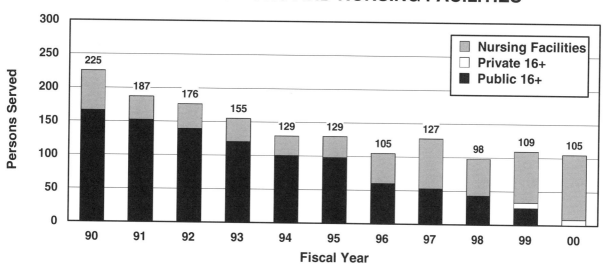

Source: The Coleman Institute and Department of Psychiatry, University of Colorado, 2002.

189

INDIVIDUAL AND FAMILY SUPPORT

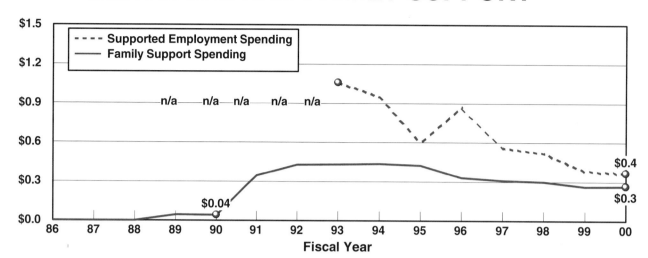

PARTICIPANTS AND SPENDING LEVELS

	1990	1991	1992	1993	1994	1995	1996	1997	1998	1999	2000
TOTAL IFS ($)	n/a	n/a	n/a	1,248,176	1,188,074	906,484	1,081,154	807,774	777,056	619,930	632,076
INDIVIDUAL SUPPORT ($)	n/a	n/a	n/a	885,976	814,074	531,484	782,154	521,180	494,388	366,866	366,866
Supported Employment ($)	n/a	n/a	n/a	885,976	814,074	531,484	782,154	521,180	494,388	366,866	366,866
# of Persons	115	125	126	133	136	105	110	69	68	53	53
Supported Living ($)	0	0	0	0	0	0	0	0	0	0	0
# of Persons	0	0	0	0	0	0	0	0	0	0	0
Personal Assistance ($)	0	0	0	0	0	0	0	0	0	0	0
# of Persons	0	0	0	0	0	0	0	0	0	0	0
FAMILY SUPPORT ($)	32,102	277,222	352,000	362,200	374,000	375,000	299,000	286,594	282,668	253,064	265,210
Total Families	68	204	375	448	634	612	671	556	565	609	632
Cash Subsidy/Payment ($)	0	0	0	0	0	0	0	0	0	0	0
# of Families	0	0	0	0	0	0	0	0	0	0	0
Other Family Support ($)	32,102	277,222	352,000	362,200	374,000	375,000	299,000	286,594	282,668	253,064	265,210
# of Families	68	204	375	448	634	612	671	556	565	609	632

PARTICIPANTS IN DAY/WORK AND SUPPORTED EMPLOYMENT

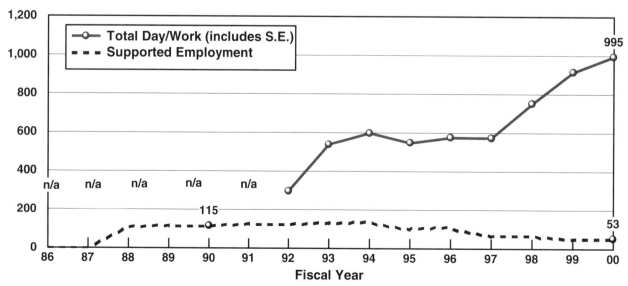

Source: The Coleman Institute and Department of Psychiatry, University of Colorado, 2002.

TRENDS IN SPENDING

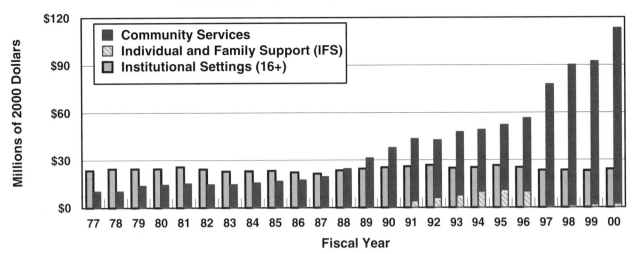

*Supported Living data for 1997-2000 were unavailable. The drop in IFS spending from 1996 to 1997 is an artifact of these missing data.

FISCAL EFFORT

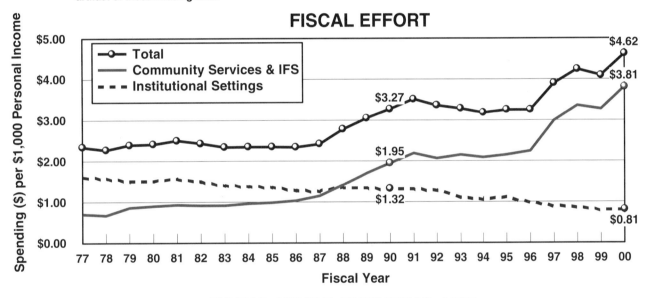

TOTAL MR/DD SPENDING AND
UNMATCHED STATE/LOCAL FUNDS

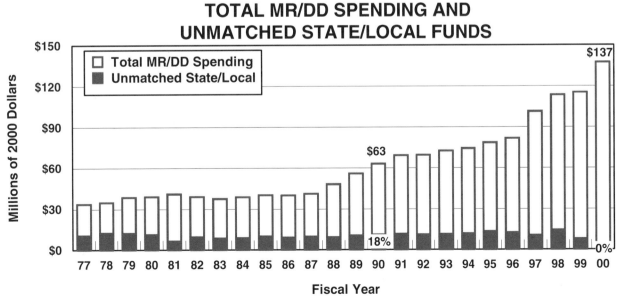

Source: The Coleman Institute and Department of Psychiatry, University of Colorado, 2002.

191

IDAHO

TRENDS IN REVENUE

COMMUNITY SERVICES REVENUE IN 2000

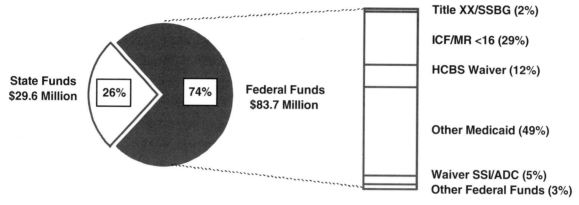

Total: $113.3 Million

COMPONENTS OF FEDERAL MR/DD MEDICAID REVENUE

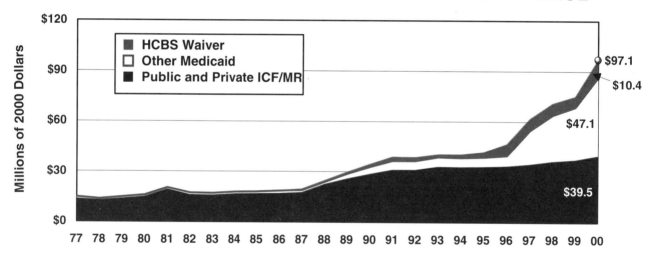

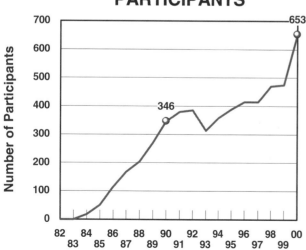

HCBS WAIVER PARTICIPANTS

WAIVER SPENDING PER PARTICIPANT

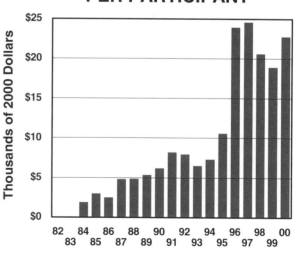

192

Source: The Coleman Institute and Department of Psychiatry, University of Colorado, 2002.

TRENDS IN RESIDENTIAL SERVICES

PERSONS SERVED BY SETTING IN 2000

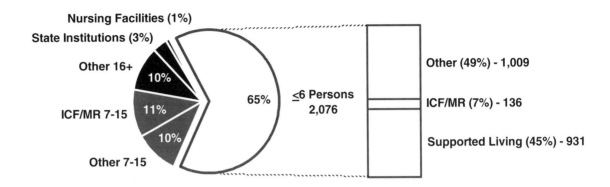

Total: 3,212

PERSONS SERVED BY SETTING

	1990	1991	1992	1993	1994	1995	1996	1997	1998	1999	2000
TOTAL	1,195	1,176	1,886	2,228	2,758	2,882	2,719	2,731	2,927	2,772	3,212
16+ PERSONS	372	313	462	471	498	517	517	506	432	415	464
Nursing Facilities	124	90	90	112	133	107	110	45	39	32	28
State Institutions	193	165	172	154	147	140	131	112	120	112	110
Private ICF/MR	55	58	58	58	58	58	58	58	0	0	0
Other Residential	0	0	142	147	160	212	218	291	273	271	326
7-15 PERSONS	823	863	526	591	617	593	540	616	647	626	672
Public ICF/MR	0	0	0	0	0	0	0	0	0	0	0
Private ICF/MR	248	281	289	296	296	296	296	369	385	353	346
Other Residential	575	582	237	295	321	297	244	247	262	273	326
≤6 PERSONS	0	0	898	1,166	1,643	1,772	1,662	1,609	1,848	1,731	2,076
Public ICF/MR	0	0	0	0	0	0	0	0	0	0	0
Private ICF/MR	0	0	12	43	43	43	43	72	107	134	136
Other Residential	0	0	886	1,123	1,600	1,729	1,619	1,537	1,741	1,597	1,940

PERSONS SERVED IN PUBLIC AND PRIVATE INSTITUTIONS AND NURSING FACILITIES

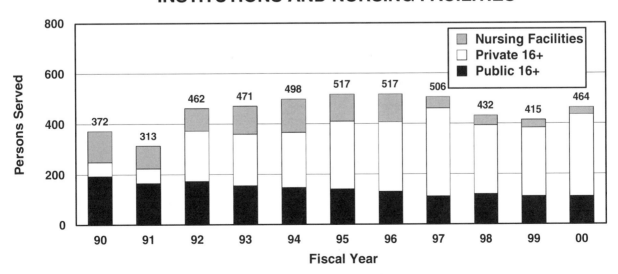

Source: The Coleman Institute and Department of Psychiatry, University of Colorado, 2002.

INDIVIDUAL AND FAMILY SUPPORT

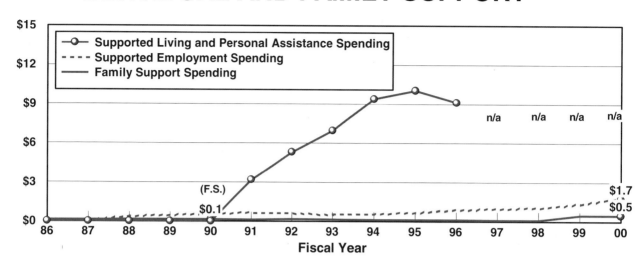

PARTICIPANTS AND SPENDING LEVELS

	1990	1991	1992	1993	1994	1995	1996	1997	1998	1999	2000
TOTAL IFS ($)	n/a	3,155,900	4,995,930	6,411,801	8,670,091	9,539,661	9,143,972	n/a	n/a	n/a	n/a
INDIVIDUAL SUPPORT ($)	n/a	3,042,400	4,848,930	6,279,601	8,549,891	9,419,461	9,024,172	n/a	n/a	n/a	n/a
Supported Employment ($)	na	492,400	502,000	454,400	502,000	555,900	771,000	865,189	923,692	1,291,323	1,747,859
# of Persons	133	168	450	206	318	315	267	326	402	n/a	n/a
Supported Living ($)	0	50,000	241,667	1,200,000	2,166,667	3,008,333	4,166,667	n/a	n/a	n/a	n/a
# of Persons	0	6	29	144	260	361	500	401	455	825	931
Personal Assistance ($)	0	2,500,000	4,105,263	4,625,201	5,881,224	5,855,228	4,086,505	n/a	n/a	n/a	n/a
# of Persons	0	380	624	703	894	890	621	438	475	n/a	n/a
FAMILY SUPPORT ($)	113,500	113,500	147,000	132,200	120,200	120,200	119,800	107,084	108,567	463,284	471,747
Total Families	438	471	468	495	535	468	545	741	840	1,047	988
Cash Subsidy/Payment ($)	0	0	0	0	0	0	0	0	0	0	0
# of Families	0	0	0	0	0	0	0	0	0	0	0
Other Family Support ($)	113,500	113,500	147,000	132,200	120,200	120,200	119,800	107,084	108,567	463,284	471,747
# of Families	438	471	468	495	535	468	545	741	840	1,047	988

PARTICIPANTS IN DAY/WORK AND SUPPORTED EMPLOYMENT

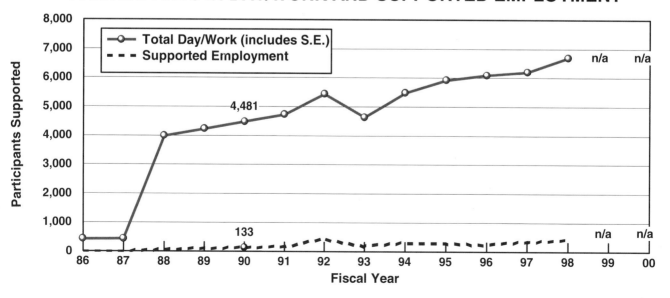

Source: The Coleman Institute and Department of Psychiatry, University of Colorado, 2002.

TRENDS IN SPENDING

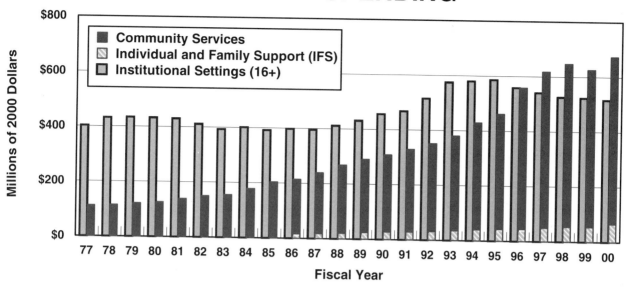

Millions of 2000 Dollars

- ■ Community Services
- ▨ Individual and Family Support (IFS)
- ▨ Institutional Settings (16+)

$800
$600
$400
$200
$0

Fiscal Year: 77 78 79 80 81 82 83 84 85 86 87 88 89 90 91 92 93 94 95 96 97 98 99 00

FISCAL EFFORT

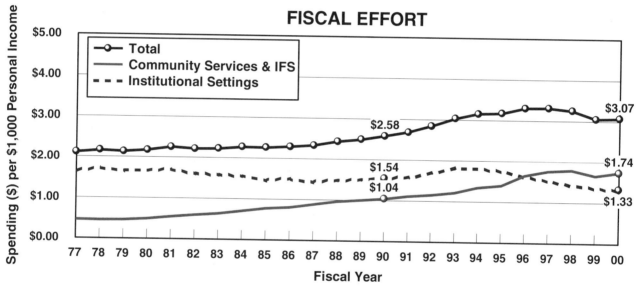

Spending ($) per $1,000 Personal Income

- ─○─ Total
- ─── Community Services & IFS
- ▬ ▬ Institutional Settings

$5.00
$4.00
$3.00
$2.00
$1.00
$0.00

$2.58 $3.07
$1.54 $1.74
$1.04 $1.33

Fiscal Year: 77 78 79 80 81 82 83 84 85 86 87 88 89 90 91 92 93 94 95 96 97 98 99 00

TOTAL MR/DD SPENDING AND
UNMATCHED STATE/LOCAL FUNDS

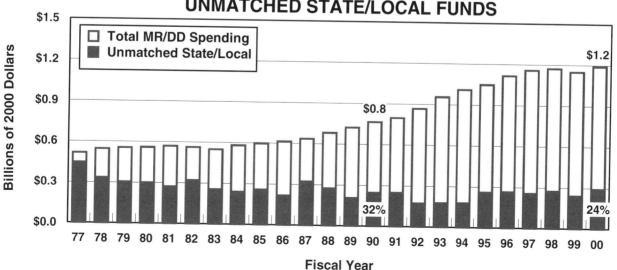

Billions of 2000 Dollars

- ☐ Total MR/DD Spending
- ■ Unmatched State/Local

$1.5
$1.2
$0.9
$0.6
$0.3
$0.0

$0.8 $1.2
32%   24%

Fiscal Year: 77 78 79 80 81 82 83 84 85 86 87 88 89 90 91 92 93 94 95 96 97 98 99 00

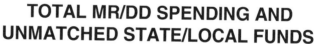

Source: The Coleman Institute and Department of Psychiatry, University of Colorado, 2002.

ILLINOIS

TRENDS IN REVENUE

COMMUNITY SERVICES REVENUE IN 2000

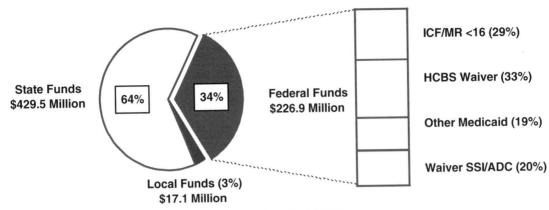

State Funds
$429.5 Million

64%

34%

Federal Funds
$226.9 Million

Local Funds (3%)
$17.1 Million

ICF/MR <16 (29%)

HCBS Waiver (33%)

Other Medicaid (19%)

Waiver SSI/ADC (20%)

Total: $673.5 Million

COMPONENTS OF FEDERAL MR/DD MEDICAID REVENUE

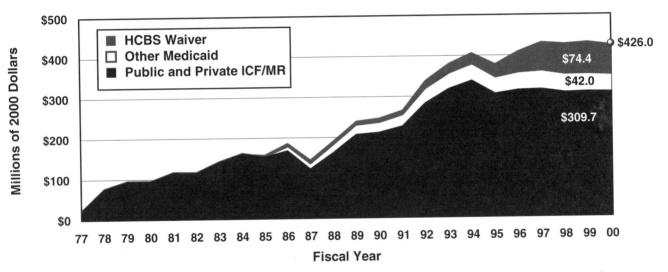

HCBS WAIVER PARTICIPANTS

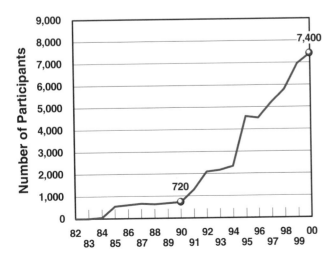

WAIVER SPENDING PER PARTICIPANT

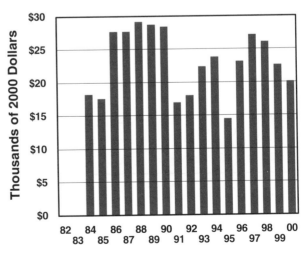

Source: The Coleman Institute and Department of Psychiatry, University of Colorado, 2002.

TRENDS IN RESIDENTIAL SERVICES

PERSONS SERVED BY SETTING IN 2000

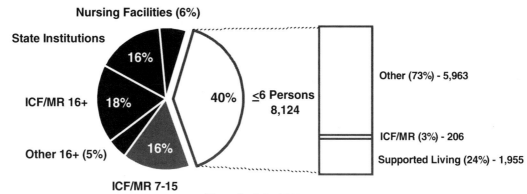

Nursing Facilities (6%)

State Institutions 16%

ICF/MR 16+ 18%

Other 16+ (5%)

ICF/MR 7-15 16%

40% ≤6 Persons 8,124

Other (73%) - 5,963

ICF/MR (3%) - 206

Supported Living (24%) - 1,955

Total: 20,405

PERSONS SERVED BY SETTING

	1990	1991	1992	1993	1994	1995	1996	1997	1998	1999	2000
TOTAL	18,303	18,683	19,295	18,551	19,039	20,031	20,025	19,990	20,197	20,099	20,405
16+ PERSONS	13,985	13,590	12,980	11,721	11,434	11,836	11,037	10,329	9,861	9,390	9,073
Nursing Facilities	3,906	3,629	2,159	1,659	1,750	2,038	1,971	1,764	1,543	1,341	1,267
State Institutions	4,473	4,348	4,348	3,980	3,790	3,714	3,645	3,582	3,405	3,304	3,221
Private ICF/MR	4,188	4,212	5,081	4,705	4,601	4,817	4,243	3,864	3,864	3,765	3,647
Other Residential	1,418	1,401	1,392	1,377	1,293	1,267	1,178	1,119	1,049	980	938
7-15 PERSONS	4,318	5,093	2,489	2,524	2,706	2,729	2,821	2,952	2,952	3,245	3,208
Public ICF/MR	0	0	0	0	0	0	0	0	0	0	0
Private ICF/MR	1,670	2,279	2,439	2,502	2,684	2,708	2,821	2,952	2,952	3,245	3,208
Other Residential	2,648	2,814	50	22	22	21	0	0	0	0	0
≤6 PERSONS	0	0	3,826	4,306	4,899	5,466	6,167	6,709	7,384	7,464	8,124
Public ICF/MR	0	0	0	0	0	0	0	0	0	0	0
Private ICF/MR	0	0	0	96	184	204	204	194	194	207	206
Other Residential	0	0	3,826	4,210	4,715	5,262	5,963	6,515	7,190	7,257	7,918

PERSONS SERVED IN PUBLIC AND PRIVATE INSTITUTIONS AND NURSING FACILITIES

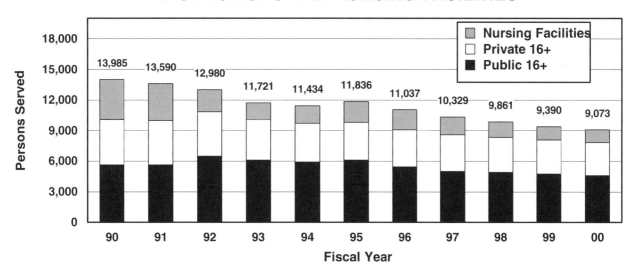

Persons Served

Legend:
- Nursing Facilities
- Private 16+
- Public 16+

13,985 13,590 12,980 11,721 11,434 11,836 11,037 10,329 9,861 9,390 9,073

Fiscal Year: 90 91 92 93 94 95 96 97 98 99 00

Source: The Coleman Institute and Department of Psychiatry, University of Colorado, 2002.

INDIVIDUAL AND FAMILY SUPPORT

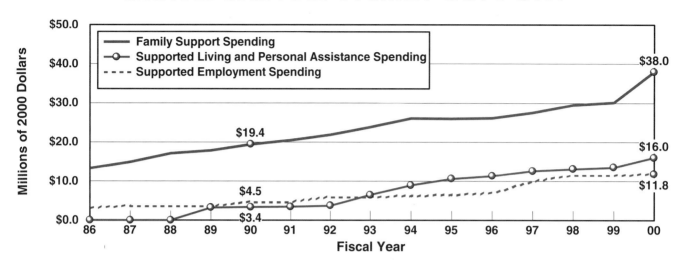

PARTICIPANTS AND SPENDING LEVELS

	1990	1991	1992	1993	1994	1995	1996	1997	1998	1999	2000
TOTAL IFS ($)	21,069,500	22,983,500	25,690,300	30,332,136	35,206,594	37,877,388	40,146,161	46,406,900	51,169,600	53,134,525	65,834,179
INDIVIDUAL SUPPORT ($)	6,098,928	6,541,062	7,776,627	10,382,890	12,879,482	14,912,821	16,471,950	20,970,200	23,351,200	24,087,414	27,860,710
Supported Employment ($)	3,488,200	3,777,200	4,723,400	4,970,867	5,222,292	5,542,311	6,204,600	9,301,800	10,930,600	11,036,394	11,819,696
# of Persons	853	1,168	1,370	1,367	1,369	1,415	1,593	2,123	2,478	2,272	2,455
Supported Living ($)	2,610,728	2,763,862	3,053,227	5,412,023	7,657,190	9,370,510	10,267,350	11,668,400	12,420,600	13,051,020	16,041,014
# of Persons	1,374	1,541	1,471	1,498	1,610	1,911	1,932	2,039	2,136	1,793	1,955
Personal Assistance ($)	0	0	0	0	0	0	0	0	0	0	0
# of Persons	0	0	0	0	0	0	0	0	0	0	0
FAMILY SUPPORT ($)	14,970,572	16,442,438	17,913,673	19,949,246	22,327,112	22,964,567	23,674,211	25,436,700	27,818,400	29,047,111	37,973,469
Total Families	14,273	15,718	15,179	14,978	14,953	14,184	13,958	16,930	17,574	14,625	16,434
Cash Subsidy/Payment ($)	0	705,900	1,202,800	2,630,200	4,147,000	4,852,000	5,409,500	5,715,800	6,631,900	8,511,317	16,545,171
# of Families	0	204	250	382	584	656	612	603	728	1,024	1,941
Other Family Support ($)	14,970,572	15,736,538	16,710,873	17,319,046	18,180,112	18,112,567	18,264,711	19,720,900	21,186,500	20,535,794	21,428,298
# of Families	14,273	15,514	14,929	14,596	14,369	13,528	13,346	16,327	16,846	13,601	14,493

PARTICIPANTS IN DAY/WORK AND SUPPORTED EMPLOYMENT

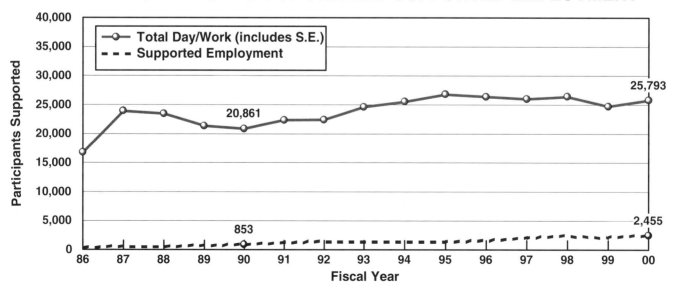

Source: The Coleman Institute and Department of Psychiatry, University of Colorado, 2002.

TRENDS IN SPENDING

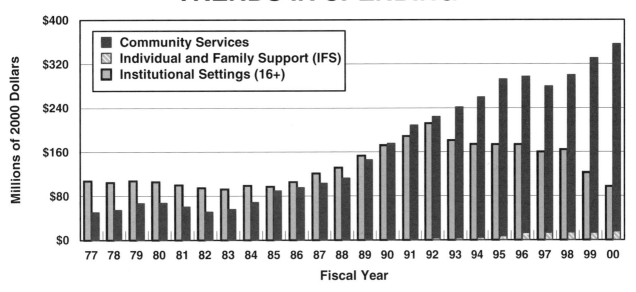

Millions of 2000 Dollars

- Community Services
- Individual and Family Support (IFS)
- Institutional Settings (16+)

Fiscal Year: 77 78 79 80 81 82 83 84 85 86 87 88 89 90 91 92 93 94 95 96 97 98 99 00

FISCAL EFFORT

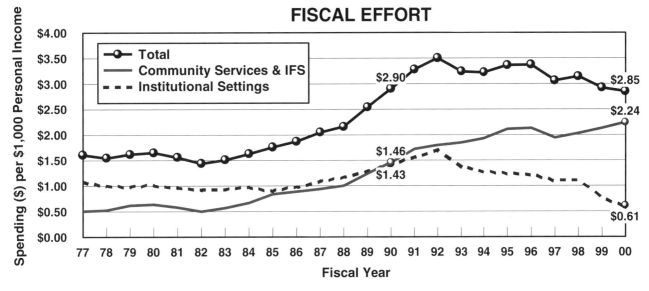

Spending ($) per $1,000 Personal Income

- Total
- Community Services & IFS
- Institutional Settings

$2.90 $2.85
$2.24
$1.46
$1.43
$0.61

Fiscal Year: 77 78 79 80 81 82 83 84 85 86 87 88 89 90 91 92 93 94 95 96 97 98 99 00

TOTAL MR/DD SPENDING AND
UNMATCHED STATE/LOCAL FUNDS

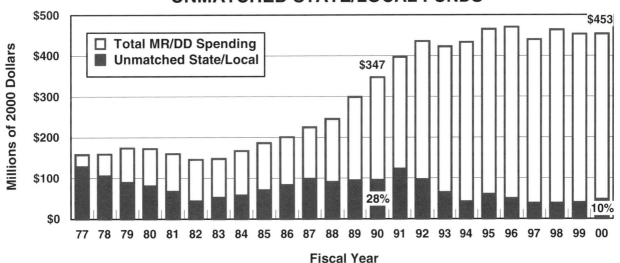

Millions of 2000 Dollars

- Total MR/DD Spending
- Unmatched State/Local

$347 $453
28%   10%

Fiscal Year: 77 78 79 80 81 82 83 84 85 86 87 88 89 90 91 92 93 94 95 96 97 98 99 00

Source: The Coleman Institute and Department of Psychiatry, University of Colorado, 2002.

TRENDS IN REVENUE

COMMUNITY SERVICES REVENUE IN 2000

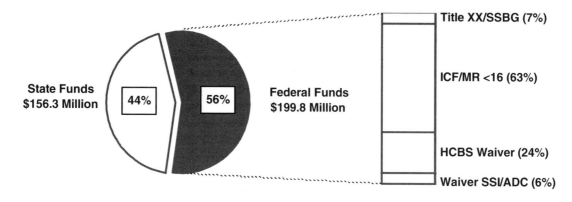

State Funds $156.3 Million 44%

56% **Federal Funds $199.8 Million**

Title XX/SSBG (7%)

ICF/MR <16 (63%)

HCBS Waiver (24%)

Waiver SSI/ADC (6%)

Total: $356.1 Million

COMPONENTS OF FEDERAL MR/DD MEDICAID REVENUE

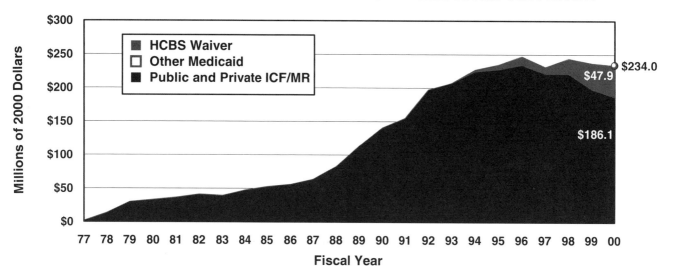

- ■ HCBS Waiver
- □ Other Medicaid
- ■ Public and Private ICF/MR

$234.0
$47.9
$186.1

Millions of 2000 Dollars

Fiscal Year

HCBS WAIVER PARTICIPANTS

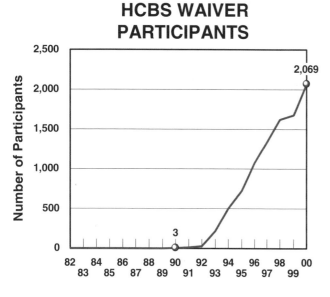

2,069

3

Number of Participants

WAIVER SPENDING PER PARTICIPANT

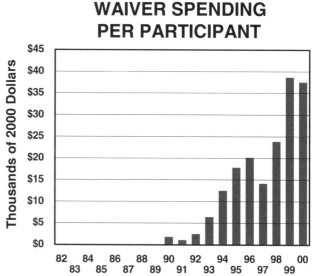

Thousands of 2000 Dollars

Source: The Coleman Institute and Department of Psychiatry, University of Colorado, 2002.

TRENDS IN RESIDENTIAL SERVICES
PERSONS SERVED BY SETTING IN 2000

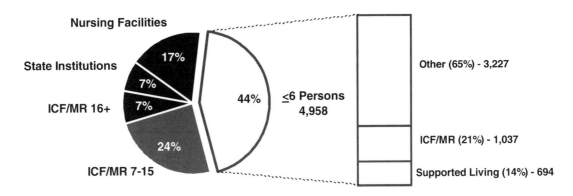

Total: 11,262

PERSONS SERVED BY SETTING

	1990	1991	1992	1993	1994	1995	1996	1997	1998	1999	2000
TOTAL	9,659	9,826	9,875	10,038	10,174	10,152	10,297	10,643	11,199	11,671	11,262
16+ PERSONS	5,132	4,997	4,835	4,641	4,639	4,507	4,313	4,009	4,177	3,961	3,550
Nursing Facilities	2,370	2,305	2,241	2,135	2,047	2,057	2,057	1,823	2,000	2,200	1,933
State Institutions	1,983	1,912	1,814	1,556	1,441	1,299	1,261	1,191	1,182	926	782
Private ICF/MR	779	780	780	950	1,151	1,151	995	995	995	835	835
Other Residential	0	0	0	0	0	0	0	0	0	0	0
7-15 PERSONS	1,327	1,474	2,716	2,724	2,757	2,767	2,767	2,763	2,763	2,754	2,754
Public ICF/MR	0	0	0	0	0	0	0	0	0	0	0
Private ICF/MR	1,327	1,474	2,716	2,724	2,757	2,767	2,767	2,763	2,763	2,754	2,754
Other Residential	0	0	0	0	0	0	0	0	0	0	0
≤6 PERSONS	3,200	3,355	2,324	2,673	2,778	2,878	3,217	3,871	4,259	4,956	4,958
Public ICF/MR	0	0	0	0	0	0	0	0	0	0	0
Private ICF/MR	2,000	2,000	934	1,023	1,028	1,028	1,028	1,032	1,032	1,037	1,037
Other Residential	1,200	1,355	1,390	1,650	1,750	1,850	2,189	2,839	3,227	3,919	3,921

PERSONS SERVED IN PUBLIC AND PRIVATE INSTITUTIONS AND NURSING FACILITIES

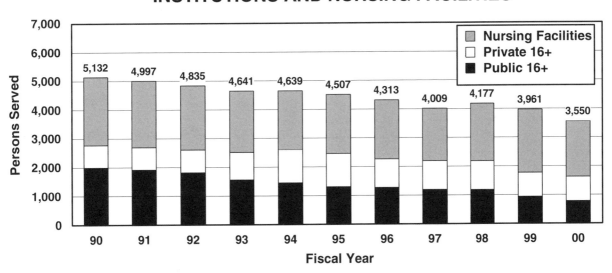

Source: The Coleman Institute and Department of Psychiatry, University of Colorado, 2002.

201

INDIVIDUAL AND FAMILY SUPPORT

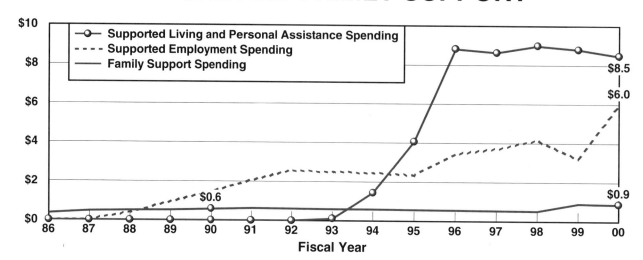

PARTICIPANTS AND SPENDING LEVELS

	1990	1991	1992	1993	1994	1995	1996	1997	1998	1999	2000
TOTAL IFS ($)	na	na	2,602,350	2,694,250	3,831,450	6,198,840	11,568,331	11,898,665	12,897,109	12,464,035	15,344,196
INDIVIDUAL SUPPORT ($)	na	na	2,100,000	2,191,900	3,329,100	5,696,490	11,065,981	11,396,315	12,394,759	11,589,035	14,469,196
Supported Employment ($)	na	na	2,100,000	2,100,000	2,100,000	2,100,000	3,091,000	3,421,333	3,916,833	3,111,107	5,991,266
# of Persons	na	na	881	1,000	1,300	1,478	1,500	1,626	1,726	1,786	1,824
Supported Living ($)	0	0	0	0	0	0	0	0	502,943	502,944	502,945
# of Persons	0	0	0	0	0	0	0	0	58	59	60
Personal Assistance ($)	0	0	0	91,900	1,229,100	3,596,490	7,974,981	7,974,982	7,974,983	7,974,984	7,974,985
# of Persons	0	0	0	40	128	391	630	631	632	633	634
FAMILY SUPPORT ($)	446,062	502,350	502,350	502,350	502,350	502,350	502,350	502,350	502,350	875,000	875,000
Total Families	na	1,500	1,500	1,500	1,500	1,500	1,500	1,500	1,500	1,500	2,400
Cash Subsidy/Payment ($)	0	0	0	0	0	0	0	0	0	0	0
# of Families	0	0	0	0	0	0	0	0	0	0	0
Other Family Support ($)	446,062	502,350	502,350	502,350	502,350	502,350	502,350	502,350	502,350	875,000	875,000
# of Families	na	1,500	1,500	1,500	1,500	1,500	1,500	1,500	1,500	1,500	2,400

PARTICIPANTS IN DAY/WORK AND SUPPORTED EMPLOYMENT

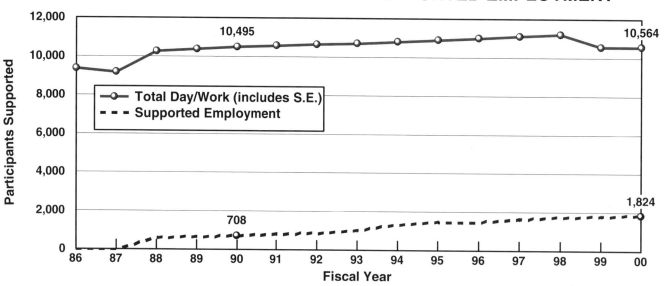

Source: The Coleman Institute and Department of Psychiatry, University of Colorado, 2002.

TRENDS IN SPENDING

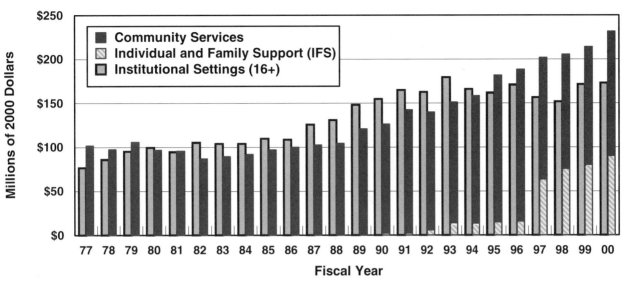

FISCAL EFFORT

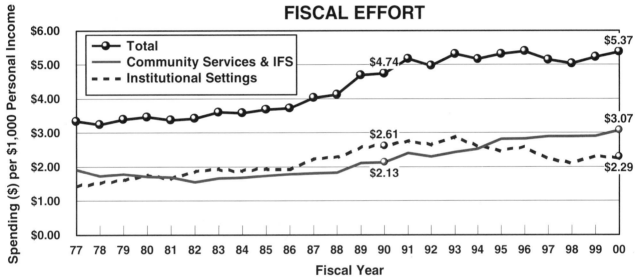

TOTAL MR/DD SPENDING AND UNMATCHED STATE/LOCAL FUNDS

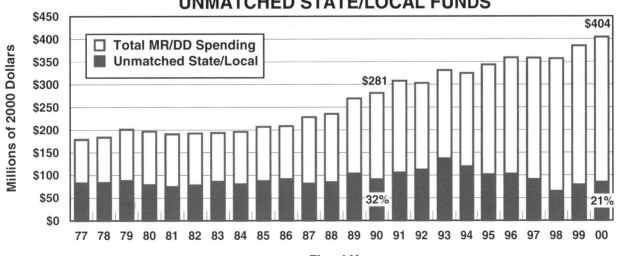

Source: The Coleman Institute and Department of Psychiatry, University of Colorado, 2002.

203

TRENDS IN REVENUE

COMMUNITY SERVICES REVENUE IN 2000

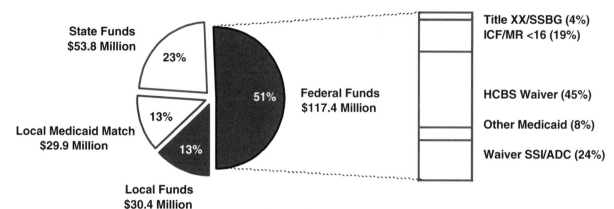

State Funds
$53.8 Million

23%

13%

Local Medicaid Match
$29.9 Million

13%

51%

Federal Funds
$117.4 Million

Local Funds
$30.4 Million

Title XX/SSBG (4%)
ICF/MR <16 (19%)

HCBS Waiver (45%)

Other Medicaid (8%)

Waiver SSI/ADC (24%)

Total: $231.5 Million

COMPONENTS OF FEDERAL MR/DD MEDICAID REVENUE

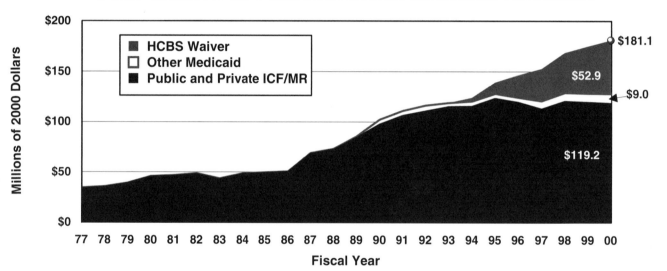

Millions of 2000 Dollars

- ■ HCBS Waiver
- □ Other Medicaid
- ■ Public and Private ICF/MR

$200

$150

$100

$50

$0

$181.1

$52.9

$9.0

$119.2

77 78 79 80 81 82 83 84 85 86 87 88 89 90 91 92 93 94 95 96 97 98 99 00

Fiscal Year

HCBS WAIVER PARTICIPANTS

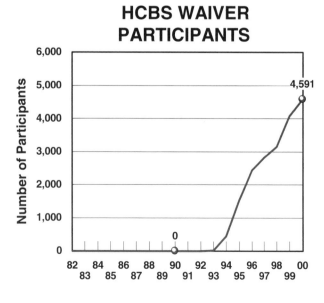

Number of Participants

6,000

5,000

4,000

3,000

2,000

1,000

0

4,591

0

82 84 86 88 90 92 94 96 98 00
83 85 87 89 91 93 95 97 99

WAIVER SPENDING PER PARTICIPANT

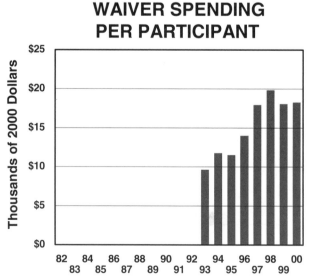

Thousands of 2000 Dollars

$25

$20

$15

$10

$5

$0

82 84 86 88 90 92 94 96 98 00
83 85 87 89 91 93 95 97 99

Source: The Coleman Institute and Department of Psychiatry, University of Colorado, 2002.

TRENDS IN RESIDENTIAL SERVICES

PERSONS SERVED BY SETTING IN 2000

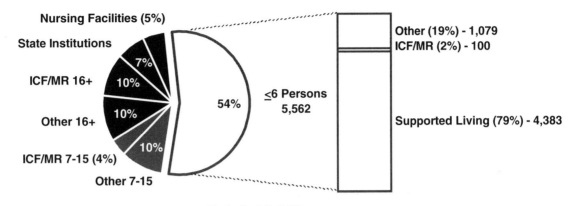

Nursing Facilities (5%)
State Institutions
ICF/MR 16+
Other 16+
ICF/MR 7-15 (4%)
Other 7-15

7%
10%
10%
10%
54%

≤6 Persons
5,562

Other (19%) - 1,079
ICF/MR (2%) - 100

Supported Living (79%) - 4,383

Total: 10,260

PERSONS SERVED BY SETTING

	1990	1991	1992	1993	1994	1995	1996	1997	1998	1999	2000
TOTAL	7,474	7,665	7,494	6,786	6,788	6,812	6,802	8,154	8,613	9,588	10,260
16+ PERSONS	4,847	4,615	4,621	3,429	3,258	2,985	2,819	3,246	3,101	3,070	3,293
Nursing Facilities	1,394	1,212	1,278	748	716	607	520	515	480	536	536
State Institutions	986	946	895	843	784	719	687	679	654	631	679
Private ICF/MR	821	837	837	963	1,002	1,110	1,128	1,030	935	836	1,008
Other Residential	1,646	1,620	1,611	875	756	549	484	1,022	1,032	1,067	1,070
7-15 PERSONS	1,598	1,709	899	1,066	1,192	1,344	1,401	1,715	1,640	1,405	1,405
Public ICF/MR	0	0	0	0	0	0	0	0	0	0	0
Private ICF/MR	189	240	224	304	352	389	396	450	433	287	403
Other Residential	1,409	1,469	675	762	840	955	1,005	1,265	1,207	1,118	1,002
≤6 PERSONS	1,029	1,341	1,974	2,291	2,338	2,483	2,582	3,193	3,872	5,113	5,562
Public ICF/MR	0	0	0	0	0	0	0	0	0	0	0
Private ICF/MR	0	0	35	40	44	49	52	106	144	122	100
Other Residential	1,029	1,341	1,939	2,251	2,294	2,434	2,530	3,087	3,728	4,991	5,462

PERSONS SERVED IN PUBLIC AND PRIVATE
INSTITUTIONS AND NURSING FACILITIES

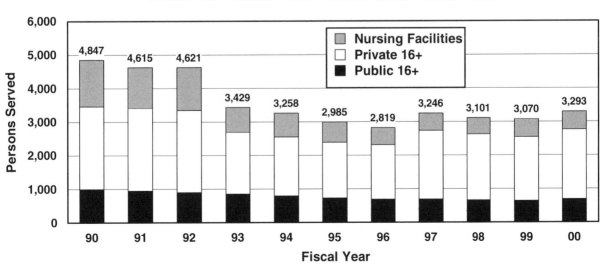

Source: The Coleman Institute and Department of Psychiatry, University of Colorado, 2002.

205

INDIVIDUAL AND FAMILY SUPPORT

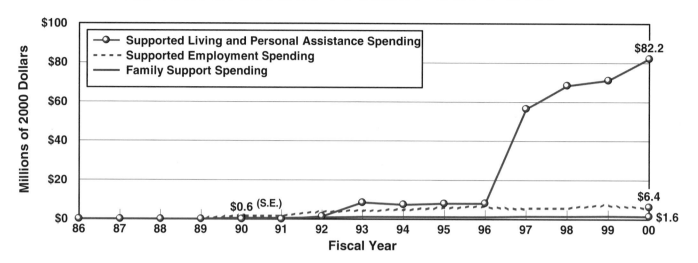

PARTICIPANTS AND SPENDING LEVELS

	1990	1991	1992	1993	1994	1995	1996	1997	1998	1999	2000
TOTAL IFS ($)	1,597,003	1,812,293	4,739,475	11,748,868	11,458,524	13,113,350	14,229,000	58,943,531	71,252,185	38,798,740	43,253,501
INDIVIDUAL SUPPORT ($)	1,167,003	1,315,293	4,031,475	10,693,868	10,353,524	11,975,800	13,064,000	57,544,531	69,727,185	34,420,948	38,788,187
Supported Employment ($)	1,167,003	1,315,293	2,860,191	3,582,396	3,960,777	4,881,921	5,700,000	5,328,514	5,182,471	6,784,166	6,400,909
# of Persons	460	653	1,052	1,318	1,457	1,795	2,096	1,567	1,823	1,855	2,379
Supported Living ($)	0	0	1,171,284	7,111,472	6,392,747	6,729,879	7,000,000	52,216,017	64,544,714	68,268,310	81,905,145
# of Persons	0	0	1,380	1,796	1,614	1,699	1,768	2,384	2,585	3,839	4,354
Personal Assistance ($)	0	0	0	0	0	364,000	364,000	0	0	252,653	298,219
# of Persons	0	0	0	0	0	35	37	0	0	26	29
FAMILY SUPPORT ($)	430,000	497,000	708,000	1,055,000	1,105,000	1,137,550	1,165,000	1,399,000	1,525,000	1,565,000	1,575,000
Total Families	166	182	235	290	301	313	347	383	452	422	417
Cash Subsidy/Payment ($)	400,000	442,000	653,000	1,000,000	1,050,000	1,082,550	1,110,000	1,344,000	1,470,000	1,510,000	1,520,000
# of Families	136	137	193	250	260	275	304	344	410	382	379
Other Family Support ($)	30,000	55,000	55,000	55,000	55,000	55,000	55,000	55,000	55,000	55,000	55,000
# of Families	30	45	42	40	41	38	43	39	42	40	38

PARTICIPANTS IN DAY/WORK AND SUPPORTED EMPLOYMENT

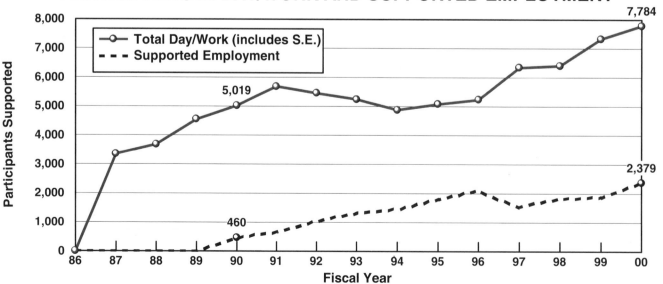

Source: The Coleman Institute and Department of Psychiatry, University of Colorado, 2002.

TRENDS IN SPENDING

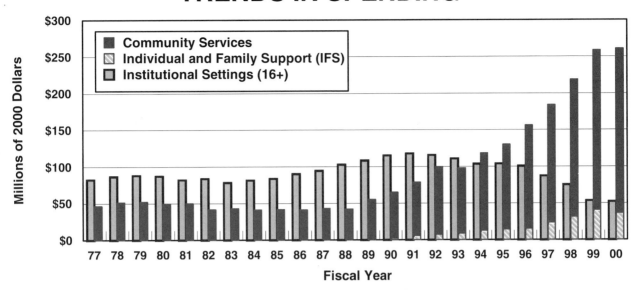

FISCAL EFFORT

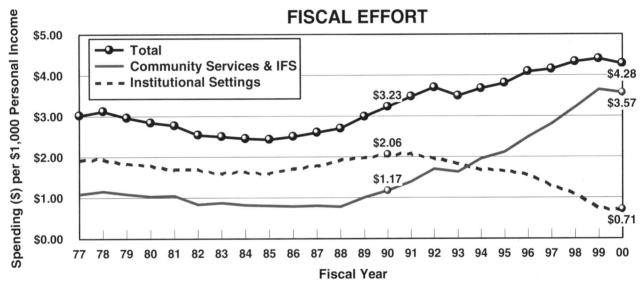

TOTAL MR/DD SPENDING AND
UNMATCHED STATE/LOCAL FUNDS

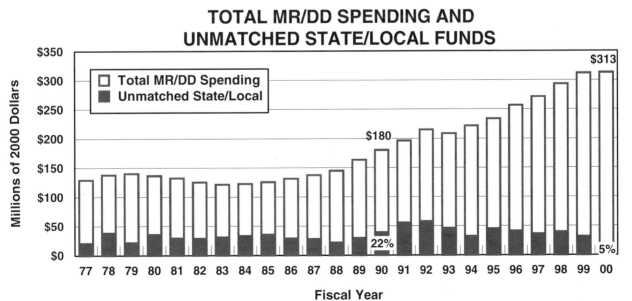

Source: The Coleman Institute and Department of Psychiatry, University of Colorado, 2002.

TRENDS IN REVENUE

COMMUNITY SERVICES REVENUE IN 2000

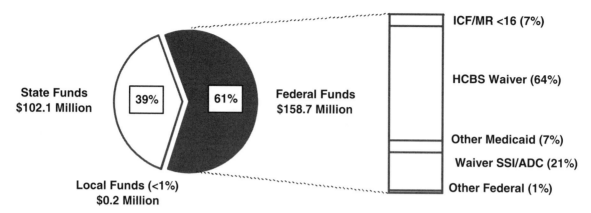

State Funds
$102.1 Million

39%

61%

Federal Funds
$158.7 Million

Local Funds (<1%)
$0.2 Million

ICF/MR <16 (7%)

HCBS Waiver (64%)

Other Medicaid (7%)

Waiver SSI/ADC (21%)

Other Federal (1%)

Total: $261.0 Million

COMPONENTS OF FEDERAL MR/DD MEDICAID REVENUE

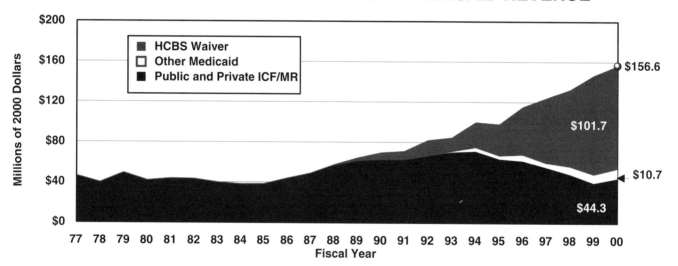

Millions of 2000 Dollars

- ■ HCBS Waiver
- □ Other Medicaid
- ■ Public and Private ICF/MR

$156.6

$101.7

$10.7

$44.3

Fiscal Year

HCBS WAIVER PARTICIPANTS

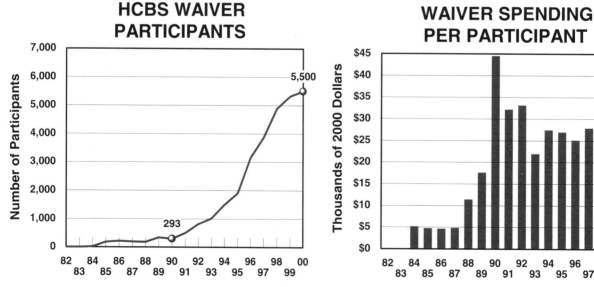

Number of Participants

5,500

293

WAIVER SPENDING PER PARTICIPANT

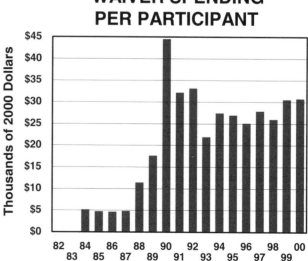

Thousands of 2000 Dollars

Source: The Coleman Institute and Department of Psychiatry, University of Colorado, 2002.

TRENDS IN RESIDENTIAL SERVICES
PERSONS SERVED BY SETTING IN 2000

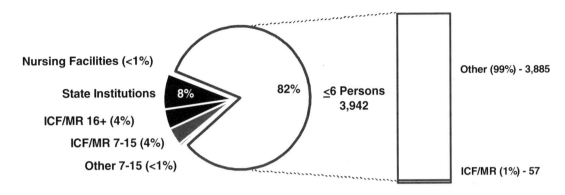

Nursing Facilities (<1%)

State Institutions 8%

ICF/MR 16+ (4%)

ICF/MR 7-15 (4%)

Other 7-15 (<1%)

82%

≤6 Persons
3,942

Other (99%) - 3,885

ICF/MR (1%) - 57

Total: 4,779

PERSONS SERVED BY SETTING

	1990	1991	1992	1993	1994	1995	1996	1997	1998	1999	2000
TOTAL	3,701	4,044	4,107	3,773	3,931	3,878	3,787	4,502	4,569	4,505	4,779
16+ PERSONS	1,662	1,692	1,614	1,552	1,491	1,361	1,316	1,147	910	610	614
Nursing Facilities*	0	0	0	0	0	0	0	0	0	0	13
State Institutions	1,017	1,015	943	897	836	741	696	601	474	395	386
Private ICF/MR	645	677	671	655	655	620	620	546	436	215	215
Other Residential	0	0	0	0	0	0	0	0	0	0	0
7-15 PERSONS	2,039	2,268	824	280	280	277	269	264	281	253	223
Public ICF/MR	0	0	0	0	0	0	0	0	0	0	0
Private ICF/MR	278	241	233	218	218	218	218	199	201	201	194
Other Residential	1,761	2,027	591	62	62	59	51	65	80	52	29
≤6 PERSONS	0	84	1,669	1,941	2,160	2,240	2,202	3,091	3,378	3,642	3,942
Public ICF/MR	0	0	0	0	0	0	0	0	0	0	0
Private ICF/MR	0	84	84	72	72	72	72	60	60	60	57
Other Residential	0	0	1,585	1,869	2,088	2,168	2,130	3,031	3,318	3,582	3,885

PERSONS SERVED IN PUBLIC AND PRIVATE INSTITUTIONS AND NURSING FACILITIES

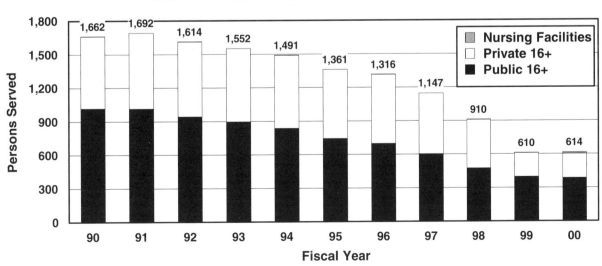

Persons Served

- Nursing Facilities
- Private 16+
- Public 16+

1,662 1,692 1,614 1,552 1,491 1,361 1,316 1,147 910 610 614

Fiscal Year

90 91 92 93 94 95 96 97 98 99 00

Source: The Coleman Institute and Department of Psychiatry, University of Colorado, 2002.

INDIVIDUAL AND FAMILY SUPPORT

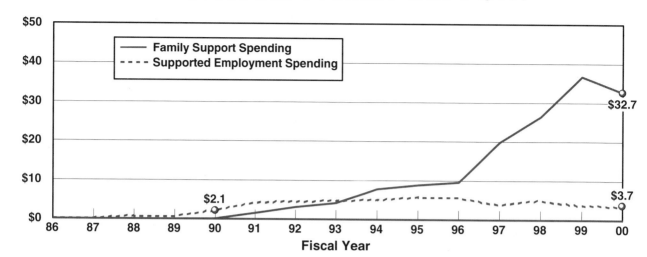

PARTICIPANTS AND SPENDING LEVELS

	1990	1991	1992	1993	1994	1995	1996	1997	1998	1999	2000
TOTAL IFS ($)	1,691,800	4,524,000	6,048,200	7,324,952	10,869,880	12,796,868	13,874,360	22,004,388	29,633,568	38,798,740	43,253,501
INDIVIDUALS SUPPORT ($)	1,600,000	3,300,000	3,500,000	3,813,345	4,221,168	4,983,816	5,226,308	3,622,950	4,710,402	34,420,948	38,788,187
Supported Employment ($)	1,600,000	3,300,000	3,500,000	3,813,345	4,221,168	4,983,816	5,226,308	3,622,950	4,710,402	3,688,891	3,686,207
# of Persons	270	561	592	645	714	843	884	415	501	446	471
Supported Living ($)	0	0	0	0	0	0	0	0	0	0	0
# of Persons	0	0	0	0	0	0	0	0	0	0	0
Personal Assistance ($)	0	0	0	0	0	0	0	0	0	0	0
# of Persons	0	0	0	0	0	0	0	0	0	0	0
FAMILY SUPPORT ($)	91,800	1,224,000	2,548,200	3,511,607	6,648,712	7,813,052	8,648,052	18,381,438	24,923,166	35,372,612	32,677,800
Total Families	9	120	441	474	1,214	1,421	1,490	2,507	3,121	3,329	3,030
Cash Subsidy/Payment ($)	0	0	600,000	732,800	1,000,000	1,150,000	1,300,000	1,300,000	1,300,000	2,100,366	2,623,200
# of Families	0	0	250	390	416	541	541	541	541	875	1,093
Other Family Support ($)	91,800	1,224,000	1,948,200	2,778,807	5,648,712	6,663,052	7,348,052	17,081,438	23,623,166	33,272,246	30,054,600
# of Families	9	120	191	84	798	880	949	1,966	2,580	2,454	1,937

PARTICIPANTS IN DAY/WORK AND SUPPORTED EMPLOYMENT

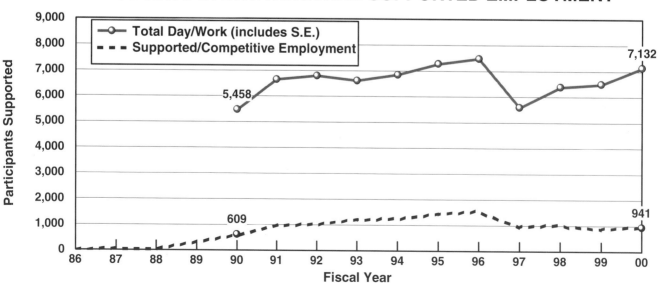

Source: The Coleman Institute and Department of Psychiatry, University of Colorado, 2002.

TRENDS IN SPENDING

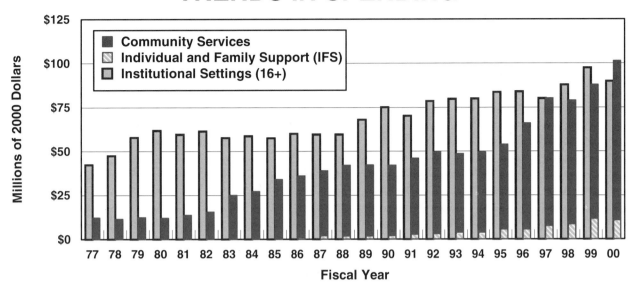

Millions of 2000 Dollars

- ■ Community Services
- ▨ Individual and Family Support (IFS)
- ▧ Institutional Settings (16+)

Fiscal Year

FISCAL EFFORT

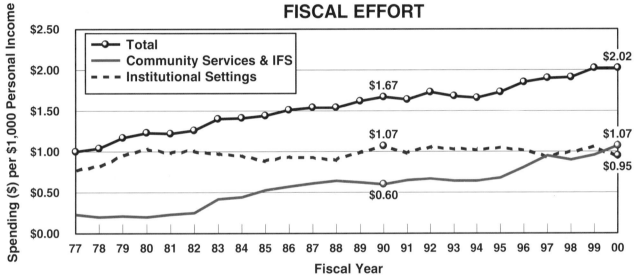

Spending ($) per $1,000 Personal Income

- —○— Total
- —— Community Services & IFS
- - - - Institutional Settings

$1.67

$1.07

$0.60

$2.02

$1.07

$0.95

Fiscal Year

TOTAL MR/DD SPENDING AND
UNMATCHED STATE/LOCAL FUNDS

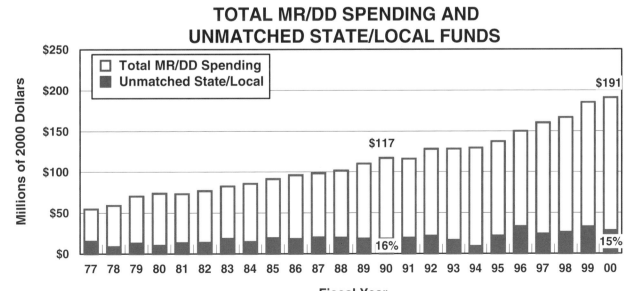

Millions of 2000 Dollars

- ☐ Total MR/DD Spending
- ■ Unmatched State/Local

$117

$191

16%

15%

Fiscal Year

Source: The Coleman Institute and Department of Psychiatry, University of Colorado, 2002.

211

TRENDS IN REVENUE

COMMUNITY SERVICES REVENUE IN 2000

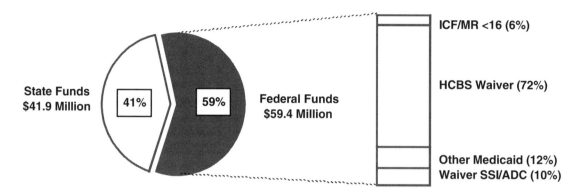

State Funds
$41.9 Million

41%

59%

Federal Funds
$59.4 Million

ICF/MR <16 (6%)

HCBS Waiver (72%)

Other Medicaid (12%)
Waiver SSI/ADC (10%)

Total: $101.3 Million

COMPONENTS OF FEDERAL MR/DD MEDICAID REVENUE

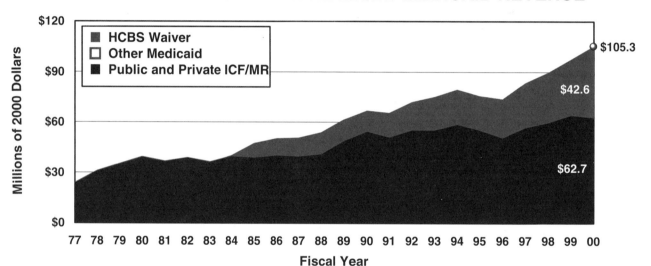

Millions of 2000 Dollars

- ■ HCBS Waiver
- □ Other Medicaid
- ■ Public and Private ICF/MR

$120

$90

$60

$30

$0

$105.3

$42.6

$62.7

77 78 79 80 81 82 83 84 85 86 87 88 89 90 91 92 93 94 95 96 97 98 99 00

Fiscal Year

HCBS WAIVER PARTICIPANTS

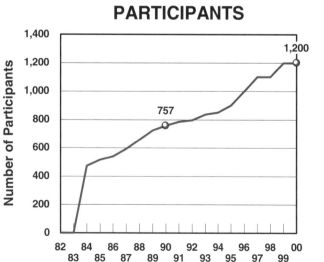

Number of Participants

1,400
1,200
1,000
800
600
400
200
0

757

1,200

82 83 84 85 86 87 88 89 90 91 92 93 94 95 96 97 98 99 00

WAIVER SPENDING PER PARTICIPANT

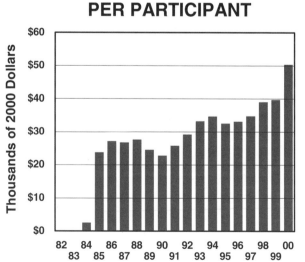

Thousands of 2000 Dollars

$60
$50
$40
$30
$20
$10
$0

82 83 84 85 86 87 88 89 90 91 92 93 94 95 96 97 98 99 00

Source: The Coleman Institute and Department of Psychiatry, University of Colorado, 2002.

TRENDS IN RESIDENTIAL SERVICES
PERSONS SERVED BY SETTING IN 2000

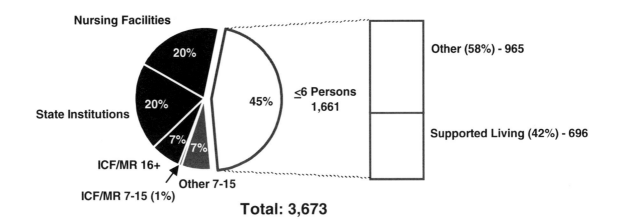

Nursing Facilities 20%

State Institutions 20%

7% 7%

ICF/MR 16+

Other 7-15

ICF/MR 7-15 (1%)

45%

≤6 Persons 1,661

Other (58%) - 965

Supported Living (42%) - 696

Total: 3,673

PERSONS SERVED BY SETTING

	1990	1991	1992	1993	1994	1995	1996	1997	1998	1999	2000
TOTAL	n/a	n/a	3,155	3,237	3,314	3,480	3,570	3,386	3,398	3,881	3,673
16+ PERSONS	2,062	2,115	2,275	2,283	2,292	2,300	2,284	1,992	1,980	1,922	1,736
Nursing Facilities	880	927	1,067	1,075	1,084	1,092	1,100	751	751	744	744
State Institutions	744	750	770	770	770	770	746	751	751	747	735
Private ICF/MR	438	438	438	438	438	438	438	490	478	431	257
Other Residential	0	0	0	0	0	0	0	0	0	0	0
7-15 PERSONS	757	786	176	197	204	244	276	284	284	276	276
Public ICF/MR	0	0	0	0	0	0	24	24	32	24	24
Private ICF/MR	0	0	0	0	0	0	0	0	0	0	0
Other Residential	757	786	176	197	204	244	252	260	252	252	252
≤6 PERSONS	n/a	n/a	704	757	818	936	1,010	1,110	1,134	1,683	1,661
Public ICF/MR	0	0	0	0	0	0	0	4	4	0	0
Private ICF/MR	0	0	0	0	0	0	0	0	0	0	0
Other Residential	n/a	n/a	704	757	818	936	1,010	1,106	1,130	1,683	1,661

PERSONS SERVED IN PUBLIC AND PRIVATE INSTITUTIONS AND NURSING FACILITIES

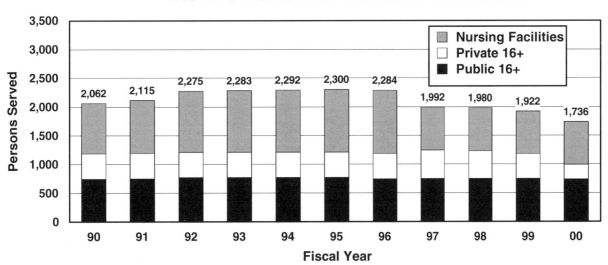

Source: The Coleman Institute and Department of Psychiatry, University of Colorado, 2002.

213

INDIVIDUAL AND FAMILY SUPPORT

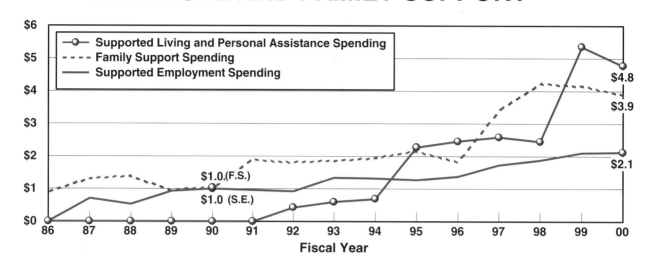

PARTICIPANTS AND SPENDING LEVELS

	1990	1991	1992	1993	1994	1995	1996	1997	1998	1999	2000
TOTAL IFS ($)	1,565,327	2,303,928	2,590,359	3,174,948	3,385,216	5,034,502	5,146,352	7,191,854	8,103,482	11,216,419	10,808,010
INDIVIDUAL SUPPORT ($)	770,698	772,709	1,107,714	1,625,977	1,724,131	3,137,581	3,477,187	4,001,924	4,095,233	7,196,923	6,906,010
Supported Employment ($)	770,698	772,709	759,365	1,126,688	1,132,540	1,126,761	1,250,496	1,609,647	1,781,761	2,035,445	2,126,512
# of Persons	n/a	n/a	n/a	507	546	545	553	570	587	615	633
Supported Living ($)	0	0	348,349	499,289	591,591	2,010,820	2,226,691	2,392,277	2,313,472	5,161,478	4,779,498
# of Persons	0	0	62	89	124	216	264	257	224	727	696
Personal Assistance ($)	0	0	0	0	0	0	0	0	0	0	0
# of Persons	0	0	0	0	0	0	0	0	0	0	0
FAMILY SUPPORT ($)	794,629	1,531,219	1,482,645	1,548,971	1,661,085	1,896,921	1,669,165	3,189,930	4,008,249	4,019,496	3,902,000
Total Families	n/a	n/a	n/a	n/a	n/a	n/a	1,000	n/a	n/a	2,000	1,950
Cash Subsidy/Payment ($)	0	0	0	0	0	0	0	0	0	0	0
# of Families	0	0	0	0	0	0	0	0	0	0	0
Other Family Support ($)	794,629	1,531,219	1,482,645	1,548,971	1,661,085	1,896,921	1,669,165	3,189,930	4,008,249	4,019,496	3,902,000
# of Families	n/a	n/a	n/a	n/a	n/a	n/a	1,924	n/a	n/a	2,000	1,950

PARTICIPANTS IN DAY/WORK AND SUPPORTED EMPLOYMENT

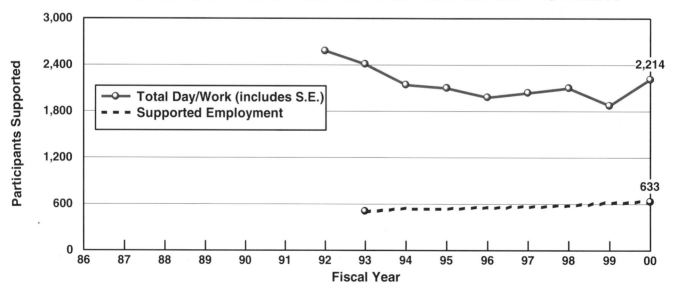

214

Source: The Coleman Institute and Department of Psychiatry, University of Colorado, 2002.

TRENDS IN SPENDING

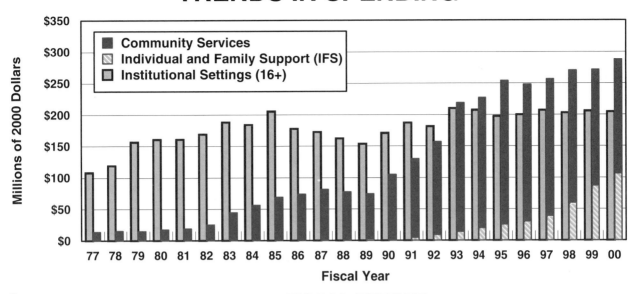

FISCAL EFFORT

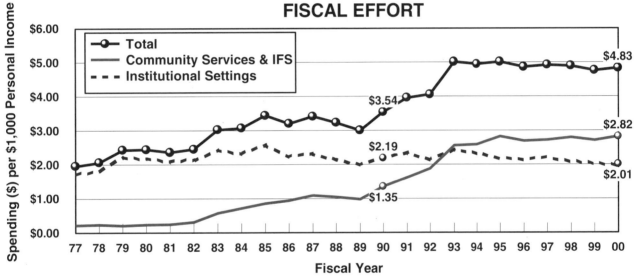

TOTAL MR/DD SPENDING AND
UNMATCHED STATE/LOCAL FUNDS

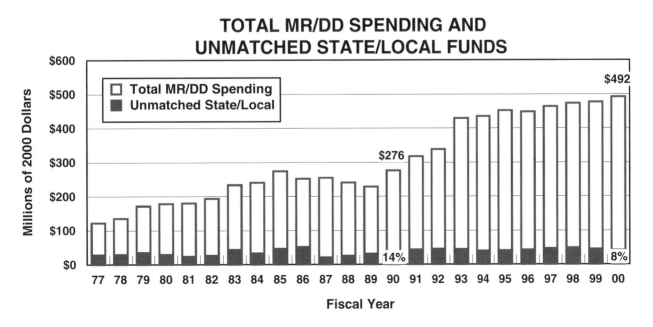

Source: The Coleman Institute and Department of Psychiatry, University of Colorado, 2002.

215

TRENDS IN REVENUE

COMMUNITY SERVICES REVENUE IN 2000

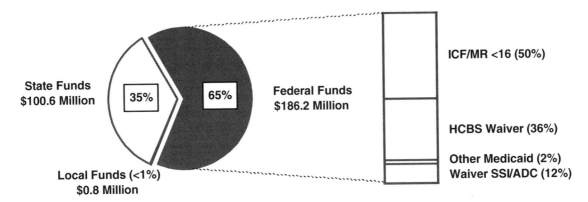

State Funds
$100.6 Million

35%

65%

Federal Funds
$186.2 Million

Local Funds (<1%)
$0.8 Million

ICF/MR <16 (50%)

HCBS Waiver (36%)

Other Medicaid (2%)
Waiver SSI/ADC (12%)

Total: $287.6 Million

COMPONENTS OF FEDERAL MR/DD MEDICAID REVENUE

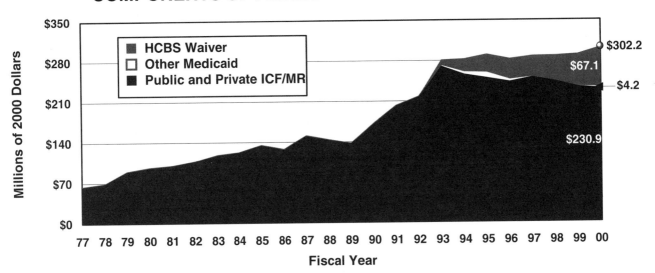

Millions of 2000 Dollars

- ■ HCBS Waiver
- □ Other Medicaid
- ■ Public and Private ICF/MR

$302.2
$67.1
$4.2
$230.9

Fiscal Year

HCBS WAIVER PARTICIPANTS

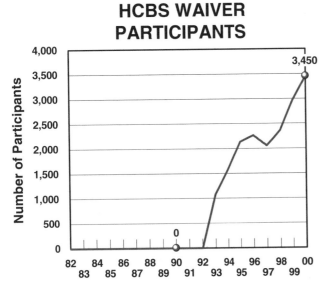

Number of Participants

3,450

0

WAIVER SPENDING PER PARTICIPANT

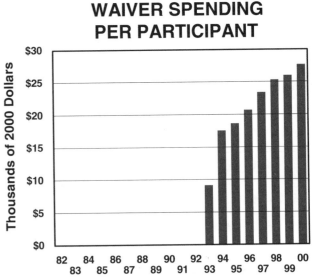

Thousands of 2000 Dollars

Source: The Coleman Institute and Department of Psychiatry, University of Colorado, 2002.

TRENDS IN RESIDENTIAL SERVICES

PERSONS SERVED BY SETTING IN 2000

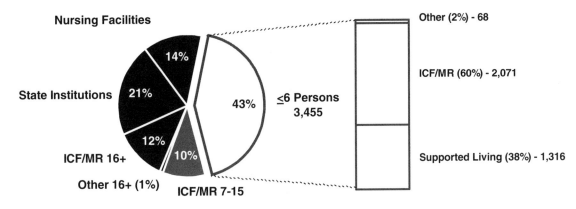

Total: 8,111

PERSONS SERVED BY SETTING

	1990	1991	1992	1993	1994	1995	1996	1997	1998	1999	2000
TOTAL	7,467	7,565	7,386	7,696	7,960	8,036	9,597	9,014	9,778	7,949	8,111
16+ PERSONS	5,286	5,069	4,907	4,840	4,749	4,526	4,419	4,240	3,865	3,894	3,861
Nursing Facilities	1,331	1,331	1,331	1,257	1,265	1,231	1,267	1,127	845	1,109	1,109
State Institutions	2,582	2,482	2,372	2,305	2,259	2,173	2,030	2,009	1,928	1,752	1,717
Private ICF/MR	1,303	1,186	1,134	1,206	1,153	1,050	1,050	1,032	1,020	968	970
Other Residential	70	70	70	72	72	72	72	72	72	65	65
7-15 PERSONS	272	272	333	413	537	693	763	771	765	787	795
Public ICF/MR	0	0	0	8	8	8	8	0	0	0	0
Private ICF/MR	272	272	333	405	529	685	755	771	765	787	795
Other Residential	0	0	0	0	0	0	0	0	0	0	0
≤6 PERSONS	1,909	2,224	2,146	2,443	2,674	2,817	4,415	4,003	5,148	3,268	3,455
Public ICF/MR	36	36	58	74	74	86	86	78	78	78	78
Private ICF/MR	1,460	1,776	1,681	1,860	1,882	1,927	1,976	1,970	2,043	2,011	1,993
Other Residential	413	412	407	509	718	804	2,353	1,955	3,027	1,179	1,384

PERSONS SERVED IN PUBLIC AND PRIVATE INSTITUTIONS AND NURSING FACILITIES

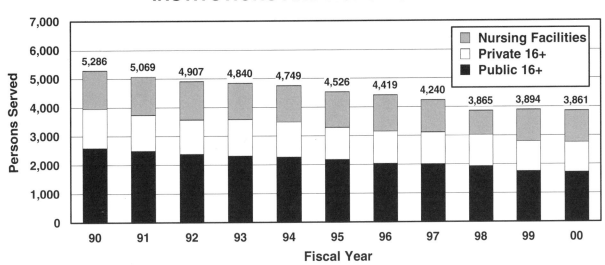

Source: The Coleman Institute and Department of Psychiatry, University of Colorado, 2002.

217

INDIVIDUAL AND FAMILY SUPPORT

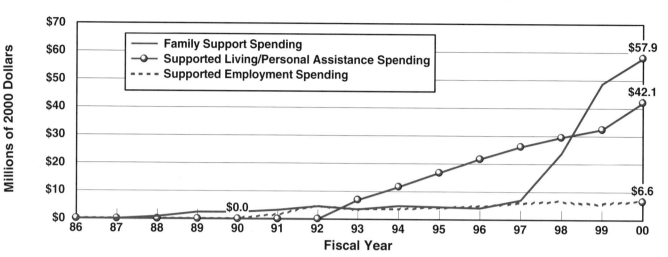

PARTICIPANTS AND SPENDING LEVELS

	1990	1991	1992	1993	1994	1995	1996	1997	1998	1999	2000
TOTAL IFS ($)	1,847,291	3,786,363	7,596,213	11,631,965	17,325,378	22,398,041	27,499,008	35,846,821	56,551,188	83,903,598	106,602,962
INDIVIDUAL SUPPORT ($)	0	1,175,450	3,860,289	8,677,019	13,195,314	18,415,515	23,792,006	29,391,802	34,122,963	36,897,141	48,655,673
Supported Employment ($)	0	1,175,450	3,829,465	2,905,068	3,236,583	3,653,705	4,145,809	5,218,029	6,290,249	5,712,454	6,597,236
# of Persons	0	265	578	436	583	542	615	693	770	992	1,208
Supported Living ($)	0	0	30,824	1,406,836	900,848	900,848	1,147,623	2,908,394	3,920,528	31,184,687	42,058,437
# of Persons	0	0	23	309	456	540	540	208	229	1,093	1,316
Personal Assistance ($)	0	0	0	4,365,115	9,057,883	13,860,962	18,498,574	21,265,379	23,912,186	0	0
# of Persons	0	0	0	489	950	1,411	1,669	1,599	1,927	0	0
FAMILY SUPPORT ($)	1,847,291	2,610,913	3,735,924	2,954,946	4,130,064	3,982,526	3,707,002	6,455,019	22,428,225	47,006,457	57,947,289
Total Families	895	980	1,480	1,662	2,241	2,040	2,022	2,141	3,108	5,016	5,629
Cash Subsidy/Payment ($)	89,170	283,218	1,043,845	681,866	743,398	1,145,815	1,145,815	2,384,436	2,711,548	4,070,468	4,405,038
# of Families	65	110	609	638	731	895	885	836	973	1,349	1,574
Other Family Support ($)	1,758,121	2,327,695	2,692,079	2,273,080	3,386,666	2,836,711	2,561,187	4,070,583	19,716,677	42,935,989	53,542,251
# of Families	830	870	871	1,024	1,510	1,145	1,137	1,305	2,135	3,667	4,055

PARTICIPANTS IN DAY/WORK AND SUPPORTED EMPLOYMENT

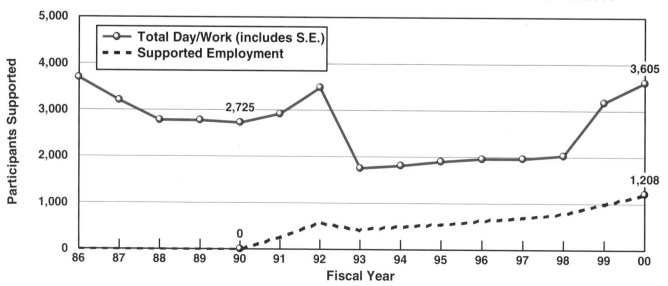

Source: The Coleman Institute and Department of Psychiatry, University of Colorado, 2002.

TRENDS IN SPENDING

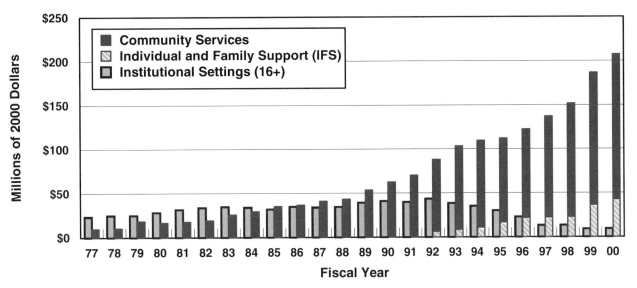

FISCAL EFFORT

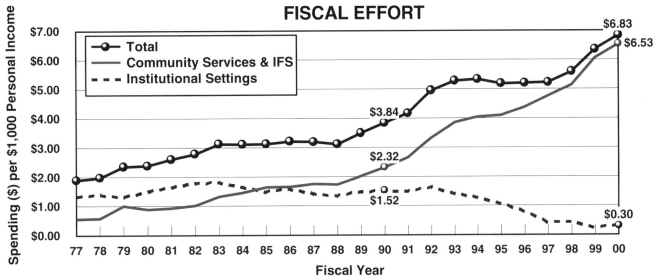

TOTAL MR/DD SPENDING AND
UNMATCHED STATE/LOCAL FUNDS

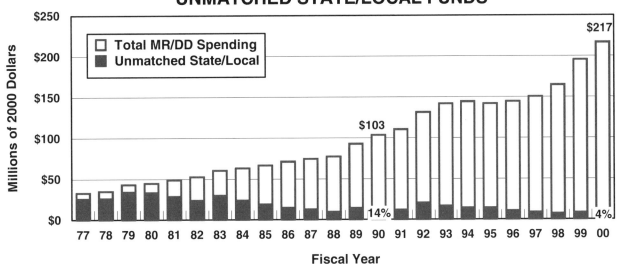

Source: The Coleman Institute and Department of Psychiatry, University of Colorado, 2002.

MAINE

TRENDS IN REVENUE

COMMUNITY SERVICES REVENUE IN 2000

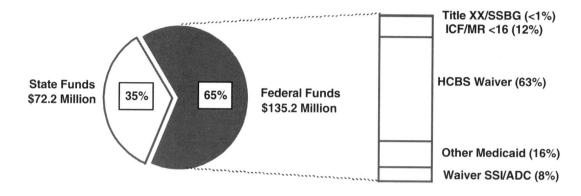

State Funds
$72.2 Million

35%

65%

Federal Funds
$135.2 Million

Title XX/SSBG (<1%)
ICF/MR <16 (12%)

HCBS Waiver (63%)

Other Medicaid (16%)

Waiver SSI/ADC (8%)

Total: $207.4 Million

COMPONENTS OF FEDERAL MR/DD MEDICAID REVENUE

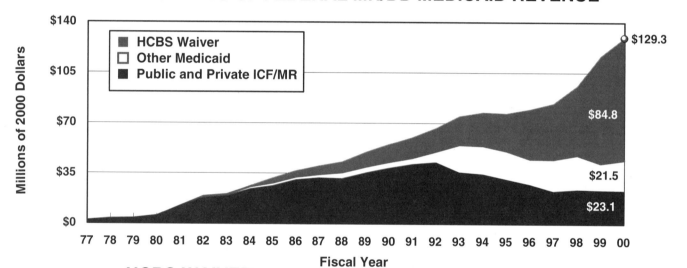

- ■ HCBS Waiver
- □ Other Medicaid
- ■ Public and Private ICF/MR

$129.3

$84.8

$21.5

$23.1

Millions of 2000 Dollars

Fiscal Year

HCBS WAIVER PARTICIPANTS
WAIVER SPENDING PER PARTICIPANT

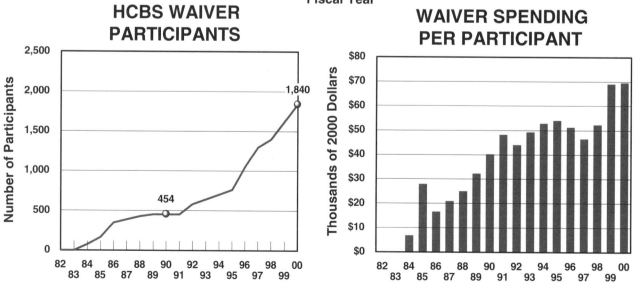

1,840

454

Number of Participants

Thousands of 2000 Dollars

220

Source: The Coleman Institute and Department of Psychiatry, University of Colorado, 2002.

TRENDS IN RESIDENTIAL SERVICES
PERSONS SERVED BY SETTING IN 2000

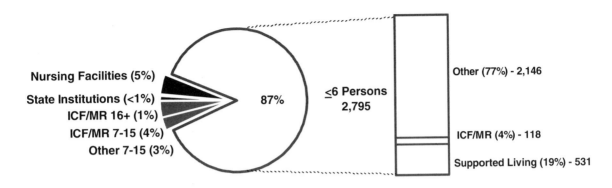

Nursing Facilities (5%)
State Institutions (<1%)
ICF/MR 16+ (1%)
ICF/MR 7-15 (4%)
Other 7-15 (3%)

87%

≤6 Persons 2,795

Other (77%) - 2,146
ICF/MR (4%) - 118
Supported Living (19%) - 531

Total: 3,204

PERSONS SERVED BY SETTING

	1990	1991	1992	1993	1994	1995	1996	1997	1998	1999	2000
TOTAL	1,255	1,313	2,448	2,394	2,363	2,499	2,637	2,632	2,902	3,087	3,204
16+ PERSONS	628	595	598	551	497	434	395	342	342	207	192
Nursing Facilities	217	212	207	207	207	207	207	200	200	144	145
State Institutions	284	265	261	232	178	115	76	25	25	10	11
Private ICF/MR	127	118	109	92	92	92	92	97	97	37	36
Other Residential	0	0	21	20	20	20	20	20	20	16	0
7-15 PERSONS	616	706	394	376	366	360	360	215	215	219	217
Public ICF/MR	0	0	0	0	0	0	0	0	0	0	0
Private ICF/MR	272	287	198	180	170	157	157	157	157	118	120
Other Residential	344	419	196	196	196	203	203	58	58	101	97
≤6 PERSONS	12	12	1,456	1,467	1,500	1,705	1,882	2,075	2,345	2,661	2,795
Public ICF/MR	12	12	12	12	12	12	12	12	12	11	11
Private ICF/MR	0	0	144	102	102	102	102	102	102	111	107
Other Residential	0	0	1,300	1,353	1,386	1,591	1,768	1,961	2,231	2,539	2,677

PERSONS SERVED IN PUBLIC AND PRIVATE INSTITUTIONS AND NURSING FACILITIES

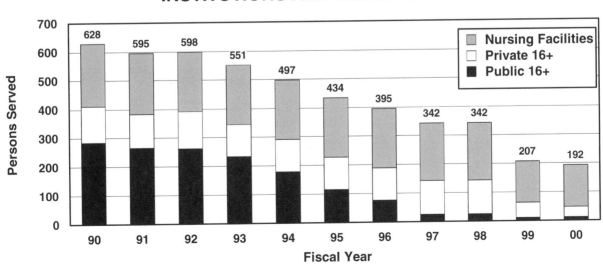

Source: The Coleman Institute and Department of Psychiatry, University of Colorado, 2002.

221

INDIVIDUAL AND FAMILY SUPPORT

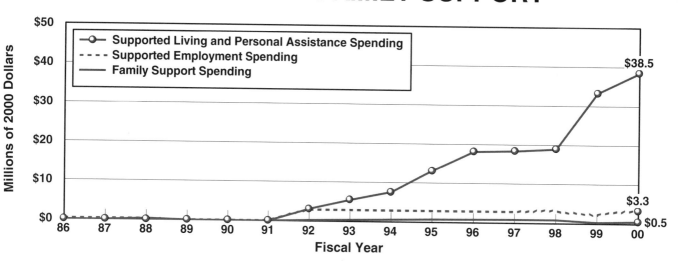

PARTICIPANTS AND SPENDING LEVELS

	1990	1991	1992	1993	1994	1995	1996	1997	1998	1999	2000
TOTAL IFS ($)	n/a	n/a	5,084,275	7,311,987	9,393,104	14,674,435	19,716,184	20,475,506	21,607,942	34,720,553	42,341,011
INDIVIDUAL SUPPORT ($)	0	0	4,884,275	6,981,955	8,933,040	14,084,340	18,996,057	19,697,552	20,772,160	34,462,985	41,808,324
Supported Employment ($)	0	0	2,384,275	2,400,000	2,460,000	2,520,000	2,580,000	2,700,000	2,880,000	2,356,870	3,280,391
# of Persons	0	0	389	400	410	420	430	450	480	612	688
Supported Living ($)	0	0	2,500,000	4,581,955	6,473,040	11,564,340	16,416,057	16,997,552	17,892,160	32,106,115	38,527,933
# of Persons	0	0	125	175	200	300	367	376	400	486	531
Personal Assistance ($)	0	0	0	0	0	0	0	0	0	0	0
# of Persons	0	0	0	0	0	0	0	0	0	0	0
FAMILY SUPPORT ($)	n/a	n/a	200,000	330,032	460,064	590,095	720,127	777,954	835,782	257,568	532,687
Total Families	n/a	n/a	10	231	453	674	895	965	1,035	350	500
Cash Subsidy/Payment ($)	0	0	0	0	0	0	0	0	0	0	0
# of Families	0	0	0	0	0	0	0	0	0	0	0
Other Family Support ($)	n/a	n/a	200,000	330,032	460,064	590,095	720,127	777,954	835,782	257,568	532,687
# of Families	n/a	n/a	10	231	453	674	895	965	1,035	350	500

PARTICIPANTS IN DAY/WORK AND SUPPORTED EMPLOYMENT

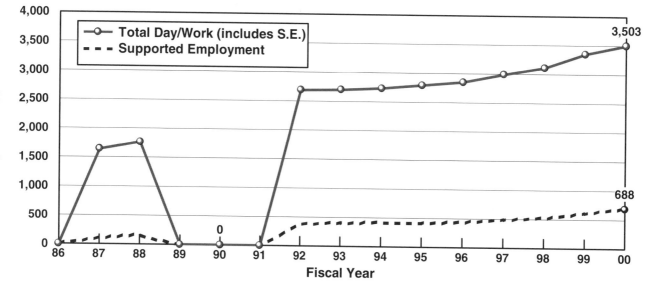

Source: The Coleman Institute and Department of Psychiatry, University of Colorado, 2002.

TRENDS IN SPENDING

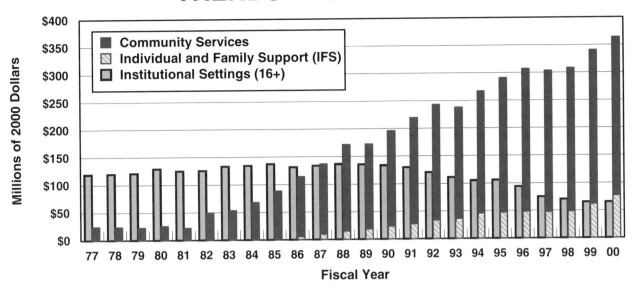

FISCAL EFFORT

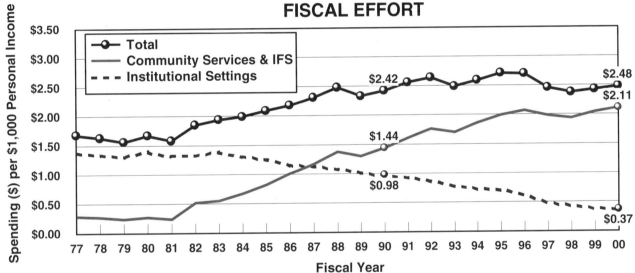

TOTAL MR/DD SPENDING AND
UNMATCHED STATE/LOCAL FUNDS

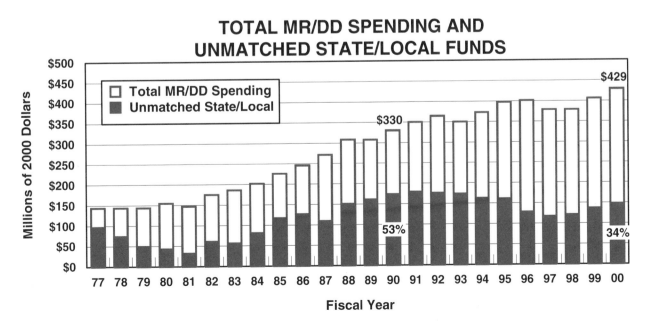

Source: The Coleman Institute and Department of Psychiatry, University of Colorado, 2002.

TRENDS IN REVENUE

COMMUNITY SERVICES REVENUE IN 2000

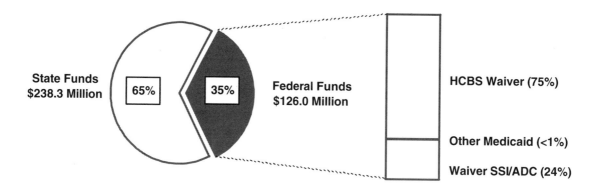

State Funds
$238.3 Million

65%

35%

Federal Funds
$126.0 Million

HCBS Waiver (75%)

Other Medicaid (<1%)

Waiver SSI/ADC (24%)

Total: $364.3 Million

COMPONENTS OF FEDERAL MR/DD MEDICAID REVENUE

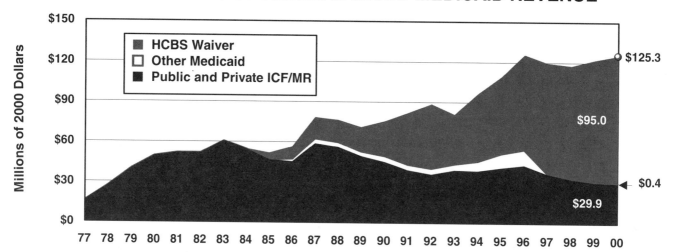

Millions of 2000 Dollars

- ■ HCBS Waiver
- □ Other Medicaid
- ■ Public and Private ICF/MR

$150

$120

$90

$60

$30

$0

$125.3

$95.0

$0.4

$29.9

77 78 79 80 81 82 83 84 85 86 87 88 89 90 91 92 93 94 95 96 97 98 99 00

Fiscal Year

HCBS WAIVER PARTICIPANTS

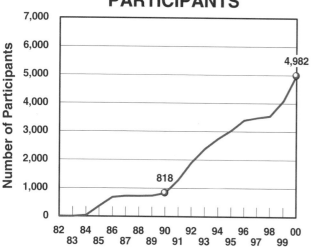

Number of Participants

7,000

6,000

5,000

4,000

3,000

2,000

1,000

0

4,982

818

82 83 84 85 86 87 88 89 90 91 92 93 94 95 96 97 98 99 00

WAIVER SPENDING PER PARTICIPANT

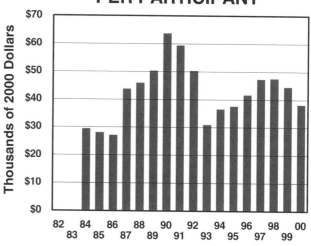

Thousands of 2000 Dollars

$70

$60

$50

$40

$30

$20

$10

$0

82 83 84 85 86 87 88 89 90 91 92 93 94 95 96 97 98 99 00

Source: The Coleman Institute and Department of Psychiatry, University of Colorado, 2002.

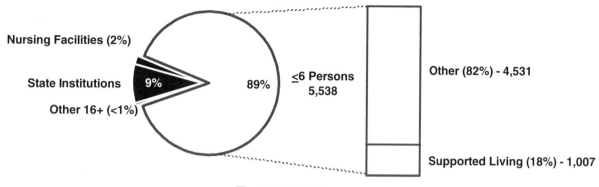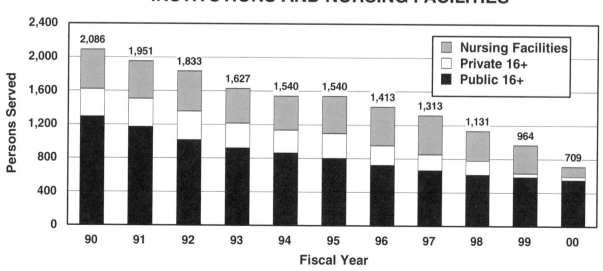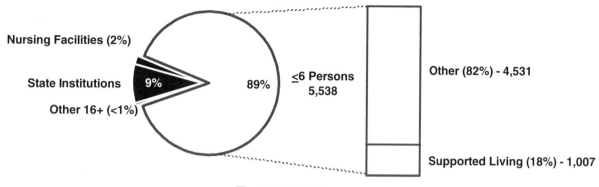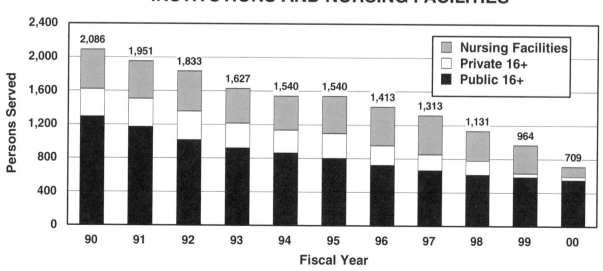

TRENDS IN RESIDENTIAL SERVICES
PERSONS SERVED BY SETTING IN 2000

Nursing Facilities (2%)

State Institutions 9%

Other 16+ (<1%)

89%

≤6 Persons
5,538

Other (82%) - 4,531

Supported Living (18%) - 1,007

Total: 6,247

PERSONS SERVED BY SETTING

	1990	1991	1992	1993	1994	1995	1996	1997	1998	1999	2000
TOTAL	4,816	4,692	4,921	4,942	5,097	5,373	5,488	5,580	5,461	6,102	6,247
16+ PERSONS	2,086	1,951	1,833	1,627	1,540	1,540	1,413	1,313	1,131	964	709
Nursing Facilities	467	448	478	413	407	445	462	464	357	336	121
State Institutions	1,291	1,168	1,014	916	858	797	720	659	607	584	548
Private ICF/MR	0	0	0	0	0	0	0	0	0	0	0
Other Residential	328	335	341	298	275	298	231	190	167	44	40
7-15 PERSONS	0	0	0	0	0	0	0	0	0	0	0
Public ICF/MR	0	0	0	0	0	0	0	0	0	0	0
Private ICF/MR	0	0	0	0	0	0	0	0	0	0	0
Other Residential	0	0	0	0	0	0	0	0	0	0	0
≤6 PERSONS	2,730	2,741	3,088	3,315	3,557	3,833	4,075	4,267	4,330	5,138	5,538
Public ICF/MR	0	0	0	0	0	0	0	0	0	0	0
Private ICF/MR	0	0	0	0	0	0	0	0	0	0	0
Other Residential	2,730	2,741	3,088	3,315	3,557	3,833	4,075	4,267	4,330	5,138	5,538

PERSONS SERVED IN PUBLIC AND PRIVATE INSTITUTIONS AND NURSING FACILITIES

Nursing Facilities / Private 16+ / Public 16+

INDIVIDUAL AND FAMILY SUPPORT

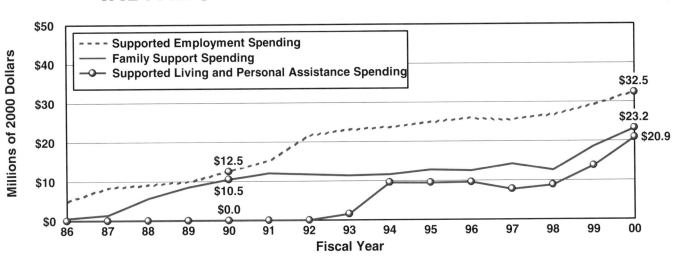

PARTICIPANTS AND SPENDING LEVELS

	1990	1991	1992	1993	1994	1995	1996	1997	1998	1999	2000
TOTAL IFS ($)	9,604,356	12,212,259	27,261,749	30,159,932	38,440,780	41,489,245	43,320,786	43,959,993	45,197,539	59,228,502	76,574,892
INDIVIDUAL SUPPORT ($)	9,604,356	12,212,259	17,671,238	20,602,519	28,456,716	30,192,552	31,999,401	30,752,635	33,311,769	41,234,613	53,337,719
Supported Employment ($)	9,604,356	12,212,259	17,671,238	19,282,032	20,288,049	21,846,715	23,341,900	23,607,168	25,025,812	28,029,258	32,455,582
# of Persons	1,111	1,467	1,767	2,025	2,204	2,583	2,728	2,604	2,745	3,123	3,390
Supported Living ($)	0	0	0	1,320,487	8,168,667	8,345,837	8,657,501	7,145,467	8,285,957	13,205,355	20,882,137
# of Persons	0	0	0	93	193	207	269	283	283	703	1,007
Personal Assistance ($)	0	0	0	0	0	0	0	0	0	0	0
# of Persons	0	0	0	0	0	0	0	0	0	0	0
FAMILY SUPPORT ($)	na	na	9,590,511	9,557,413	9,984,064	11,296,693	11,321,385	13,207,358	11,885,770	17,993,889	23,237,173
Total Families	na	na	785	800	815	875	1,000	1,038	1,104	6,026	5,383
Cash Subsidy/Payment ($)			0	0	0	0	0	0	0	0	0
# of Families			0	0	0	0	0	0	0	0	0
Other Family Support ($)			9,590,511	9,557,413	9,984,064	11,296,693	11,321,385	13,207,358	11,885,770	17,993,889	23,237,173
# of Families			785	800	815	875	1,000	1,038	1,104	6,026	5,383

PARTICIPANTS IN DAY/WORK AND SUPPORTED EMPLOYMENT

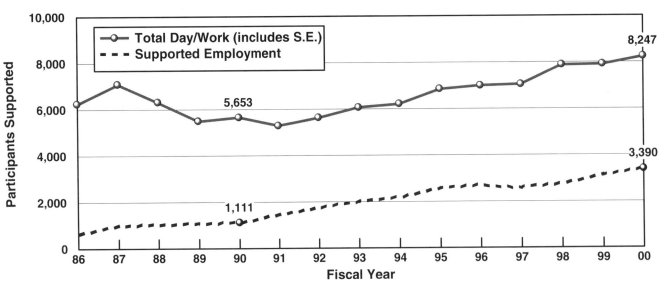

Source: The Coleman Institute and Department of Psychiatry, University of Colorado, 2002.

TRENDS IN SPENDING

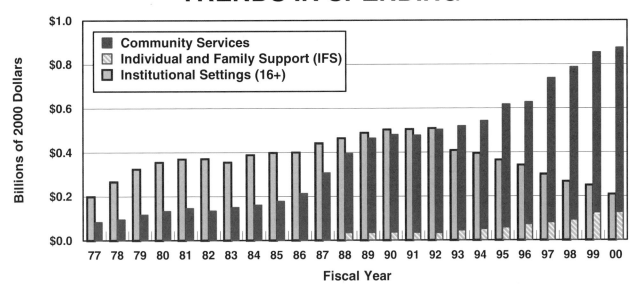

FISCAL EFFORT

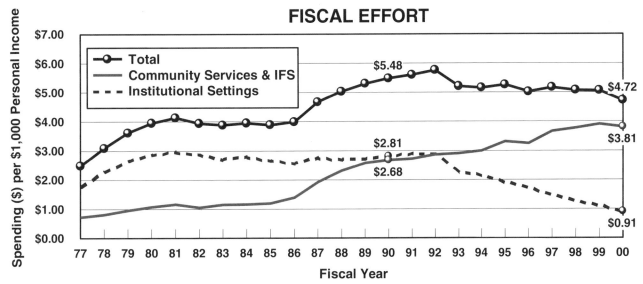

TOTAL MR/DD SPENDING AND
UNMATCHED STATE/LOCAL FUNDS

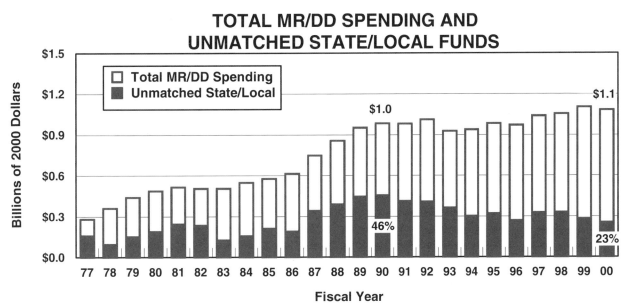

Source: The Coleman Institute and Department of Psychiatry, University of Colorado, 2002.

TRENDS IN REVENUE

COMMUNITY SERVICES REVENUE IN 2000

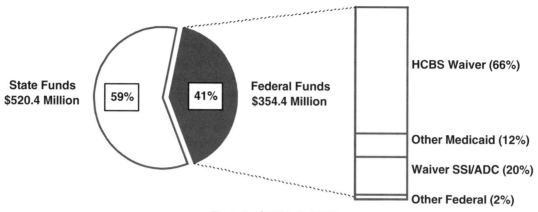

State Funds
$520.4 Million

59%

41%

Federal Funds
$354.4 Million

HCBS Waiver (66%)

Other Medicaid (12%)

Waiver SSI/ADC (20%)

Other Federal (2%)

Total: $874.8 Million

COMPONENTS OF FEDERAL MR/DD MEDICAID REVENUE

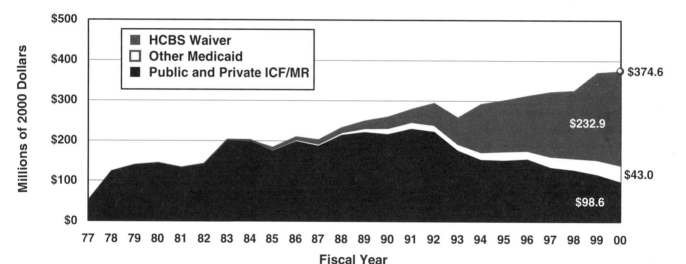

Millions of 2000 Dollars

- ■ HCBS Waiver
- □ Other Medicaid
- ■ Public and Private ICF/MR

$374.6

$232.9

$43.0

$98.6

Fiscal Year

HCBS WAIVER PARTICIPANTS

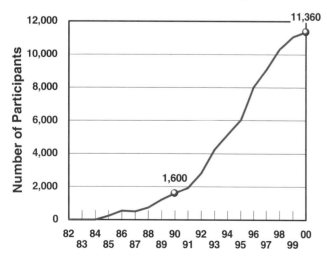

Number of Participants

11,360

1,600

WAIVER SPENDING PER PARTICIPANT

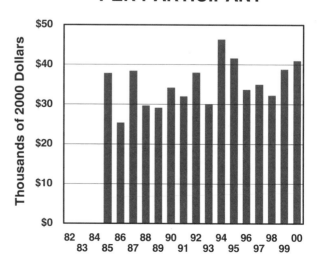

Thousands of 2000 Dollars

Source: The Coleman Institute and Department of Psychiatry, University of Colorado, 2002.

TRENDS IN RESIDENTIAL SERVICES

PERSONS SERVED BY SETTING IN 2000

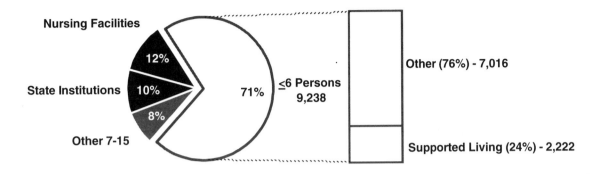

Nursing Facilities — 12%
State Institutions — 10%
Other 7-15 — 8%
71% ≤6 Persons 9,238

Other (76%) - 7,016
Supported Living (24%) - 2,222

Total: 13,030

PERSONS SERVED BY SETTING

	1990	1991	1992	1993	1994	1995	1996	1997	1998	1999	2000
TOTAL	10,248	10,172	10,007	10,172	10,124	10,881	11,332	12,036	12,050	12,619	13,030
16+ PERSONS	4,775	4,580	4,364	4,069	4,043	3,878	3,661	3,444	3,140	2,924	2,792
Nursing Facilities	1,870	1,802	1,750	1,735	1,823	1,769	1,777	1,714	1,617	1,559	1,499
State Institutions	2,905	2,778	2,614	2,334	2,220	2,109	1,884	1,730	1,523	1,365	1,293
Private ICF/MR	0	0	0	0	0	0	0	0	0	0	0
Other Residential	0	0	0	0	0	0	0	0	0	0	0
7-15 PERSONS	5,473	5,592	2,532	2,298	1,511	1,485	1,205	1,294	1,006	1,000	1,000
Public ICF/MR	232	232	232	232	0	0	0	0	0	0	0
Private ICF/MR	309	320	320	320	0	0	0	0	0	0	0
Other Residential	4,932	5,040	1,980	1,746	1,511	1,485	1,205	1,294	1,006	1,000	1,000
≤6 PERSONS	0	0	3,111	3,805	4,570	5,518	6,466	7,298	7,904	8,695	9,238
Public ICF/MR	0	0	0	0	0	0	0	0	0	0	0
Private ICF/MR	0	0	0	0	0	0	0	0	0	0	0
Other Residential	0	0	3,111	3,805	4,570	5,518	6,466	7,298	7,904	8,695	9,238

PERSONS SERVED IN PUBLIC AND PRIVATE INSTITUTIONS AND NURSING FACILITIES

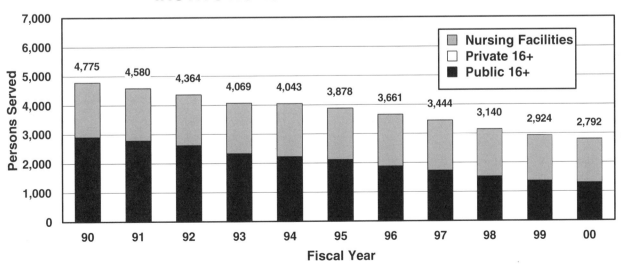

Legend:
- Nursing Facilities
- Private 16+
- Public 16+

Values above bars: 4,775 (90), 4,580 (91), 4,364 (92), 4,069 (93), 4,043 (94), 3,878 (95), 3,661 (96), 3,444 (97), 3,140 (98), 2,924 (99), 2,792 (00)

Y-axis: Persons Served
X-axis: Fiscal Year

Source: The Coleman Institute and Department of Psychiatry, University of Colorado, 2002.

INDIVIDUAL AND FAMILY SUPPORT

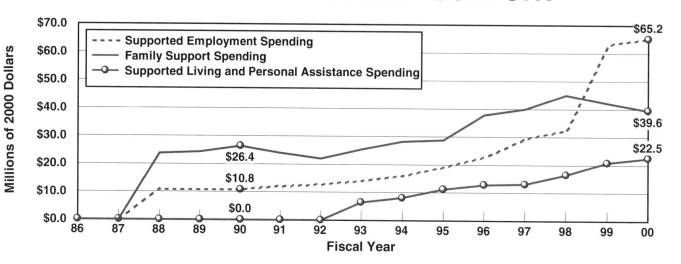

PARTICIPANTS AND SPENDING LEVELS

	1990	1991	1992	1993	1994	1995	1996	1997	1998	1999	2000
TOTAL IFS ($)	28,600,000	28,800,000	28,100,000	38,160,761	44,581,753	51,965,695	66,105,716	76,132,469	88,361,437	121,499,470	127,244,701
INDIVIDUAL SUPPORT ($)	8,300,000	9,600,000	10,100,000	17,007,684	20,428,676	26,538,117	31,954,131	39,136,150	45,886,564	80,828,375	87,669,310
Supported Employment ($)	8,300,000	9,600,000	10,100,000	11,660,032	13,550,845	16,651,244	20,400,000	27,069,933	30,360,000	60,767,221	65,187,598
# of Persons	1,053	1,225	1,325	2,628	2,538	2,659	2,721	2,970	3,037	5,012	5,100
Supported Living ($)	0	0	0	5,347,652	6,877,831	9,886,873	11,554,131	12,066,217	15,526,564	20,061,154	22,481,712
# of Persons	0	0	0	840	884	1,030	1,176	1,500	1,800	2,000	2,222
Personal Assistance ($)	0	0	0	0	0	0	0	0	0	0	0
# of Persons	0	0	0	0	0	0	0	0	0	0	0
FAMILY SUPPORT ($)	20,300,000	19,200,000	18,000,000	21,153,077	24,153,077	25,427,578	34,151,585	36,996,319	42,474,873	40,671,095	39,575,391
Total Families	na	na	na	10,384	10,384	11,134	12,672	13,483	14,313	14,518	15,010
Cash Subsidy/Payment ($)	0	0	0	0	0	0	0	0	0	0	0
# of Families	0	0	0	0	0	0	0	0	0	0	0
Other Family Support ($)	20,300,000	19,200,000	18,000,000	21,153,077	24,153,077	25,427,578	34,151,585	36,996,319	42,474,873	40,671,095	39,575,391
# of Families	na	na	na	10,384	10,384	11,134	12,672	13,483	14,313	14,518	15,010

PARTICIPANTS IN DAY/WORK AND SUPPORTED EMPLOYMENT

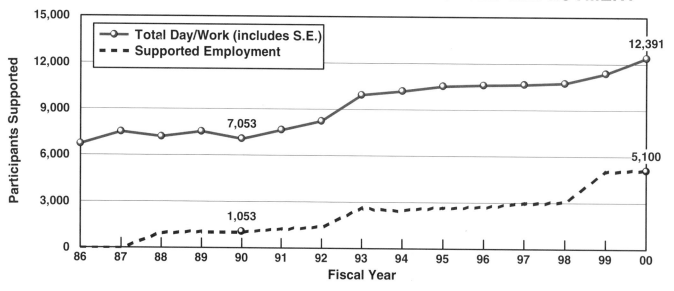

Source: The Coleman Institute and Department of Psychiatry, University of Colorado, 2002.

TRENDS IN SPENDING

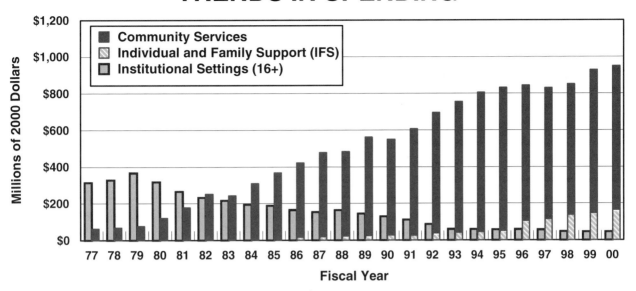

Millions of 2000 Dollars

- ■ Community Services
- ▨ Individual and Family Support (IFS)
- ▤ Institutional Settings (16+)

Fiscal Year

FISCAL EFFORT

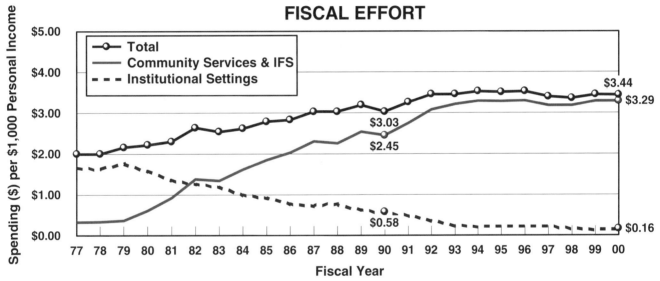

Spending ($) per $1,000 Personal Income

- —○— Total
- —— Community Services & IFS
- - - - Institutional Settings

$3.44
$3.29
$3.03
$2.45
$0.58
$0.16

Fiscal Year

TOTAL MR/DD SPENDING AND
UNMATCHED STATE/LOCAL FUNDS

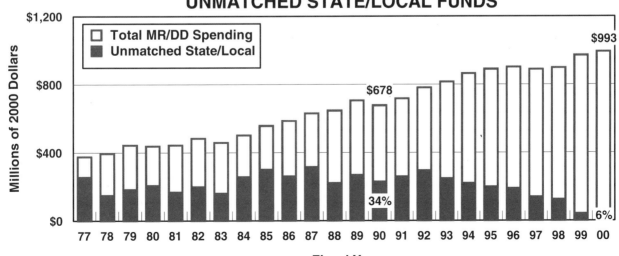

Millions of 2000 Dollars

- □ Total MR/DD Spending
- ■ Unmatched State/Local

$993
$678
34%
6%

Fiscal Year

Source: The Coleman Institute and Department of Psychiatry, University of Colorado, 2002.

MICHIGAN

TRENDS IN REVENUE
COMMUNITY SERVICES REVENUE IN 2000

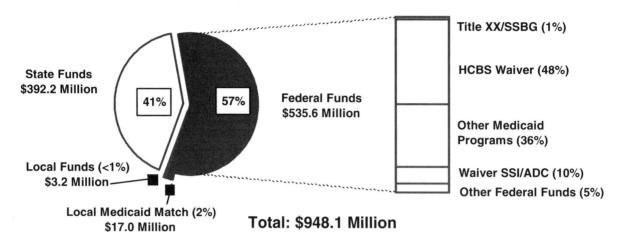

State Funds $392.2 Million — 41%

Federal Funds $535.6 Million — 57%

Local Funds (<1%) $3.2 Million

Local Medicaid Match (2%) $17.0 Million

Title XX/SSBG (1%)
HCBS Waiver (48%)
Other Medicaid Programs (36%)
Waiver SSI/ADC (10%)
Other Federal Funds (5%)

Total: $948.1 Million

COMPONENTS OF FEDERAL MR/DD MEDICAID REVENUE

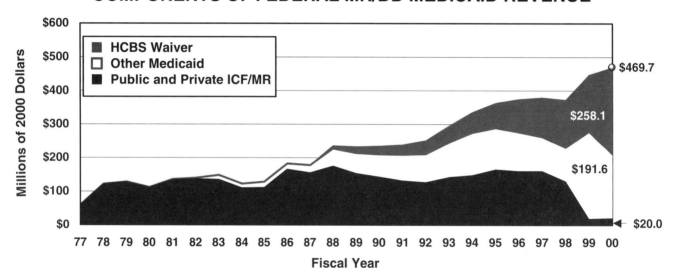

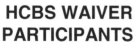

HCBS WAIVER PARTICIPANTS

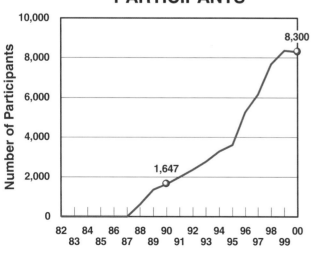

WAIVER SPENDING PER PARTICIPANT

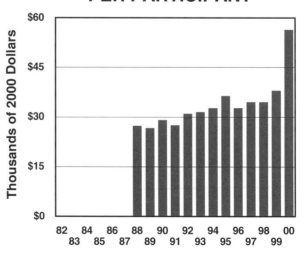

232

Source: The Coleman Institute and Department of Psychiatry, University of Colorado, 2002.

TRENDS IN RESIDENTIAL SERVICES

PERSONS SERVED BY SETTING IN 2000

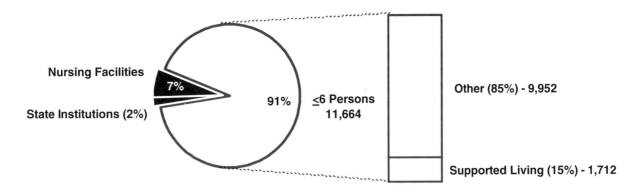

Nursing Facilities 7%

State Institutions (2%)

91% ≤6 Persons 11,664

Other (85%) - 9,952

Supported Living (15%) - 1,712

Total: 12,752

PERSONS SERVED BY SETTING

	1990	1991	1992	1993	1994	1995	1996	1997	1998	1999	2000
TOTAL	10,341	10,515	9,981	9,225	9,164	9,462	9,833	10,318	10,150	12,999	12,752
16+ PERSONS	3,537	3,136	2,594	2,297	2,058	1,983	1,231	1,194	1,120	1,110	1,088
Nursing Facilities	2,482	2,266	1,938	1,804	1,620	1,586	869	888	840	838	838
State Institutions	1,055	870	656	493	438	397	362	306	280	272	250
Private ICF/MR	0	0	0	0	0	0	0	0	0	0	0
Other Residential	0	0	0	0	0	0	0	0	0	0	0
7-15 PERSONS	450	462	404	0	0	0	0	0	0	0	0
Public ICF/MR	0	0	0	0	0	0	0	0	0	0	0
Private ICF/MR	0	112	104	0	0	0	0	0	0	0	0
Other Residential	450	350	300	0	0	0	0	0	0	0	0
≤6 PERSONS	6,354	6,917	6,983	6,928	7,106	7,479	8,602	9,124	9,030	11,889	11,664
Public ICF/MR	0	0	0	0	0	0	0	0	0	0	0
Private ICF/MR	2,025	1,967	1,932	1,841	1,916	2,181	2,286	2,590	2,152	0	0
Other Residential	4,329	4,950	5,051	5,087	5,190	5,298	6,316	6,534	6,878	11,889	11,664

PERSONS SERVED IN PUBLIC AND PRIVATE INSTITUTIONS AND NURSING FACILITIES

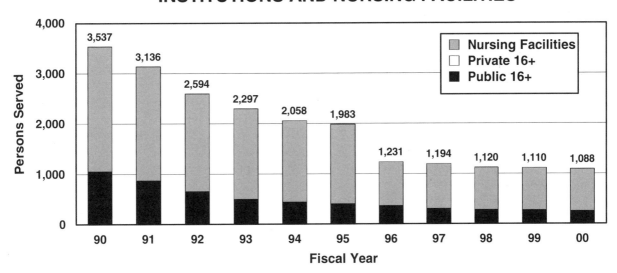

Source: The Coleman Institute and Department of Psychiatry, University of Colorado, 2002.

INDIVIDUAL AND FAMILY SUPPORT

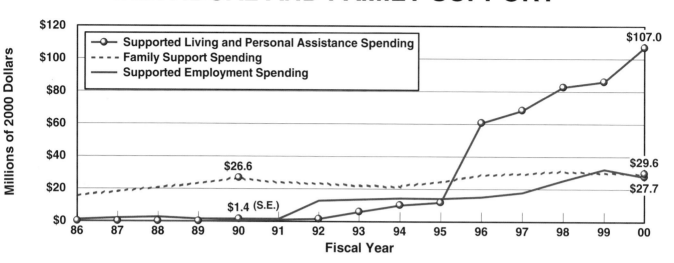

PARTICIPANTS AND SPENDING LEVELS

	1990	1991	1992	1993	1994	1995	1996	1997	1998	1999	2000
TOTAL IFS ($)	n/a	n/a	30,879,299	35,015,819	39,148,835	44,088,425	94,353,816	106,004,036	130,743,748	142,770,746	164,301,050
INDIVIDUAL SUPPORT ($)	n/a	n/a	11,642,381	16,259,370	20,728,029	22,775,513	68,472,770	79,529,570	101,874,543	113,851,179	134,661,096
Supported Employment ($)	1,113,000	1,113,000	10,433,014	11,331,396	12,195,968	12,452,083	13,572,770	16,362,726	23,834,338	30,943,489	27,673,589
# of Persons	993	2,645	3,000	3,167	3,333	3,275	3,613	4,372	4,379	5,539	5,648
Supported Living ($)	n/a	n/a	1,209,366	4,927,974	8,532,061	10,323,430	54,900,000	63,166,844	78,040,205	82,907,690	106,987,507
# of Persons	n/a	n/a	125	495	643	725	1,057	1,582	1,760	1,937	1,712
Personal Assistance ($)	0	0	0	0	0	0	0	0	0	0	0
# of Persons	0	0	0	0	0	0	0	0	0	0	0
FAMILY SUPPORT ($)	20,497,776	19,290,662	19,236,918	18,756,449	18,420,806	21,312,912	25,881,046	26,474,466	28,869,205	28,919,567	29,639,954
Total Families	12,549	13,604	13,684	12,206	10,663	10,946	11,555	11,504	12,046	12,683	13,207
Cash Subsidy/Payment ($)	11,174,100	10,467,881	10,414,137	10,809,899	11,350,487	11,662,551	12,071,234	12,551,658	12,880,159	13,325,489	13,720,845
# of Families	3,687	3,842	3,922	4,176	4,365	4,461	4,645	4,794	4,936	5,156	5,264
Other Family Support ($)	9,323,676	8,822,781	8,822,781	7,946,550	7,070,319	9,650,361	13,809,812	13,922,808	15,989,046	15,594,078	15,919,109
# of Families	8,862	9,762	9,762	8,030	6,298	6,485	6,910	6,710	7,110	7,527	7,943

PARTICIPANTS IN DAY/WORK AND SUPPORTED EMPLOYMENT

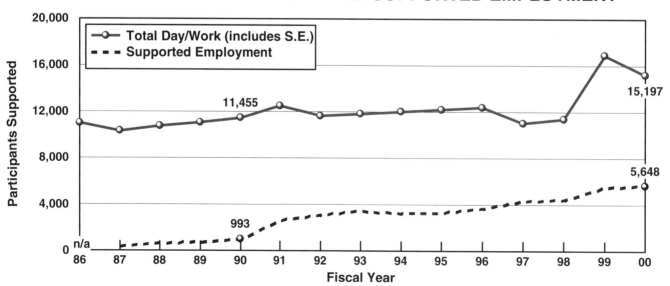

Source: The Coleman Institute and Department of Psychiatry, University of Colorado, 2002.

TRENDS IN SPENDING

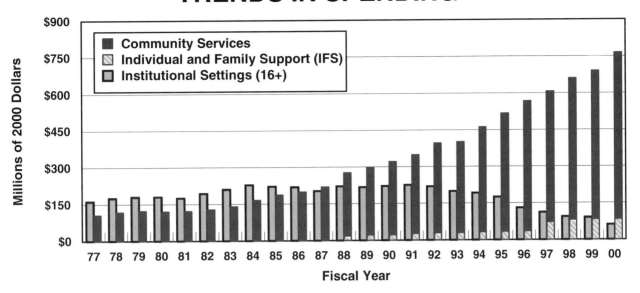

FISCAL EFFORT

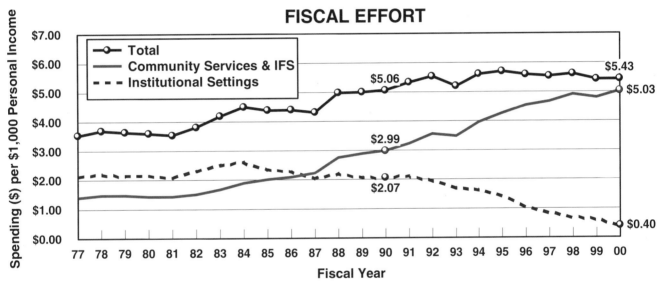

TOTAL MR/DD SPENDING AND
UNMATCHED STATE/LOCAL FUNDS

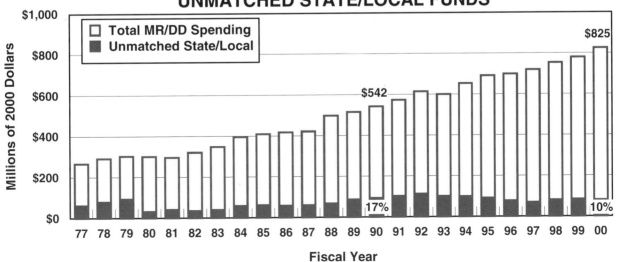

Source: The Coleman Institute and Department of Psychiatry, University of Colorado, 2002.

TRENDS IN REVENUE

COMMUNITY SERVICES REVENUE IN 2000

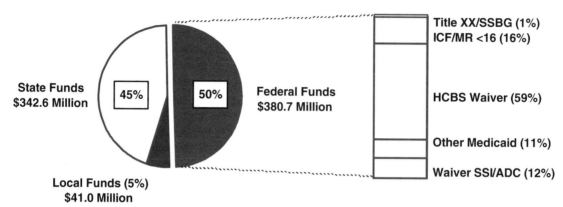

State Funds
$342.6 Million

45%

50%

Federal Funds
$380.7 Million

Local Funds (5%)
$41.0 Million

Title XX/SSBG (1%)
ICF/MR <16 (16%)

HCBS Waiver (59%)

Other Medicaid (11%)

Waiver SSI/ADC (12%)

Total: $764.3 Million

COMPONENTS OF FEDERAL MR/DD MEDICAID REVENUE

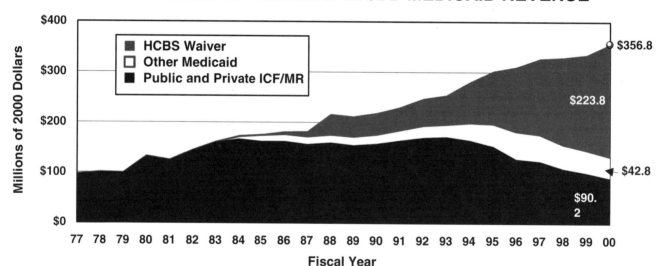

Millions of 2000 Dollars

- ■ HCBS Waiver
- □ Other Medicaid
- ■ Public and Private ICF/MR

$400
$300
$200
$100
$0

$356.8

$223.8

$42.8

$90.2

77 78 79 80 81 82 83 84 85 86 87 88 89 90 91 92 93 94 95 96 97 98 99 00

Fiscal Year

HCBS WAIVER PARTICIPANTS

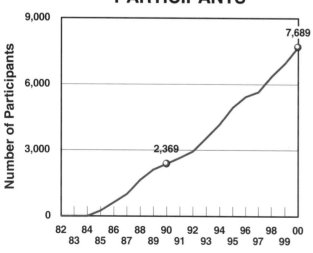

Number of Participants

9,000

6,000

3,000

0

7,689

2,369

82 83 84 85 86 87 88 89 90 91 92 93 94 95 96 97 98 99 00

WAIVER SPENDING PER PARTICIPANT

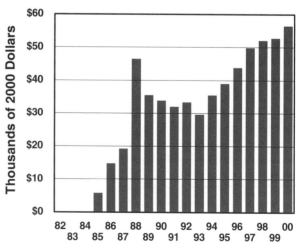

Thousands of 2000 Dollars

$60
$50
$40
$30
$20
$10
$0

82 83 84 85 86 87 88 89 90 91 92 93 94 95 96 97 98 99 00

Source: The Coleman Institute and Department of Psychiatry, University of Colorado, 2002.

TRENDS IN RESIDENTIAL SERVICES
PERSONS SERVED BY SETTING IN 2000

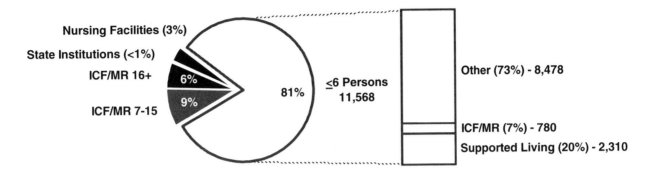

Nursing Facilities (3%)
State Institutions (<1%)
ICF/MR 16+
6%
ICF/MR 7-15
9%
81%
≤6 Persons
11,568

Other (73%) - 8,478
ICF/MR (7%) - 780
Supported Living (20%) - 2,310

Total: 14,212

PERSONS SERVED BY SETTING

	1990	1991	1992	1993	1994	1995	1996	1997	1998	1999	2000
TOTAL	n/a	n/a	10,840	11,961	11,838	12,242	12,366	14,306	14,639	13,908	14,212
16+ PERSONS	3,971	3,652	3,367	3,567	3,209	2,942	2,617	2,114	2,048	1,663	1,403
Nursing Facilities	802	827	845	1,000	1,000	1,000	1,074	746	736	568	491
State Institutions	1,352	1,177	1,033	929	760	610	442	281	194	111	59
Private ICF/MR	1,747	1,588	1,444	1,596	1,409	1,299	1,074	1,087	1,118	984	853
Other Residential	70	60	45	42	40	33	27	0	0	0	0
7-15 PERSONS	5,760	5,843	1,884	1,822	1,779	1,740	1,663	1,436	1,344	1,256	1,241
Public ICF/MR	0	0	0	0	0	0	0	0	0	0	0
Private ICF/MR	2,369	2,301	1,884	1,822	1,779	1,740	1,663	1,436	1,344	1,256	1,241
Other Residential	3,391	3,542	0	0	0	0	0	0	0	0	0
≤6 PERSONS	n/a	n/a	5,589	6,572	6,850	7,560	8,086	10,756	11,247	10,989	11,568
Public ICF/MR	0	0	18	90	90	90	90	90	90	90	90
Private ICF/MR	0	0	834	781	837	896	947	747	729	699	690
Other Residential	n/a	n/a	4,737	5,701	5,923	6,574	7,049	9,919	10,428	10,200	10,788

PERSONS SERVED IN PUBLIC AND PRIVATE INSTITUTIONS AND NURSING FACILITIES

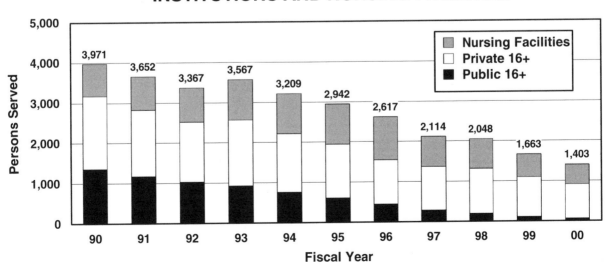

Legend:
- Nursing Facilities
- Private 16+
- Public 16+

Persons Served / Fiscal Year

3,971 · 3,652 · 3,367 · 3,567 · 3,209 · 2,942 · 2,617 · 2,114 · 2,048 · 1,663 · 1,403

Source: The Coleman Institute and Department of Psychiatry, University of Colorado, 2002.

INDIVIDUAL AND FAMILY SUPPORT

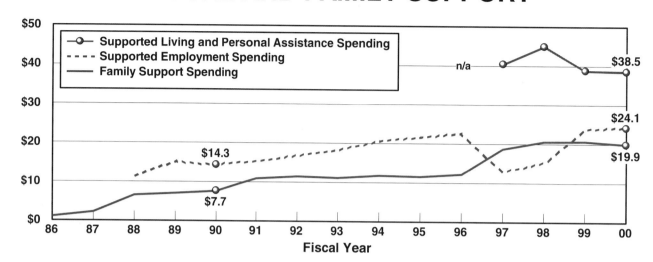

PARTICIPANTS AND SPENDING LEVELS

	1990	1991	1992	1993	1994	1995	1996	1997	1998	1999	2000
TOTAL IFS ($)	16,927,241	20,809,976	22,980,905	24,467,648	27,559,384	29,116,039	31,310,703	66,539,262	76,075,700	80,192,221	82,568,761
INDIVIDUAL SUPPORT ($)	11,038,415	12,113,633	13,584,625	15,161,965	17,490,285	18,933,432	20,285,894	49,191,317	56,612,391	60,280,767	62,657,307
Supported Employment ($)	11,038,415	12,113,633	13,584,625	15,161,965	17,490,285	18,933,432	20,285,894	11,831,277	14,226,033	22,920,397	24,118,966
# of Persons*	4,026	4,342	4,458	4,760	5,253	5,440	5,576	4,471	4,831	4,831	4,831
Supported Living ($)	0	0	0	0	0	0	0	0	0	0	0
# of Persons	0	0	0	0	0	0	0	0	0	0	0
Personal Assistance ($)	0	0	0	0	0	0	0	37,360,040	42,386,358	37,360,370	38,538,341
# of Persons	0	0	0	0	0	0	0	2,607	2,779	2,136	2,310
FAMILY SUPPORT ($)	5,888,826	8,696,343	9,396,280	9,305,683	10,069,099	10,182,607	11,024,809	17,347,945	19,463,309	19,911,454	19,911,454
Total Families	2,331	2,795	2,981	2,990	3,150	3,280	3,476	2,624	2,824	2,546	2,546
Cash Subsidy/Payment ($)	1,128,700	1,195,000	1,410,000	1,483,948	1,511,196	1,232,607	1,674,809	1,669,647	1,650,855	2,099,000	2,099,000
# of Families	435	455	641	690	700	680	726	719	755	1,118	1,118
Other Family Support ($)	4,760,126	7,501,343	7,986,280	7,821,735	8,557,903	8,950,000	9,350,000	15,678,298	17,812,454	17,812,454	17,812,454
# of Families	1,896	2,340	2,340	2,300	2,450	2,600	2,750	1,905	2,069	1,428	1,428

PARTICIPANTS IN DAY/WORK AND SUPPORTED EMPLOYMENT

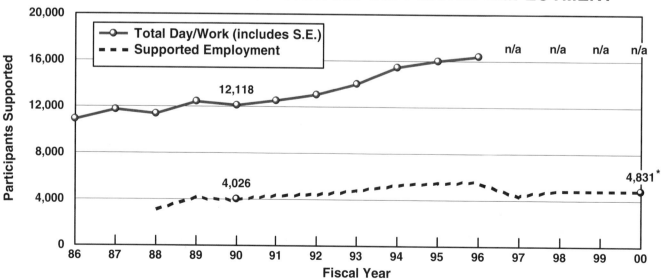

*FY98 data used for FY 1999 and FY 2000 supported employment data.

Source: The Coleman Institute and Department of Psychiatry, University of Colorado, 2002.

TRENDS IN SPENDING

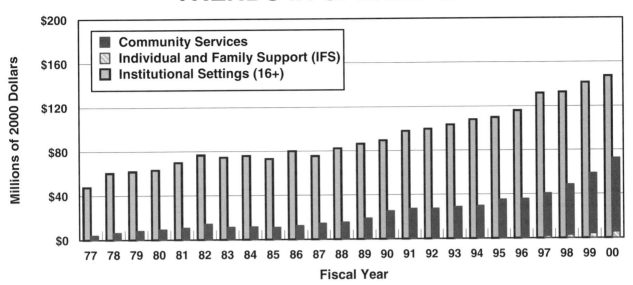

FISCAL EFFORT

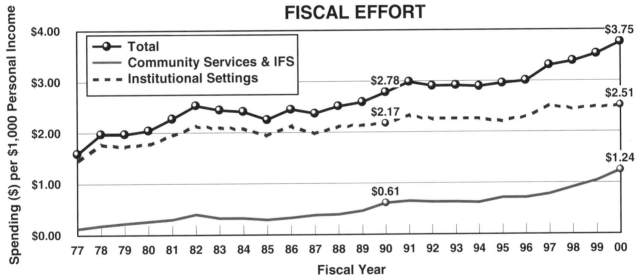

TOTAL MR/DD SPENDING AND
UNMATCHED STATE/LOCAL FUNDS

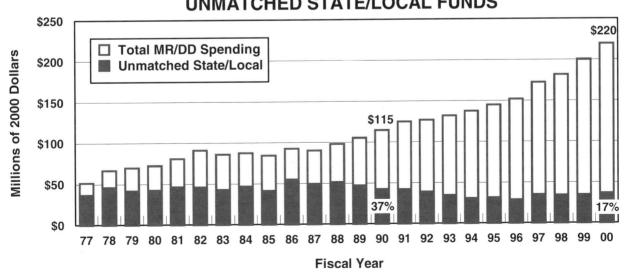

Source: The Coleman Institute and Department of Psychiatry, University of Colorado, 2002.

TRENDS IN REVENUE

COMMUNITY SERVICES REVENUE IN 2000

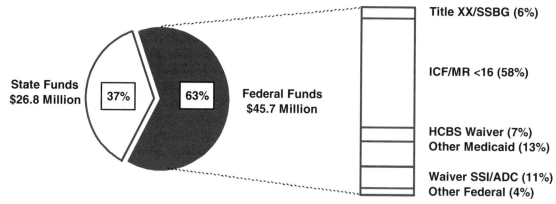

State Funds
$26.8 Million

37%

63%

Federal Funds
$45.7 Million

Title XX/SSBG (6%)

ICF/MR <16 (58%)

HCBS Waiver (7%)
Other Medicaid (13%)

Waiver SSI/ADC (11%)
Other Federal (4%)

Total: $72.4 Million

COMPONENTS OF FEDERAL MR/DD MEDICAID REVENUE

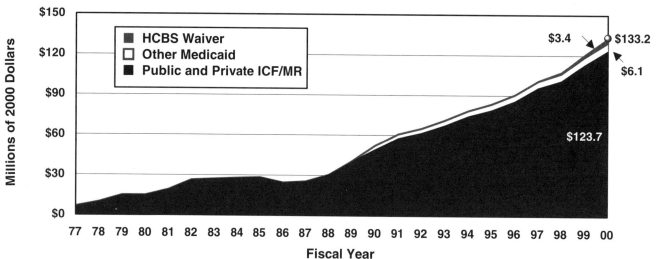

HCBS WAIVER PARTICIPANTS

WAIVER SPENDING PER PARTICIPANT

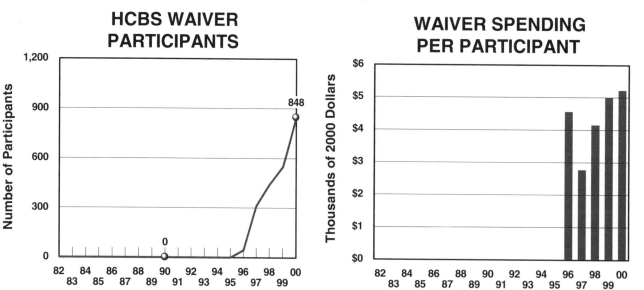

Source: The Coleman Institute and Department of Psychiatry, University of Colorado, 2002.

TRENDS IN RESIDENTIAL SERVICES

PERSONS SERVED BY SETTING IN 2000

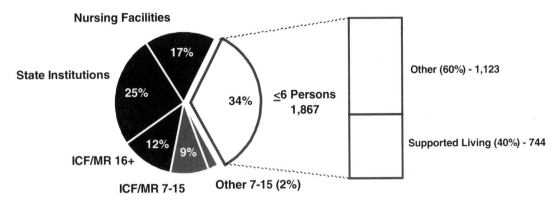

Total: 5,427

PERSONS SERVED BY SETTING

	1990	1991	1992	1993	1994	1995	1996	1997	1998	1999	2000
TOTAL	2,554	2,842	3,135	3,623	3,912	4,169	4,428	4,730	4,953	5,046	5,427
16+ PERSONS	2,286	2,583	2,806	2,891	2,958	3,015	3,019	2,959	2,830	2,911	2,943
Nursing Facilities	200	480	718	800	882	964	1,046	972	900	900	900
State Institutions	1,491	1,508	1,493	1,483	1,458	1,458	1,442	1,424	1,403	1,359	1,382
Private ICF/MR	595	595	595	608	618	593	531	563	527	652	661
Other Residential	0	0	0	0	0	0	0	0	0	0	0
7-15 PERSONS	268	259	82	168	220	221	255	334	441	502	617
Public ICF/MR	0	0	20	106	158	159	193	220	338	399	489
Private ICF/MR	0	0	0	0	0	0	0	0	0	0	0
Other Residential	268	259	62	62	62	62	62	114	103	103	128
≤6 PERSONS	0	0	247	564	734	933	1,154	1,437	1,682	1,633	1,867
Public ICF/MR	0	0	0	0	0	0	0	0	0	0	0
Private ICF/MR	0	0	0	0	0	0	0	0	0	0	0
Other Residential	0	0	247	564	734	933	1,154	1,437	1,682	1,633	1,867

PERSONS SERVED IN PUBLIC AND PRIVATE INSTITUTIONS AND NURSING FACILITIES

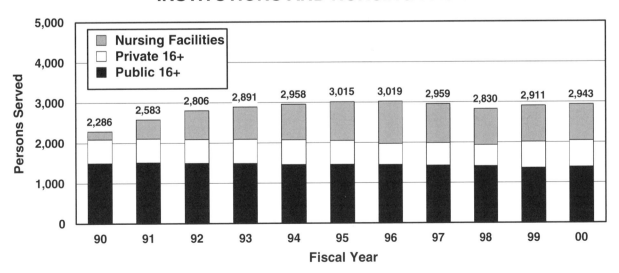

Source: The Coleman Institute and Department of Psychiatry, University of Colorado, 2002.

241

INDIVIDUAL AND FAMILY SUPPORT

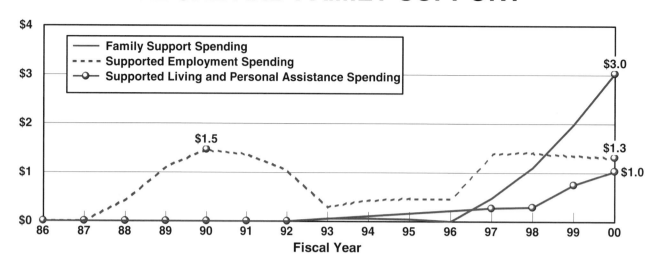

PARTICIPANTS AND SPENDING LEVELS

	1990	1991	1992	1993	1994	1995	1996	1997	1998	1999	2000
TOTAL IFS ($)	1,128,067	1,106,424	860,959	na	na	na	na	1,954,520	2,622,727	3,924,410	5,370,213
INDIVIDUAL SUPPORT ($)	1,128,067	1,106,424	860,959	na	na	na	na	1,516,420	1,581,912	2,015,857	2,342,085
Supported Employment ($)	1,128,067	1,106,424	860,959	246,316	352,233	394,063	419,988	1,267,929	1,309,919	1,296,374	1,310,894
# of Persons	461	508	451	150	157	170	173	303	362	307	300
Supported Living ($)	0	0	0	na	na	na	na	225,700	226,685	396,618	471,281
# of Persons	0	0	0	120	116	123	122	90	100	404	462
Personal Assistance ($)	0	0	0	0	0	0	0	22,791	45,308	322,865	559,910
# of Persons	0	0	0	0	0	0	0	39	80	172	282
FAMILY SUPPORT ($)	0	0	0	47,562	47,628	35,978	0	438,100	1,040,815	1,908,553	3,028,128
Total Families	0	0	0	41	45	41	0	170	279	434	640
Cash Subsidy/Payment ($)	0	0	0	0	0	0	0	0	0	0	0
# of Families	0	0	0	0	0	0	0	0	0	0	0
Other Family Support ($)	0	0	0	47,562	47,628	35,978	0	438,100	1,040,815	1,908,553	3,028,128
# of Families	0	0	0	41	45	41	0	170	279	434	640

PARTICIPANTS IN DAY/WORK AND SUPPORTED EMPLOYMENT

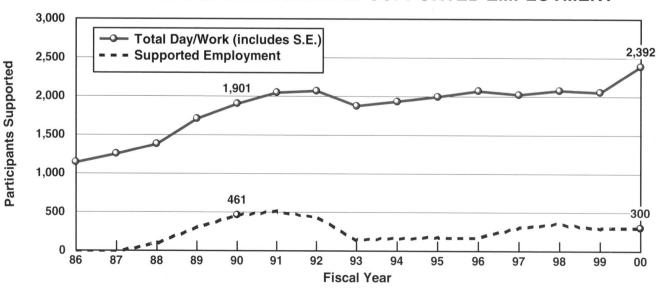

Source: The Coleman Institute and Department of Psychiatry, University of Colorado, 2002.

TRENDS IN SPENDING

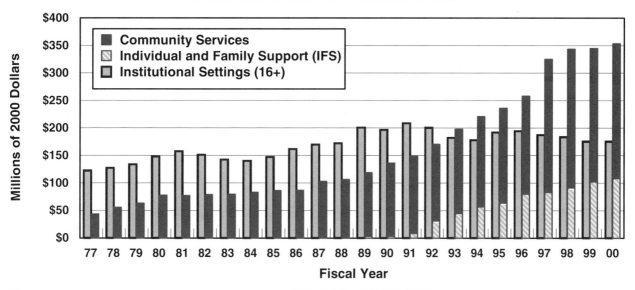

Community Services
Individual and Family Support (IFS)
Institutional Settings (16+)

Millions of 2000 Dollars

Fiscal Year
77 78 79 80 81 82 83 84 85 86 87 88 89 90 91 92 93 94 95 96 97 98 99 00

FISCAL EFFORT

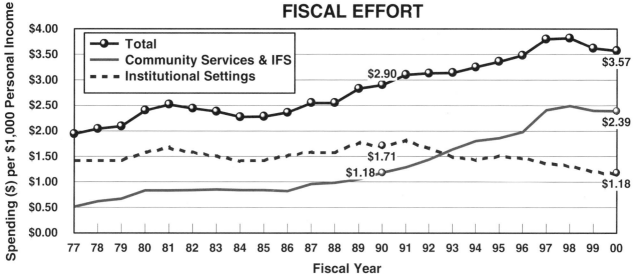

Spending ($) per $1,000 Personal Income

Total
Community Services & IFS
Institutional Settings

$2.90
$1.71
$1.18
$3.57
$2.39
$1.18

Fiscal Year
77 78 79 80 81 82 83 84 85 86 87 88 89 90 91 92 93 94 95 96 97 98 99 00

TOTAL MR/DD SPENDING AND
UNMATCHED STATE/LOCAL FUNDS

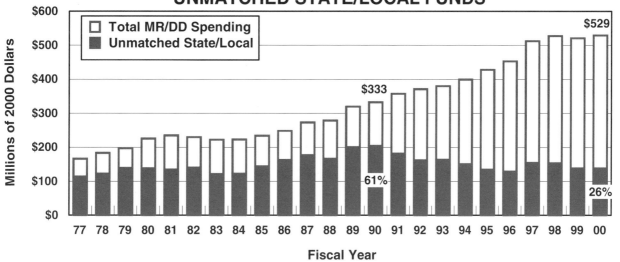

Millions of 2000 Dollars

Total MR/DD Spending
Unmatched State/Local

$333
$529
61%
26%

Fiscal Year
77 78 79 80 81 82 83 84 85 86 87 88 89 90 91 92 93 94 95 96 97 98 99 00

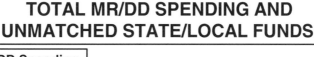

TRENDS IN REVENUE

COMMUNITY SERVICES REVENUE IN 2000

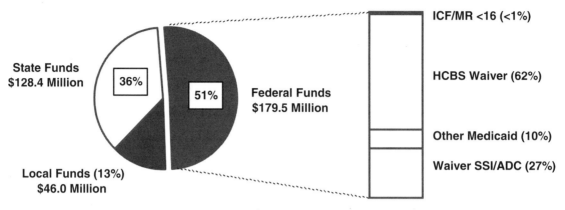

State Funds
$128.4 Million

36%

51%

Federal Funds
$179.5 Million

Local Funds (13%)
$46.0 Million

ICF/MR <16 (<1%)

HCBS Waiver (62%)

Other Medicaid (10%)

Waiver SSI/ADC (27%)

Total: $353.9 Million

COMPONENTS OF FEDERAL MR/DD MEDICAID REVENUE

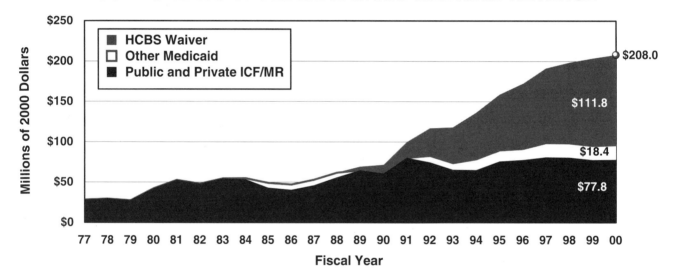

Millions of 2000 Dollars

- HCBS Waiver
- Other Medicaid
- Public and Private ICF/MR

$208.0

$111.8

$18.4

$77.8

Fiscal Year

HCBS WAIVER PARTICIPANTS

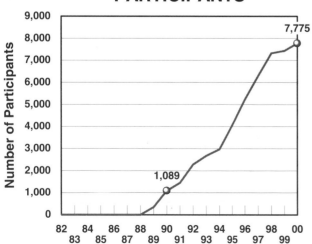

Number of Participants

7,775

1,089

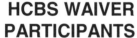

WAIVER SPENDING PER PARTICIPANT

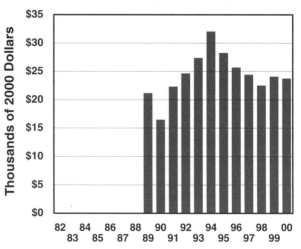

Thousands of 2000 Dollars

244

Source: The Coleman Institute and Department of Psychiatry, University of Colorado, 2002.

TRENDS IN RESIDENTIAL SERVICES

PERSONS SERVED BY SETTING IN 2000

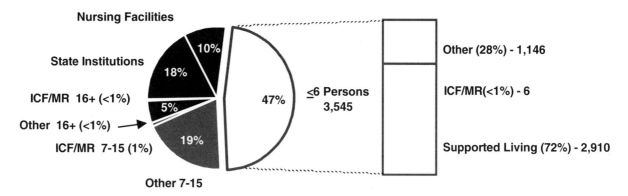

Nursing Facilities

State Institutions

ICF/MR 16+ (<1%)

Other 16+ (<1%)

ICF/MR 7-15 (1%)

Other 7-15

Other (28%) - 1,146

ICF/MR(<1%) - 6

Supported Living (72%) - 2,910

Total: 8,584

PERSONS SERVED BY SETTING

	1990	1991	1992	1993	1994	1995	1996	1997	1998	1999	2000
TOTAL	8,714	8,673	9,252	8,681	8,347	8,329	8,586	8,797	9,077	8,775	8,584
16+ PERSONS	6,474	5,894	5,513	4,763	4,500	4,348	4,215	3,693	3,574	3,028	2,798
Nursing Facilities	2,600	2,244	2,230	2,064	1,832	1,751	1,657	1,444	1,278	1,025	830
State Institutions	1,898	1,708	1,554	1,480	1,490	1,494	1,494	1,523	1,516	1,524	1,509
Private ICF/MR	176	192	84	64	64	67	64	84	84	32	27
Other Residential	1,800	1,750	1,645	1,155	1,114	1,036	1,000	642	696	447	432
7-15 PERSONS	1,351	1,576	2,085	1,862	1,463	1,441	1,427	1,638	1,560	1,704	1,724
Public ICF/MR	16	8	0	0	0	0	0	0	0	0	0
Private ICF/MR	157	120	105	127	127	127	127	78	78	87	73
Other Residential	1,178	1,448	1,980	1,735	1,336	1,314	1,300	1,560	1,482	1,617	1,651
≤6 PERSONS	889	1,203	1,654	2,056	2,384	2,540	2,944	3,466	3,943	4,043	4,062
Public ICF/MR	0	0	0	0	0	0	0	0	0	0	0
Private ICF/MR	36	36	24	24	16	0	0	0	0	6	6
Other Residential	853	1,167	1,630	2,032	2,368	2,540	2,944	3,466	3,943	4,037	4,056

PERSONS SERVED IN PUBLIC AND PRIVATE INSTITUTIONS AND NURSING FACILITIES

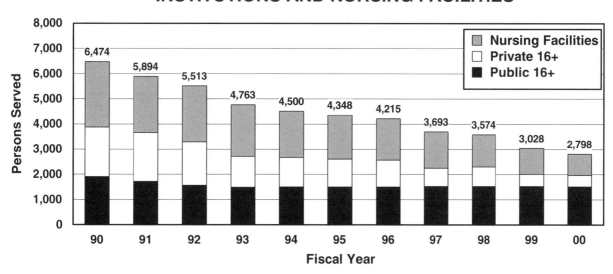

Source: The Coleman Institute and Department of Psychiatry, University of Colorado, 2002.

245

INDIVIDUAL AND FAMILY SUPPORT

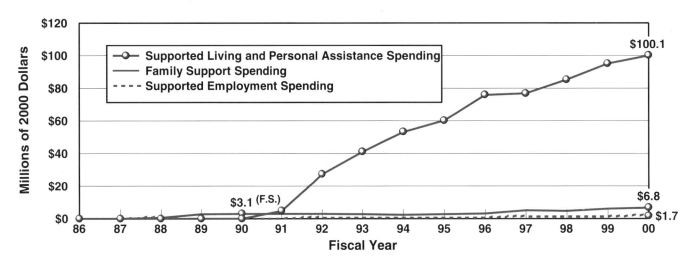

PARTICIPANTS AND SPENDING LEVELS

	1990	1991	1992	1993	1994	1995	1996	1997	1998	1999	2000
TOTAL IFS ($)	2,595,318	6,616,535	25,274,270	37,204,982	48,393,016	56,291,791	72,378,182	77,041,108	86,089,186	98,824,918	108,529,181
INDIVIDUAL SUPPORT ($)	197,875	4,148,210	22,761,360	34,829,225	46,214,411	53,818,978	69,505,012	72,296,139	81,536,740	92,942,487	101,737,960
Supported Employment ($)	197,875	235,095	393,936	472,519	551,103	644,349	753,888	1,230,894	1,015,379	1,309,078	1,654,936
# of Persons	105	105	131	175	220	280	336	229	256	437	480
Supported Living ($)	0	3,913,115	22,367,424	34,356,706	45,663,308	53,174,629	68,751,124	70,266,772	78,450,183	88,043,705	94,866,472
# of Persons	0	118	661	995	1,296	1,479	1,874	2,262	2,392	2,352	2,393
Personal Assistance ($)	0	0	0	0	0	0	0	798,473	2,071,178	3,589,704	5,216,552
# of Persons	0	0	0	0	0	0	0	231	595	428	517
FAMILY SUPPORT ($)	2,397,443	2,468,325	2,512,910	2,375,757	2,178,605	2,472,813	2,873,170	4,744,969	4,552,446	5,882,431	6,791,221
Total Families	2,538	2,329	2,429	2,507	2,585	2,398	2,425	3,652	4,228	4,742	5,018
Cash Subsidy/Payment ($)	0	0	0	0	0	286,442	687,455	687,456	873,916	1,042,666	1,042,666
# of Families	0	0	0	0	0	327	469	561	611	740	901
Other Family Support ($)	2,397,443	2,468,325	2,512,910	2,375,757	2,178,605	2,186,371	2,185,715	4,057,513	3,678,530	4,839,765	5,748,555
# of Families	2,538	2,329	2,429	2,507	2,585	2,290	2,270	3,091	3,617	4,002	4,117

PARTICIPANTS IN DAY/WORK AND SUPPORTED EMPLOYMENT

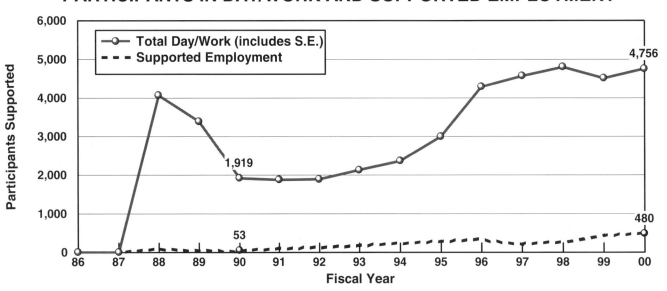

Source: The Coleman Institute and Department of Psychiatry, University of Colorado, 2002.

TRENDS IN SPENDING

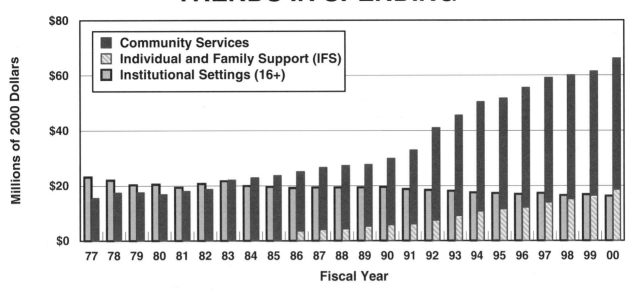

FISCAL EFFORT

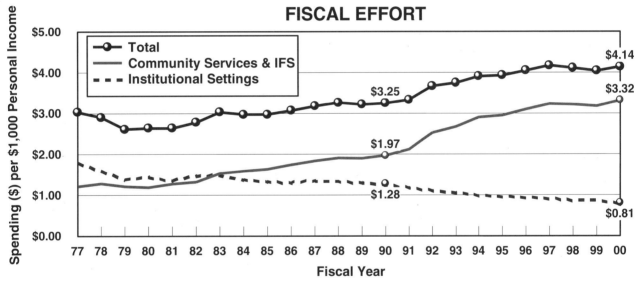

TOTAL MR/DD SPENDING AND
UNMATCHED STATE/LOCAL FUNDS

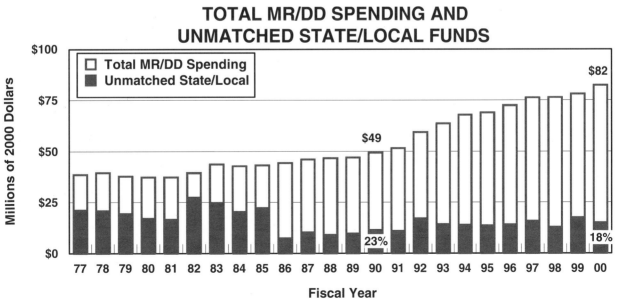

Source: The Coleman Institute and Department of Psychiatry, University of Colorado, 2002.

247

TRENDS IN REVENUE

COMMUNITY SERVICES REVENUE IN 2000

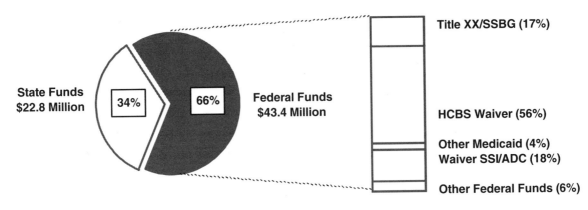

State Funds
$22.8 Million

34% **66%**

Federal Funds
$43.4 Million

Title XX/SSBG (17%)

HCBS Waiver (56%)

Other Medicaid (4%)
Waiver SSI/ADC (18%)

Other Federal Funds (6%)

Total: $66.2 Million

COMPONENTS OF FEDERAL MR/DD MEDICAID REVENUE

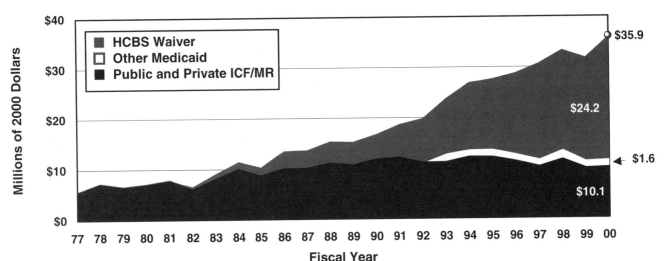

- ■ HCBS Waiver
- □ Other Medicaid
- ■ Public and Private ICF/MR

Millions of 2000 Dollars

$40

$30

$20

$10

$0

$35.9

$24.2

$1.6

$10.1

77 78 79 80 81 82 83 84 85 86 87 88 89 90 91 92 93 94 95 96 97 98 99 00

Fiscal Year

HCBS WAIVER PARTICIPANTS

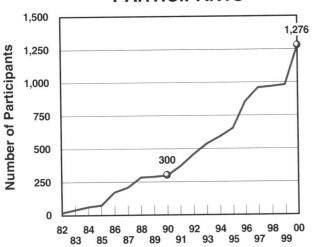

Number of Participants

1,500

1,250

1,000

750

500

250

0

1,276

300

82 83 84 85 86 87 88 89 90 91 92 93 94 95 96 97 98 99 00

WAIVER SPENDING PER PARTICIPANT

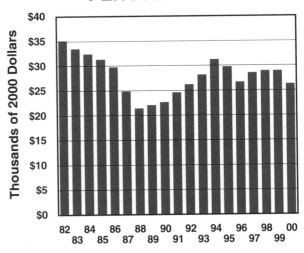

Thousands of 2000 Dollars

$40
$35
$30
$25
$20
$15
$10
$5
$0

82 83 84 85 86 87 88 89 90 91 92 93 94 95 96 97 98 99 00

Source: The Coleman Institute and Department of Psychiatry, University of Colorado, 2002.

TRENDS IN RESIDENTIAL SERVICES

PERSONS SERVED BY SETTING IN 2000

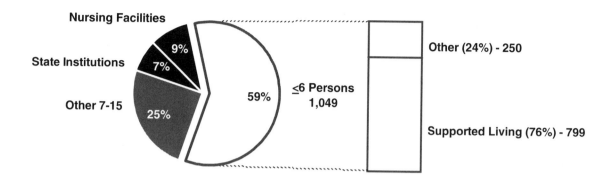

Total: 1,778

PERSONS SERVED BY SETTING

	1990	1991	1992	1993	1994	1995	1996	1997	1998	1999	2000
TOTAL	1,385	1,373	1,564	1,603	1,629	1,637	1,666	1,721	1,706	1,488	1,778
16+ PERSONS	473	444	404	330	330	324	326	333	298	288	292
Nursing Facilities	238	237	230	171	166	167	169	183	163	163	162
State Institutions	235	207	174	159	164	157	157	150	135	125	130
Private ICF/MR	0	0	0	0	0	0	0	0	0	0	0
Other Residential	0	0	0	0	0	0	0	0	0	0	0
7-15 PERSONS	553	523	486	494	503	496	501	485	488	437	437
Public ICF/MR	0	0	0	0	0	0	0	0	0	0	0
Private ICF/MR	10	10	8	8	8	8	8	8	8	0	0
Other Residential	543	513	478	486	495	488	493	477	480	437	437
≤6 PERSONS	359	406	674	779	796	817	839	903	920	763	1,049
Public ICF/MR	0	0	0	0	0	0	0	0	0	0	0
Private ICF/MR	0	0	0	0	0	0	0	0	0	0	0
Other Residential	359	406	674	779	796	817	839	903	920	763	1,049

PERSONS SERVED IN PUBLIC AND PRIVATE INSTITUTIONS AND NURSING FACILITIES

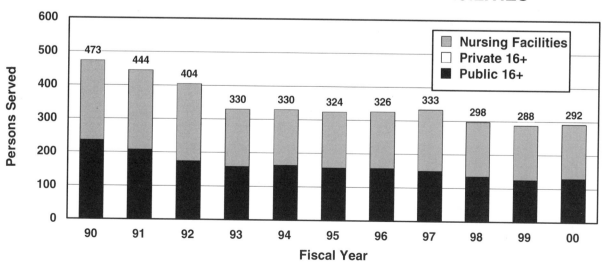

Source: The Coleman Institute and Department of Psychiatry, University of Colorado, 2002.

INDIVIDUAL AND FAMILY SUPPORT

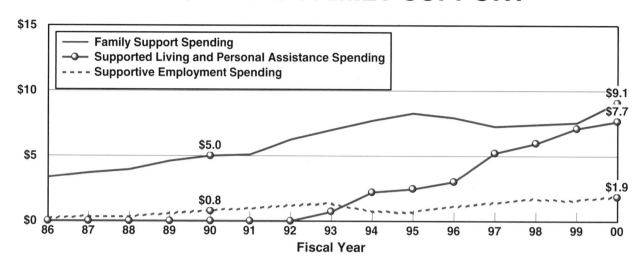

PARTICIPANTS AND SPENDING LEVELS

	1990	1991	1992	1993	1994	1995	1996	1997	1998	1999	2000
TOTAL IFS ($)	4,428,039	4,846,014	6,088,809	7,524,654	9,148,232	10,099,374	10,856,190	12,823,520	14,226,311	15,725,251	18,609,425
INDIVIDUAL SUPPORT ($)	579,922	758,119	973,367	1,669,718	2,550,113	2,804,401	3,678,647	6,105,675	7,237,863	8,440,608	9,520,611
Supported Employment ($)	579,922	758,119	973,367	1,071,784	661,769	630,934	957,372	1,283,810	1,610,248	1,598,931	1,857,808
# of Persons	162	198	233	193	158	150	221	240	260	220	249
Supported Living ($)	0	0	0	597,934	1,888,344	2,173,467	2,721,275	4,821,865	5,627,615	6,841,677	7,662,803
# of Persons	0	0	0	64	74	87	70	516	538	515	799
Personal Assistance ($)	0	0	0	0	0	0	0	0	0	0	0
# of Persons	0	0	0	0	0	0	0	0	0	0	0
FAMILY SUPPORT ($)	3,848,117	4,087,895	5,115,442	5,854,936	6,598,119	7,294,973	7,177,543	6,717,845	6,988,448	7,284,643	9,088,814
Total Families	1,024	1,200	1,753	2,015	2,495	2,775	2,639	1,645	1,633	1,970	2,762
Cash Subsidy/Payment ($)	0	0	0	0	0	0	0	0	0	0	0
# of Families	0	0	0	0	0	0	0	0	0	0	0
Other Family Support ($)	3,848,117	4,087,895	5,115,442	5,854,936	6,598,119	7,294,973	7,177,543	6,717,845	6,988,448	7,284,643	9,088,814
# of Families	1,509	1,831	2,352	2,697	3,027	3,238	2,639	1,615	1,633	1,970	2,762

PARTICIPANTS IN DAY/WORK AND SUPPORTED EMPLOYMENT

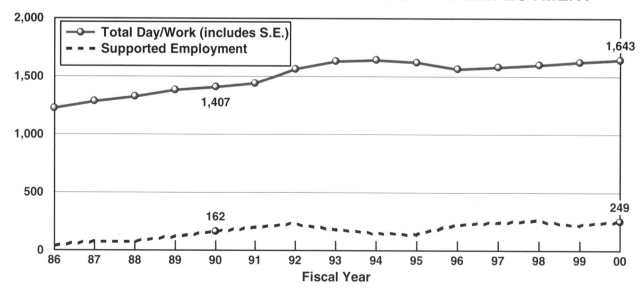

Source: The Coleman Institute and Department of Psychiatry, University of Colorado, 2002.

TRENDS IN SPENDING

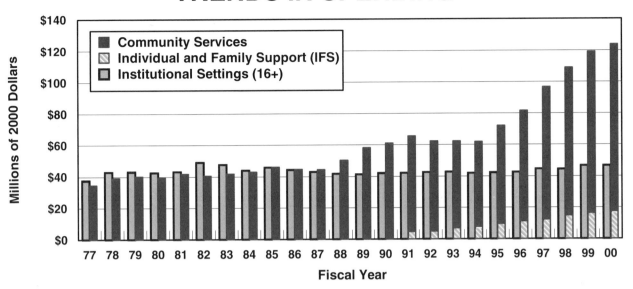

FISCAL EFFORT

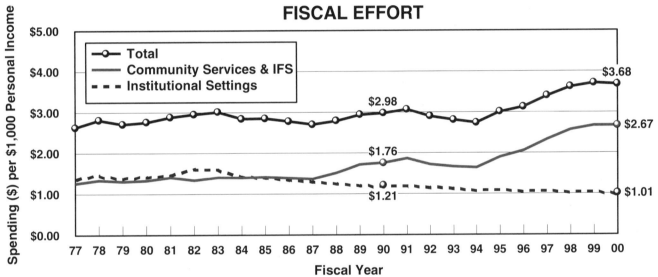

TOTAL MR/DD SPENDING AND
UNMATCHED STATE/LOCAL FUNDS

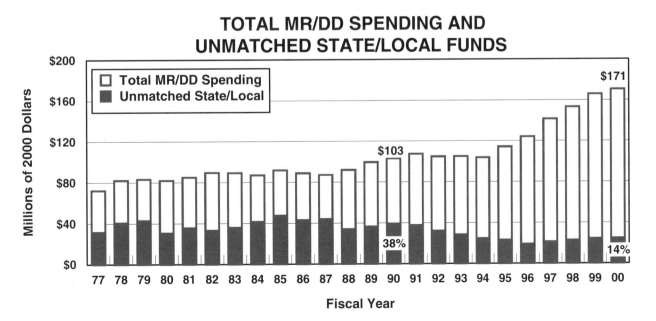

Source: The Coleman Institute and Department of Psychiatry, University of Colorado, 2002.

TRENDS IN REVENUE

COMMUNITY SERVICES REVENUE IN 2000

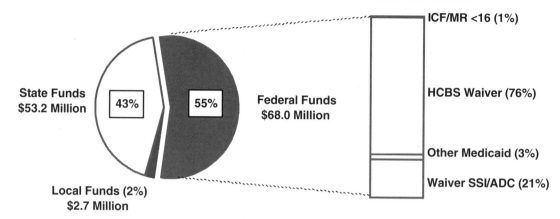

State Funds
$53.2 Million

43%

55%

Federal Funds
$68.0 Million

Local Funds (2%)
$2.7 Million

ICF/MR <16 (1%)

HCBS Waiver (76%)

Other Medicaid (3%)

Waiver SSI/ADC (21%)

Total: $123.9 Million

COMPONENTS OF FEDERAL MR/DD MEDICAID REVENUE

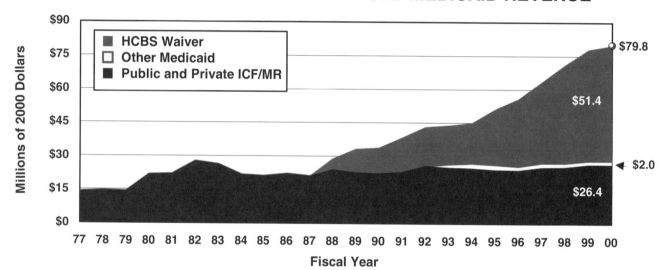

Millions of 2000 Dollars

- HCBS Waiver
- Other Medicaid
- Public and Private ICF/MR

$90
$75
$60
$45
$30
$15
$0

$79.8
$51.4
$2.0
$26.4

77 78 79 80 81 82 83 84 85 86 87 88 89 90 91 92 93 94 95 96 97 98 99 00

Fiscal Year

HCBS WAIVER PARTICIPANTS

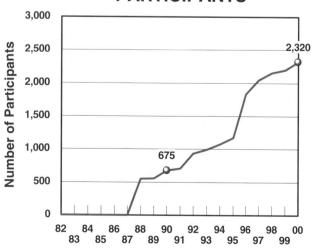

Number of Participants

3,000
2,500
2,000
1,500
1,000
500
0

2,320

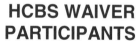675

82 83 84 85 86 87 88 89 90 91 92 93 94 95 96 97 98 99 00

WAIVER SPENDING PER PARTICIPANT

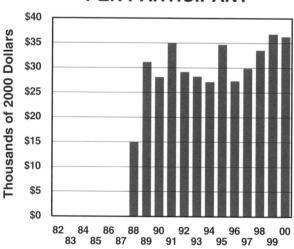

Thousands of 2000 Dollars

$40
$35
$30
$25
$20
$15
$10
$5
$0

82 83 84 85 86 87 88 89 90 91 92 93 94 95 96 97 98 99 00

Source: The Coleman Institute and Department of Psychiatry, University of Colorado, 2002.

TRENDS IN RESIDENTIAL SERVICES

PERSONS SERVED BY SETTING IN 2000

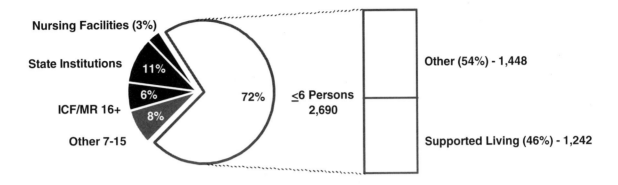

Nursing Facilities (3%)

State Institutions 11%

6%

ICF/MR 16+ 8%

Other 7-15

72%

≤6 Persons 2,690

Other (54%) - 1,448

Supported Living (46%) - 1,242

Total: 3,744

PERSONS SERVED BY SETTING

	1990	1991	1992	1993	1994	1995	1996	1997	1998	1999	2000
TOTAL	2,928	3,041	3,055	3,101	3,059	3,115	3,439	3,434	3,430	3,422	3,744
16+ PERSONS	1,146	1,185	1,190	1,198	1,138	1,119	1,110	947	849	796	754
Nursing Facilities	437	461	476	490	445	432	454	316	215	155	115
State Institutions	466	466	458	452	444	433	404	394	393	401	399
Private ICF/MR	243	258	256	256	249	254	252	237	241	240	240
Other Residential	0	0	0	0	0	0	0	0	0	0	0
7-15 PERSONS	1,087	1,142	8	8	9	8	259	262	287	228	300
Public ICF/MR	0	0	0	0	0	0	0	0	0	0	0
Private ICF/MR	8	8	8	8	9	8	9	9	9	9	0
Other Residential	1,079	1,134	0	0	0	0	250	253	278	219	300
≤6 PERSONS	695	714	1,857	1,895	1,912	1,988	2,070	2,225	2,294	2,398	2,690
Public ICF/MR	0	0	0	0	0	0	0	0	0	0	0
Private ICF/MR	0	0	0	0	0	0	0	0	0	0	0
Other Residential	695	714	1,857	1,895	1,912	1,988	2,070	2,225	2,294	2,398	2,690

PERSONS SERVED IN PUBLIC AND PRIVATE INSTITUTIONS AND NURSING FACILITIES

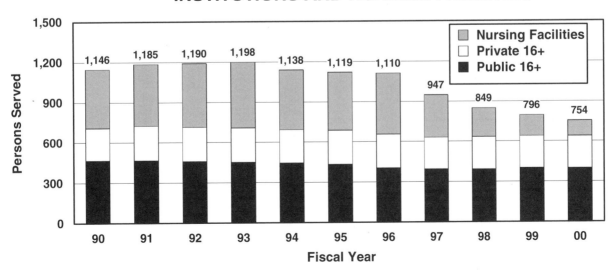

Persons Served / Fiscal Year

Legend: Nursing Facilities, Private 16+, Public 16+

1,146 1,185 1,190 1,198 1,138 1,119 1,110 947 849 796 754

Source: The Coleman Institute and Department of Psychiatry, University of Colorado, 2002.

INDIVIDUAL AND FAMILY SUPPORT

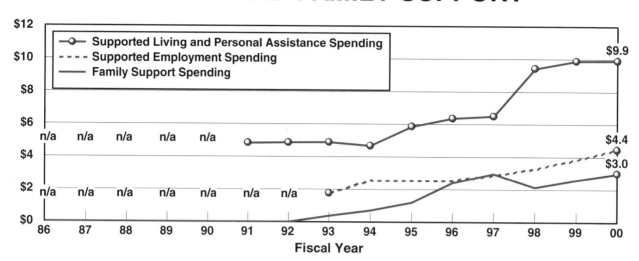

PARTICIPANTS AND SPENDING LEVELS

	1990	1991	1992	1993	1994	1995	1996	1997	1998	1999	2000
TOTAL IFS ($)	n/a	n/a	n/a	5,846,096	6,733,508	8,439,289	10,198,113	11,333,796	13,956,391	15,658,195	17,312,363
INDIVIDUAL SUPPORT ($)	n/a	n/a	n/a	5,549,488	6,132,687	7,386,465	8,024,118	8,608,457	11,946,337	13,165,577	14,337,648
Supported Employment ($)	n/a	n/a	n/a	1,469,012	2,139,144	2,225,706	2,279,478	2,615,629	3,055,758	3,651,774	4,440,912
# of Persons	382	367	397	445	648	678	718	739	724	797	890
Supported Living ($)	n/a	3,866,542	3,967,394	4,080,476	3,993,543	5,160,759	5,744,640	5,992,828	8,890,579	9,513,803	9,896,736
# of Persons	695	713	714	751	735	760	977	1,056	1,091	1,201	1,242
Personal Assistance ($)	0	0	0	0	0	0	0	0	0	0	0
# of Persons	0	0	0	0	0	0	0	0	0	0	0
FAMILY SUPPORT ($)	0	0	0	296,608	600,821	1,052,824	2,173,995	2,725,339	2,010,054	2,492,618	2,974,715
Total Families	0	0	0	118	267	309	606	666	728	758	753
Cash Subsidy/Payment ($)	0	0	0	0	0	0	0	0	0	0	0
# of Families	0	0	0	0	0	0	0	0	0	0	0
Other Family Support ($)	0	0	0	296,608	600,821	1,052,824	2,173,995	2,725,339	2,010,054	2,492,618	2,974,715
# of Families	0	0	0	118	267	309	606	666	728	758	753

PARTICIPANTS IN DAY/WORK AND SUPPORTED EMPLOYMENT

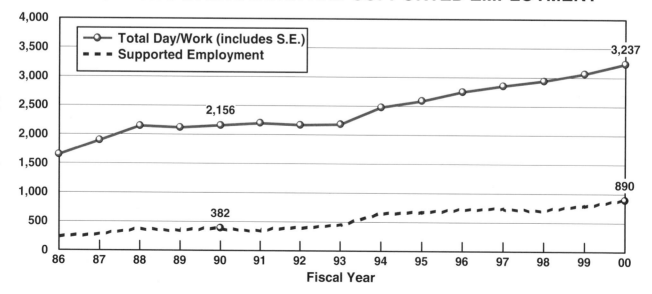

Source: The Coleman Institute and Department of Psychiatry, University of Colorado, 2002.

TRENDS IN SPENDING

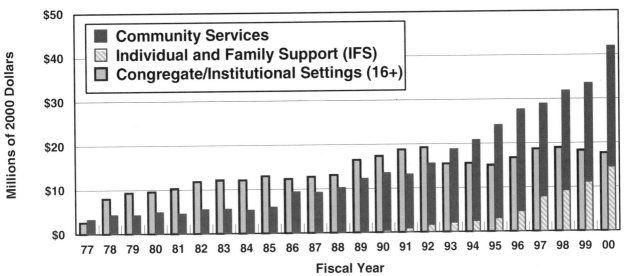

Millions of 2000 Dollars

- Community Services
- Individual and Family Support (IFS)
- Congregate/Institutional Settings (16+)

Fiscal Year

FISCAL EFFORT

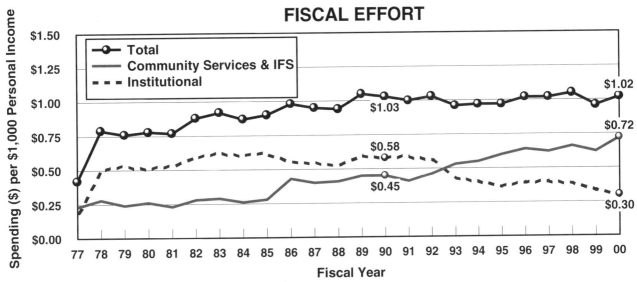

Spending ($) per $1,000 Personal Income

- Total
- Community Services & IFS
- Institutional

$1.03 $1.02
$0.58 $0.72
$0.45 $0.30

Fiscal Year

TOTAL MR/DD SPENDING AND
UNMATCHED STATE/LOCAL FUNDS

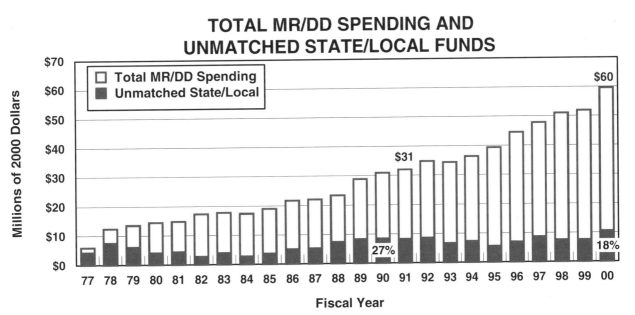

Millions of 2000 Dollars

- Total MR/DD Spending
- Unmatched State/Local

$60
$31
27%   18%

Fiscal Year

Source: The Coleman Institute and Department of Psychiatry, University of Colorado, 2002.

NEVADA

TRENDS IN REVENUE

COMMUNITY SERVICES REVENUE IN 2000

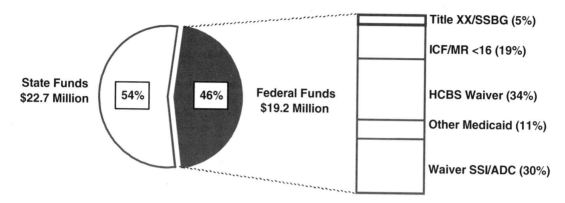

State Funds $22.7 Million — 54%

Federal Funds $19.2 Million — 46%

Title XX/SSBG (5%)
ICF/MR <16 (19%)
HCBS Waiver (34%)
Other Medicaid (11%)
Waiver SSI/ADC (30%)

Total: $41.9 Million

COMPONENTS OF FEDERAL MR/DD MEDICAID REVENUE

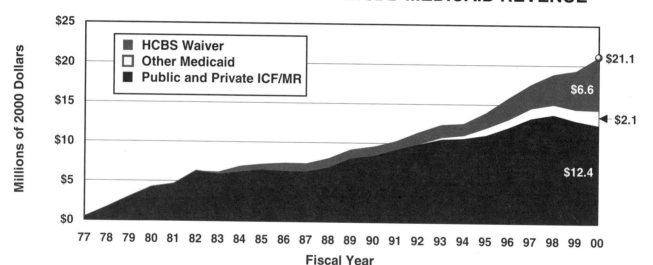

Millions of 2000 Dollars

- HCBS Waiver
- Other Medicaid
- Public and Private ICF/MR

$21.1
$6.6
$2.1
$12.4

Fiscal Year

HCBS WAIVER PARTICIPANTS

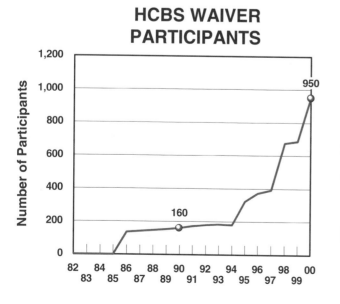

Number of Participants

950

160

WAIVER SPENDING PER PARTICIPANT

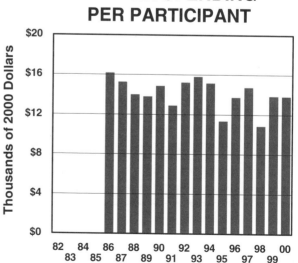

Thousands of 2000 Dollars

Source: The Coleman Institute and Department of Psychiatry, University of Colorado, 2002.

TRENDS IN RESIDENTIAL SERVICES

PERSONS SERVED BY SETTING IN 2000

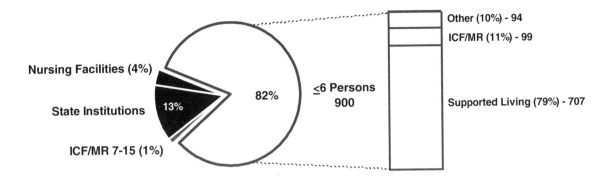

Nursing Facilities (4%)

State Institutions 13%

ICF/MR 7-15 (1%)

82%

≤6 Persons 900

Other (10%) - 94

ICF/MR (11%) - 99

Supported Living (79%) - 707

Total: 1,096

PERSONS SERVED BY SETTING

	1990	1991	1992	1993	1994	1995	1996	1997	1998	1999	2000
TOTAL	557	564	683	718	737	741	786	821	951	886	1,096
16+ PERSONS	274	290	268	272	270	256	254	273	275	208	181
Nursing Facilities	100	117	118	122	125	115	104	105	106	40	40
State Institutions	174	173	150	150	145	141	150	168	169	168	141
Private ICF/MR	0	0	0	0	0	0	0	0	0	0	0
Other Residential	0	0	0	0	0	0	0	0	0	0	0
7-15 PERSONS	0	0	0	15	15	15	27	15	15	15	15
Public ICF/MR	0	0	0	0	0	0	12	0	0	0	0
Private ICF/MR	0	0	0	15	15	15	15	15	15	15	15
Other Residential	0	0	0	0	0	0	0	0	0	0	0
≤6 PERSONS	283	274	415	431	452	470	505	533	661	663	900
Public ICF/MR	0	0	24	23	24	30	17	18	18	6	3
Private ICF/MR	0	13	24	24	32	40	60	65	77	96	96
Other Residential	283	261	367	384	396	400	428	450	566	561	801

PERSONS SERVED IN PUBLIC AND PRIVATE INSTITUTIONS AND NURSING FACILITIES

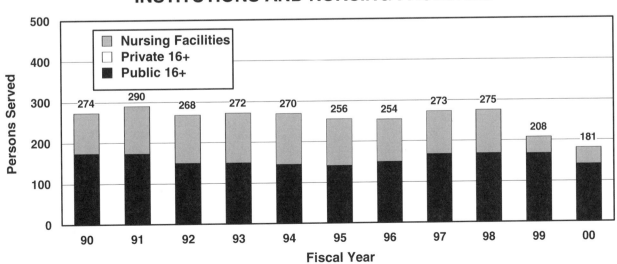

Persons Served

Legend:
- Nursing Facilities
- Private 16+
- Public 16+

274, 290, 268, 272, 270, 256, 254, 273, 275, 208, 181

Fiscal Year: 90, 91, 92, 93, 94, 95, 96, 97, 98, 99, 00

Source: The Coleman Institute and Department of Psychiatry, University of Colorado, 2002.

257

INDIVIDUAL AND FAMILY SUPPORT

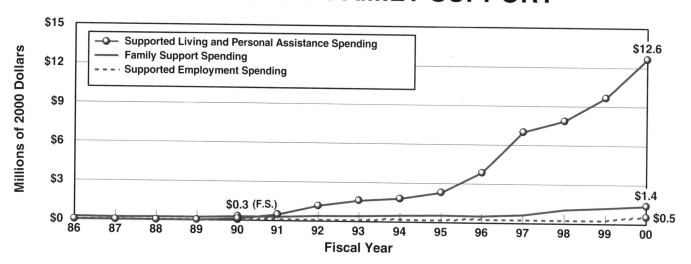

PARTICIPANTS AND SPENDING LEVELS

	1990	1991	1992	1993	1994	1995	1996	1997	1998	1999	2000
TOTAL IFS ($)	366,147	688,343	1,361,128	1,779,637	2,111,451	2,683,840	4,189,089	7,328,278	8,722,718	10,757,896	14,562,588
INDIVIDUAL SUPPORT ($)	129,577	441,420	1,043,311	1,425,341	1,683,018	2,196,517	3,722,883	6,742,187	7,709,985	9,583,728	13,183,788
Supported Employment ($)	35,230	63,635	76,292	80,508	147,396	163,678	236,067	243,262	257,785	264,000	540,000
# of Persons	18	22	35	45	120	187	196	203	215	220	450
Supported Living ($)	94,347	377,785	967,019	1,344,833	1,535,622	2,032,839	3,486,816	6,498,925	7,452,200	9,319,728	12,643,788
# of Persons	56	81	128	157	184	216	241	341	453	460	707
Personal Assistance ($)	0	0	0	0	0	0	0	0	0	0	0
# of Persons	0	0	0	0	0	0	0	0	0	0	0
FAMILY SUPPORT ($)	236,570	246,923	317,817	354,296	428,433	487,323	466,206	586,091	1,012,733	1,174,168	1,378,800
Total Families	115	200	336	322	325	308	365	463	818	1,074	1,296
Cash Subsidy/Payment ($)	178,478	188,688	266,740	280,800	353,908	395,533	371,186	381,180	484,884	649,146	752,975
# of Families	81	99	108	117	119	128	132	127	140	226	278
Other Family Support ($)	58,092	58,235	51,077	73,496	74,525	91,790	95,020	204,911	527,849	525,022	625,825
# of Families	115	200	228	205	206	180	233	336	678	848	1,018

PERSONS SERVED IN DAY/WORK AND SUPPORTED EMPLOYMENT

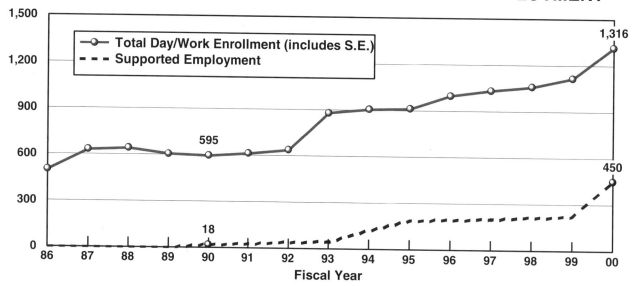

Source: The Coleman Institute and Department of Psychiatry, University of Colorado, 2002.

TRENDS IN SPENDING

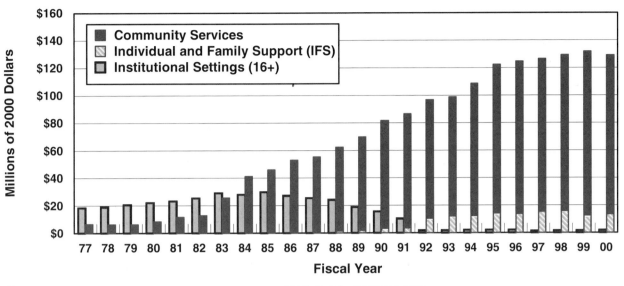

FISCAL EFFORT

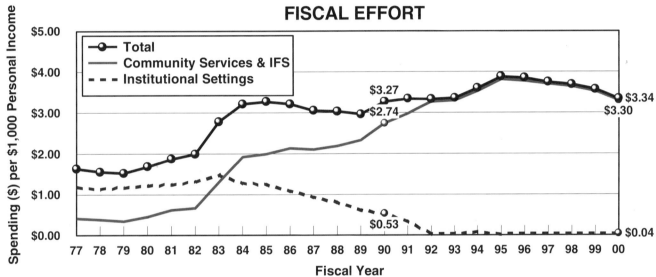

TOTAL MR/DD SPENDING AND
UNMATCHED STATE/LOCAL FUNDS

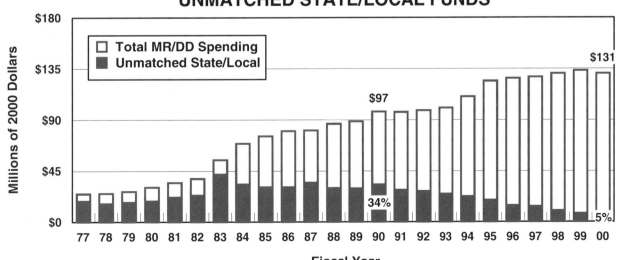

Source: The Coleman Institute and Department of Psychiatry, University of Colorado, 2002.

TRENDS IN REVENUE

COMMUNITY SERVICES REVENUE IN 2000

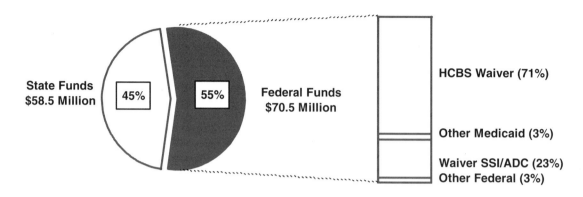

State Funds
$58.5 Million

45%

55%

Federal Funds
$70.5 Million

HCBS Waiver (71%)

Other Medicaid (3%)

Waiver SSI/ADC (23%)
Other Federal (3%)

Total: $129.1 Million

COMPONENTS OF FEDERAL MR/DD MEDICAID REVENUE

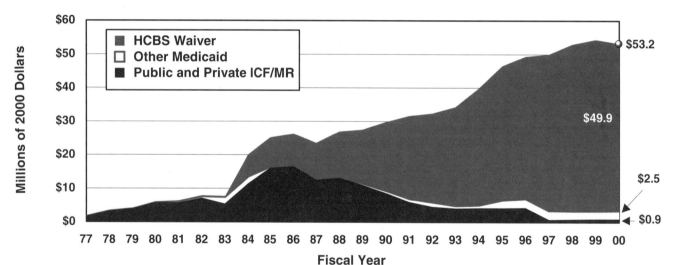

Millions of 2000 Dollars

■ HCBS Waiver
□ Other Medicaid
■ Public and Private ICF/MR

$60
$50
$40
$30
$20
$10
$0

$53.2
$49.9
$2.5
$0.9

77 78 79 80 81 82 83 84 85 86 87 88 89 90 91 92 93 94 95 96 97 98 99 00

Fiscal Year

HCBS WAIVER PARTICIPANTS

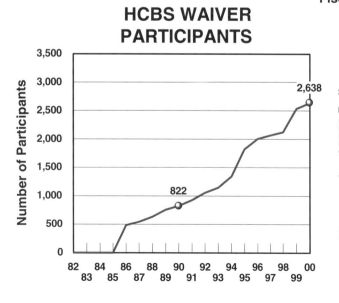

Number of Participants

3,500
3,000
2,500
2,000
1,500
1,000
500
0

2,638
822

82 84 86 88 90 92 94 96 98 00
83 85 87 89 91 93 95 97 99

WAIVER SPENDING PER PARTICIPANT

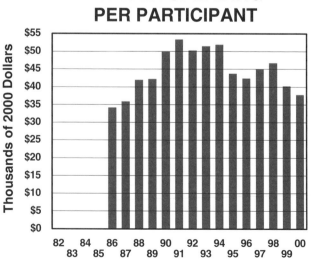

Thousands of 2000 Dollars

$55
$50
$45
$40
$35
$30
$25
$20
$15
$10
$5
$0

82 84 86 88 90 92 94 96 98 00
83 85 87 89 91 93 95 97 99

Source: The Coleman Institute and Department of Psychiatry, University of Colorado, 2002.

TRENDS IN RESIDENTIAL SERVICES
PERSONS SERVED BY SETTING IN 2000

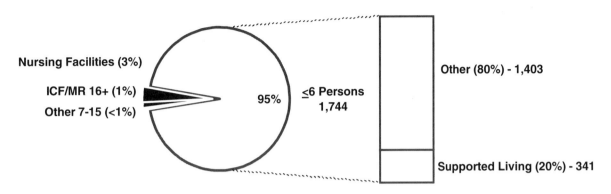

Nursing Facilities (3%)

ICF/MR 16+ (1%)

Other 7-15 (<1%)

95%

≤6 Persons
1,744

Other (80%) - 1,403

Supported Living (20%) - 341

Total: 1,840

PERSONS SERVED BY SETTING

	1990	1991	1992	1993	1994	1995	1996	1997	1998	1999	2000
TOTAL	1,068	1,194	1,274	1,443	1,505	1,572	1,663	1,651	1,694	1,784	1,840
16+ PERSONS	77	42	45	122	117	122	132	70	62	90	88
Nursing Facilities	9	9	20	97	92	97	107	48	38	64	64
State Institutions	45	10	0	0	0	0	0	0	0	0	0
Private ICF/MR	23	23	25	25	25	25	25	22	24	26	24
Other Residential	0	0	0	0	0	0	0	0	0	0	0
7-15 PERSONS	991	1,152	322	125	108	91	90	43	43	25	8
Public ICF/MR	0	0	0	0	0	0	0	0	0	0	0
Private ICF/MR	54	66	48	40	38	37	37	0	0	0	0
Other Residential	937	1,086	274	85	70	54	53	43	43	25	8
≤6 PERSONS	0	0	907	1,196	1,280	1,359	1,441	1,538	1,589	1,669	1,744
Public ICF/MR	0	0	0	0	0	0	0	0	0	0	0
Private ICF/MR	0	0	18	18	12	12	12	0	0	0	0
Other Residential	0	0	889	1,178	1,268	1,347	1,429	1,538	1,589	1,669	1,744

PERSONS SERVED IN PUBLIC AND PRIVATE INSTITUTIONS AND NURSING FACILITIES

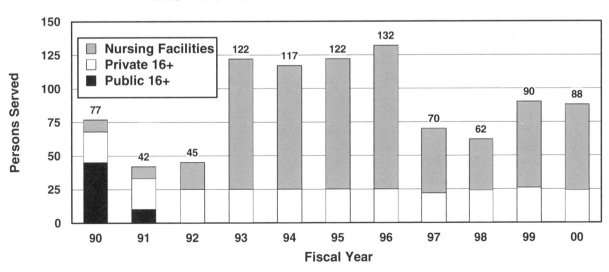

Legend:
- Nursing Facilities
- Private 16+
- Public 16+

Y-axis: Persons Served (0, 25, 50, 75, 100, 125, 150)
X-axis: Fiscal Year (90, 91, 92, 93, 94, 95, 96, 97, 98, 99, 00)

Values: 77, 42, 45, 122, 117, 122, 132, 70, 62, 90, 88

Source: The Coleman Institute and Department of Psychiatry, University of Colorado, 2002.

INDIVIDUAL AND FAMILY SUPPORT

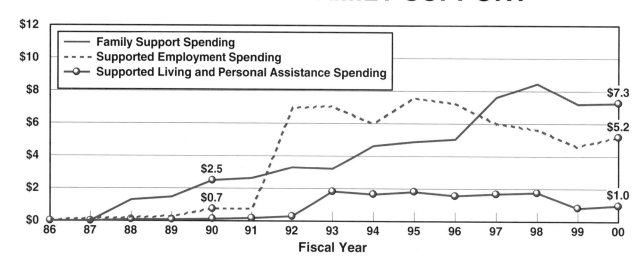

PARTICIPANTS AND SPENDING LEVELS

	1990	1991	1992	1993	1994	1995	1996	1997	1998	1999	2000
TOTAL IFS ($)	2,571,072	2,872,477	8,625,824	10,084,039	10,573,723	12,616,444	12,513,863	14,170,306	14,996,762	12,174,117	13,433,504
INDIVIDUAL SUPPORT ($)	659,910	756,017	5,932,775	7,390,497	6,608,331	8,297,772	7,960,488	7,124,844	7,007,400	5,225,802	6,163,849
Supported Employment ($)	562,410	616,017	5,692,775	5,863,148	5,188,428	6,695,468	6,542,061	5,563,756	5,340,151	4,422,345	5,181,673
# of Persons	695	590	550	501	541	523	499	442	409	472	483
Supported Living ($)	0	0	0	1,527,349	1,419,903	1,602,304	1,418,427	1,561,088	1,667,249	803,457	982,176
# of Persons	0	0	0	209	222	231	220	256	290	306	341
Personal Assistance ($)	97,500	140,000	240,000	0	0	0	0	0	0	0	0
# of Persons	15	20	30	0	0	0	0	0	0	0	0
FAMILY SUPPORT ($)	1,911,162	2,116,460	2,693,049	2,693,542	3,965,392	4,318,672	4,553,375	7,045,462	7,989,362	6,948,315	7,269,655
Total Families	n/a	n/a	n/a	3,071	3,258	3,716	3,034	4,536	5,902	5,289	4,917
Cash Subsidy/Payment ($)	0	0	0	0	0	0	0	0	0	0	0
# of Families	0	0	0	0	0	0	0	0	0	0	0
Other Family Support ($)	1,911,162	2,116,460	2,693,049	2,693,542	3,965,392	4,318,672	4,553,375	7,045,462	7,989,362	6,948,315	7,269,655
# of Families	n/a	n/a	n/a	3,071	3,258	3,716	3,034	4,536	5,902	5,289	4,917

PARTICIPANTS IN DAY/WORK AND SUPPORTED EMPLOYMENT

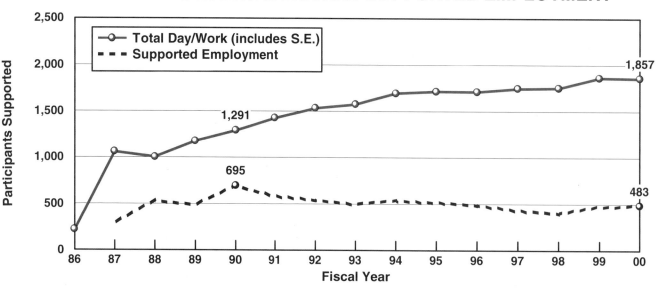

Source: The Coleman Institute and Department of Psychiatry, University of Colorado, 2002.

TRENDS IN SPENDING

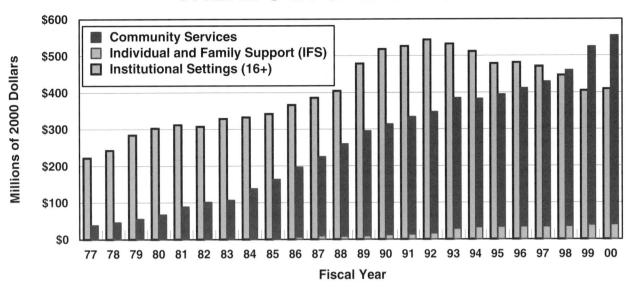

Millions of 2000 Dollars

- Community Services
- Individual and Family Support (IFS)
- Institutional Settings (16+)

Fiscal Year

FISCAL EFFORT

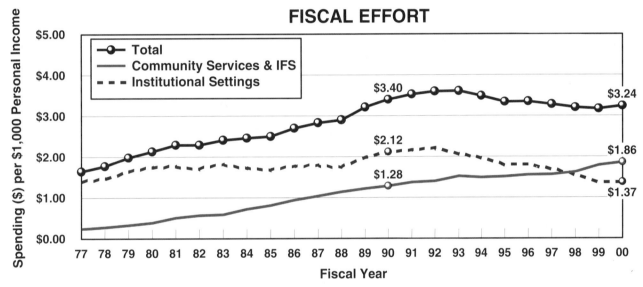

Spending ($) per $1,000 Personal Income

- Total
- Community Services & IFS
- Institutional Settings

$3.40 $3.24
$2.12 $1.86
$1.28 $1.37

Fiscal Year

TOTAL MR/DD SPENDING AND
UNMATCHED STATE/LOCAL FUNDS

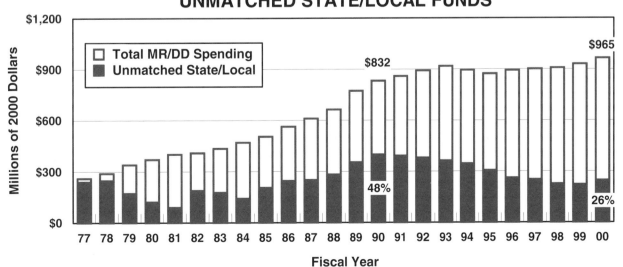

Millions of 2000 Dollars

- Total MR/DD Spending
- Unmatched State/Local

$832 $965
48%   26%

Fiscal Year

Source: The Coleman Institute and Department of Psychiatry, University of Colorado, 2002.

TRENDS IN REVENUE

COMMUNITY SERVICES REVENUE IN 2000

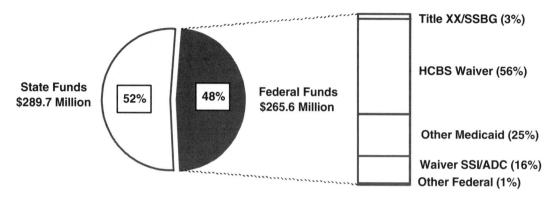

State Funds
$289.7 Million

52%

48%

Federal Funds
$265.6 Million

Title XX/SSBG (3%)

HCBS Waiver (56%)

Other Medicaid (25%)

Waiver SSI/ADC (16%)

Other Federal (1%)

Total: $555.3 Million

COMPONENTS OF FEDERAL MR/DD MEDICAID REVENUE

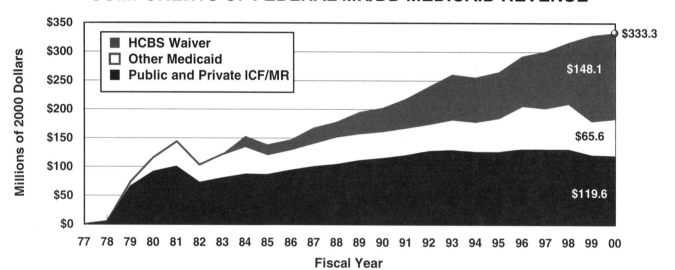

Millions of 2000 Dollars

- ■ HCBS Waiver
- □ Other Medicaid
- ■ Public and Private ICF/MR

$333.3

$148.1

$65.6

$119.6

Fiscal Year

HCBS WAIVER PARTICIPANTS

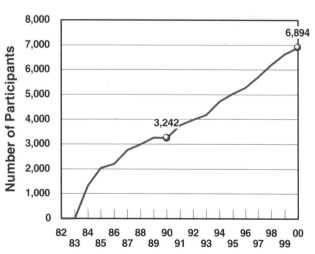

Number of Participants

6,894

3,242

WAIVER SPENDING PER PARTICIPANT

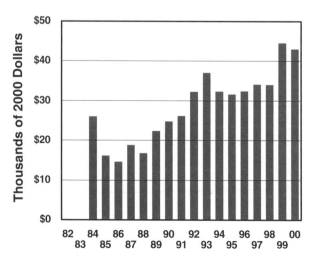

Thousands of 2000 Dollars

Source: The Coleman Institute and Department of Psychiatry, University of Colorado, 2002.

TRENDS IN RESIDENTIAL SERVICES

PERSONS SERVED BY SETTING IN 2000

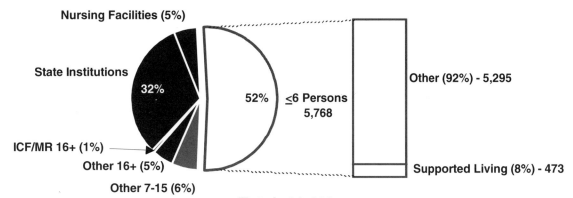

Nursing Facilities (5%)

State Institutions

32%

ICF/MR 16+ (1%)

Other 16+ (5%)

Other 7-15 (6%)

52%   ≤6 Persons
5,768

Other (92%) - 5,295

Supported Living (8%) - 473

Total: 11,199

PERSONS SERVED BY SETTING

	1990	1991	1992	1993	1994	1995	1996	1997	1998	1999	2000
TOTAL	9,328	9,722	10,395	10,723	10,918	11,049	11,216	11,257	11,502	10,951	11,199
16+ PERSONS	6,103	6,009	6,504	6,421	6,343	6,259	6,039	5,798	5,538	4,705	4,757
Nursing Facilities*	na	na	746	771	796	821	847	872	898	468	593
State Institutions	5,110	4,988	4,737	4,643	4,520	4,402	4,338	4,267	4,025	3,636	3,556
Private ICF/MR	72	72	72	72	72	72	73	73	73	73	73
Other Residential	921	949	949	935	955	964	781	586	542	528	535
7-15 PERSONS	0	0	533	533	533	533	533	685	742	688	674
Public ICF/MR	0	0	0	0	0	0	0	0	0	0	0
Private ICF/MR	0	0	0	0	0	0	0	0	0	0	0
Other Residential	0	0	533	533	533	533	533	685	742	688	674
≤6 PERSONS	3,225	3,713	3,358	3,769	4,042	4,257	4,644	4,774	5,222	5,558	5,768
Public ICF/MR	0	0	0	0	0	0	0	0	0	0	0
Private ICF/MR	0	0	0	0	0	0	0	0	0	0	0
Other Residential	3,225	3,713	3,358	3,769	4,042	4,257	4,644	4,774	5,222	5,558	5,768

*The numbers of nursing facility residents with mental retardation and related conditions receiving services from the NJ Division of Developmental Disabilities during 1996-98 were 571, 617, and 553, respectively.

PERSONS SERVED IN PUBLIC AND PRIVATE INSTITUTIONS AND NURSING FACILITIES

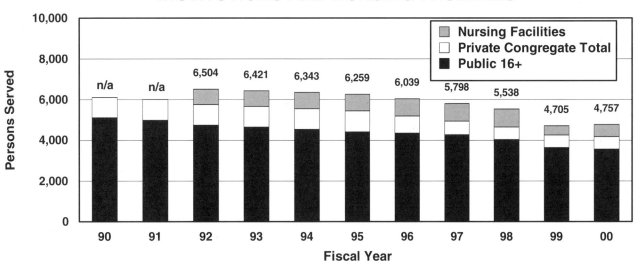

Persons Served

- Nursing Facilities
- Private Congregate Total
- Public 16+

n/a n/a 6,504 6,421 6,343 6,259 6,039 5,798 5,538 4,705 4,757

Fiscal Year

Source: The Coleman Institute and Department of Psychiatry, University of Colorado, 2002.

INDIVIDUAL AND FAMILY SUPPORT

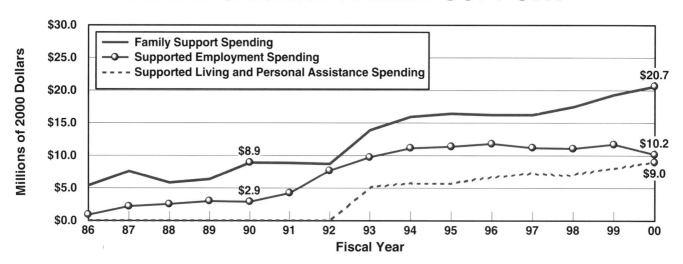

PARTICIPANTS AND SPENDING LEVELS

	1990	1991	1992	1993	1994	1995	1996	1997	1998	1999	2000
TOTAL IFS ($)	9,116,038	10,538,249	13,438,249	24,012,043	28,067,784	29,556,865	31,315,540	32,009,760	33,557,469	37,653,637	39,837,057
INDIVIDUAL SUPPORT ($)	2,235,000	3,400,000	6,300,000	12,409,043	14,412,784	15,061,865	16,612,540	17,003,100	17,070,693	19,035,576	19,172,115
Supported Employment ($)	2,235,000	3,400,000	6,300,000	8,156,432	9,561,436	10,053,184	10,669,455	10,344,852	10,458,107	11,274,902	10,185,335
# of Persons	566	632	823	1,164	1,128	1,635	1,783	1,506	1,660	1,565	1,623
Supported Living ($)	0	0	0	4,252,611	4,851,348	5,008,681	5,943,085	6,658,248	6,612,586	7,760,674	8,986,780
# of Persons	0	0	252	291	335	335	382	431	439	460	473
Personal Assistance ($)	0	0	0	0	0	0	0	0	0	0	0
# of Persons	0	0	0	0	0	0	0	0	0	0	0
FAMILY SUPPORT ($)	6,881,038	7,138,249	7,138,249	11,603,000	13,655,000	14,495,000	14,703,000	15,006,660	16,486,776	18,618,061	20,664,942
Total Families	n/a	n/a	1,739	2,009	2,670	3,460	3,897	4,393	4,491	4,851	4,590
Cash Subsidy/Payment ($)	na	na	na	na	na	na	na	2,624,456	2,082,947	3,322,376	3,361,930
# of Families	n/a	n/a	n/a	n/a	n/a	n/a	n/a	693	1,609	2,278	1,852
Other Family Support ($)	6,881,038	7,138,249	7,138,249	11,603,000	13,655,000	14,495,000	14,703,000	12,382,204	14,403,829	15,295,685	17,303,012
# of Families	n/a	n/a	1,739	2,009	2,670	3,460	3,897	4,393	4,491	4,851	4,590

PARTICIPANTS IN DAY/WORK AND SUPPORTED EMPLOYMENT

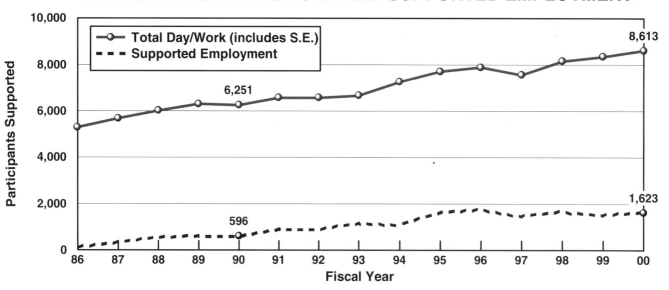

Source: The Coleman Institute and Department of Psychiatry, University of Colorado, 2002.

TRENDS IN SPENDING

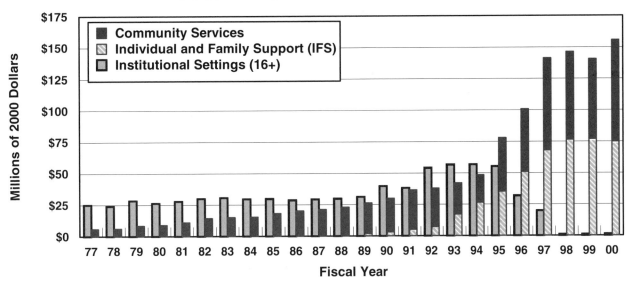

FISCAL EFFORT

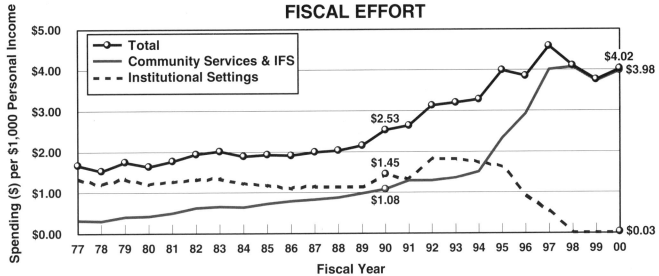

TOTAL MR/DD SPENDING AND
UNMATCHED STATE/LOCAL FUNDS

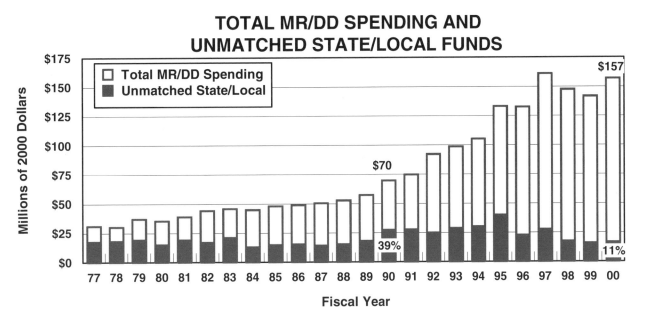

Source: The Coleman Institute and Department of Psychiatry, University of Colorado, 2002.

TRENDS IN REVENUE

COMMUNITY SERVICES REVENUE IN 2000

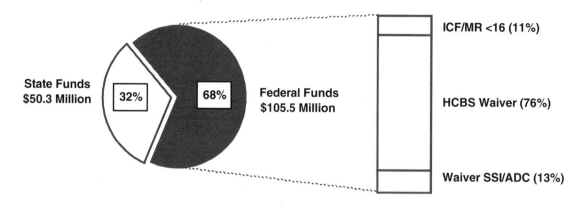

State Funds
$50.3 Million
32%

68%
Federal Funds
$105.5 Million

ICF/MR <16 (11%)

HCBS Waiver (76%)

Waiver SSI/ADC (13%)

Total: $155.8 Million

COMPONENTS OF FEDERAL MR/DD MEDICAID REVENUE

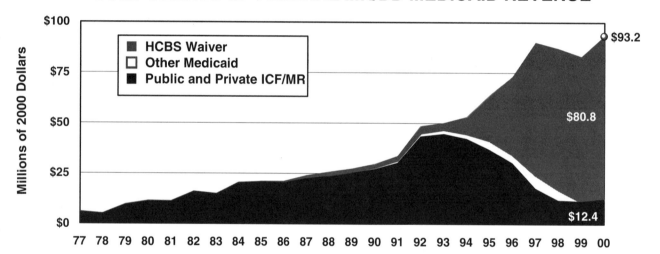

- ■ HCBS Waiver
- □ Other Medicaid
- ■ Public and Private ICF/MR

$93.2
$80.8
$12.4

Millions of 2000 Dollars

Fiscal Year

HCBS WAIVER PARTICIPANTS

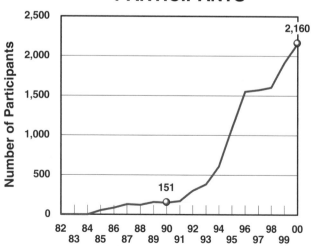

2,160
151

Number of Participants

WAIVER SPENDING PER PARTICIPANT

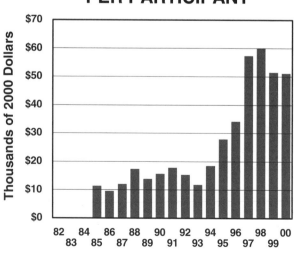

Thousands of 2000 Dollars

Source: The Coleman Institute and Department of Psychiatry, University of Colorado, 2002.

TRENDS IN RESIDENTIAL SERVICES
PERSONS SERVED BY SETTING IN 2000

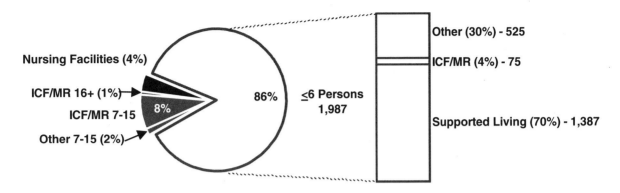

Nursing Facilities (4%)
ICF/MR 16+ (1%)
ICF/MR 7-15
Other 7-15 (2%)
8%
86%
≤6 Persons 1,987

Other (30%) - 525
ICF/MR (4%) - 75
Supported Living (70%) - 1,387

Total: 2,314

PERSONS SERVED BY SETTING

	1990	1991	1992	1993	1994	1995	1996	1997	1998	1999	2000
TOTAL	1,384	1,465	1,479	1,872	1,911	1,927	1,912	2,062	1,956	2,236	2,314
16+ PERSONS	618	617	735	741	674	574	435	316	178	110	110
Nursing Facilities	125	128	188	178	165	151	148	153	153	94	94
State Institutions	493	489	484	474	403	314	177	94	9	0	0
Private ICF/MR	0	0	63	89	106	109	110	69	16	16	16
Other Residential	0	0	0	0	0	0	0	0	0	0	0
7-15 PERSONS	766	848	198	189	187	167	208	219	236	245	217
Public ICF/MR	0	0	0	0	0	0	0	0	0	0	0
Private ICF/MR	282	339	178	189	187	167	181	188	206	214	182
Other Residential	484	509	20	0	0	0	27	31	30	31	35
≤6 PERSONS	0	0	546	942	1,050	1,186	1,269	1,527	1,542	1,881	1,987
Public ICF/MR	0	0	0	0	0	0	0	0	0	0	0
Private ICF/MR	0	0	13	13	13	33	49	49	49	52	75
Other Residential	0	0	533	929	1,037	1,153	1,220	1,478	1,493	1,829	1,912

PERSONS SERVED IN PUBLIC AND PRIVATE INSTITUTIONS AND NURSING FACILITIES

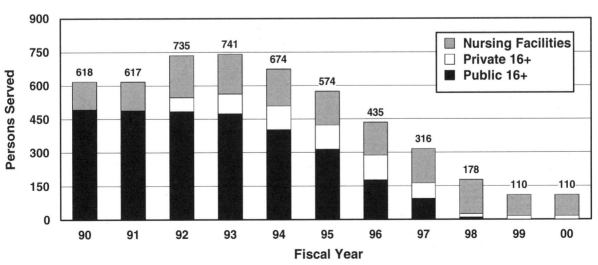

Source: The Coleman Institute and Department of Psychiatry, University of Colorado, 2002.

INDIVIDUAL AND FAMILY SUPPORT

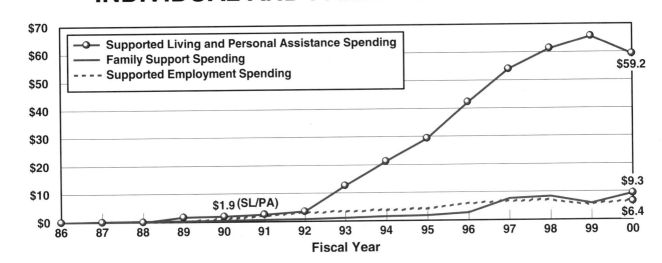

PARTICIPANTS AND SPENDING LEVELS

	1990	1991	1992	1993	1994	1995	1996	1997	1998	1999	2000
TOTAL IFS ($)	2,343,653	4,043,107	5,887,541	14,304,491	22,721,441	31,138,391	45,989,312	62,877,036	71,976,232	74,101,667	74,873,463
INDIVIDUAL SUPPORT ($)	2,011,055	3,528,769	5,270,366	13,355,953	21,441,539	29,527,126	43,586,443	55,792,001	64,096,679	68,500,879	65,545,796
Supported Employment ($)	557,334	1,546,096	2,413,636	2,827,183	3,240,730	3,654,277	5,360,443	5,898,344	6,314,294	5,317,608	6,363,632
# of Persons	131	320	436	627	818	1,009	639	787	677	1,002	1,122
Supported Living ($)	1,453,721	1,982,673	2,856,730	10,528,770	18,200,809	25,872,849	38,226,000	49,893,657	57,782,385	63,183,271	59,182,164
# of Persons	270	316	370	734	809	892	960	1,057	1,072	1,384	1,387
Personal Assistance ($)	0	0	0	0	0	0	0	0	0	0	0
# of Persons	0	0	0	0	0	0	0	0	0	0	0
FAMILY SUPPORT ($)	332,598	514,338	617,175	948,538	1,279,902	1,611,265	2,402,869	7,085,035	7,879,553	5,600,788	9,327,667
Total Families	321	508	610	937	1,265	1,592	1,027	1,309	1,351	1,311	1,737
Cash Subsidy/Payment ($)	0	0	0	0	0	0	0	0	0	0	0
# of Families	0	0	0	0	0	0	0	0	0	0	0
Other Family Support ($)	332,598	514,338	617,175	948,538	1,279,902	1,611,265	2,402,869	7,085,035	7,879,553	5,600,788	9,327,667
# of Families	321	508	610	937	1,265	1,592	1,027	1,309	1,351	1,311	1,737

PARTICIPANTS IN DAY/WORK AND SUPPORTED EMPLOYMENT

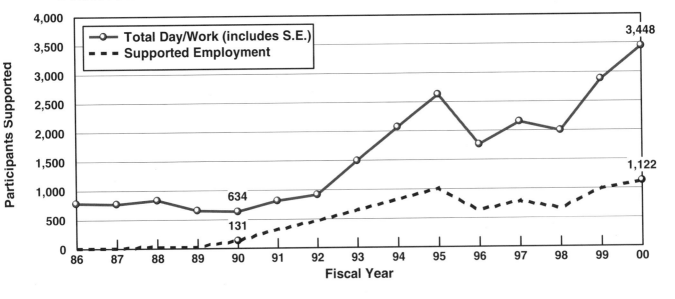

Source: The Coleman Institute and Department of Psychiatry, University of Colorado, 2002.

TRENDS IN SPENDING

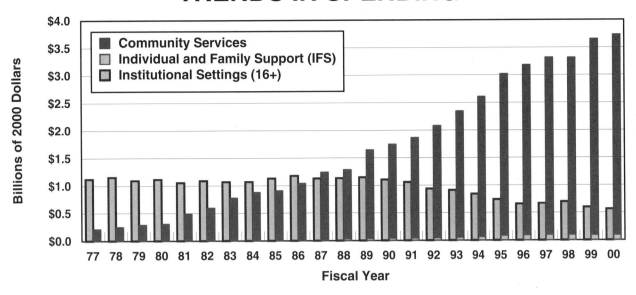

FISCAL EFFORT

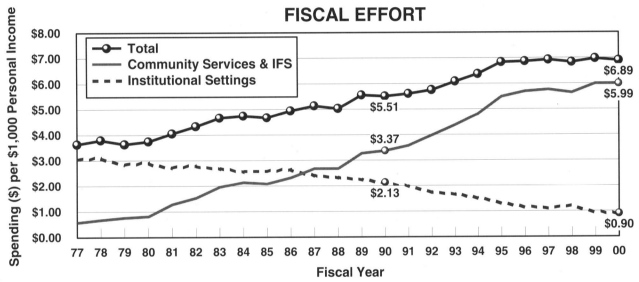

TOTAL MR/DD SPENDING AND
UNMATCHED STATE/LOCAL FUNDS

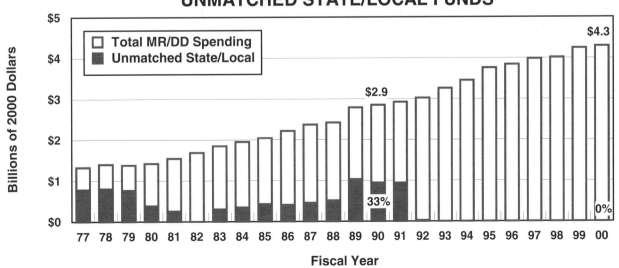

Source: The Coleman Institute and Department of Psychiatry, University of Colorado, 2002.

271

TRENDS IN REVENUE

COMMUNITY SERVICES REVENUE IN 2000

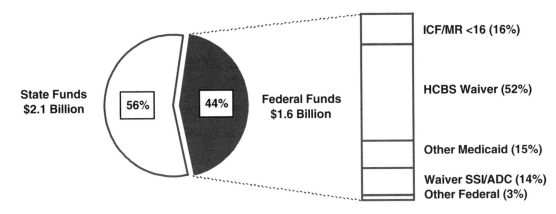

State Funds $2.1 Billion 56% 44% **Federal Funds $1.6 Billion**

ICF/MR <16 (16%)

HCBS Waiver (52%)

Other Medicaid (15%)

Waiver SSI/ADC (14%)
Other Federal (3%)

Total: $3.7 Billion

COMPONENTS OF FEDERAL MR/DD MEDICAID REVENUE

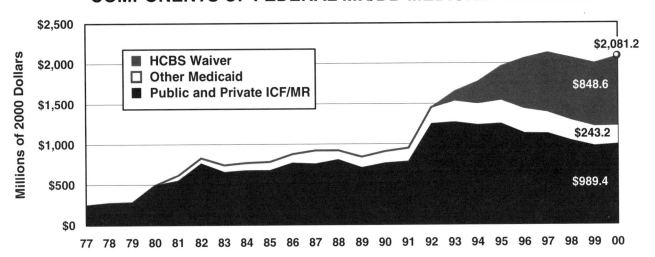

Millions of 2000 Dollars

- ■ HCBS Waiver
- □ Other Medicaid
- ■ Public and Private ICF/MR

$2,081.2

$848.6

$243.2

$989.4

Fiscal Year

HCBS WAIVER PARTICIPANTS

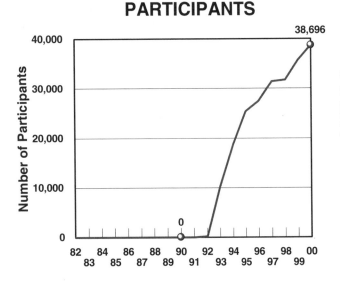

Number of Participants

38,696

0

WAIVER SPENDING PER PARTICIPANT

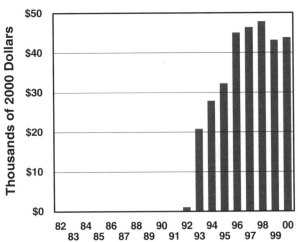

Thousands of 2000 Dollars

Source: The Coleman Institute and Department of Psychiatry, University of Colorado, 2002.

TRENDS IN RESIDENTIAL SERVICES

PERSONS SERVED BY SETTING IN 2000

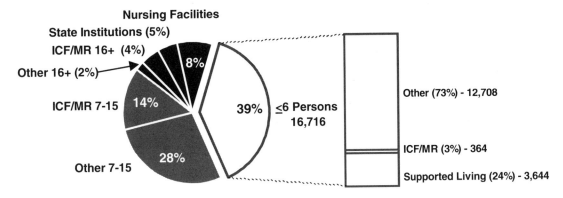

Total: 43,224

PERSONS SERVED BY SETTING

	1990	1991	1992	1993	1994	1995	1996	1997	1998	1999	2000
TOTAL	29,632	30,499	35,725	36,434	37,886	38,583	39,937	42,185	42,182	42,643	43,224
16+ PERSONS	13,718	13,250	12,670	11,980	11,158	10,152	9,311	9,065	8,694	8,682	8,340
Nursing Facilities	2,763	2,823	2,882	2,941	3,000	3,055	3,055	3,505	3,497	3,497	3,497
State Institutions	8,519	7,964	7,257	6,439	5,536	4,455	3,589	2,973	2,613	2,331	2,009
Private ICF/MR	1,782	1,814	1,886	1,598	1,620	1,640	1,665	1,651	1,643	1,944	1,923
Other Residential	654	649	645	1,002	1,002	1,002	1,002	936	941	910	911
7-15 PERSONS	13,299	14,240	15,137	15,041	16,077	16,616	17,180	17,708	17,813	17,990	18,168
Public ICF/MR	2,630	2,838	3,011	3,118	3,227	3,277	102	101	79	77	76
Private ICF/MR	4,953	5,447	5,797	5,676	6,057	6,237	6,410	6,459	6,387	6,046	6,047
Other Residential	5,716	5,955	6,329	6,247	6,793	7,102	10,668	11,148	11,347	11,867	12,045
≤6 PERSONS	2,615	3,009	7,918	9,413	10,651	11,815	13,446	15,412	15,675	15,971	16,716
Public ICF/MR	130	140	140	137	142	142	49	45	45	45	45
Private ICF/MR	555	561	575	545	557	557	557	532	538	323	319
Other Residential	1,930	2,308	7,203	8,731	9,952	11,116	12,840	14,835	15,092	15,603	16,352

PERSONS SERVED IN PUBLIC AND PRIVATE INSTITUTIONS AND NURSING FACILITIES

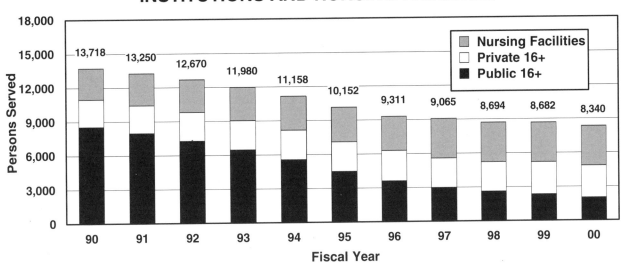

Source: The Coleman Institute and Department of Psychiatry, University of Colorado, 2002.

INDIVIDUAL AND FAMILY SUPPORT

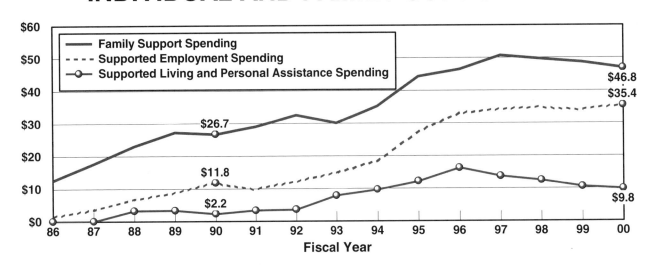

Millions of 2000 Dollars

- Family Support Spending
- Supported Employment Spending
- Supported Living and Personal Assistance Spending

$26.7

$11.8

$2.2

$46.8

$35.4

$9.8

Fiscal Year

PARTICIPANTS AND SPENDING LEVELS

	1990	1991	1992	1993	1994	1995	1996	1997	1998	1999	2000
TOTAL IFS ($)	31,352,000	33,708,000	39,226,800	44,161,000	54,347,000	74,138,000	86,445,000	90,960,720	91,421,060	89,756,740	92,057,014
INDIVIDUAL SUPPORT ($)	10,809,000	10,466,000	12,595,000	18,979,000	24,057,000	34,962,000	44,388,000	44,115,720	44,576,060	42,911,740	45,212,014
Supported Employment ($)	9,088,000	7,852,000	9,725,000	12,479,000	15,826,000	24,230,000	29,705,000	31,468,000	32,882,000	32,882,000	35,442,000
# of Persons	4,519	4,718	4,917	5,802	6,326	7,947	9,882	8,727	8,955	9,762	10,420
Supported Living ($)	0	832,000	1,231,000	1,200,000	1,951,000	4,502,000	8,453,000	5,681,000	5,313,000	6,935,000	6,594,740
# of Persons	0	130	140	270	315	912	1,336	1,314	1,263	1,235	1,463
Personal Assistance ($)	1,721,000	1,782,000	1,639,000	5,300,000	6,280,000	6,230,000	6,230,000	6,966,720	6,381,060	3,094,740	3,175,274
# of Persons	1,746	1,826	1,922	1,842	2,180	2,165	2,165	2,462	2,333	2,180	2,181
FAMILY SUPPORT ($)	20,543,000	23,242,000	26,631,800	25,182,000	30,290,000	39,176,000	42,057,000	46,845,000	46,845,000	46,845,000	46,845,000
Total Families	33,000	35,000	35,000	29,686	33,780	40,722	46,708	49,753	50,226	57,945	63,343
Cash Subsidy/Payment ($)	0	317,200	700,000	0	0	0	0	0	0	0	0
# of Families	0	100	500	0	0	0	0	0	0	0	0
Other Family Support ($)	20,543,000	22,924,800	25,931,800	25,182,000	30,290,000	39,176,000	42,057,000	46,845,000	46,845,000	46,845,000	46,845,000
# of Families	33,000	34,900	34,500	29,686	33,780	40,722	46,708	49,753	50,226	57,945	63,343

PARTICIPANTS IN DAY/WORK AND SUPPORTED EMPLOYMENT

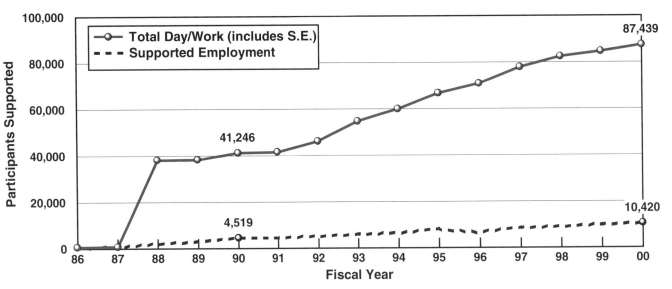

Participants Supported

- Total Day/Work (includes S.E.)
- Supported Employment

87,439

41,246

4,519

10,420

Fiscal Year

Source: The Coleman Institute and Department of Psychiatry, University of Colorado, 2002.

TRENDS IN SPENDING

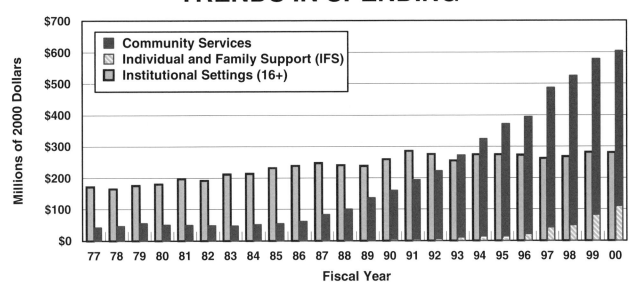

Millions of 2000 Dollars

- Community Services
- Individual and Family Support (IFS)
- Institutional Settings (16+)

Fiscal Year

FISCAL EFFORT

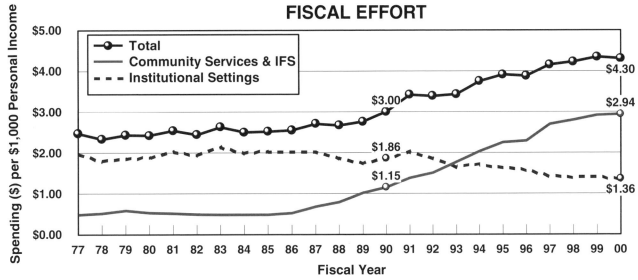

Spending ($) per $1,000 Personal Income

- Total
- Community Services & IFS
- Institutional Settings

$4.30
$3.00
$2.94
$1.86
$1.15
$1.36

Fiscal Year

TOTAL MR/DD SPENDING AND
UNMATCHED STATE/LOCAL FUNDS

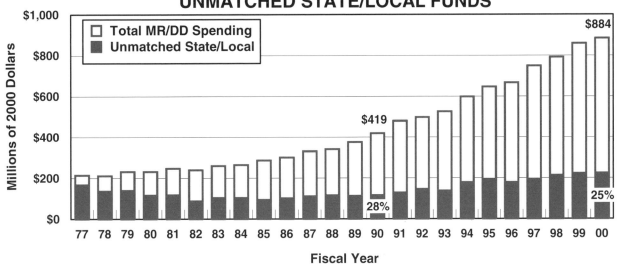

Millions of 2000 Dollars

- Total MR/DD Spending
- Unmatched State/Local

$884
$419
28%
25%

Fiscal Year

Source: The Coleman Institute and Department of Psychiatry, University of Colorado, 2002.

TRENDS IN REVENUE

COMMUNITY SERVICES REVENUE IN 2000

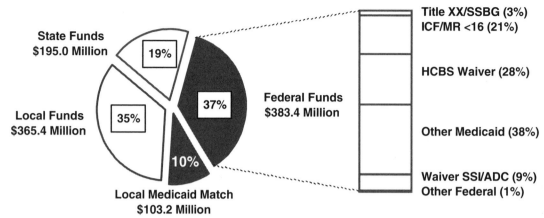

Total: $1,047.0 Million

COMPONENTS OF FEDERAL MR/DD MEDICAID REVENUE

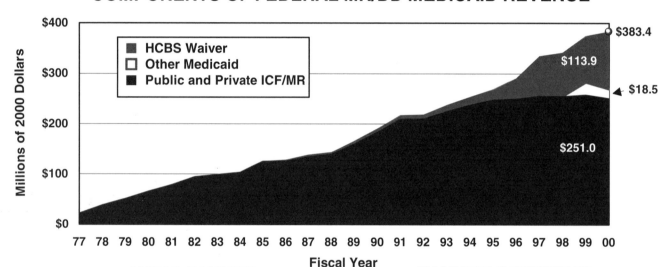

HCBS WAIVER PARTICIPANTS

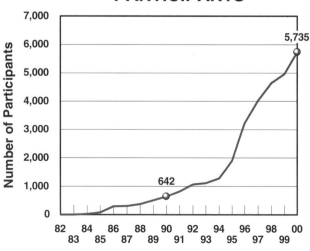

WAIVER SPENDING PER PARTICIPANT

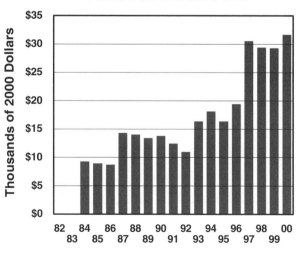

Source: The Coleman Institute and Department of Psychiatry, University of Colorado, 2002.

TRENDS IN RESIDENTIAL SERVICES

PERSONS SERVED BY SETTING IN 2000

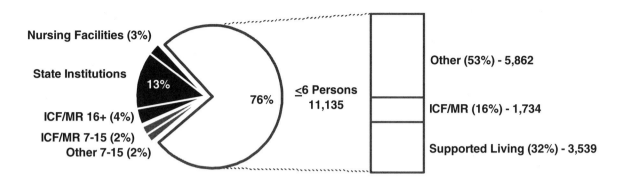

Total: 14,668

PERSONS SERVED BY SETTING

	1990	1991	1992	1993	1994	1995	1996	1997	1998	1999	2000
TOTAL	5,962	6,420	6,517	6,828	7,444	7,575	7,594	8,946	9,542	14,678	14,668
16+ PERSONS	3,514	3,421	3,342	3,335	3,417	3,283	3,180	3,069	3,027	2,996	2,937
Nursing Facilities	316	316	316	315	453	419	385	360	396	391	397
State Institutions	2,669	2,581	2,502	2,454	2,398	2,298	2,229	2,143	2,065	1,996	1,933
Private ICF/MR	445	445	445	539	539	539	539	539	539	539	539
Other Residential	84	79	79	27	27	27	27	27	27	70	68
7-15 PERSONS	267	267	276	333	333	333	334	573	556	562	596
Public ICF/MR	0	0	0	0	0	0	0	0	0	0	0
Private ICF/MR	217	217	226	283	283	283	284	286	289	306	311
Other Residential	50	50	50	50	50	50	50	287	267	256	285
≤6 PERSONS	2,181	2,732	2,899	3,160	3,694	3,959	4,080	5,304	5,959	11,120	11,135
Public ICF/MR	98	125	137	138	140	142	143	115	77	0	0
Private ICF/MR	729	1,055	1,174	1,256	1,374	1,523	1,523	1,605	1,627	1,752	1,734
Other Residential	1,354	1,552	1,588	1,766	2,180	2,294	2,414	3,584	4,255	9,368	9,401

PERSONS SERVED IN PUBLIC AND PRIVATE INSTITUTIONS AND NURSING FACILITIES

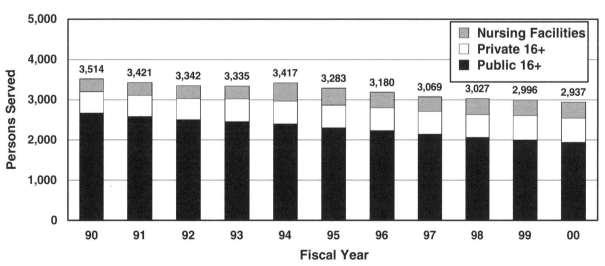

Source: The Coleman Institute and Department of Psychiatry, University of Colorado, 2002.

INDIVIDUAL AND FAMILY SUPPORT

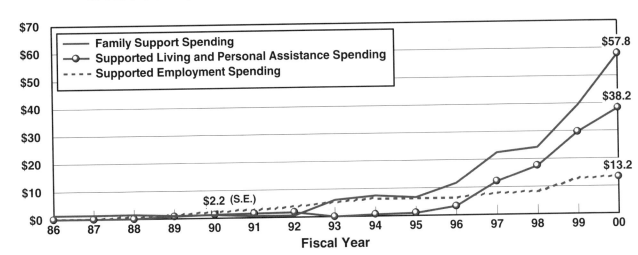

Family Support Spending
Supported Living and Personal Assistance Spending
Supported Employment Spending

PARTICIPANTS AND SPENDING LEVELS

TOTAL IFS ($)	3,544,755	3,691,260	5,031,526	9,480,097	12,189,574	11,979,133	19,034,659	39,107,667	46,999,593	78,650,307	109,213,792
INDIVIDUAL SUPPORT ($)	2,672,875	3,225,794	4,552,200	4,404,128	5,856,110	6,191,959	8,564,251	18,287,684	24,112,150	40,808,159	51,381,481
Supported Employment ($)	1,681,966	2,001,600	3,089,400	4,404,128	5,290,110	5,338,625	5,658,056	7,145,633	7,576,677	12,237,249	13,218,570
# of Persons	523	900	950	1,098	931	1,179	1,238	1,320	1,400	1,955	2,148
Supported Living ($)	0	0	0	0	566,000	853,334	2,906,195	3,972,986	7,528,120	13,480,988	14,582,583
# of Persons	0	0	0	0	65	85	205	356	844	532	594
Personal Assistance ($)	990,909	1,224,194	1,462,800	0	0	0	0	7,169,065	9,007,353	15,089,922	23,580,328
# of Persons	212	270	318	0	0	0	0	1,000	1,146	2,932	2,945
FAMILY SUPPORT ($)	871,880	465,466	479,326	5,075,969	6,333,464	5,787,174	10,470,408	20,819,983	22,887,443	37,842,148	57,832,311
Total Families	1,799	1,933	2,039	1,817	2,393	2,221	2,522	2,772	3,752	3,752	4,248
Cash Subsidy/Payment ($)	0	0	0	0	67,500	90,000	320,000	623,127	793,127	313,733	351,069
# of Families	0	0	0	0	150	200	400	650	1,000	926	1,001
Other Family Support ($)	871,880	465,466	479,326	5,075,969	6,265,964	5,697,174	10,150,408	20,196,856	22,094,316	37,528,415	57,481,242
# of Families	1,799	1,933	2,039	1,817	2,243	2,021	2,122	4,844	6,484	2,826	3,247

PARTICIPANTS IN DAY/WORK AND SUPPORTED EMPLOYMENT

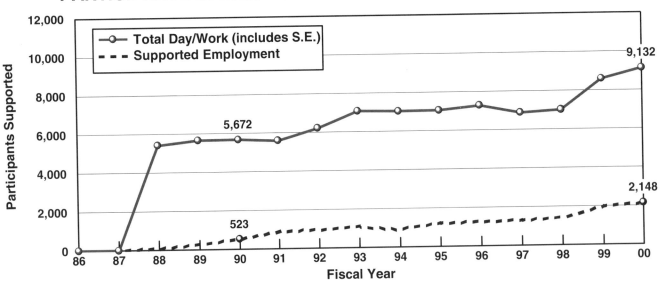

Total Day/Work (includes S.E.)
Supported Employment

Source: The Coleman Institute and Department of Psychiatry, University of Colorado, 2002.

TRENDS IN SPENDING

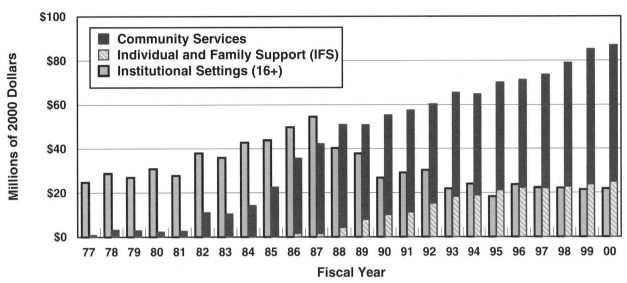

Community Services
Individual and Family Support (IFS)
Institutional Settings (16+)

FISCAL EFFORT

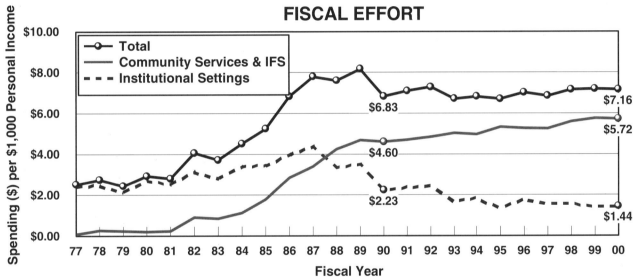

Total
Community Services & IFS
Institutional Settings

$6.83
$7.16
$5.72
$4.60
$2.23
$1.44

TOTAL MR/DD SPENDING AND
UNMATCHED STATE/LOCAL FUNDS

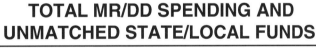
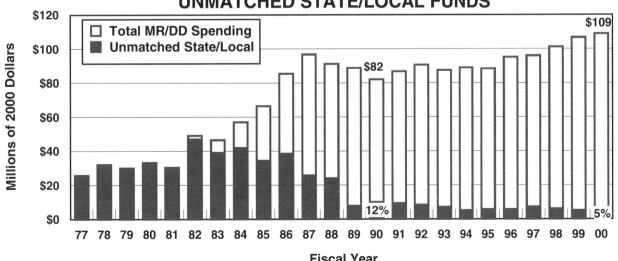

Total MR/DD Spending
Unmatched State/Local

$109
$82
12%
5%

Source: The Coleman Institute and Department of Psychiatry, University of Colorado, 2002.

TRENDS IN REVENUE

COMMUNITY SERVICES REVENUE IN 2000

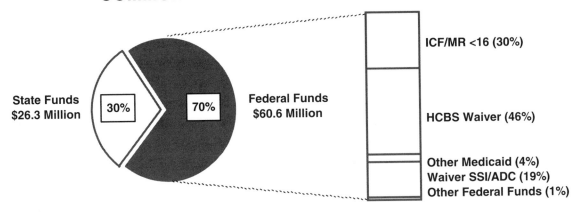

State Funds
$26.3 Million

30%

70%

Federal Funds
$60.6 Million

ICF/MR <16 (30%)

HCBS Waiver (46%)

Other Medicaid (4%)
Waiver SSI/ADC (19%)
Other Federal Funds (1%)

Total: $87.0 Million

COMPONENTS OF FEDERAL MR/DD MEDICAID REVENUE

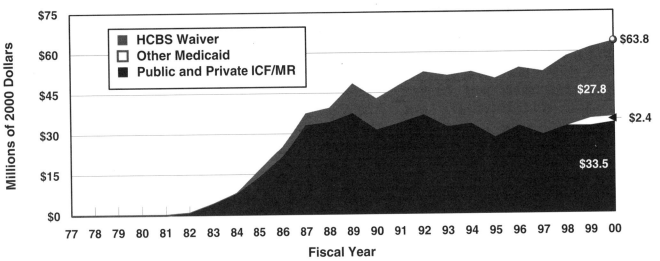

Millions of 2000 Dollars

- ■ HCBS Waiver
- □ Other Medicaid
- ■ Public and Private ICF/MR

$75
$60
$45
$30
$15
$0

$63.8
$27.8
$2.4
$33.5

77 78 79 80 81 82 83 84 85 86 87 88 89 90 91 92 93 94 95 96 97 98 99 00

Fiscal Year

HCBS WAIVER PARTICIPANTS

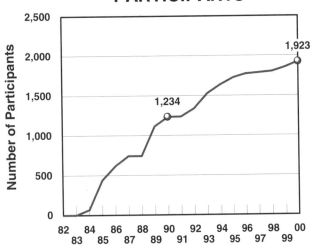

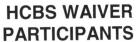

Number of Participants

2,500
2,000
1,500
1,000
500
0

1,923

1,234

82 83 84 85 86 87 88 89 90 91 92 93 94 95 96 97 98 99 00

WAIVER SPENDING PER PARTICIPANT

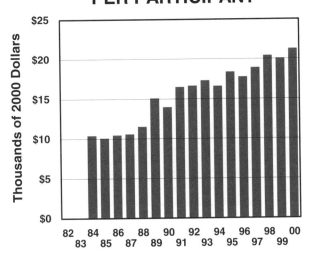

Thousands of 2000 Dollars

$25
$20
$15
$10
$5
$0

82 83 84 85 86 87 88 89 90 91 92 93 94 95 96 97 98 99 00

Source: The Coleman Institute and Department of Psychiatry, University of Colorado, 2002.

TRENDS IN RESIDENTIAL SERVICES

PERSONS SERVED BY SETTING IN 2000

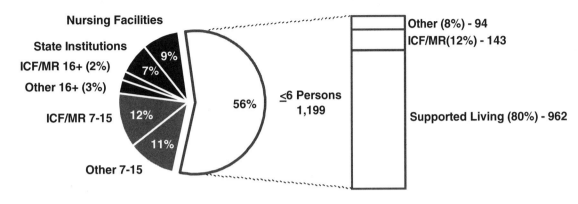

Nursing Facilities
State Institutions
ICF/MR 16+ (2%)
Other 16+ (3%)
ICF/MR 7-15
Other 7-15

9%
7%
12%
11%
56%

≤6 Persons
1,199

Other (8%) - 94
ICF/MR(12%) - 143
Supported Living (80%) - 962

Total: 2,150

PERSONS SERVED BY SETTING

	1990	1991	1992	1993	1994	1995	1996	1997	1998	1999	2000
TOTAL	1,942	1,944	2,040	2,007	2,000	1,999	2,091	2,106	2,167	2,172	2,150
16+ PERSONS	489	458	424	395	368	361	421	464	464	441	445
Nursing Facilities	192	186	175	169	169	159	191	212	220	190	184
State Institutions	251	226	203	180	153	140	148	150	142	142	152
Private ICF/MR	0	0	0	0	0	0	20	40	40	44	44
Other Residential	46	46	46	46	46	62	62	62	62	65	65
7-15 PERSONS	1,453	1,486	431	635	673	631	647	600	607	506	506
Public ICF/MR	0	0	0	0	0	0	0	0	0	0	0
Private ICF/MR	420	410	240	358	405	384	414	359	366	267	267
Other Residential	1,033	1,076	191	277	268	247	233	241	241	239	239
≤6 PERSONS	0	0	1,185	977	959	1,007	1,023	1,042	1,096	1,225	1,199
Public ICF/MR	0	0	0	0	0	0	0	0	0	0	0
Private ICF/MR	0	0	156	65	69	78	80	45	51	143	143
Other Residential	0	0	1,029	912	890	929	943	997	1,045	1,082	1,056

PERSONS SERVED IN PUBLIC AND PRIVATE INSTITUTIONS AND NURSING FACILITIES

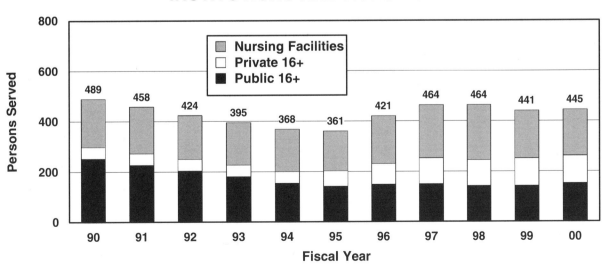

INDIVIDUAL AND FAMILY SUPPORT

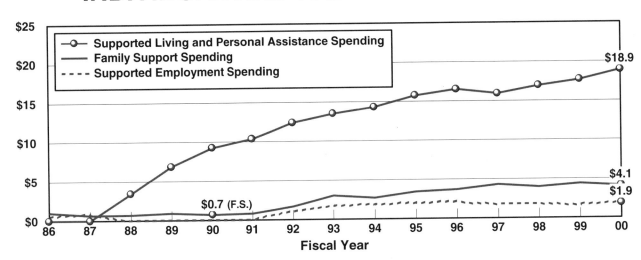

PARTICIPANTS AND SPENDING LEVELS

	1990	1991	1992	1993	1994	1995	1996	1997	1998	1999	2000
TOTAL IFS ($)	7,665,713	8,972,971	12,422,495	15,201,099	16,106,287	18,696,793	20,127,052	20,443,094	21,411,256	22,926,376	24,877,181
INDIVIDUAL SUPPORT ($)	7,119,604	8,295,270	11,033,541	12,671,397	13,777,974	15,643,232	16,773,452	16,463,059	17,657,073	18,707,387	20,782,480
Supported Employment ($)	0	0	908,963	1,374,246	1,508,300	1,727,020	1,837,829	1,723,006	1,671,361	1,673,906	1,863,883
# of Persons	0	0	127	254	260	264	268	330	321	331	326
Supported Living ($)	7,119,604	8,295,270	10,124,578	11,046,463	11,875,810	13,388,946	14,320,199	14,138,238	15,351,224	16,390,695	18,263,136
# of Persons	654	726	800	837	822	856	868	881	903	893	897
Personal Assistance ($)	0	0	0	250,688	393,864	527,266	615,424	601,815	634,488	642,786	655,461
# of Persons	0	0	0	21	33	45	52	65	65	65	65
FAMILY SUPPORT ($)	546,109	677,701	1,388,954	2,529,702	2,328,313	3,053,561	3,353,600	3,980,035	3,754,183	4,218,989	4,094,701
Total Families	360	475	732	538	503	594	517	538	543	844	895
Cash Subsidy/Payment ($)	109,173	319,646	378,563	505,130	237,490	400,880	395,561	616,416	527,457	686,974	589,417
# of Families	106	197	226	118	63	105	98	106	115	387	387
Other Family Support ($)	436,936	358,055	1,010,391	2,024,572	2,090,823	2,652,681	2,958,039	3,363,619	3,226,726	3,532,015	3,505,284
# of Families	254	278	506	420	440	489	419	432	428	457	508

PARTICIPANTS IN DAY/WORK AND SUPPORTED EMPLOYMENT

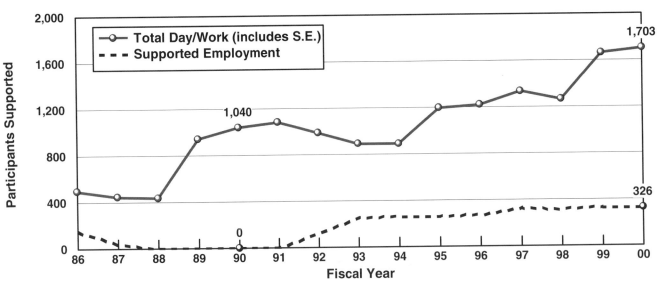

Source: The Coleman Institute and Department of Psychiatry, University of Colorado, 2002.

TRENDS IN SPENDING

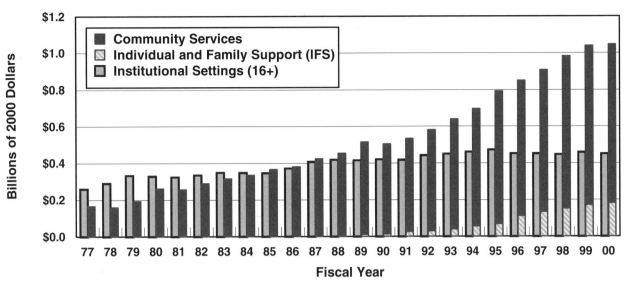

Legend:
- ■ Community Services
- ▨ Individual and Family Support (IFS)
- ▧ Institutional Settings (16+)

Y-axis: Billions of 2000 Dollars

X-axis: Fiscal Year (77–00)

FISCAL EFFORT

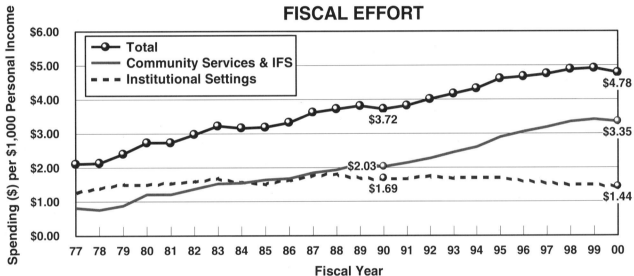

Legend:
- —○— Total
- —— Community Services & IFS
- – – – Institutional Settings

Y-axis: Spending ($) per $1,000 Personal Income

X-axis: Fiscal Year (77–00)

Data labels: $3.72, $2.03, $1.69, $4.78, $3.35, $1.44

TOTAL MR/DD SPENDING AND UNMATCHED STATE/LOCAL FUNDS

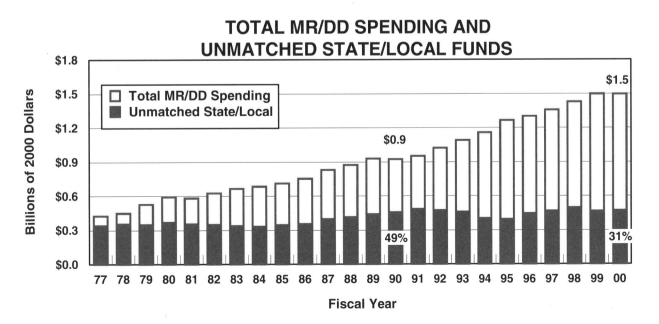

Legend:
- ☐ Total MR/DD Spending
- ■ Unmatched State/Local

Y-axis: Billions of 2000 Dollars

X-axis: Fiscal Year (77–00)

Data labels: $0.9, 49%, $1.5, 31%

Source: The Coleman Institute and Department of Psychiatry, University of Colorado, 2002.

TRENDS IN REVENUE

COMMUNITY SERVICES REVENUE IN 2000

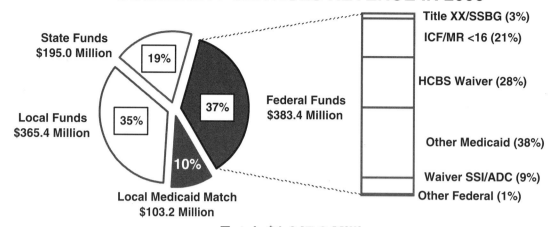

State Funds
$195.0 Million

19%

Local Funds
$365.4 Million

35%

37%

Federal Funds
$383.4 Million

10%

Local Medicaid Match
$103.2 Million

Title XX/SSBG (3%)
ICF/MR <16 (21%)
HCBS Waiver (28%)
Other Medicaid (38%)
Waiver SSI/ADC (9%)
Other Federal (1%)

Total: $1,047.0 Million

COMPONENTS OF FEDERAL MR/DD MEDICAID REVENUE

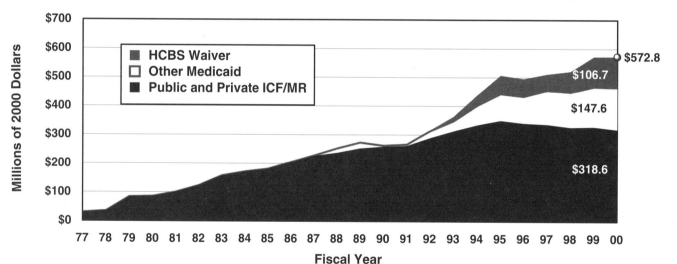

Millions of 2000 Dollars

$700
$600
$500
$400
$300
$200
$100
$0

- ■ HCBS Waiver
- □ Other Medicaid
- ■ Public and Private ICF/MR

$572.8
$106.7
$147.6
$318.6

77 78 79 80 81 82 83 84 85 86 87 88 89 90 91 92 93 94 95 96 97 98 99 00

Fiscal Year

HCBS WAIVER PARTICIPANTS

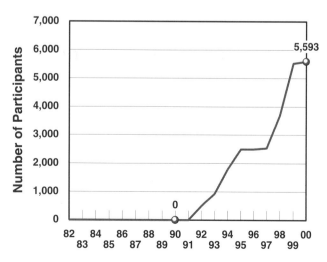

Number of Participants

7,000
6,000
5,000
4,000
3,000
2,000
1,000
0

5,593

0

82 83 84 85 86 87 88 89 90 91 92 93 94 95 96 97 98 99 00

WAIVER SPENDING PER PARTICIPANT

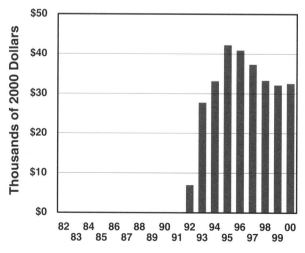

Thousands of 2000 Dollars

$50
$40
$30
$20
$10
$0

82 83 84 85 86 87 88 89 90 91 92 93 94 95 96 97 98 99 00

Source: The Coleman Institute and Department of Psychiatry, University of Colorado, 2002.

TRENDS IN RESIDENTIAL SERVICES

PERSONS SERVED BY SETTING IN 2000

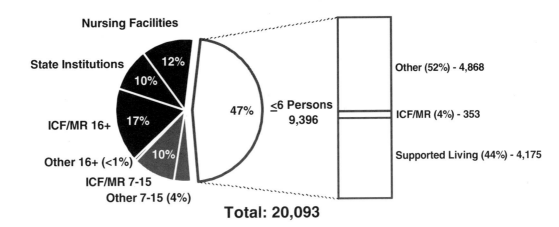

Total: 20,093

PERSONS SERVED BY SETTING

	1990	1991	1992	1993	1994	1995	1996	1997	1998	1999	2000
TOTAL	16,899	16,854	17,046	16,940	16,822	16,420	17,662	19,144	19,518	19,368	20,093
16+ PERSONS	11,087	10,544	9,890	9,291	8,645	8,231	7,946	7,884	8,075	7,975	7,925
Nursing Facilities	3,828	3,439	3,000	2,684	2,402	2,288	2,173	2,231	2,430	2,430	2,430
State Institutions	2,656	2,540	2,434	2,261	2,184	2,131	2,087	2,039	2,019	2,004	1,990
Private ICF/MR	4,024	4,090	4,160	4,101	3,851	3,633	3,498	3,386	3,421	3,400	3,374
Other Residential	579	475	296	245	208	179	188	228	205	141	131
7-15 PERSONS	2,879	2,962	3,113	3,188	3,068	3,027	3,099	3,110	3,011	2,892	2,772
Public ICF/MR	0	0	0	0	0	0	0	0	0	0	0
Private ICF/MR	1,325	1,432	1,619	1,769	1,811	1,848	1,978	1,949	1,996	1,975	1,974
Other Residential	1,554	1,530	1,494	1,419	1,257	1,179	1,121	1,161	1,015	917	798
≤6 PERSONS	2,933	3,348	4,043	4,461	5,109	5,162	6,617	8,150	8,432	8,501	9,396
Public ICF/MR	0	0	0	0	0	0	0	0	0	0	0
Private ICF/MR	86	102	120	133	149	166	193	239	283	285	353
Other Residential	2,847	3,246	3,923	4,328	4,960	4,996	6,424	7,911	8,149	8,216	9,043

PERSONS SERVED IN PUBLIC AND PRIVATE INSTITUTIONS AND NURSING FACILITIES

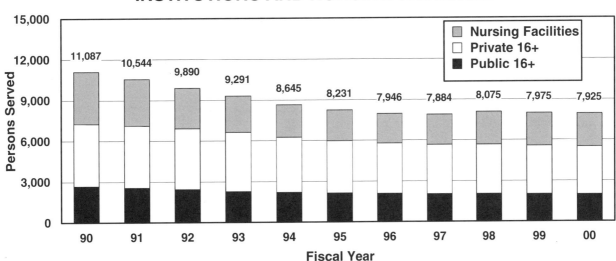

Source: The Coleman Institute and Department of Psychiatry, University of Colorado, 2002.

INDIVIDUAL AND FAMILY SUPPORT

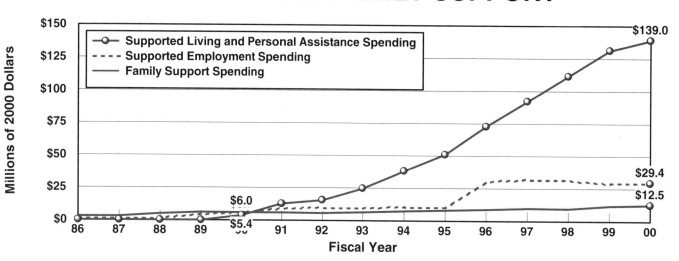

PARTICIPANTS AND SPENDING LEVELS

	1990	1991	1992	1993	1994	1995	1996	1997	1998	1999	2000
TOTAL IFS ($)	11,686,675	21,746,659	24,963,265	33,915,211	47,731,827	61,150,367	100,991,816	122,995,993	143,790,727	165,854,065	181,032,454
INDIVIDUAL SUPPORT ($)	7,048,515	16,969,354	20,185,960	28,588,131	41,385,097	54,016,266	93,030,394	113,921,782	134,602,404	154,440,458	168,488,487
Supported Employment ($)	4,183,200	6,740,400	7,473,600	7,944,261	8,660,071	8,953,216	27,287,410	28,956,509	29,515,500	28,036,169	29,443,769
# of Persons	3,486	5,617	6,228	6,368	6,221	6,305	7,069	7,886	8,193	8,119	8,538
Supported Living ($)	2,865,315	10,228,954	12,712,360	20,643,871	32,725,027	45,063,050	65,742,984	84,965,273	105,086,904	126,404,289	139,044,718
# of Persons	260	698	1,099	1,168	1,749	2,667	3,056	4,143	4,292	4,313	4,175
Personal Assistance ($)	0	0	0	0	0	0	0	0	0	0	0
# of Persons	0	0	0	0	0	0	0	0	0	0	0
FAMILY SUPPORT ($)	4,638,160	4,777,305	4,777,305	5,327,080	6,346,730	7,134,101	7,961,422	9,074,211	9,188,323	11,413,607	12,543,967
Total Families	5,349	6,908	7,258	7,363	8,572	10,289	11,507	11,135	9,883	11,762	12,110
Cash Subsidy/Payment ($)	0	0	0	0	0	0	0	0	0	0	0
# of Families	0	0	0	0	0	0	0	0	0	0	0
Other Family Support ($)	4,638,160	4,777,305	4,777,305	5,327,080	6,346,730	7,134,101	7,961,422	9,074,211	9,188,323	11,413,607	12,543,967
# of Families	5,349	6,908	7,258	7,363	8,572	10,289	11,507	11,135	9,883	11,762	12,110

PARTICIPANTS IN DAY/WORK AND SUPPORTED EMPLOYMENT

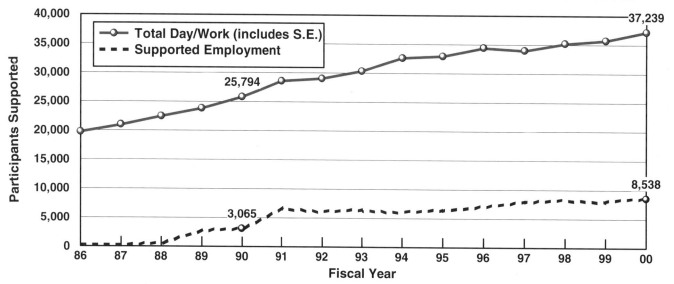

Source: The Coleman Institute and Department of Psychiatry, University of Colorado, 2002.

TRENDS IN SPENDING

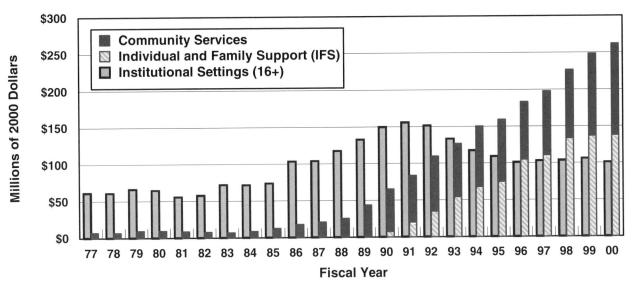

FISCAL EFFORT

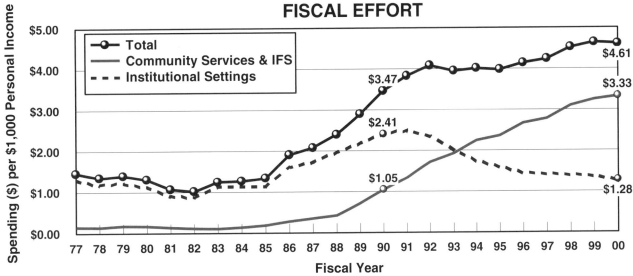

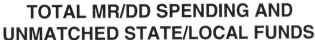

TOTAL MR/DD SPENDING AND
UNMATCHED STATE/LOCAL FUNDS

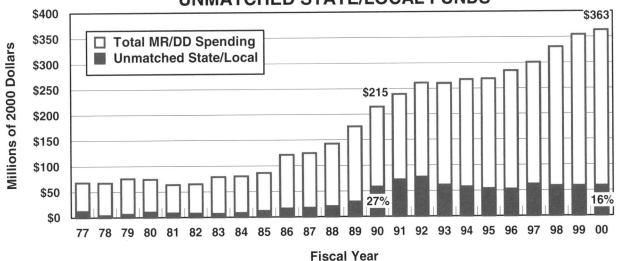

Source: The Coleman Institute and Department of Psychiatry, University of Colorado, 2002.

287

TRENDS IN REVENUE

COMMUNITY SERVICES REVENUE IN 2000

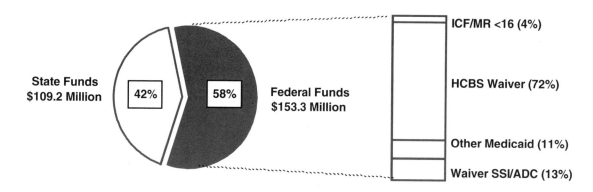

State Funds
$109.2 Million

42%   58%

Federal Funds
$153.3 Million

ICF/MR <16 (4%)

HCBS Waiver (72%)

Other Medicaid (11%)

Waiver SSI/ADC (13%)

Total: $262.5 Million

COMPONENTS OF FEDERAL MR/DD MEDICAID REVENUE

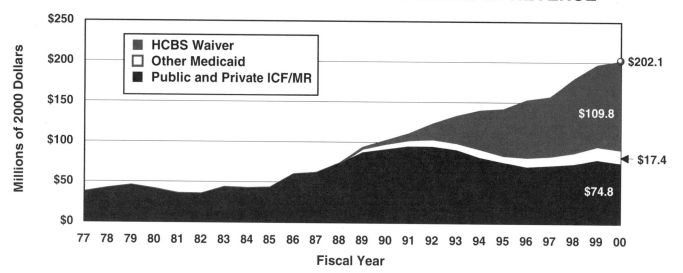

Millions of 2000 Dollars

- ■ HCBS Waiver
- □ Other Medicaid
- ■ Public and Private ICF/MR

$202.1
$109.8
$17.4
$74.8

Fiscal Year

HCBS WAIVER PARTICIPANTS

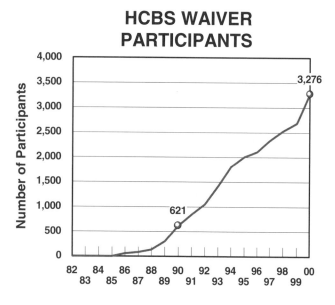

Number of Participants

3,276

621

WAIVER SPENDING PER PARTICIPANT

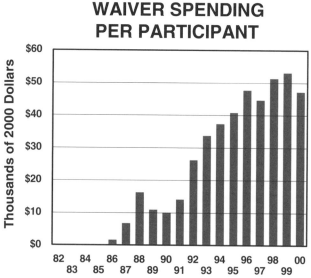

Thousands of 2000 Dollars

Source: The Coleman Institute and Department of Psychiatry, University of Colorado, 2002.

TRENDS IN RESIDENTIAL SERVICES

PERSONS SERVED BY SETTING IN 2000

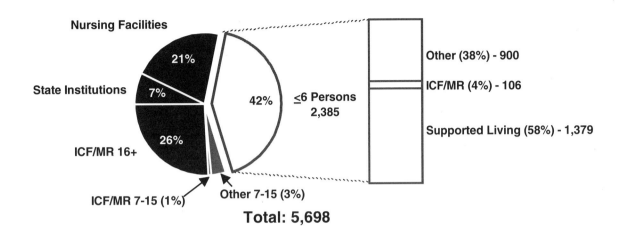

Nursing Facilities 21%

State Institutions 7%

ICF/MR 16+ 26%

ICF/MR 7-15 (1%)

Other 7-15 (3%)

≤6 Persons 2,385 — 42%

Other (38%) - 900

ICF/MR (4%) - 106

Supported Living (58%) - 1,379

Total: 5,698

PERSONS SERVED BY SETTING

	1990	1991	1992	1993	1994	1995	1996	1997	1998	1999	2000
TOTAL	5,804	5,886	5,881	5,568	5,328	5,467	5,172	5,206	5,274	5,596	5,698
16+ PERSONS	4,914	4,753	4,579	4,105	3,758	3,719	3,043	2,906	2,752	3,043	3,082
Nursing Facilities	1,955	1,854	1,767	1,644	1,486	1,391	912	946	902	1,092	1,210
State Institutions	1,010	910	839	765	662	618	548	508	447	422	407
Private ICF/MR	1,949	1,989	1,973	1,696	1,610	1,710	1,583	1,452	1,403	1,529	1,465
Other Residential	0	0	0	0	0	0	0	0	0	0	0
7-15 PERSONS	675	834	395	267	249	237	218	213	213	224	231
Public ICF/MR	0	0	0	0	0	0	0	0	0	0	0
Private ICF/MR	0	0	0	0	0	0	24	23	23	34	41
Other Residential	675	834	395	267	249	237	194	190	190	190	190
≤6 PERSONS	215	299	907	1,196	1,321	1,511	1,911	2,087	2,309	2,329	2,385
Public ICF/MR	0	0	0	0	0	0	0	0	0	0	0
Private ICF/MR	0	0	0	0	0	0	12	23	61	79	106
Other Residential	215	299	907	1,196	1,321	1,511	1,899	2,064	2,248	2,250	2,279

PERSONS SERVED IN PUBLIC AND PRIVATE INSTITUTIONS AND NURSING FACILITIES

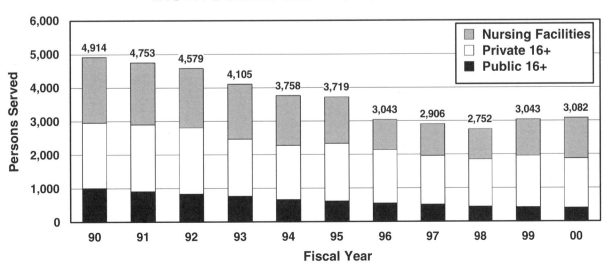

Legend: Nursing Facilities, Private 16+, Public 16+

Persons Served values by Fiscal Year: 4,914 (90), 4,753 (91), 4,579 (92), 4,105 (93), 3,758 (94), 3,719 (95), 3,043 (96), 2,906 (97), 2,752 (98), 3,043 (99), 3,082 (00)

Source: The Coleman Institute and Department of Psychiatry, University of Colorado, 2002.

289

INDIVIDUAL AND FAMILY SUPPORT

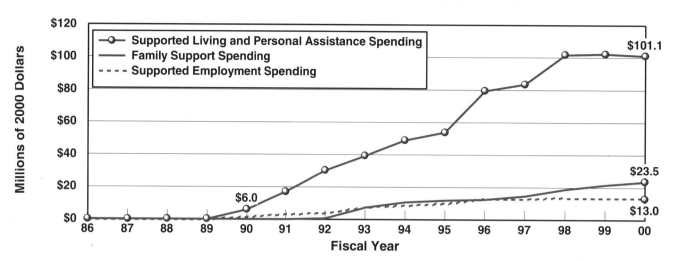

PARTICIPANTS AND SPENDING LEVELS

	1990	1991	1992	1993	1994	1995	1996	1997	1998	1999	2000
TOTAL IFS ($)	5,591,987	15,999,093	28,172,937	45,012,095	58,172,473	66,153,106	94,870,835	102,247,971	125,966,890	131,615,549	137,564,271
INDIVIDUAL SUPPORT ($)	5,541,003	15,919,973	27,668,930	38,828,305	49,093,824	55,756,483	83,572,470	88,754,293	108,244,132	110,954,750	114,047,868
Supported Employment ($)	917,715	2,325,279	2,968,297	5,935,105	7,245,534	8,317,254	11,653,345	11,529,709	12,250,048	12,507,587	12,955,420
# of Persons	125	258	392	651	889	1,577	1,550	1,627	1,579	1,590	1,630
Supported Living ($)	4,535,788	13,493,894	24,573,133	32,763,200	41,718,290	47,309,229	58,448,094	61,951,559	71,117,282	73,397,126	74,673,486
# of Persons	87	220	349	442	583	660	685	700	720	725	734
Personal Assistance ($)	87,500	100,800	127,500	130,000	130,000	130,000	13,471,031	15,273,025	24,876,802	25,050,037	26,418,962
# of Persons	35	40	50	55	55	55	349	477	609	625	645
FAMILY SUPPORT ($)	50,984	79,120	504,007	6,183,790	9,078,649	10,396,623	11,298,365	13,493,678	17,722,758	20,660,799	23,516,403
Total Families	124	155	385	733	1,325	1,428	986	1,450	1,495	1,765	1,990
Cash Subsidy/Payment ($)	0	0	0	0	1,338,650	1,470,500	1,484,300	2,621,000	2,684,350	2,696,700	2,690,100
# of Families	0	0	0	0	479	492	490	868	883	982	997
Other Family Support ($)	50,984	79,120	504,007	6,183,790	7,739,999	8,926,123	9,814,065	10,872,678	15,038,408	17,964,099	20,826,303
# of Families	124	155	385	733	846	936	742	771	766	783	993

PARTICIPANTS IN DAY/WORK AND SUPPORTED EMPLOYMENT

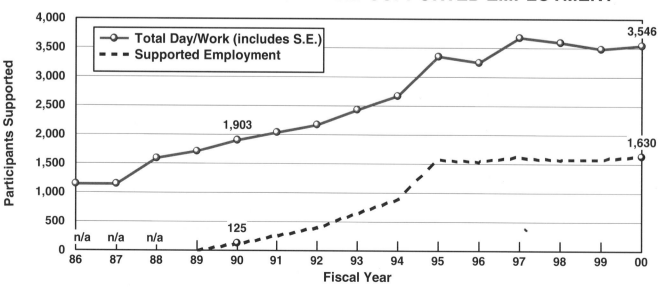

Source: The Coleman Institute and Department of Psychiatry, University of Colorado, 2002.

TRENDS IN SPENDING

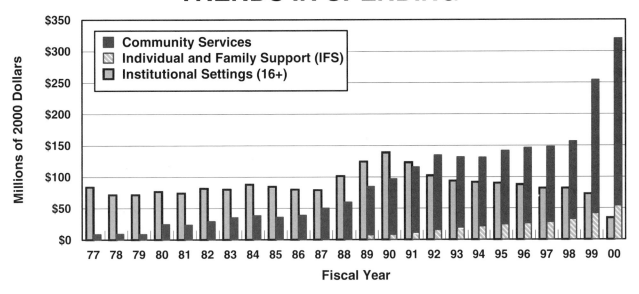

Millions of 2000 Dollars

- ■ Community Services
- ▨ Individual and Family Support (IFS)
- ▧ Institutional Settings (16+)

Fiscal Year

FISCAL EFFORT

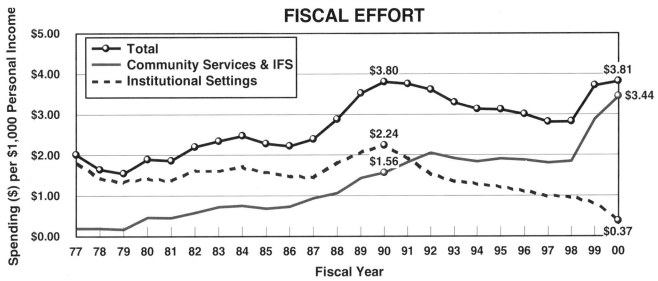

Spending ($) per $1,000 Personal Income

- —○— Total
- —— Community Services & IFS
- - - - Institutional Settings

$3.80 $3.81
$3.44
$2.24
$1.56
$0.37

Fiscal Year

TOTAL MR/DD SPENDING AND
UNMATCHED STATE/LOCAL FUNDS

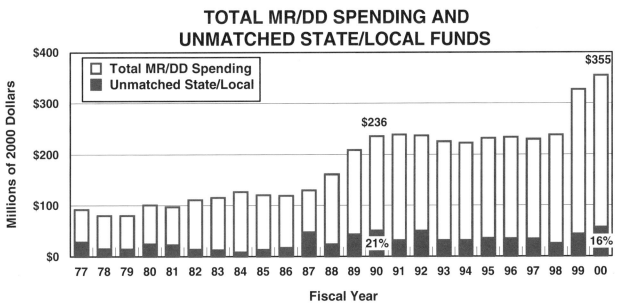

Millions of 2000 Dollars

- ☐ Total MR/DD Spending
- ■ Unmatched State/Local

$355
$236
21%   16%

Fiscal Year

Source: The Coleman Institute and Department of Psychiatry, University of Colorado, 2002.

TRENDS IN REVENUE

COMMUNITY SERVICES REVENUE IN 2000

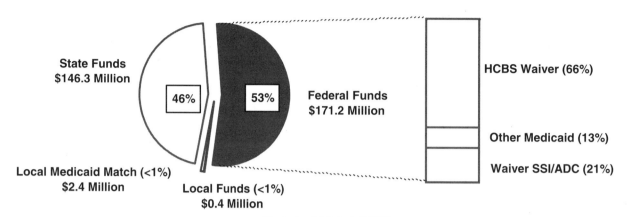

State Funds
$146.3 Million

46%

53%

Federal Funds
$171.2 Million

Local Medicaid Match (<1%)
$2.4 Million

Local Funds (<1%)
$0.4 Million

HCBS Waiver (66%)

Other Medicaid (13%)

Waiver SSI/ADC (21%)

Total: $320.3 Million

COMPONENTS OF FEDERAL MR/DD MEDICAID REVENUE

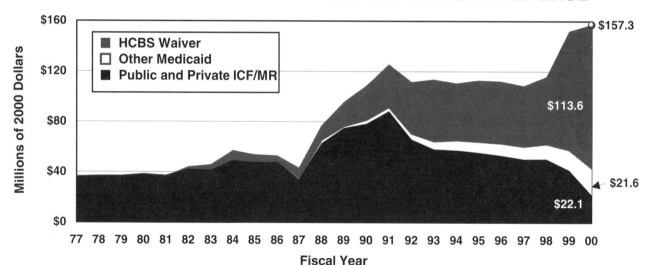

HCBS WAIVER PARTICIPANTS

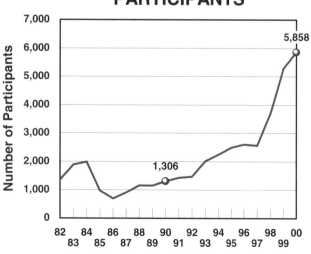

WAIVER SPENDING PER PARTICIPANT

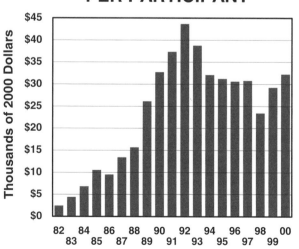

Source: The Coleman Institute and Department of Psychiatry, University of Colorado, 2002.

TRENDS IN RESIDENTIAL SERVICES

PERSONS SERVED BY SETTING IN 2000

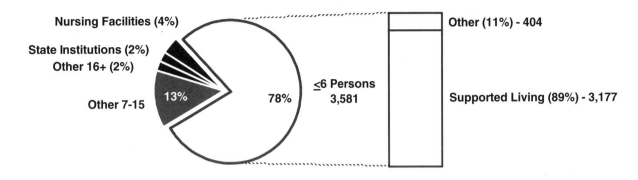

Nursing Facilities (4%)
State Institutions (2%)
Other 16+ (2%)
Other 7-15
13%
78%
≤6 Persons
3,581

Other (11%) - 404
Supported Living (89%) - 3,177

Total: 4,562

PERSONS SERVED BY SETTING

	1990	1991	1992	1993	1994	1995	1996	1997	1998	1999	2000
TOTAL	4,168	4,233	4,332	4,296	4,235	4,239	4,258	3,981	4,200	4,556	4,562
16+ PERSONS	1,556	1,422	1,248	1,135	987	904	836	741	680	575	384
Nursing Facilities	443	435	420	380	340	300	260	240	220	200	180
State Institutions	840	754	603	530	506	463	435	403	361	276	105
Private ICF/MR	140	100	100	100	0	0	0	0	0	0	0
Other Residential	133	133	125	125	141	141	141	98	99	99	99
7-15 PERSONS	697	622	611	600	600	600	600	437	441	597	597
Public ICF/MR	0	0	0	0	0	0	0	0	0	0	0
Private ICF/MR	22	22	11	0	0	0	0	0	0	0	0
Other Residential	675	600	600	600	600	600	600	437	441	597	597
≤6 PERSONS	1,915	2,189	2,473	2,561	2,648	2,735	2,822	2,803	3,079	3,384	3,581
Public ICF/MR	0	0	0	0	0	0	0	0	0	0	0
Private ICF/MR	0	0	0	0	0	0	0	0	0	0	0
Other Residential	1,915	2,189	2,473	2,561	2,648	2,735	2,822	2,803	3,079	3,384	3,581

PERSONS SERVED IN PUBLIC AND PRIVATE INSTITUTIONS AND NURSING FACILITIES

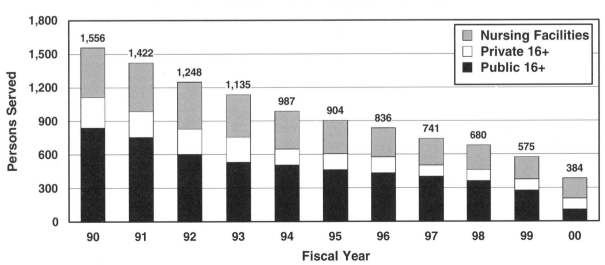

Legend:
■ Nursing Facilities
□ Private 16+
■ Public 16+

Source: The Coleman Institute and Department of Psychiatry, University of Colorado, 2002.

293

INDIVIDUAL AND FAMILY SUPPORT

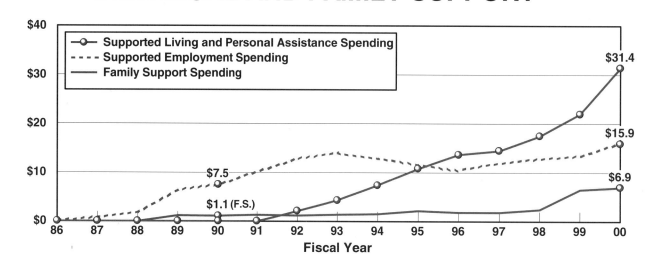

PARTICIPANTS AND SPENDING LEVELS

	1990	1991	1992	1993	1994	1995	1996	1997	1998	1999	2000
TOTAL IFS ($)	6,586,571	9,072,877	12,995,899	16,400,574	18,623,224	21,749,326	23,417,286	26,017,184	30,784,641	40,294,486	54,166,028
INDIVIDUAL SUPPORT ($)	5,762,215	8,031,275	12,054,793	15,282,396	17,361,097	19,876,991	21,790,122	24,386,542	28,542,241	34,057,199	47,263,818
Supported Employment ($)	5,762,215	8,031,275	10,354,739	11,699,734	11,065,507	10,347,010	9,459,968	11,031,137	12,078,731	12,918,516	15,884,054
# of Persons	1,230	1,392	1,617	1,630	1,898	1,699	1,602	1,487	1,509	1,474	1,500
Supported Living ($)	0	0	0	620,972	1,968,373	4,327,825	5,890,156	6,346,312	7,722,594	10,069,327	13,597,250
# of Persons	0	0	0	158	215	273	330	333	346	1,925	2,013
Personal Assistance ($)	0	0	1,700,054	2,961,690	4,327,217	5,202,156	6,439,998	7,009,093	8,740,916	11,069,356	17,782,514
# of Persons	0	0	477	527	577	626	676	672	708	1,039	1,164
FAMILY SUPPORT ($)	824,356	1,041,602	941,106	1,118,178	1,262,127	1,872,335	1,627,164	1,630,642	2,242,400	6,237,287	6,902,210
Total Families	334	435	435	327	279	448	393	1,011	1,034	889	999
Cash Subsidy/Payment ($)	390,085	416,959	466,542	530,220	565,406	390,622	389,507	302,226	265,826	0	0
# of Families	183	183	183	195	159	124	84	85	79	0	0
Other Family Support ($)	434,271	624,643	474,564	587,958	696,721	1,481,713	1,237,657	1,328,416	1,976,574	6,237,287	6,902,210
# of Families	151	252	252	132	120	324	309	926	955	889	999

PARTICIPANTS IN DAY/WORK AND SUPPORTED EMPLOYMENT

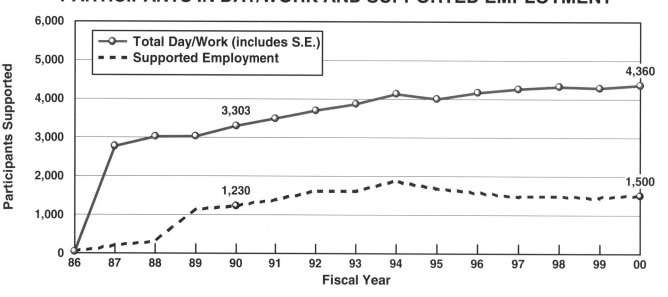

Source: The Coleman Institute and Department of Psychiatry, University of Colorado, 2002.

TRENDS IN SPENDING

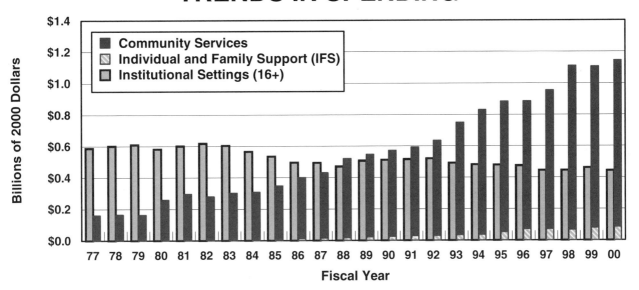

FISCAL EFFORT

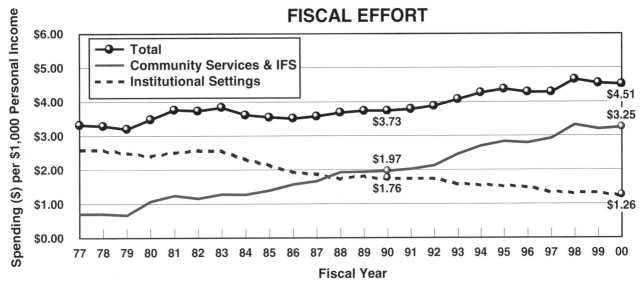

TOTAL MR/DD SPENDING AND
UNMATCHED STATE/LOCAL FUNDS

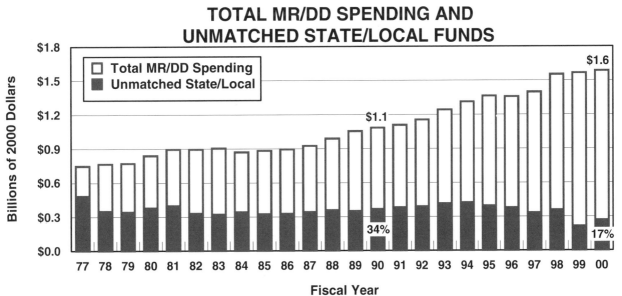

Source: The Coleman Institute and Department of Psychiatry, University of Colorado, 2002.

TRENDS IN REVENUE
COMMUNITY SERVICES REVENUE IN 2000

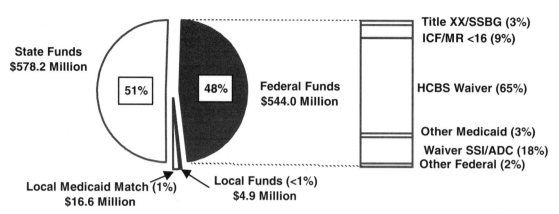

State Funds $578.2 Million — 51%
48% — **Federal Funds $544.0 Million**

Title XX/SSBG (3%)
ICF/MR <16 (9%)
HCBS Waiver (65%)
Other Medicaid (3%)
Waiver SSI/ADC (18%)
Other Federal (2%)

Local Medicaid Match (1%) $16.6 Million
Local Funds (<1%) $4.9 Million

Total: $1.144 Billion

COMPONENTS OF FEDERAL MR/DD MEDICAID REVENUE

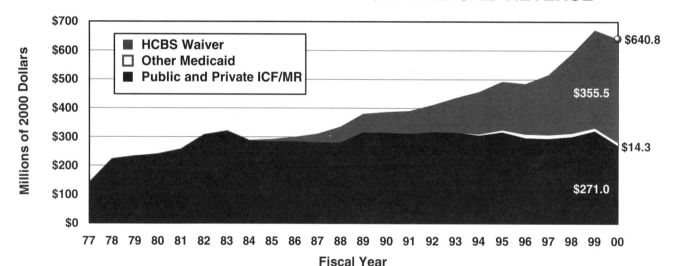

- HCBS Waiver
- Other Medicaid
- Public and Private ICF/MR

$640.8
$355.5
$14.3
$271.0

Millions of 2000 Dollars / **Fiscal Year**

HCBS WAIVER PARTICIPANTS

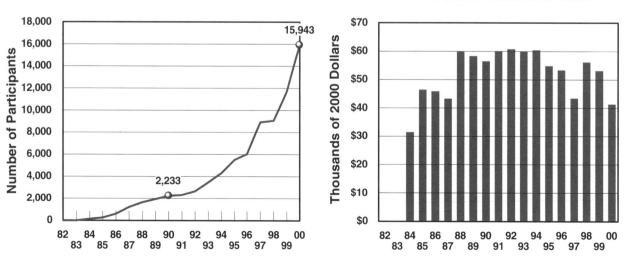

15,943
2,233

Number of Participants

WAIVER SPENDING PER PARTICIPANT

Thousands of 2000 Dollars

Source: The Coleman Institute and Department of Psychiatry, University of Colorado, 2002.

TRENDS IN RESIDENTIAL SERVICES
PERSONS SERVED BY SETTING IN 2000

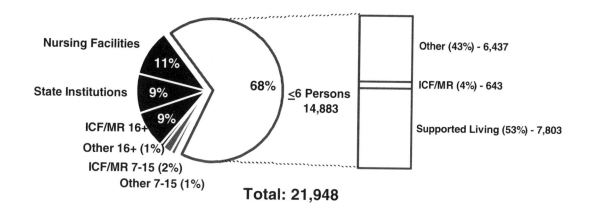

Nursing Facilities
State Institutions
ICF/MR 16+
Other 16+ (1%)
ICF/MR 7-15 (2%)
Other 7-15 (1%)

68%   ≤6 Persons 14,883

Other (43%) - 6,437
ICF/MR (4%) - 643
Supported Living (53%) - 7,803

Total: 21,948

PERSONS SERVED BY SETTING

	1990	1991	1992	1993	1994	1995	1996	1997	1998	1999	2000
TOTAL	15,007	14,976	18,191	16,381	16,667	19,051	19,768	20,314	20,950	20,570	21,948
16+ PERSONS	6,567	6,354	9,513	8,930	8,642	8,000	8,010	7,539	6,928	6,271	6,376
Nursing Facilities	na	na	2,925	2,695	2,465	2,235	2,353	2,359	2,350	2,350	2,350
State Institutions	4,043	3,925	3,807	3,739	3,616	3,460	3,272	2,875	2,533	2,241	1,969
Private ICF/MR	2,041	2,097	2,097	1,879	1,985	1,989	1,949	1,906	1,895	1,527	1,869
Other Residential	483	332	684	617	576	316	436	399	150	153	188
7-15 PERSONS	1,429	1,680	1,423	642	834	1,078	728	759	896	817	689
Public ICF/MR	0	0	0	0	0	0	0	0	0	0	0
Private ICF/MR	1,135	1,143	1,359	570	756	724	661	662	630	383	463
Other Residential	294	537	64	72	78	354	67	97	266	434	226
≤6 PERSONS	7,011	6,942	7,255	6,809	7,191	9,973	11,030	12,016	13,126	13,482	14,883
Public ICF/MR	0	0	0	0	0	0	0	0	0	0	0
Private ICF/MR	0	0	0	648	646	695	695	702	689	942	643
Other Residential	7,011	6,942	7,255	6,161	6,545	9,278	10,335	11,314	12,437	12,540	14,240

PERSONS SERVED IN PUBLIC AND PRIVATE INSTITUTIONS AND NURSING FACILITIES

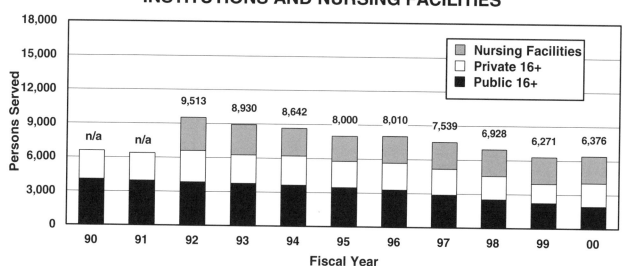

Source: The Coleman Institute and Department of Psychiatry, University of Colorado, 2002.

297

PENNSYLVANIA

INDIVIDUAL AND FAMILY SUPPORT

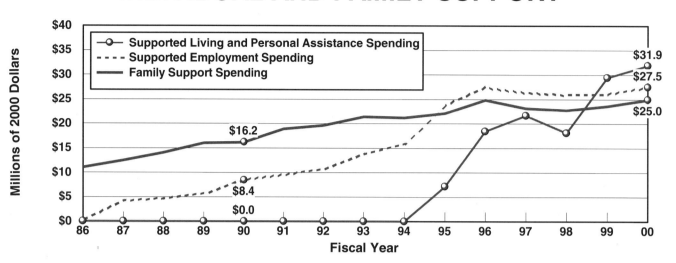

PARTICIPANTS AND SPENDING LEVELS

	1990	1991	1992	1993	1994	1995	1996	1997	1998	1999	2000
TOTAL IFS ($)	18,948,198	22,780,320	24,860,915	29,385,745	31,791,437	46,852,214	63,854,444	65,839,999	63,031,063	76,178,359	84,388,585
INDIVIDUAL SUPPORT ($)	6,492,690	7,634,880	8,787,213	11,504,508	13,606,884	27,344,464	41,383,293	44,434,928	41,517,875	53,422,070	59,431,178
Supported Employment ($)	6,492,690	7,634,880	8,787,213	11,504,508	13,606,884	21,057,032	24,726,962	24,413,821	24,449,531	25,068,475	27,515,147
# of Persons	2,502	2,651	2,841	3,358	3,786	5,135	5,954	3,164	3,930	6,511	6,803
Supported Living ($)	0	0	0	0	0	6,287,432	16,656,331	20,021,107	17,068,344	28,353,595	31,916,031
# of Persons	0	0	0	0	0	589	1,203	1,389	1,460	7,467	7,803
Personal Assistance ($)	0	0	0	0	0	0	0	0	0	0	0
# of Persons	0	0	0	0	0	0	0	0	0	0	0
FAMILY SUPPORT ($)	12,455,508	15,145,440	16,073,702	17,881,237	18,184,553	19,507,750	22,471,151	21,405,071	21,513,188	22,756,289	24,957,407
Total Families	15,328	15,757	16,288	17,664	17,523	18,348	20,657	22,976	18,863	18,949	21,500
Cash Subsidy/Payment ($)	0	0	0	0	0	0	0	0	0	0	0
# of Families	0	0	0	0	0	0	0	0	0	0	0
Other Family Support ($)	12,455,508	15,145,440	16,073,702	17,881,237	18,184,553	19,507,750	22,471,151	21,405,071	21,513,188	22,756,289	24,957,407
# of Families	15,328	15,757	16,288	17,664	17,523	18,348	20,657	22,976	18,863	18,949	21,500

PARTICIPANTS IN DAY/WORK AND SUPPORTED EMPLOYMENT

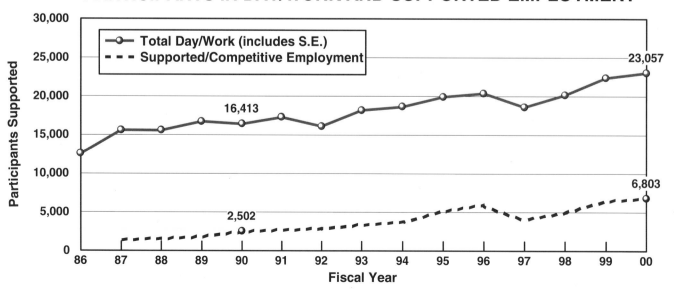

298

Source: The Coleman Institute and Department of Psychiatry, University of Colorado, 2002.

TRENDS IN SPENDING

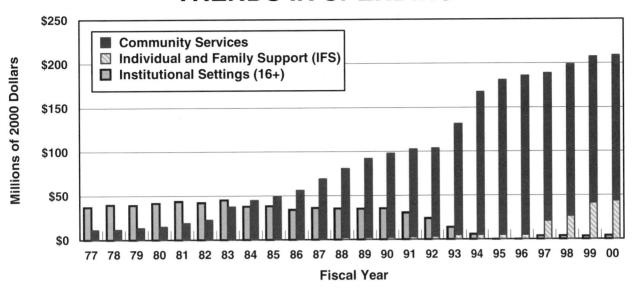

FISCAL EFFORT

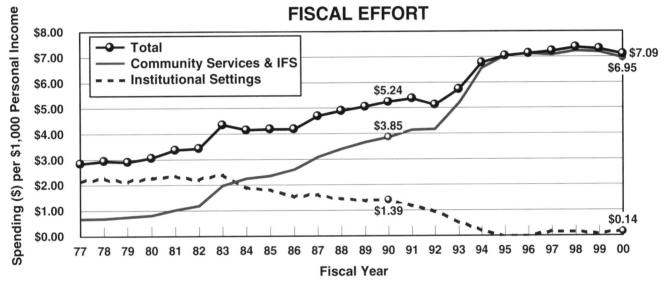

TOTAL MR/DD SPENDING AND
UNMATCHED STATE/LOCAL FUNDS

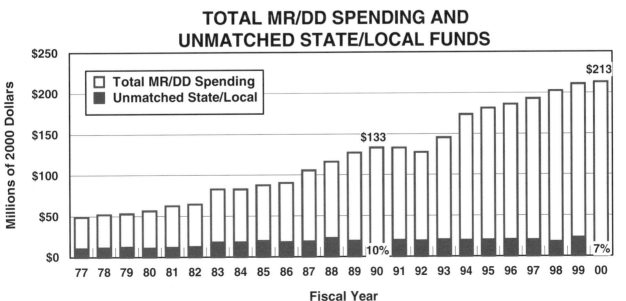

Source: The Coleman Institute and Department of Psychiatry, University of Colorado, 2002.

299

TRENDS IN REVENUE

COMMUNITY SERVICES REVENUE IN 2000

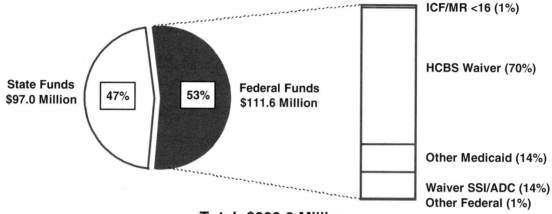

State Funds
$97.0 Million

47%

53%

Federal Funds
$111.6 Million

ICF/MR <16 (1%)

HCBS Waiver (70%)

Other Medicaid (14%)

Waiver SSI/ADC (14%)
Other Federal (1%)

Total: $208.6 Million

COMPONENTS OF FEDERAL MR/DD MEDICAID REVENUE

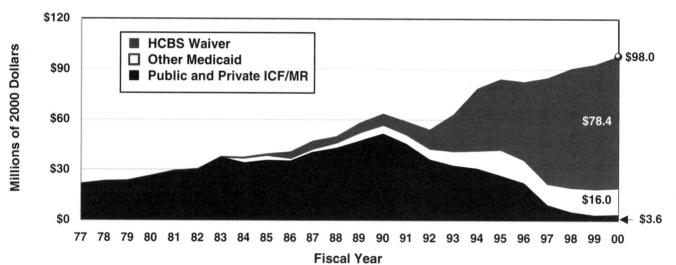

- ■ HCBS Waiver
- □ Other Medicaid
- ■ Public and Private ICF/MR

$98.0

$78.4

$16.0

$3.6

Millions of 2000 Dollars

Fiscal Year

HCBS WAIVER PARTICIPANTS

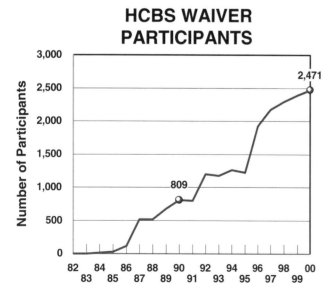

2,471

809

Number of Participants

WAIVER SPENDING PER PARTICIPANT

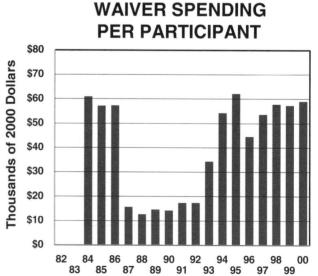

Thousands of 2000 Dollars

Source: The Coleman Institute and Department of Psychiatry, University of Colorado, 2002.

TRENDS IN RESIDENTIAL SERVICES
PERSONS SERVED BY SETTING IN 2000

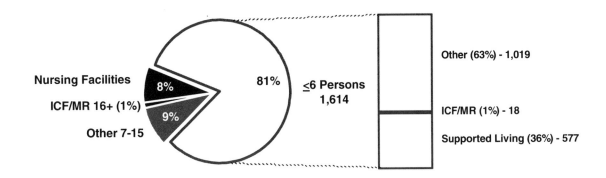

Total: 1,981

PERSONS SERVED BY SETTING

	1990	1991	1992	1993	1994	1995	1996	1997	1998	1999	2000
TOTAL	1,513	1,484	1,483	1,588	1,483	1,536	1,530	1,706	1,807	1,962	1,981
16+ PERSONS	364	313	265	324	236	193	184	206	202	163	187
Nursing Facilities	147	123	100	206	201	193	184	181	177	138	162
State Institutions	217	190	165	118	35	0	0	0	0	0	0
Private ICF/MR	0	0	0	0	0	0	0	25	25	25	25
Other Residential	0	0	0	0	0	0	0	0	0	0	0
7-15 PERSONS	362	345	278	354	315	361	337	314	305	178	180
Public ICF/MR	0	0	0	29	45	43	0	0	0	0	0
Private ICF/MR	144	144	54	75	74	37	32	9	0	0	0
Other Residential	218	201	224	250	196	281	305	305	305	178	180
≤6 PERSONS	787	826	940	910	932	982	1,009	1,186	1,300	1,621	1,614
Public ICF/MR	24	0	14	17	19	19	19	19	19	18	18
Private ICF/MR	450	440	390	265	234	224	193	40	0	0	0
Other Residential	313	386	536	628	679	739	797	1,127	1,281	1,603	1,596

PERSONS SERVED IN PUBLIC AND PRIVATE INSTITUTIONS AND NURSING FACILITIES

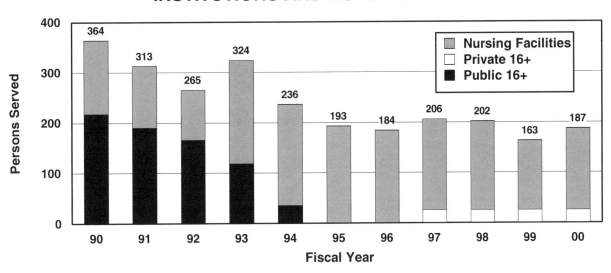

INDIVIDUAL AND FAMILY SUPPORT

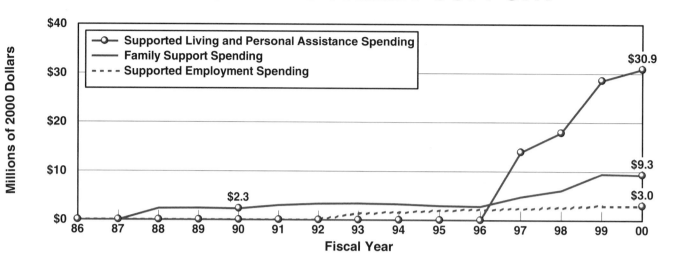

PARTICIPANTS AND SPENDING LEVELS

	1990	1991	1992	1993	1994	1995	1996	1997	1998	1999	2000
TOTAL IFS ($)	1,772,185	2,403,423	2,735,176	3,961,780	4,026,474	4,299,245	4,377,910	19,430,576	24,965,764	39,530,557	43,223,045
INDIVIDUAL SUPPORT ($)	0	0	0	1,110,000	1,261,750	1,692,136	1,857,635	15,039,324	19,232,929	30,430,901	33,918,472
Supported Employment ($)	0	0	0	1,110,000	1,261,750	1,692,136	1,857,635	2,175,770	2,341,038	2,879,886	2,996,597
# of Persons	0	0	0	222	245	319	340	435	458	486	497
Supported Living ($)	0	0	0	0	0	0	0	12,863,554	16,891,891	27,551,015	30,921,875
# of Persons	0	0	0	0	0	0	0	0	335	530	577
Personal Assistance ($)	0	0	0	0	0	0	0	0	0	0	0
# of Persons	0	0	0	0	0	0	0	0	0	0	0
FAMILY SUPPORT ($)	1,772,185	2,403,423	2,735,176	2,851,780	2,764,724	2,607,109	2,520,275	4,391,252	5,732,835	9,099,656	9,304,573
Total Families	0	0	n/a	575	549	499	597	789	796	933	965
Cash Subsidy/Payment ($)	336,185	305,094	273,244	264,821	249,663	230,183	208,441	204,638	196,329	190,068	184,448
# of Families	0	0	n/a	76	71	65	61	64	59	55	54
Other Family Support ($)	1,436,000	2,098,329	2,461,932	2,586,959	2,515,061	2,376,926	2,311,834	4,186,614	5,536,506	8,909,588	9,120,125
# of Families	0	0	n/a	499	478	434	536	725	737	878	911

PARTICIPANTS IN DAY/WORK AND SUPPORTED EMPLOYMENT

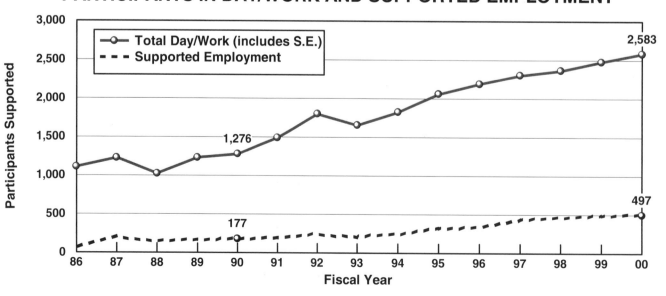

Source: The Coleman Institute and Department of Psychiatry, University of Colorado, 2002.

TRENDS IN SPENDING

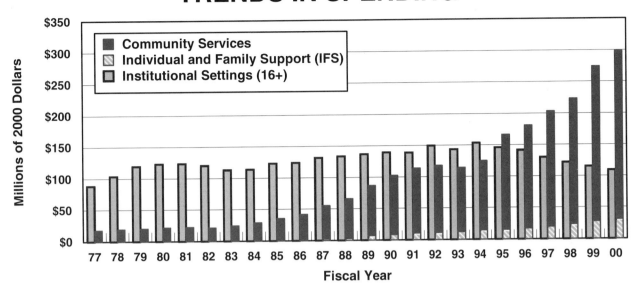

FISCAL EFFORT

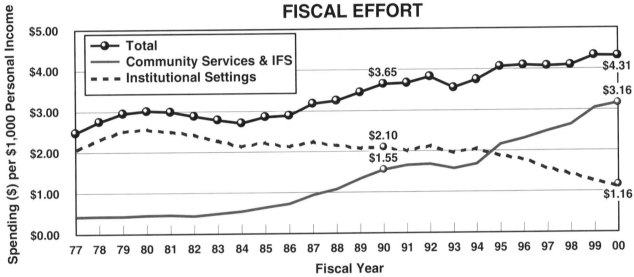

TOTAL MR/DD SPENDING AND
UNMATCHED STATE/LOCAL FUNDS

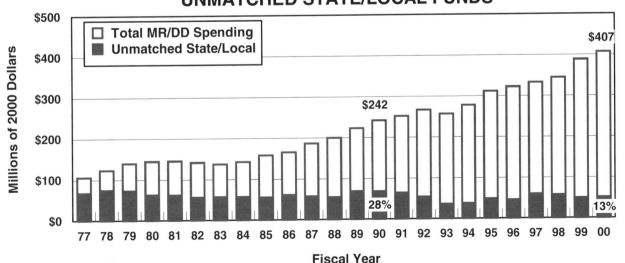

Source: The Coleman Institute and Department of Psychiatry, University of Colorado, 2002.

TRENDS IN REVENUE

COMMUNITY SERVICES REVENUE IN 2000

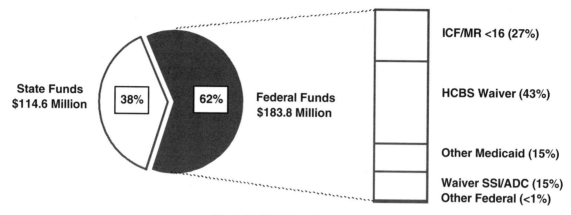

State Funds
$114.6 Million

38%

62%

Federal Funds
$183.8 Million

ICF/MR <16 (27%)

HCBS Waiver (43%)

Other Medicaid (15%)

Waiver SSI/ADC (15%)
Other Federal (<1%)

Total: $298.4 Million

COMPONENTS OF FEDERAL MR/DD MEDICAID REVENUE

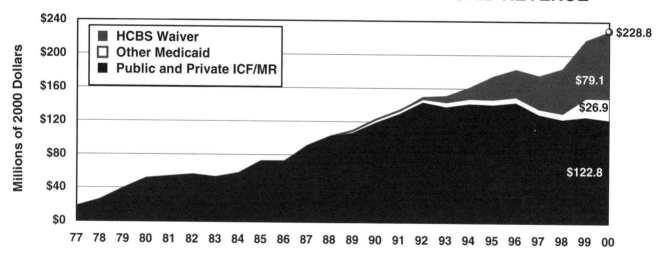

Millions of 2000 Dollars

- ■ HCBS Waiver
- □ Other Medicaid
- ■ Public and Private ICF/MR

$240
$200
$160
$120
$80
$40
$0

$228.8
$79.1
$26.9
$122.8

77 78 79 80 81 82 83 84 85 86 87 88 89 90 91 92 93 94 95 96 97 98 99 00

Fiscal Year

HCBS WAIVER PARTICIPANTS

Number of Participants

6,000
5,000
4,000
3,000
2,000
1,000
0

4,489

82 83 84 85 86 87 88 89 90 91 92 93 94 95 96 97 98 99 00

WAIVER SPENDING PER PARTICIPANT

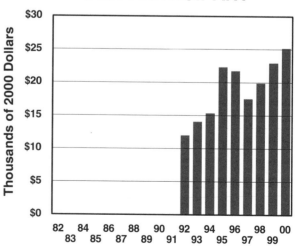

Thousands of 2000 Dollars

$30
$25
$20
$15
$10
$5
$0

82 83 84 85 86 87 88 89 90 91 92 93 94 95 96 97 98 99 00

Source: The Coleman Institute and Department of Psychiatry, University of Colorado, 2002.

TRENDS IN RESIDENTIAL SERVICES

PERSONS SERVED BY SETTING IN 2000

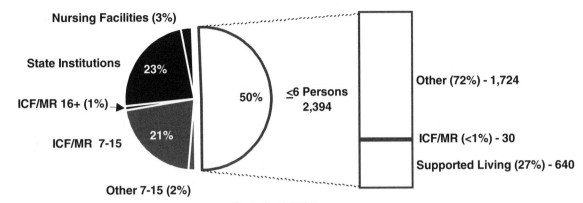

Nursing Facilities (3%)
State Institutions 23%
ICF/MR 16+ (1%)
ICF/MR 7-15 21%
Other 7-15 (2%)
50%
≤6 Persons 2,394
Other (72%) - 1,724
ICF/MR (<1%) - 30
Supported Living (27%) - 640

Total: 4,747

	1990	1991	1992	1993	1994	1995	1996	1997	1998	1999	2000
TOTAL	3,990	4,199	4,280	4,322	4,661	4,802	4,980	4,560	4,444	4,577	4,747
16+ PERSONS	2,418	2,350	2,252	2,200	2,014	1,879	1,724	1,640	1,511	1,324	1,280
Nursing Facilities	117	100	72	76	80	96	104	99	121	121	121
State Institutions	2,254	2,205	2,135	2,080	1,890	1,740	1,574	1,497	1,346	1,159	1,115
Private ICF/MR	47	45	45	44	44	43	46	44	44	44	44
Other Residential	0	0	0	0	0	0	0	0	0	0	0
7-15 PERSONS	1,572	1,849	1,109	1,049	1,095	1,111	1,089	1,099	1,080	1,088	1,073
Public ICF/MR	480	547	608	629	607	609	603	601	582	547	544
Private ICF/MR	414	452	456	382	444	458	446	434	428	460	455
Other Residential	678	850	45	38	44	44	40	64	70	81	74
≤6 PERSONS	0	0	919	1,073	1,552	1,812	2,167	1,821	1,853	2,165	2,394
Public ICF/MR	0	0	8	8	4	5	5	56	51	0	6
Private ICF/MR	0	0	0	9	36	69	59	9	5	24	24
Other Residential	0	0	911	1,056	1,512	1,738	2,103	1,756	1,797	2,141	2,364

PERSONS SERVED IN PUBLIC AND PRIVATE INSTITUTIONS AND NURSING FACILITIES

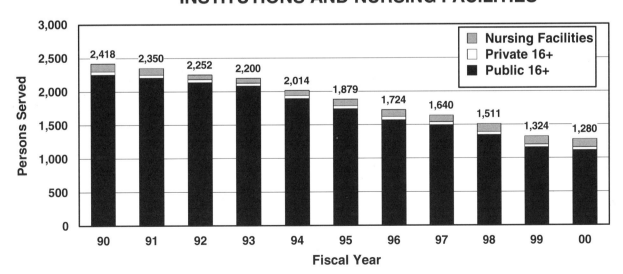

Legend: Nursing Facilities, Private 16+, Public 16+

Values by Fiscal Year: 2,418 (90), 2,350 (91), 2,252 (92), 2,200 (93), 2,014 (94), 1,879 (95), 1,724 (96), 1,640 (97), 1,511 (98), 1,324 (99), 1,280 (00)

X-axis: Fiscal Year
Y-axis: Persons Served

Source: The Coleman Institute and Department of Psychiatry, University of Colorado, 2002.

INDIVIDUAL AND FAMILY SUPPORT

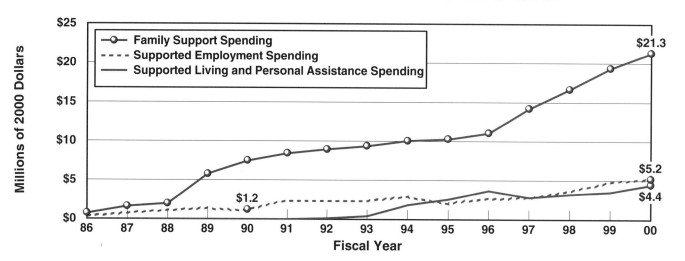

PARTICIPANTS AND SPENDING LEVELS

	1990	1991	1992	1993	1994	1995	1996	1997	1998	1999	2000
TOTAL IFS ($)	6,684,290	8,618,812	9,243,520	10,098,100	12,580,800	13,181,500	15,548,500	18,159,100	22,106,067	26,575,000	30,939,000
INDIVIDUAL SUPPORT ($)	927,078	1,875,126	1,939,261	2,276,500	3,983,000	4,128,000	5,576,000	5,051,100	6,387,867	7,947,000	9,639,000
Supported Employment ($)	927,078	1,875,126	1,867,761	1,941,000	2,408,000	1,878,000	2,276,000	2,458,500	3,354,467	4,577,000	5,190,000
# of Persons	844	973	1,148	1,200	1,264	1,440	1,662	1,641	1,987	1,193	1,187
Supported Living ($)	0	0	0	0	0	0	0	0	0	0	0
# of Persons	0	0	0	0	0	0	0	0	0	0	0
Personal Assistance ($)	0	0	71,500	335,500	1,575,000	2,250,000	3,300,000	2,592,600	3,033,400	3,370,000	4,449,000
# of Persons	0	0	13	61	350	450	600	447	523	623	640
FAMILY SUPPORT ($)	5,757,212	6,743,686	7,304,259	7,821,600	8,597,800	9,053,500	9,972,500	13,108,000	15,718,200	18,628,000	21,300,000
Total Families	1,155	1,326	1,359	1,659	2,537	4,082	5,282	6,077	6,092	6,223	6,749
Cash Subsidy/Payment ($)	440,934	490,041	509,293	683,600	931,800	717,500	711,500	1,235,850	1,362,350	2,028,000	2,600,000
# of Families	413	476	375	225	241	275	263	314	348	456	544
Other Family Support ($)	5,316,278	6,253,645	6,794,966	7,138,000	7,666,000	8,336,000	9,261,000	11,872,150	14,355,850	16,600,000	18,700,000
# of Families	742	850	984	1,434	2,296	3,807	5,019	5,763	5,744	5,956	6,459

PARTICIPANTS IN DAY/WORK AND SUPPORTED EMPLOYMENT

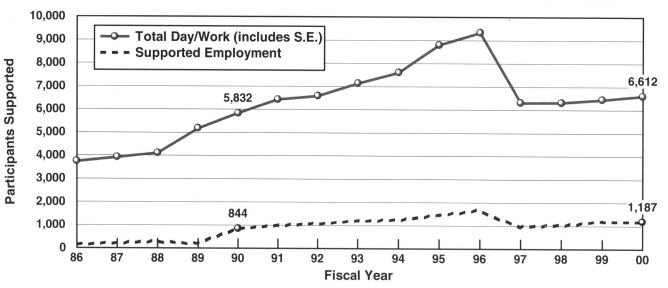

Source: The Coleman Institute and Department of Psychiatry, University of Colorado, 2002.

TRENDS IN SPENDING

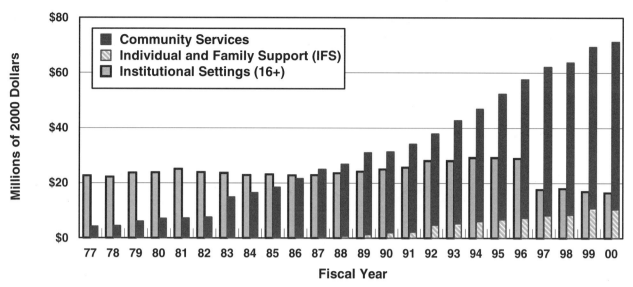

Legend:
- Community Services
- Individual and Family Support (IFS)
- Institutional Settings (16+)

Y-axis: Millions of 2000 Dollars ($0–$80)
X-axis: Fiscal Year (77–00)

FISCAL EFFORT

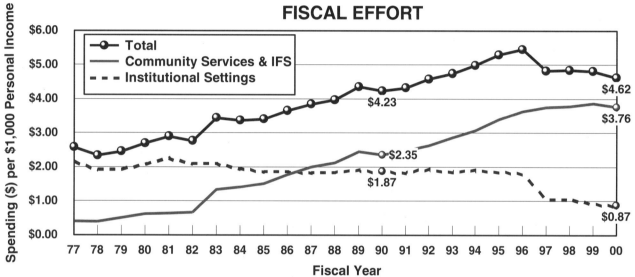

Y-axis: Spending ($) per $1,000 Personal Income ($0.00–$6.00)
X-axis: Fiscal Year (77–00)

Legend:
- Total
- Community Services & IFS
- Institutional Settings

Labels: $4.23, $2.35, $1.87, $4.62, $3.76, $0.87

TOTAL MR/DD SPENDING AND
UNMATCHED STATE/LOCAL FUNDS

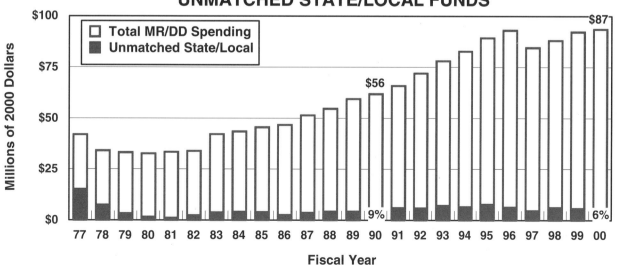

Legend:
- Total MR/DD Spending
- Unmatched State/Local

Y-axis: Millions of 2000 Dollars ($0–$100)
X-axis: Fiscal Year (77–00)

Labels: $56, $87, 9%, 6%

Source: The Coleman Institute and Department of Psychiatry, University of Colorado, 2002.

TRENDS IN REVENUE
COMMUNITY SERVICES REVENUE IN 2000

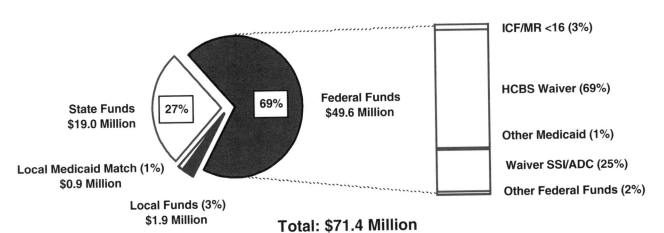

State Funds $19.0 Million

27%

69%

Federal Funds $49.6 Million

Local Medicaid Match (1%) $0.9 Million

Local Funds (3%) $1.9 Million

Total: $71.4 Million

ICF/MR <16 (3%)
HCBS Waiver (69%)
Other Medicaid (1%)
Waiver SSI/ADC (25%)
Other Federal Funds (2%)

COMPONENTS OF FEDERAL MR/DD MEDICAID REVENUE

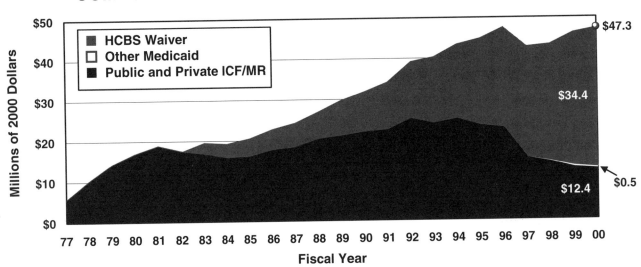

Legend: HCBS Waiver; Other Medicaid; Public and Private ICF/MR

Millions of 2000 Dollars — Fiscal Year

$47.3 / $34.4 / $12.4 / $0.5

HCBS WAIVER PARTICIPANTS

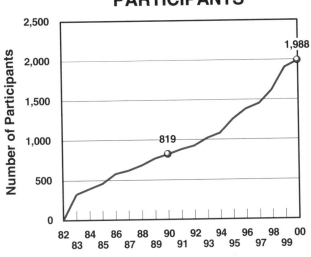
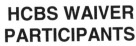

1,988 / 819

WAIVER SPENDING PER PARTICIPANT

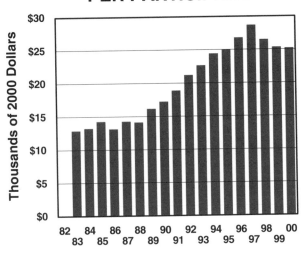

Source: The Coleman Institute and Department of Psychiatry, University of Colorado, 2002.

TRENDS IN RESIDENTIAL SERVICES

PERSONS SERVED BY SETTING IN 2000

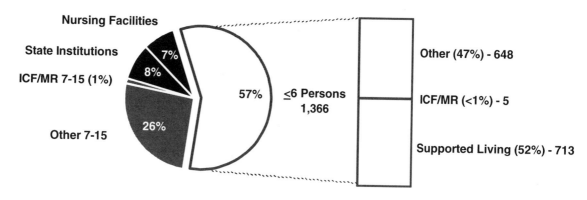

Nursing Facilities

State Institutions

ICF/MR 7-15 (1%)

Other 7-15

7%

8%

26%

57%

≤6 Persons
1,366

Other (47%) - 648

ICF/MR (<1%) - 5

Supported Living (52%) - 713

Total: 2,382

PERSONS SERVED BY SETTING

	1990	1991	1992	1993	1994	1995	1996	1997	1998	1999	2000
TOTAL	1,546	1,543	2,005	1,920	1,831	2,232	2,162	2,116	2,263	2,406	2,382
16+ PERSONS	532	517	522	533	495	513	492	422	415	397	373
Nursing Facilities	141	139	137	163	144	175	169	190	187	186	177
State Institutions	391	378	385	370	351	338	323	232	228	211	196
Private ICF/MR	0	0	0	0	0	0	0	0	0	0	0
Other Residential	0	0	0	0	0	0	0	0	0	0	0
7-15 PERSONS	715	707	664	637	653	679	684	660	672	647	643
Public ICF/MR	0	0	0	0	0	0	0	0	0	0	0
Private ICF/MR	184	178	167	152	151	102	97	92	84	30	29
Other Residential	531	529	497	485	502	577	587	568	588	617	614
≤6 PERSONS	299	319	819	750	683	1,040	986	1,034	1,176	1,362	1,366
Public ICF/MR	0	0	0	0	0	0	0	0	0	0	0
Private ICF/MR	0	0	0	0	0	0	0	0	5	5	5
Other Residential	299	319	819	750	683	1,040	986	1,034	1,171	1,357	1,361

PERSONS SERVED IN PUBLIC AND PRIVATE INSTITUTIONS AND NURSING FACILITIES

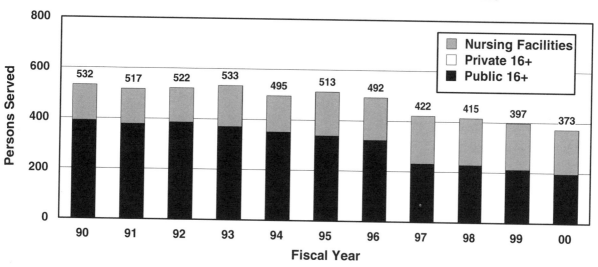

Persons Served

800

600

400

200

0

Nursing Facilities
Private 16+
Public 16+

532 517 522 533 495 513 492 422 415 397 373

90 91 92 93 94 95 96 97 98 99 00

Fiscal Year

Source: The Coleman Institute and Department of Psychiatry, University of Colorado, 2002.

INDIVIDUAL AND FAMILY SUPPORT

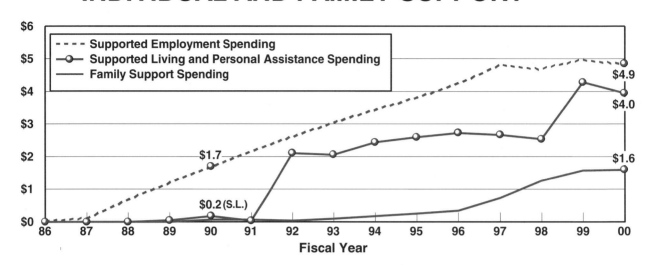

PARTICIPANTS AND SPENDING LEVELS

	1990	1991	1992	1993	1994	1995	1996	1997	1998	1999	2000
TOTAL IFS ($)	1,503,609	1,806,159	3,897,090	4,358,633	5,205,069	5,894,123	6,611,652	7,614,877	8,032,932	10,446,460	10,410,307
INDIVIDUAL SUPPORT ($)	1,451,575	1,754,511	3,863,404	4,275,482	5,053,319	5,667,657	6,298,652	6,929,080	6,841,850	8,927,635	8,808,735
Supported Employment ($)	1,312,647	1,724,725	2,136,802	2,548,880	2,960,957	3,373,035	3,830,449	4,460,877	4,444,917	4,799,557	4,856,723
# of Persons	242	301	402	449	553	575	660	745	760	767	745
Supported Living ($)	138,928	29,786	1,726,602	1,726,602	2,092,362	2,294,622	2,468,203	2,468,203	2,396,933	4,128,078	3,952,012
# of Persons	14	4	321	321	389	693	658	658	689	755	713
Personal Assistance ($)	0	0	0	0	0	0	0	0	0	0	0
# of Persons	0	0	0	0	0	0	0	0	0	0	0
FAMILY SUPPORT ($)	52,034	51,648	33,686	83,151	151,750	226,466	313,000	685,797	1,191,082	1,518,825	1,601,572
Total Families	6	28	785	800	815	875	1,000	1,038	1,104	1,285	1,613
Cash Subsidy/Payment ($)	0	0	0	0	0	0	0	0	0	0	0
# of Families	0	0	0	0	0	0	0	0	0	0	0
Other Family Support ($)	52,034	51,648	33,686	83,151	151,750	226,466	313,000	685,797	1,191,082	1,518,825	1,601,572
# of Families	6	28	50	116	144	476	693	898	1,106	1,285	1,613

PARTICIPANTS IN DAY/WORK AND SUPPORTED EMPLOYMENT

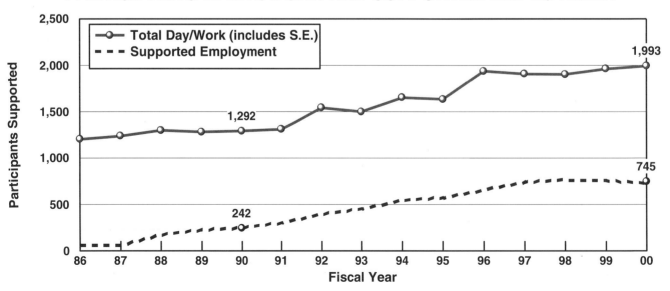

Source: The Coleman Institute and Department of Psychiatry, University of Colorado, 2002.

TRENDS IN SPENDING

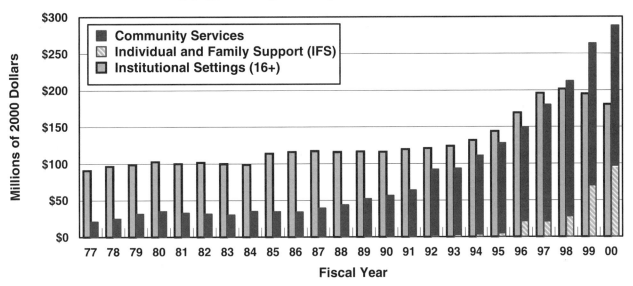

Millions of 2000 Dollars

- ■ Community Services
- ▨ Individual and Family Support (IFS)
- ▧ Institutional Settings (16+)

Fiscal Year

FISCAL EFFORT

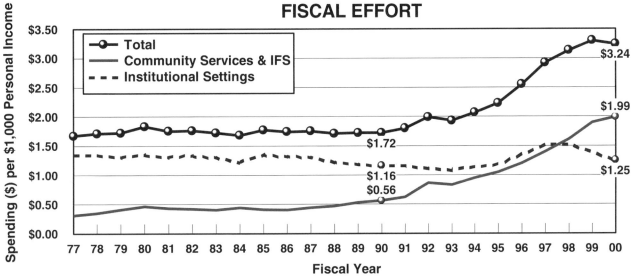

Spending ($) per $1,000 Personal Income

- ─○─ Total
- ─── Community Services & IFS
- ─ ─ Institutional Settings

$3.24

$1.99

$1.72

$1.16

$1.25

$0.56

Fiscal Year

TOTAL MR/DD SPENDING AND
UNMATCHED STATE/LOCAL FUNDS

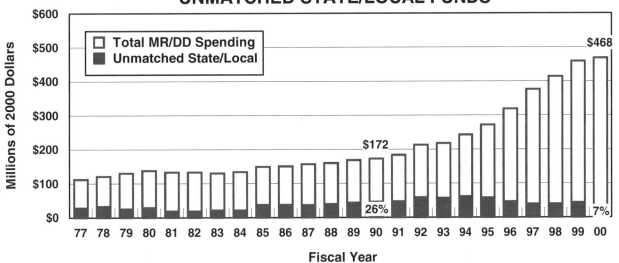

Millions of 2000 Dollars

- ☐ Total MR/DD Spending
- ■ Unmatched State/Local

$468

$172

26%

7%

Fiscal Year

Source: The Coleman Institute and Department of Psychiatry, University of Colorado, 2002.

TRENDS IN REVENUE

COMMUNITY SERVICES REVENUE IN 2000

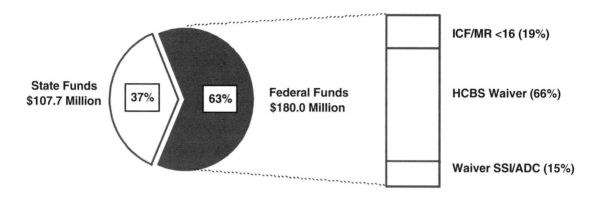

State Funds
$107.7 Million

37%

63%

Federal Funds
$180.0 Million

ICF/MR <16 (19%)

HCBS Waiver (66%)

Waiver SSI/ADC (15%)

Total: $287.7 Million

COMPONENTS OF FEDERAL MR/DD MEDICAID REVENUE

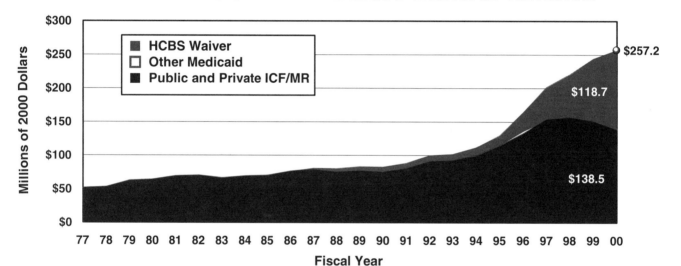

Millions of 2000 Dollars

- ■ HCBS Waiver
- □ Other Medicaid
- ■ Public and Private ICF/MR

$300
$250 — $257.2
$200
$150 — $118.7
$100
$50 — $138.5
$0

77 78 79 80 81 82 83 84 85 86 87 88 89 90 91 92 93 94 95 96 97 98 99 00

Fiscal Year

HCBS WAIVER PARTICIPANTS

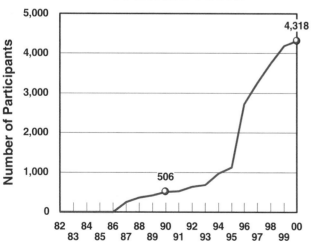

Number of Participants

5,000
4,000 — 4,318
3,000
2,000
1,000 — 506
0

82 83 84 85 86 87 88 89 90 91 92 93 94 95 96 97 98 99 00

WAIVER SPENDING PER PARTICIPANT

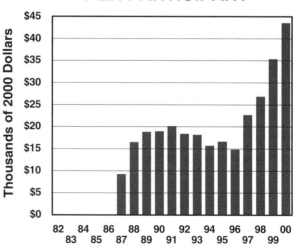

Thousands of 2000 Dollars

$45
$40
$35
$30
$25
$20
$15
$10
$5
$0

82 83 84 85 86 87 88 89 90 91 92 93 94 95 96 97 98 99 00

Source: The Coleman Institute and Department of Psychiatry, University of Colorado, 2002.

TRENDS IN RESIDENTIAL SERVICES
PERSONS SERVED BY SETTING IN 2000

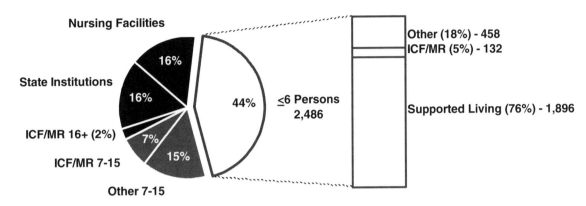

Nursing Facilities 16%

State Institutions 16%

ICF/MR 16+ (2%)

ICF/MR 7-15 7%

Other 7-15 15%

44% ≤6 Persons 2,486

Other (18%) - 458
ICF/MR (5%) - 132
Supported Living (76%) - 1,896

Total: 5,662

PERSONS SERVED BY SETTING

	1990	1991	1992	1993	1994	1995	1996	1997	1998	1999	2000
TOTAL	5,029	5,219	5,210	5,230	5,450	5,874	5,762	5,906	6,036	5,623	5,662
16+ PERSONS	3,237	3,250	3,170	3,085	3,043	2,998	3,008	2,704	2,472	1,965	1,939
Nursing Facilities	1,006	1,044	1,080	1,014	1,003	1,177	1,351	1,262	1,172	846	892
State Institutions	1,947	1,930	1,890	1,871	1,800	1,669	1,513	1,298	1,156	975	903
Private ICF/MR	284	276	200	200	240	152	144	144	144	144	144
Other Residential	0	0	0	0	0	0	0	0	0	0	0
7-15 PERSONS	1,331	1,489	1,633	1,725	1,918	2,306	1,773	1,484	1,440	1,266	1,237
Public ICF/MR	0	0	0	0	0	0	0	0	0	0	0
Private ICF/MR	30	182	270	286	374	385	376	376	376	392	392
Other Residential	1,301	1,307	1,363	1,439	1,544	1,921	1,397	1,108	1,064	874	845
≤6 PERSONS	461	480	407	420	489	570	981	1,718	2,124	2,392	2,486
Public ICF/MR	0	0	0	0	0	0	0	0	0	0	0
Private ICF/MR	0	0	0	0	0	0	0	132	132	132	132
Other Residential	461	480	407	420	489	570	981	1,586	1,992	2,260	2,354

PERSONS SERVED IN PUBLIC AND PRIVATE INSTITUTIONS AND NURSING FACILITIES

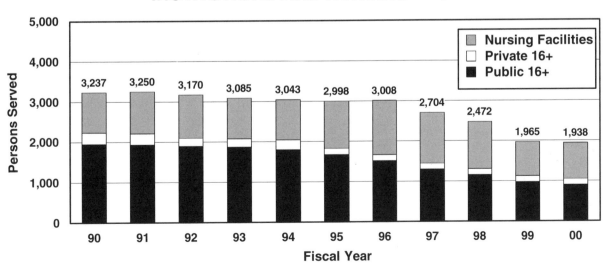

Source: The Coleman Institute and Department of Psychiatry, University of Colorado, 2002.

313

INDIVIDUAL AND FAMILY SUPPORT

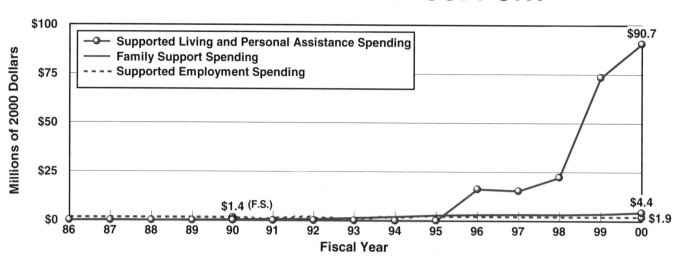

PARTICIPANTS AND SPENDING LEVELS

	1990	1991	1992	1993	1994	1995	1996	1997	1998	1999	2000
TOTAL IFS ($)	1,392,103	1,644,420	1,978,230	2,314,666	3,260,470	4,273,758	19,356,540	19,282,441	26,217,800	76,471,362	96,974,979
INDIVIDUAL SUPPORT ($)	1,061,751	1,084,800	1,334,760	1,176,746	1,462,290	1,815,318	16,567,970	16,163,741	23,005,500	72,912,671	92,563,447
Supported Employment ($)	1,061,751	1,084,800	1,283,800	1,118,246	1,399,890	1,725,318	1,910,982	1,932,741	1,954,500	2,072,434	1,898,370
# of Persons	318	322	425	430	476	542	577	592	644	767	801
Supported Living ($)	0	0	50,960	58,500	62,400	90,000	14,656,988	14,231,000	21,051,000	63,280,587	83,858,421
# of Persons	0	0	196	225	240	346	772	1,056	1,467	1,586	1,724
Personal Assistance ($)	0	0	0	0	0	0	0	0	0	7,559,650	6,806,656
# of Persons	0	0	0	0	0	0	0	0	0	191	172
FAMILY SUPPORT ($)	330,352	559,620	643,470	1,137,920	1,798,180	2,458,440	2,788,570	3,118,700	3,212,300	3,558,691	4,411,532
Total Families	642	905	875	871	1,324	1,776	1,995	2,214	1,902	2,679	3,048
Cash Subsidy/Payment ($)	0	0	0	0	0	0	0	0	0	0	0
# of Families	0	0	0	0	0	0	0	0	0	0	0
Other Family Support ($)	330,352	559,620	643,470	1,137,920	1,798,180	2,458,440	2,788,570	3,118,700	3,212,300	3,558,691	4,411,532
# of Families	642	905	875	871	1,324	1,776	1,995	2,214	1,902	2,679	3,048

PARTICIPANTS IN DAY/WORK AND SUPPORTED EMPLOYMENT

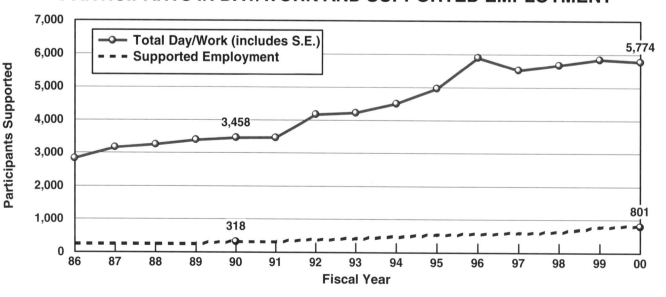

Source: The Coleman Institute and Department of Psychiatry, University of Colorado, 2002.

TRENDS IN SPENDING

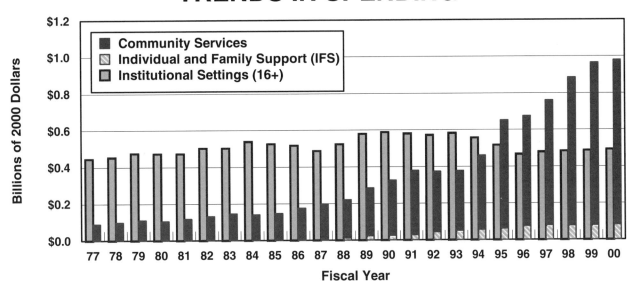

FISCAL YEAR

Legend:
- Community Services
- Individual and Family Support (IFS)
- Institutional Settings (16+)

Y-axis: Billions of 2000 Dollars

FISCAL EFFORT

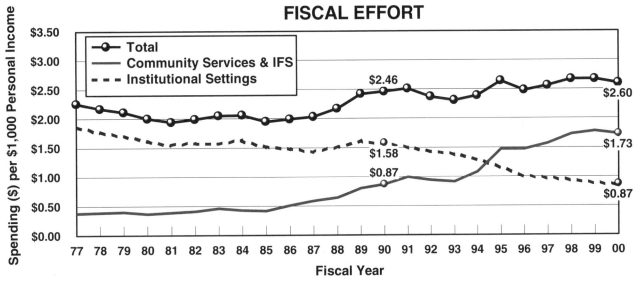

Legend:
- Total
- Community Services & IFS
- Institutional Settings

$2.46
$2.60
$1.58
$1.73
$0.87
$0.87

Y-axis: Spending ($) per $1,000 Personal Income

Fiscal Year

TOTAL MR/DD SPENDING AND
UNMATCHED STATE/LOCAL FUNDS

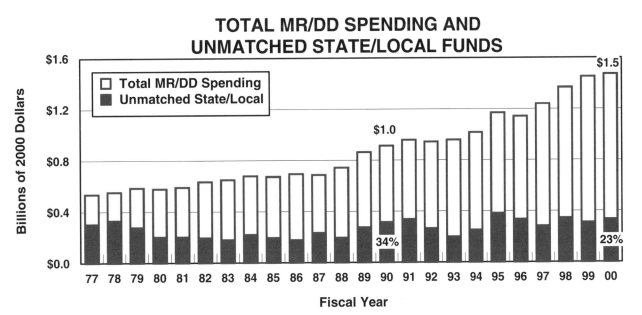

Legend:
- Total MR/DD Spending
- Unmatched State/Local

$1.0
$1.5
34%
23%

Y-axis: Billions of 2000 Dollars

Fiscal Year

Source: The Coleman Institute and Department of Psychiatry, University of Colorado, 2002.

TRENDS IN REVENUE

COMMUNITY SERVICES REVENUE IN 2000

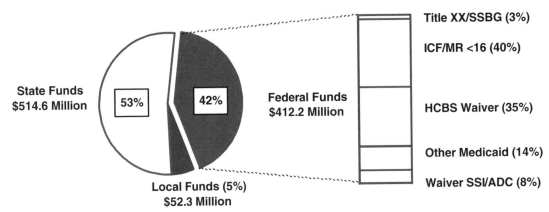

State Funds
$514.6 Million

53%

42%

Federal Funds
$412.2 Million

Local Funds (5%)
$52.3 Million

Title XX/SSBG (3%)

ICF/MR <16 (40%)

HCBS Waiver (35%)

Other Medicaid (14%)

Waiver SSI/ADC (8%)

Total: $979.1 Million

COMPONENTS OF FEDERAL MR/DD MEDICAID REVENUE

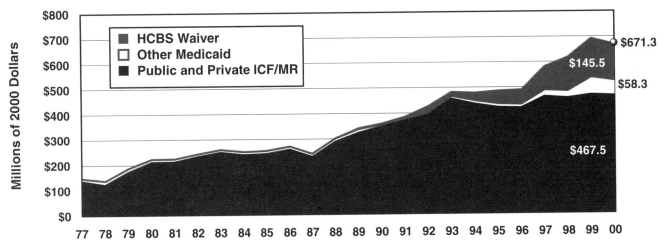

HCBS Waiver
Other Medicaid
Public and Private ICF/MR

$671.3
$145.5
$58.3
$467.5

Fiscal Year

HCBS WAIVER PARTICIPANTS

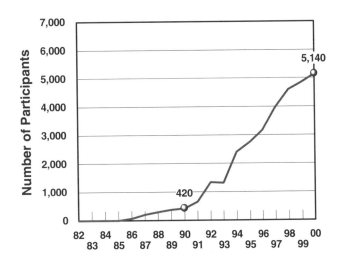

5,140

420

WAIVER SPENDING PER PARTICIPANT

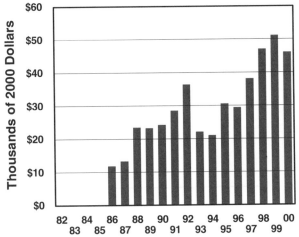

Source: The Coleman Institute and Department of Psychiatry, University of Colorado, 2002.

TRENDS IN RESIDENTIAL SERVICES

PERSONS SERVED BY SETTING IN 2000

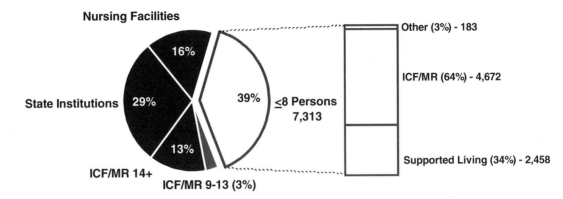

Total: 18,584

PERSONS SERVED BY SETTING*

	1990	1991	1992	1993	1994	1995	1996	1997	1998	1999	2000
TOTAL	17,624	18,131	18,605	18,321	17,678	17,478	17,544	17,987	18,649	17,762	18,584
16+ PERSONS	13,148	13,009	12,941	12,472	11,667	11,205	10,700	10,722	10,452	10,395	10,721
Nursing Facilities	3,281	3,338	3,355	3,232	3,110	2,987	2,864	2,741	2,619	2,619	2,919
State Institutions	7,290	7,094	7,041	6,580	6,242	5,879	5,517	5,673	5,525	5,296	5,338
Private ICF/MR	2,577	2,577	2,545	2,660	2,315	2,339	2,319	2,308	2,308	2,480	2,464
Other Residential	0	0	0	0	0	0	0	0	0	0	0
7-15 PERSONS	4,476	5,122	3,195	2,398	1,576	1,112	953	929	833	514	550
Public ICF/MR	24	24	24	43	35	35	333	354	273	154	177
Private ICF/MR	2,095	2,534	1,267	913	560	558	563	575	560	360	373
Other Residential	2,357	2,564	1,904	1,442	981	519	57	0	0	0	0
≤6 PERSONS	0	0	2,469	3,450	4,436	5,161	5,891	6,336	7,364	6,853	7,313
Public ICF/MR	0	0	0	0	6	180	507	767	768	823	878
Private ICF/MR	0	0	1,987	2,647	3,306	3,536	3,618	3,635	3,640	3,770	3,794
Other Residential	0	0	482	803	1,124	1,445	1,766	1,934	2,956	2,260	2,641

*Texas' classification categories were <8 persons, 9-13 persons, and 14+ persons.

PERSONS SERVED IN PUBLIC AND PRIVATE INSTITUTIONS AND NURSING FACILITIES

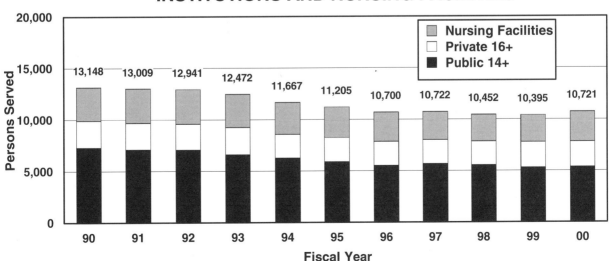

Source: The Coleman Institute and Department of Psychiatry, University of Colorado, 2002.

INDIVIDUAL AND FAMILY SUPPORT

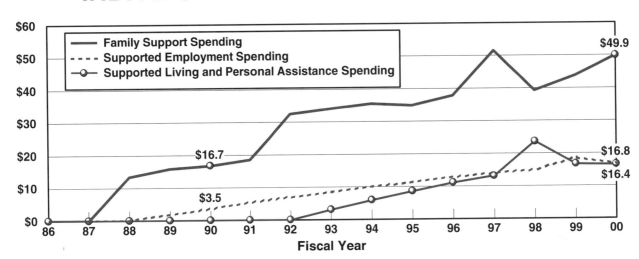

PARTICIPANTS AND SPENDING LEVELS

	1990	1991	1992	1993	1994	1995	1996	1997	1998	1999	2000
TOTAL IFS ($)	15,569,182	19,003,794	32,153,375	38,025,787	43,898,199	48,208,743	55,643,023	72,435,108	73,335,533	75,965,609	83,124,615
INDIVIDUAL SUPPORT ($)	2,692,198	4,134,395	5,576,593	9,525,215	13,473,838	17,422,460	21,371,083	24,870,044	36,214,033	33,787,773	33,241,882
Supported Employment ($)	2,692,198	4,134,395	5,576,593	7,018,790	8,460,988	9,903,185	11,345,383	12,787,580	13,969,963	17,734,541	16,792,498
# of Persons	587	924	1,260	1,597	1,934	2,271	2,607	2,944	2,991	3,659	3,971
Supported Living ($)	0	0	0	2,506,425	5,012,850	7,519,275	10,025,700	12,082,464	22,244,070	16,053,232	16,449,384
# of Persons	0	0	0	363	727	1,090	1,453	1,530	2,501	1,955	2,458
Personal Assistance ($)	0	0	0	0	0	0	0	0	0	0	0
# of Persons	0	0	0	0	0	0	0	0	0	0	0
FAMILY SUPPORT ($)	12,876,984	14,869,399	26,576,782	28,500,572	30,424,361	30,786,283	34,271,940	47,565,064	37,121,500	42,177,836	49,882,733
Total Families	6,781	6,791	9,624	10,209	10,794	10,317	11,963	11,961	9,999	10,129	10,395
Cash Subsidy/Payment ($)	3,500,000	4,500,000	7,600,000	8,753,956	9,907,912	9,500,000	12,215,824	10,659,401	9,177,518	10,838,739	12,707,989
# of Families	1,726	1,987	3,450	3,713	3,977	3,582	4,503	4,689	4,519	4,466	5,148
Other Family Support ($)	9,376,984	10,369,399	18,976,782	19,746,616	20,516,449	21,286,283	22,056,116	36,905,663	27,943,982	31,339,097	37,174,744
# of Families	5,055	4,804	6,174	6,496	6,817	6,735	7,460	7,272	5,480	5,663	5,247

PARTICIPANTS IN DAY/WORK AND SUPPORTED EMPLOYMENT

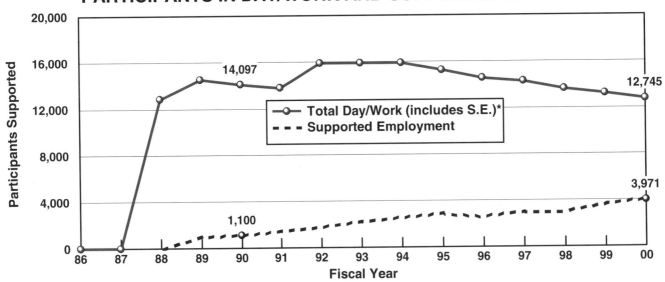

*In 1999 and 2000 respectively, data were available for only 9,711 and 9,914 total day/work clients; data were not available for a number of day habilitation clients supported by the Waiver. In the chart, 1999 and 2000 day/work totals were estimated based on the 1996-98 trend.

Source: The Coleman Institute and Department of Psychiatry, University of Colorado, 2002.

TRENDS IN SPENDING

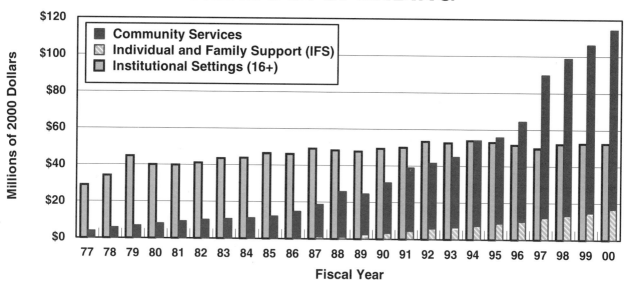

FISCAL EFFORT

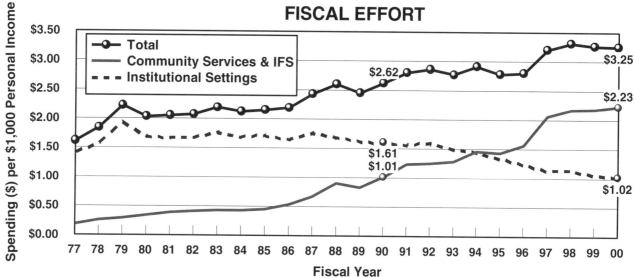

TOTAL MR/DD SPENDING AND
UNMATCHED STATE/LOCAL FUNDS

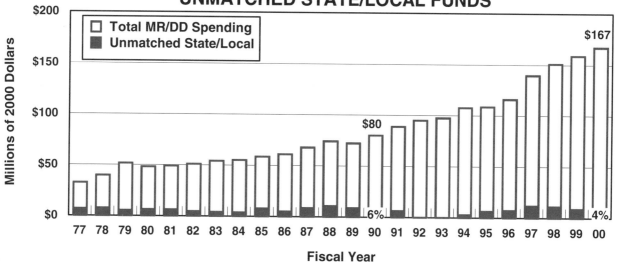

Source: The Coleman Institute and Department of Psychiatry, University of Colorado, 2002.

TRENDS IN REVENUE

COMMUNITY SERVICES REVENUE IN 2000

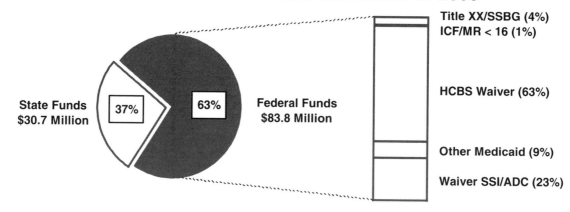

State Funds
$30.7 Million

37%

63%

Federal Funds
$83.8 Million

Title XX/SSBG (4%)
ICF/MR < 16 (1%)

HCBS Waiver (63%)

Other Medicaid (9%)

Waiver SSI/ADC (23%)

Total: $114.5 Million

COMPONENTS OF FEDERAL MR/DD MEDICAID REVENUE

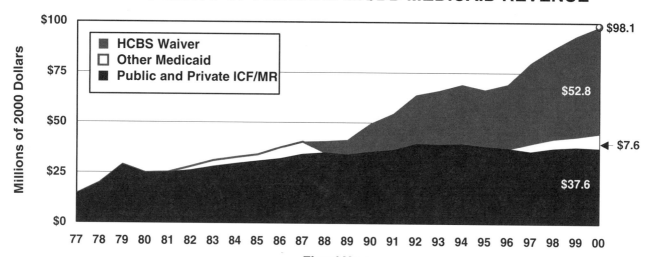

Millions of 2000 Dollars

- ■ HCBS Waiver
- □ Other Medicaid
- ■ Public and Private ICF/MR

$98.1

$52.8

$7.6

$37.6

Fiscal Year

HCBS WAIVER PARTICIPANTS

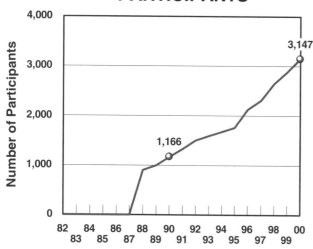

Number of Participants

3,147

1,166

WAIVER SPENDING PER PARTICIPANT

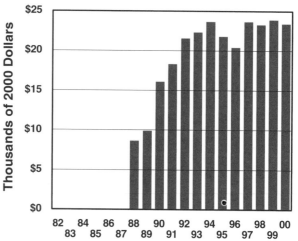

Thousands of 2000 Dollars

Source: The Coleman Institute and Department of Psychiatry, University of Colorado, 2002.

TRENDS IN RESIDENTIAL SERVICES

PERSONS SERVED BY SETTING IN 2000

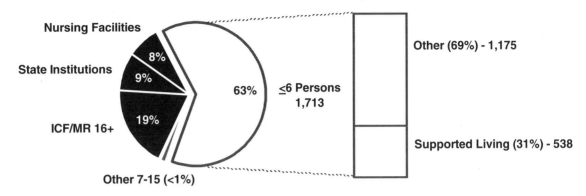

Nursing Facilities 8%

State Institutions 9%

ICF/MR 16+ 19%

63% ≤6 Persons 1,713

Other 7-15 (<1%)

Other (69%) - 1,175

Supported Living (31%) - 538

Total: 2,702

PERSONS SERVED BY SETTING

	1990	1991	1992	1993	1994	1995	1996	1997	1998	1999	2000
TOTAL	2,010	2,044	2,277	2,309	2,280	2,384	2,400	2,375	2,441	2,580	2,702
16+ PERSONS	1,238	1,195	1,161	1,118	1,061	1,035	1,025	1,010	1,041	944	945
Nursing Facilities	306	279	279	245	210	203	218	236	253	170	203
State Institutions	464	434	384	373	350	329	303	284	263	250	236
Private ICF/MR	468	482	498	500	501	503	504	490	525	524	506
Other Residential	0	0	0	0	0	0	0	0	0	0	0
7-15 PERSONS	378	370	229	203	174	143	122	87	50	48	44
Public ICF/MR	0	0	0	0	0	0	0	0	0	0	0
Private ICF/MR	12	11	11	12	12	12	12	12	12	12	12
Other Residential	366	359	218	191	162	131	110	75	38	36	32
≤6 PERSONS	394	479	887	988	1,045	1,206	1,253	1,278	1,350	1,588	1,713
Public ICF/MR	0	0	0	0	0	0	0	0	0	0	0
Private ICF/MR	0	0	0	0	0	0	0	0	0	0	0
Other Residential	394	479	887	988	1,045	1,206	1,253	1,278	1,350	1,588	1,713

PERSONS SERVED IN PUBLIC AND PRIVATE INSTITUTIONS AND NURSING FACILITIES

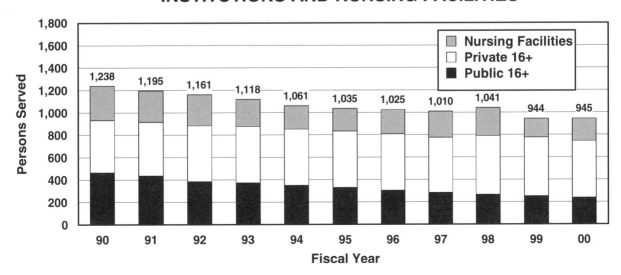

Source: The Coleman Institute and Department of Psychiatry, University of Colorado, 2002.

321

INDIVIDUAL AND FAMILY SUPPORT

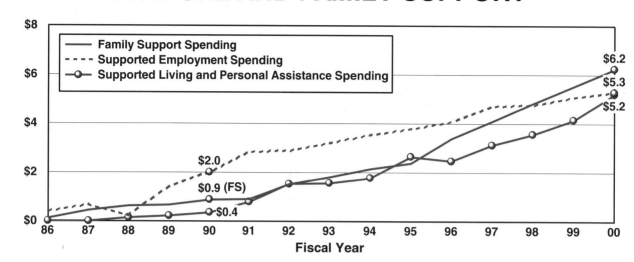

PARTICIPANTS AND SPENDING LEVELS

	1990	1991	1992	1993	1994	1995	1996	1997	1998	1999	2000
TOTAL IFS ($)	2,505,143	3,628,802	4,853,040	5,476,130	6,367,900	7,788,900	8,967,000	11,033,521	12,390,924	14,240,100	16,746,400
INDIVIDUAL SUPPORT ($)	1,827,417	2,900,212	3,606,928	3,964,300	4,523,000	5,680,500	5,898,000	7,250,835	7,841,320	8,905,300	10,501,000
Supported Employment ($)	1,549,658	2,265,832	2,355,343	2,658,100	3,006,300	3,344,100	3,662,000	4,362,099	4,483,565	4,903,300	5,292,000
# of Persons	240	372	664	690	753	809	927	742	755	833	860
Supported Living ($)	151,980	361,280	927,900	975,000	1,257,500	2,025,000	1,796,000	2,415,536	2,866,665	3,385,200	4,252,000
# of Persons	105	149	188	198	219	317	289	324	373	392	441
Personal Assistance ($)	125,779	273,100	323,685	331,200	259,200	311,400	440,000	473,200	491,090	616,800	957,000
# of Persons	32	50	51	67	50	59	60	60	60	74	97
FAMILY SUPPORT ($)	677,726	728,590	1,246,112	1,511,830	1,844,900	2,108,400	3,069,000	3,782,686	4,549,604	5,334,800	6,245,400
Total Families	n/a	n/a	497	733	928	1,080	1,478	1,498	1,630	1,797	2,366
Cash Subsidy/Payment ($)	45,348	44,579	44,250	44,730	114,600	164,600	219,000	213,167	453,178	594,700	932,100
# of Families	140	137	123	258	381	549	475	455	727	886	1,573
Other Family Support ($)	632,378	684,011	1,201,862	1,467,100	1,730,300	1,943,800	2,850,000	3,569,519	4,096,426	4,740,100	5,313,300
# of Families	n/a	n/a	827	1,005	1,427	1,680	1,703	1,712	1,769	1,300	1,528

PARTICIPANTS IN DAY/WORK AND SUPPORTED EMPLOYMENT

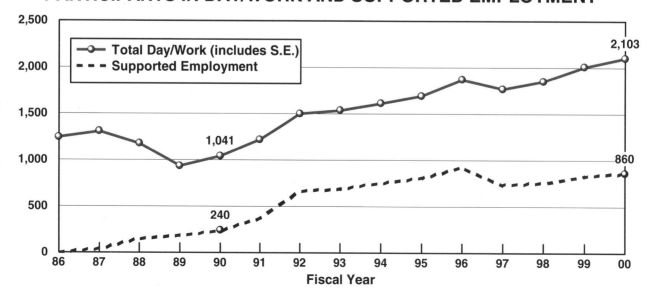

   Source: The Coleman Institute and Department of Psychiatry, University of Colorado, 2002.

TRENDS IN SPENDING

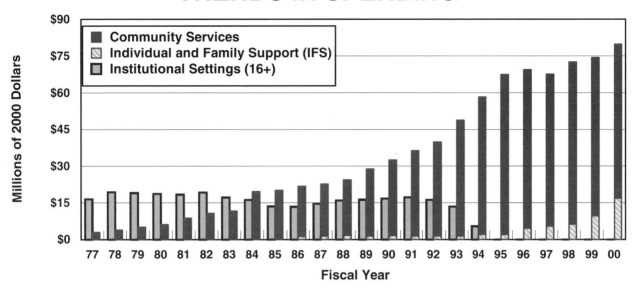

FISCAL EFFORT

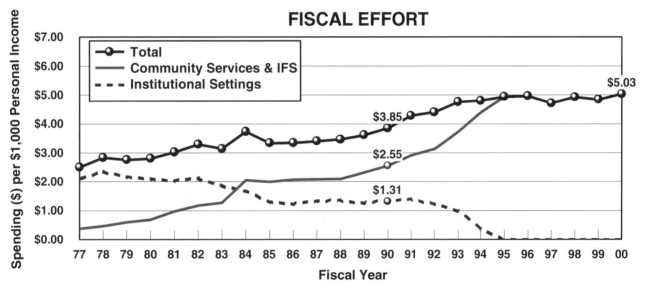

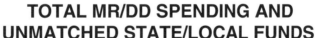

TOTAL MR/DD SPENDING AND
UNMATCHED STATE/LOCAL FUNDS

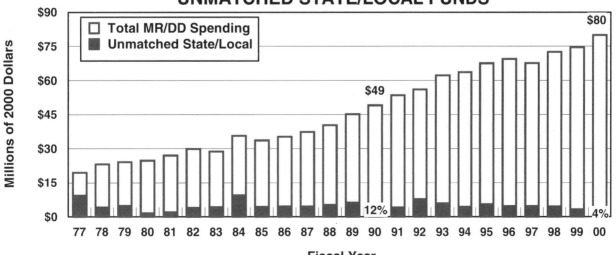

Source: The Coleman Institute and Department of Psychiatry, University of Colorado, 2002.

TRENDS IN REVENUE

COMMUNITY SERVICES REVENUE IN 2000

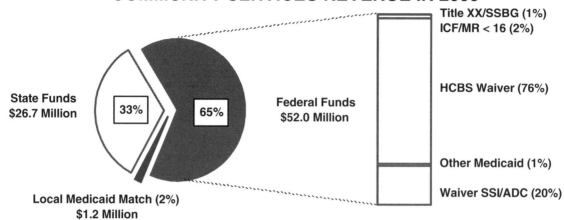

State Funds
$26.7 Million

33%

65%

Local Medicaid Match (2%)
$1.2 Million

Federal Funds
$52.0 Million

Title XX/SSBG (1%)
ICF/MR < 16 (2%)

HCBS Waiver (76%)

Other Medicaid (1%)

Waiver SSI/ADC (20%)

Total: $79.9 Million

COMPONENTS OF FEDERAL MR/DD MEDICAID REVENUE

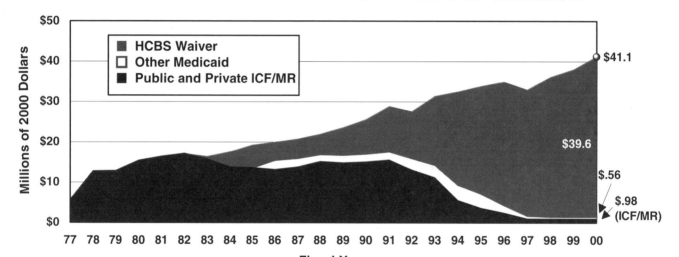

- ■ HCBS Waiver
- □ Other Medicaid
- ■ Public and Private ICF/MR

$41.1
$39.6
$.56
$.98
(ICF/MR)

Fiscal Year

HCBS WAIVER PARTICIPANTS

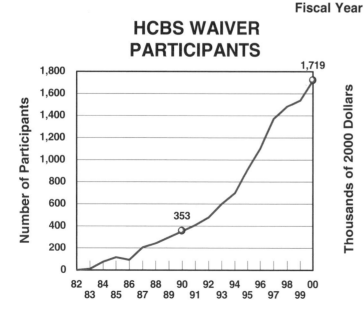

1,719

353

WAIVER SPENDING PER PARTICIPANT

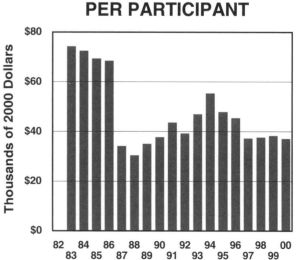

Source: The Coleman Institute and Department of Psychiatry, University of Colorado, 2002.

TRENDS IN RESIDENTIAL SERVICES
PERSONS SERVED BY SETTING IN 2000

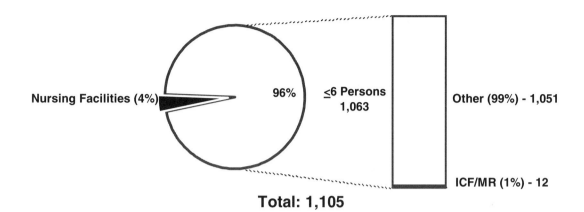

Nursing Facilities (4%) 96% ≤6 Persons 1,063 Other (99%) - 1,051

ICF/MR (1%) - 12

Total: 1,105

PERSONS SERVED BY SETTING

	1990	1991	1992	1993	1994	1995	1996	1997	1998	1999	2000
TOTAL	794	801	910	903	882	858	890	976	1,068	1,097	1,105
16+ PERSONS	268	262	226	151	105	76	68	61	61	56	42
Nursing Facilities	89	92	91	89	82	76	68	61	61	56	42
State Institutions	179	170	135	62	23	0	0	0	0	0	0
Private ICF/MR	0	0	0	0	0	0	0	0	0	0	0
Other Residential	0	0	0	0	0	0	0	0	0	0	0
7-15 PERSONS	0	0	0	0	0	0	0	0	0	0	0
Public ICF/MR	0	0	0	0	0	0	0	0	0	0	0
Private ICF/MR	0	0	0	0	0	0	0	0	0	0	0
Other Residential	0	0	0	0	0	0	0	0	0	0	0
≤6 PERSONS	526	539	684	752	777	782	822	915	1,007	1,041	1,063
Public ICF/MR	0	0	0	0	0	0	0	0	0	0	0
Private ICF/MR	51	50	48	54	45	42	27	12	12	12	12
Other Residential	475	490	636	698	732	740	795	903	995	1,029	1,051

PERSONS SERVED IN PUBLIC AND PRIVATE INSTITUTIONS AND NURSING FACILITIES

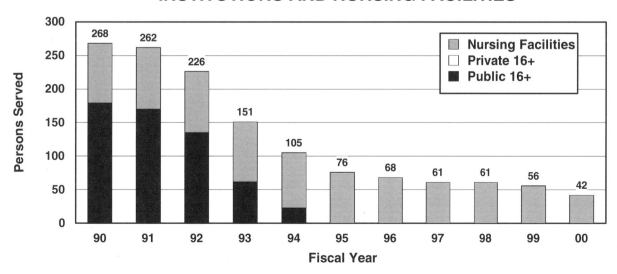

Source: The Coleman Institute and Department of Psychiatry, University of Colorado, 2002.

INDIVIDUAL AND FAMILY SUPPORT

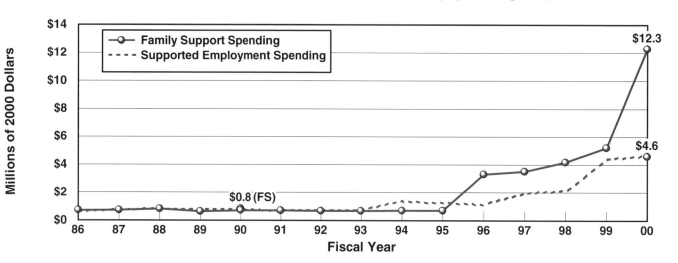

PARTICIPANTS AND SPENDING LEVELS

	1990	1991	1992	1993	1994	1995	1996	1997	1998	1999	2000
TOTAL IFS ($)	1,181,388	1,152,231	1,163,684	1,198,498	1,779,264	1,788,657	4,047,643	5,061,232	5,911,833	9,234,607	16,865,173
INDIVIDUAL SUPPORT ($)	633,133	591,254	615,093	629,948	1,181,505	1,166,251	1,052,178	1,813,749	1,974,034	4,215,201	4,580,753
Supported Employment ($)	633,133	591,254	615,093	629,948	1,181,505	1,166,251	1,052,178	1,813,749	1,974,034	4,215,201	4,580,753
# of Persons	224	205	209	255	270	268	263	481	534	661	698
Supported Living ($)	0	0	0	0	0	0	0	0	0	0	0
# of Persons	0	0	0	0	0	0	0	0	0	0	0
Personal Assistance ($)	0	0	0	0	0	0	0	0	0	0	0
# of Persons	0	0	0	0	0	0	0	0	0	0	0
FAMILY SUPPORT ($)	548,255	560,977	548,591	568,550	597,759	622,406	2,995,465	3,247,483	3,937,799	5,019,406	12,284,420
Total Families	481	450	450	450	450	500	602	690	756	796	1,003
Cash Subsidy/Payment ($)	0	0	0	0	0	0	0	0	0	0	0
# of Families	0	0	0	0	0	0	0	0	0	0	0
Other Family Support ($)	548,255	560,977	548,591	568,550	597,759	622,406	2,995,465	3,247,483	3,937,799	5,019,406	12,284,420
# of Families	481	450	450	450	450	500	602	690	756	796	1,003

PARTICIPANTS IN DAY/WORK AND SUPPORTED EMPLOYMENT

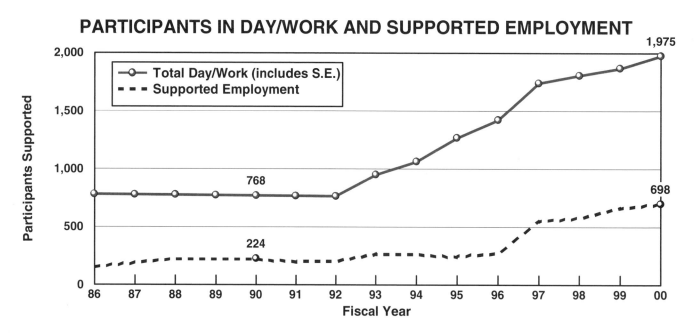

Source: The Coleman Institute and Department of Psychiatry, University of Colorado, 2002.

TRENDS IN SPENDING

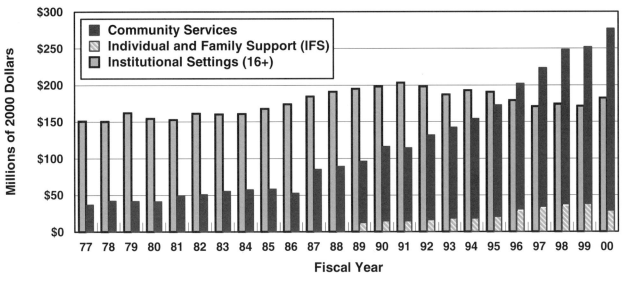

Millions of 2000 Dollars

- Community Services
- Individual and Family Support (IFS)
- Institutional Settings (16+)

Fiscal Year

FISCAL EFFORT

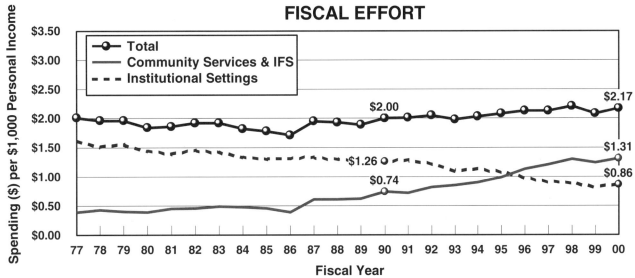

Spending ($) per $1,000 Personal Income

- Total
- Community Services & IFS
- Institutional Settings

$2.00 $2.17

$1.31

$1.26 $1.31

$0.74 $0.86

Fiscal Year

TOTAL MR/DD SPENDING AND
UNMATCHED STATE/LOCAL FUNDS

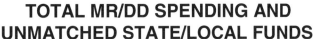
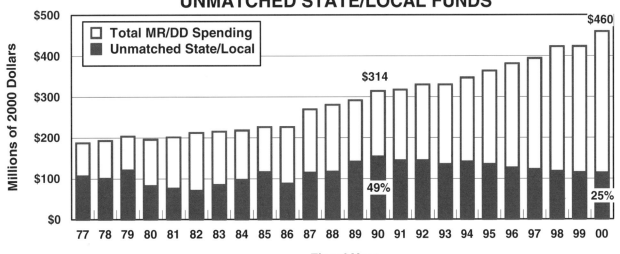

Millions of 2000 Dollars

- Total MR/DD Spending
- Unmatched State/Local

$460

$314

49%   25%

Fiscal Year

Source: The Coleman Institute and Department of Psychiatry, University of Colorado, 2002.

TRENDS IN REVENUE

COMMUNITY SERVICES REVENUE IN 2000

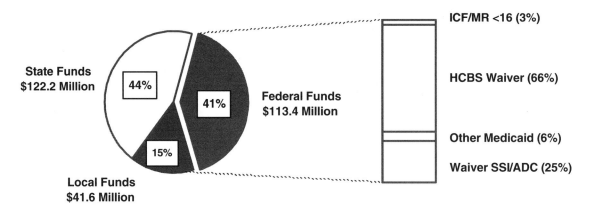

State Funds
$122.2 Million

44%

41%

15%

Federal Funds
$113.4 Million

Local Funds
$41.6 Million

ICF/MR <16 (3%)

HCBS Waiver (66%)

Other Medicaid (6%)

Waiver SSI/ADC (25%)

Total: $277.1 Million

COMPONENTS OF FEDERAL MR/DD MEDICAID REVENUE

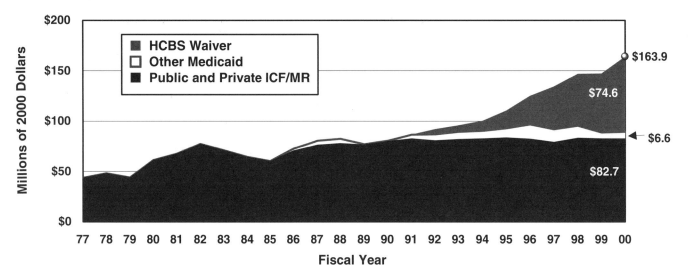

- ■ HCBS Waiver
- □ Other Medicaid
- ■ Public and Private ICF/MR

Millions of 2000 Dollars

$200 | $150 | $100 | $50 | $0

77 78 79 80 81 82 83 84 85 86 87 88 89 90 91 92 93 94 95 96 97 98 99 00

Fiscal Year

$163.9

$74.6

$6.6

$82.7

HCBS WAIVER PARTICIPANTS

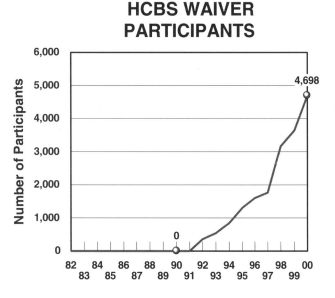

Number of Participants

6,000 | 5,000 | 4,000 | 3,000 | 2,000 | 1,000 | 0

4,698

0

82 83 84 85 86 87 88 89 90 91 92 93 94 95 96 97 98 99 00

WAIVER SPENDING PER PARTICIPANT

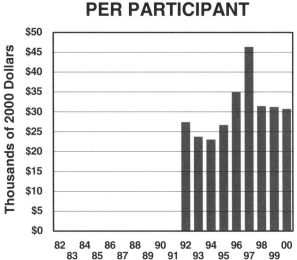

Thousands of 2000 Dollars

$50 | $45 | $40 | $35 | $30 | $25 | $20 | $15 | $10 | $5 | $0

82 83 84 85 86 87 88 89 90 91 92 93 94 95 96 97 98 99 00

Source: The Coleman Institute and Department of Psychiatry, University of Colorado, 2002.

TRENDS IN RESIDENTIAL SERVICES

PERSONS SERVED BY SETTING IN 2000

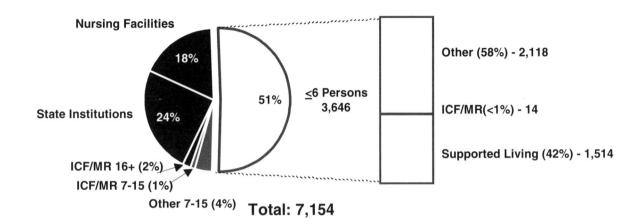

Nursing Facilities 18%

State Institutions 24%

ICF/MR 16+ (2%)
ICF/MR 7-15 (1%)
Other 7-15 (4%)

51% ≤6 Persons 3,646

Other (58%) - 2,118

ICF/MR(<1%) - 14

Supported Living (42%) - 1,514

Total: 7,154

PERSONS SERVED BY SETTING

	1990	1991	1992	1993	1994	1995	1996	1997	1998	1999	2000
TOTAL	6,568	6,652	6,361	6,537	6,159	6,216	6,957	6,694	7,015	7,086	7,154
16+ PERSONS	3,912	3,996	3,706	3,525	3,731	3,533	3,366	3,133	3,272	3,216	3,148
Nursing Facilities	1,114	1,247	1,020	958	1,225	1,152	1,086	1,012	1,249	1,272	1,272
State Institutions	2,677	2,618	2,554	2,435	2,374	2,249	2,148	1,989	1,891	1,812	1,744
Private ICF/MR	121	131	132	132	132	132	132	132	132	132	132
Other Residential	0	0	0	0	0	0	0	0	0	0	0
7-15 PERSONS	869	606	343	468	498	520	497	480	452	253	360
Public ICF/MR	0	0	0	0	0	0	0	0	0	0	0
Private ICF/MR	95	90	85	85	85	85	75	75	75	75	75
Other Residential	774	516	258	383	413	435	422	405	377	178	285
≤6 PERSONS	1,787	2,050	2,312	2,544	1,930	2,163	3,094	3,081	3,291	3,617	3,646
Public ICF/MR	0	0	0	0	0	0	0	0	0	0	0
Private ICF/MR	0	0	0	14	14	14	14	14	14	14	14
Other Residential	1,787	2,050	2,312	2,530	1,916	2,149	3,080	3,067	3,277	3,603	3,632

PERSONS SERVED IN PUBLIC AND PRIVATE INSTITUTIONS AND NURSING FACILITIES

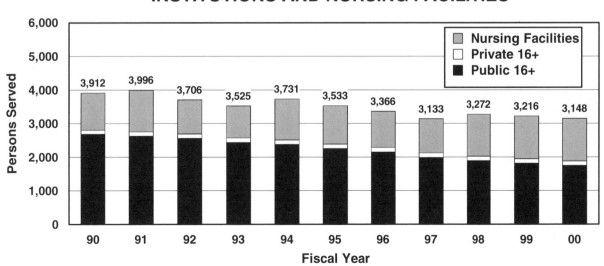

Legend: Nursing Facilities, Private 16+, Public 16+

Values: 3,912 | 3,996 | 3,706 | 3,525 | 3,731 | 3,533 | 3,366 | 3,133 | 3,272 | 3,216 | 3,148

Fiscal Year: 90, 91, 92, 93, 94, 95, 96, 97, 98, 99, 00

Persons Served

INDIVIDUAL AND FAMILY SUPPORT

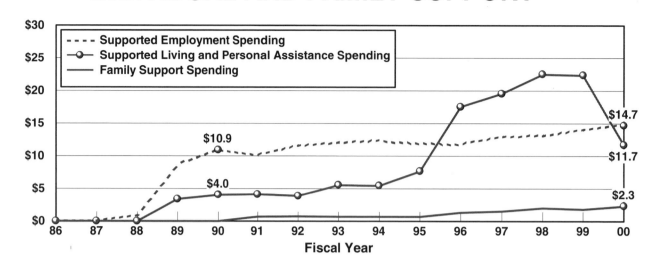

PARTICIPANTS AND SPENDING LEVELS

	1990	1991	1992	1993	1994	1995	1996	1997	1998	1999	2000
TOTAL IFS ($)	11,519,554	12,069,376	13,226,595	15,233,489	15,799,591	18,008,948	27,843,984	31,476,009	35,509,990	36,757,433	28,743,788
INDIVIDUAL SUPPORT ($)	11,519,554	11,519,376	12,626,595	14,633,489	15,199,591	17,408,948	26,647,989	30,045,633	33,581,825	35,006,908	26,419,708
Supported Employment ($)	8,415,117	8,206,656	9,453,032	9,984,103	10,525,439	10,624,339	10,753,513	11,942,300	12,311,930	13,435,248	14,699,870
# of Persons	1,870	925	1,783	2,196	2,190	2,128	2,134	2,267	2,360	2,218	2,312
Supported Living ($)	3,104,437	3,312,720	3,173,563	4,649,386	4,674,152	6,784,609	9,888,654	10,915,748	13,082,800	12,047,024	4,141,653
# of Persons	1,421	807	1,418	1,502	839	1,026	1,538	1,575	1,768	1,660	1,212
Personal Assistance ($)	0	0	0	0	0	0	6,005,822	7,187,585	8,187,095	9,524,636	7,578,185
# of Persons	0	0	0	0	0	0	452	475	516	295	302
FAMILY SUPPORT ($)	0	550,000	600,000	600,000	600,000	600,000	1,195,995	1,430,376	1,928,165	1,750,525	2,324,080
Total Families	0	565	600	600	600	600	1,431	1,850	1,988	1,967	2,164
Cash Subsidy/Payment ($)	0	0	0	0	0	0	0	0	0	0	0
# of Families	0	0	0	0	0	0	0	0	0	0	0
Other Family Support ($)	0	550,000	600,000	600,000	600,000	600,000	1,195,995	1,430,376	1,928,165	1,750,525	2,324,080
# of Families	0	565	600	600	600	600	1,431	1,850	1,988	1,967	2,164

*The decline in supported living spending in 2000 was largely attributable to a decline in the number of relatively higher cost in-home provider staff.

PARTICIPANTS IN DAY/WORK AND SUPPORTED EMPLOYMENT

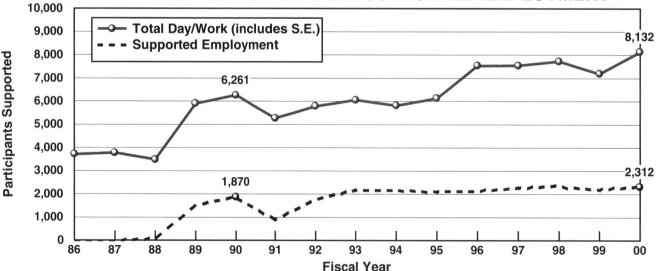

*Day/Work totals for 1991-98 do not include data for some private provider day programs; these data were not available.

Source: The Coleman Institute and Department of Psychiatry, University of Colorado, 2002.

TRENDS IN SPENDING

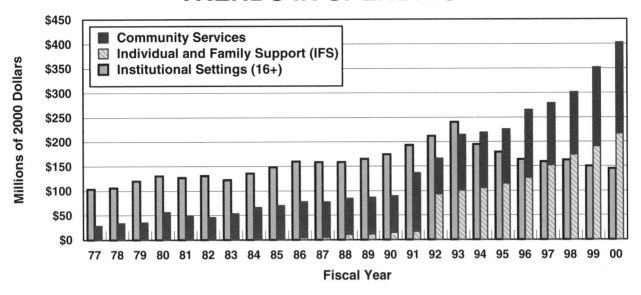

FISCAL EFFORT

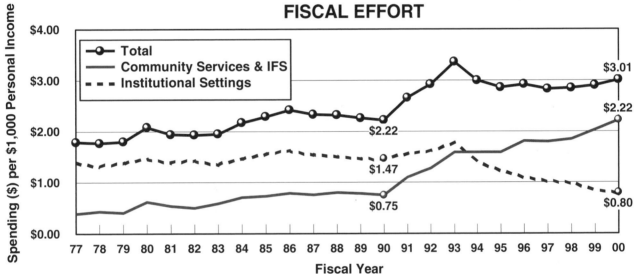

TOTAL MR/DD SPENDING AND
UNMATCHED STATE/LOCAL FUNDS

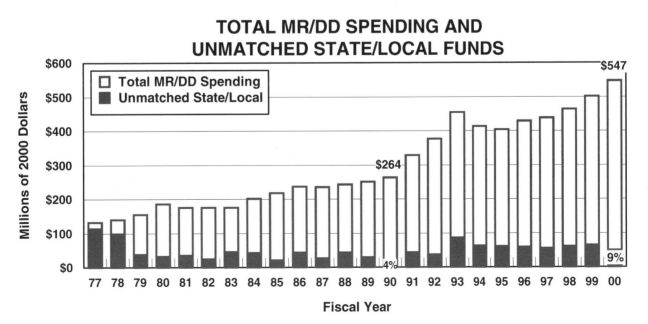

Source: The Coleman Institute and Department of Psychiatry, University of Colorado, 2002.

331

TRENDS IN REVENUE

COMMUNITY SERVICES REVENUE IN 2000

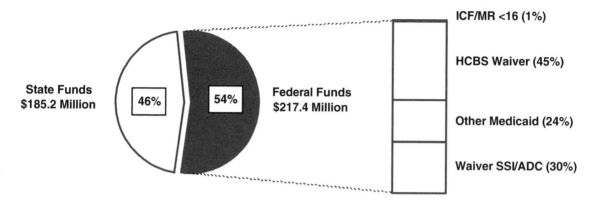

State Funds
$185.2 Million

46%

54%

Federal Funds
$217.4 Million

ICF/MR <16 (1%)

HCBS Waiver (45%)

Other Medicaid (24%)

Waiver SSI/ADC (30%)

Total: $402.5 Million

COMPONENTS OF FEDERAL MR/DD MEDICAID REVENUE

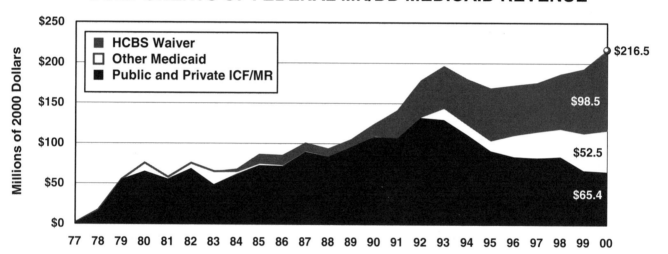

- HCBS Waiver
- Other Medicaid
- Public and Private ICF/MR

$216.5

$98.5

$52.5

$65.4

Millions of 2000 Dollars

Fiscal Year

HCBS WAIVER PARTICIPANTS

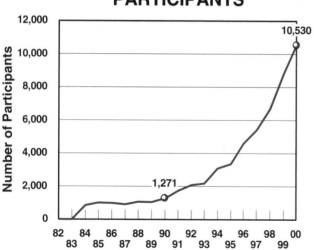

Number of Participants

10,530

1,271

WAIVER SPENDING PER PARTICIPANT

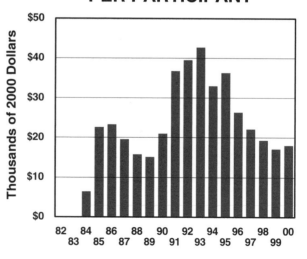

Thousands of 2000 Dollars

Source: The Coleman Institute and Department of Psychiatry, University of Colorado, 2002.

TRENDS IN RESIDENTIAL SERVICES

PERSONS SERVED BY SETTING IN 2000

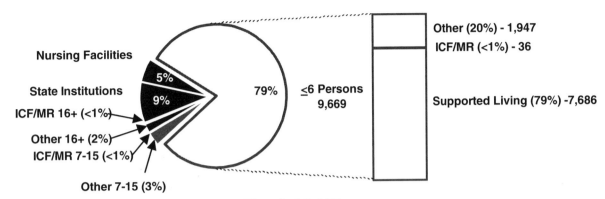

Total: 12,167

PERSONS SERVED BY SETTING

	1990	1991	1992	1993	1994	1995	1996	1997	1998	1999	2000
TOTAL	5,333	5,441	5,328	5,874	6,149	6,441	10,516	10,846	11,460	11,531	12,167
16+ PERSONS	2,743	2,633	2,476	2,416	2,217	2,200	2,476	2,398	2,338	2,190	2,089
Nursing Facilities	523	627	571	594	580	609	646	665	652	659	659
State Institutions	1,605	1,535	1,498	1,464	1,346	1,307	1,295	1,260	1,232	1,189	1,138
Private ICF/MR	397	252	215	190	140	137	114	108	93	40	37
Other Residential	218	219	192	168	151	147	421	365	361	302	255
7-15 PERSONS	461	437	440	404	411	380	400	380	358	390	409
Public ICF/MR	0	0	0	0	0	0	0	0	0	0	0
Private ICF/MR	56	48	50	50	42	42	24	24	16	22	18
Other Residential	405	389	390	354	369	338	376	356	342	368	391
≤6 PERSONS	2,129	2,371	2,412	3,054	3,521	3,861	7,640	8,068	8,764	8,951	9,669
Public ICF/MR	0	0	0	0	0	0	0	0	0	0	0
Private ICF/MR	72	76	76	70	70	70	41	41	36	36	36
Other Residential	2,057	2,295	2,336	2,984	3,451	3,791	7,599	8,027	8,728	8,915	9,633

PERSONS SERVED IN PUBLIC AND PRIVATE INSTITUTIONS AND NURSING FACILITIES

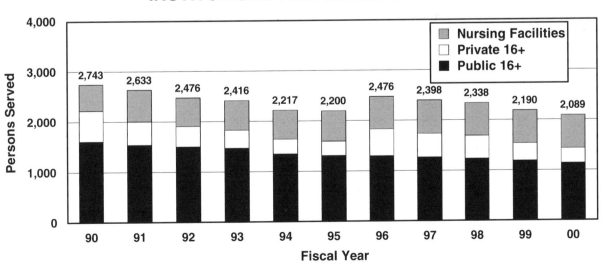

Source: The Coleman Institute and Department of Psychiatry, University of Colorado, 2002.

INDIVIDUAL AND FAMILY SUPPORT

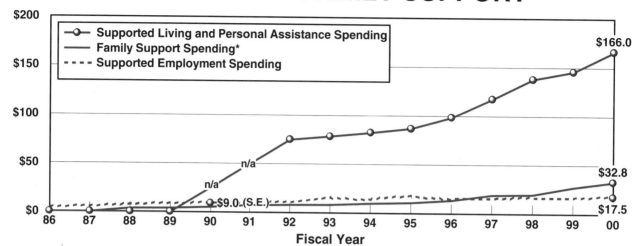

*Family Support includes the Family Support Program, MPC Child, and Voluntary Placement Program services to persons in-home.

PARTICIPANTS AND SPENDING LEVELS

	1990	1991	1992	1993	1994	1995	1996	1997	1998	1999	2000
TOTAL IFS ($)	n/a	n/a	76,289,536	84,915,652	90,927,590	101,715,246	114,707,057	140,419,205	164,031,295	182,882,694	216,289,718
INDIVIDUAL SUPPORT ($)	n/a	n/a	69,884,051	78,087,466	82,656,347	92,250,109	102,488,336	122,892,583	145,573,666	156,738,693	183,538,519
Supported Employment ($)	6,950,054	7,566,180	8,822,954	12,675,344	12,120,706	15,711,436	13,630,345	14,449,178	15,514,970	16,421,163	17,505,588
# of Persons	1,988	2,014	2,606	2,157	2,410	2,585	2,764	2,877	3,017	3,149	3,247
Supported Living ($)	n/a	n/a	61,061,097	65,412,122	70,535,641	76,538,673	74,843,035	85,790,657	102,680,375	105,951,973	125,480,390
# of Persons	n/a	n/a	2,172	2,259	2,450	2,511	2,731	2,746	2,753	3,558	3,713
Personal Assistance ($)	0	0	0	0	0	0	14,014,956	22,652,748	27,378,321	34,365,557	40,552,541
# of Persons	0	0	0	0	0	0	2,342	2,781	3,108	3,453	3,973
FAMILY SUPPORT ($)	4,028,173	5,685,558	6,405,485	6,828,186	8,271,243	9,465,137	12,218,721	17,526,622	18,457,629	26,144,001	32,751,199
Total Families	1,549	1,817	1,754	2,083	2,446	2,599	3,695	4,509	4,782	5,795	7,095
Cash Subsidy/Payment ($)	0	0	0	0	0	0	0	0	0	0	0
# of Families	0	0	0	0	0	0	0	0	0	0	0
Other Family Support ($)	4,028,173	5,685,558	6,405,485	6,828,186	8,271,243	9,465,137	12,218,721	17,526,622	18,457,629	26,144,001	32,751,199
# of Families	1,549	1,817	1,754	2,083	2,446	2,599	3,695	4,509	4,782	5,795	7,095

PARTICIPANTS IN DAY/WORK AND SUPPORTED EMPLOYMENT

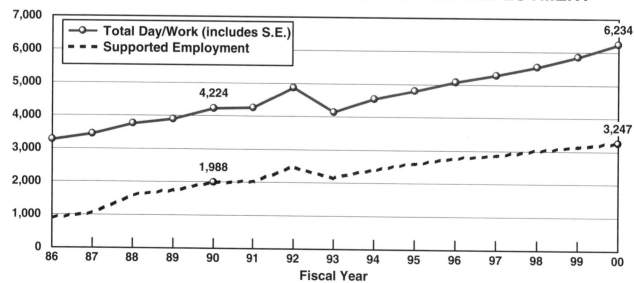

* In FY 1993 the reporting changed from authorizations to payment data.

Source: The Coleman Institute and Department of Psychiatry, University of Colorado, 2002.

TRENDS IN SPENDING

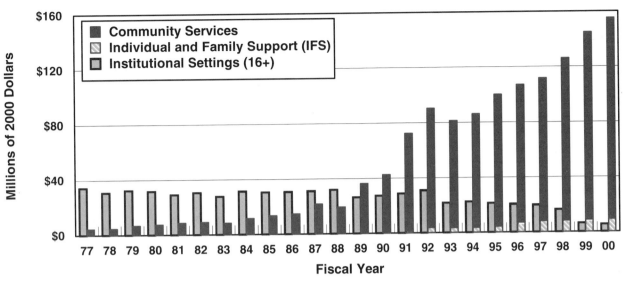

FISCAL EFFORT

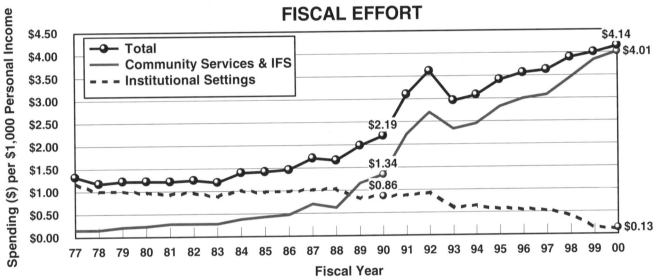

TOTAL MR/DD SPENDING AND
UNMATCHED STATE/LOCAL FUNDS

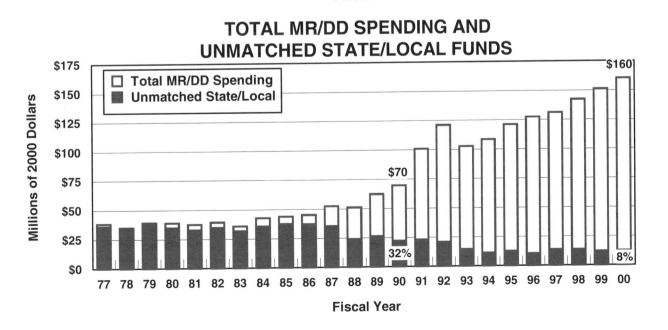

Source: The Coleman Institute and Department of Psychiatry, University of Colorado, 2002.

TRENDS IN REVENUE

COMMUNITY SERVICES REVENUE IN 2000

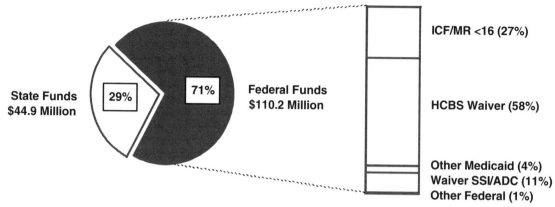

State Funds
$44.9 Million

29%

71%

Federal Funds
$110.2 Million

ICF/MR <16 (27%)

HCBS Waiver (58%)

Other Medicaid (4%)
Waiver SSI/ADC (11%)
Other Federal (1%)

Total: $155.2 Million

COMPONENTS OF FEDERAL MR/DD MEDICAID REVENUE

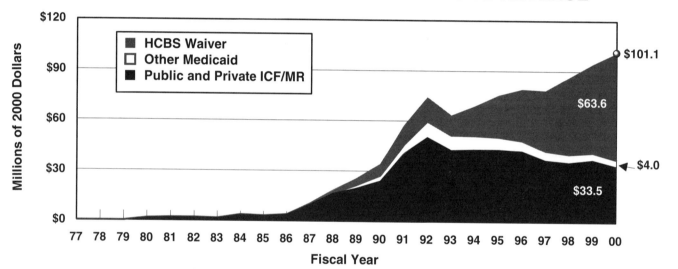

Millions of 2000 Dollars

- ■ HCBS Waiver
- □ Other Medicaid
- ■ Public and Private ICF/MR

$120

$90

$60

$30

$0

$101.1

$63.6

$4.0

$33.5

77 78 79 80 81 82 83 84 85 86 87 88 89 90 91 92 93 94 95 96 97 98 99 00

Fiscal Year

HCBS WAIVER PARTICIPANTS

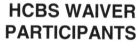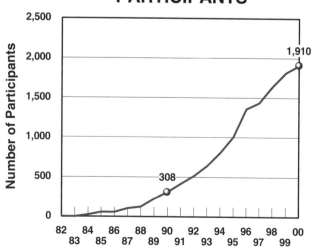

Number of Participants

2,500

2,000

1,500

1,000

500

0

1,910

308

82 83 84 85 86 87 88 89 90 91 92 93 94 95 96 97 98 99 00

WAIVER SPENDING PER PARTICIPANT

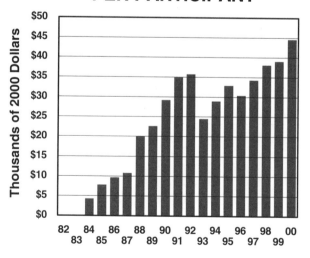

Thousands of 2000 Dollars

$50
$45
$40
$35
$30
$25
$20
$15
$10
$5
$0

82 83 84 85 86 87 88 89 90 91 92 93 94 95 96 97 98 99 00

Source: The Coleman Institute and Department of Psychiatry, University of Colorado, 2002.

TRENDS IN RESIDENTIAL SERVICES

PERSONS SERVED BY SETTING IN 2000

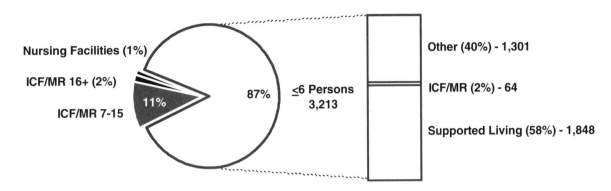

Nursing Facilities (1%)

ICF/MR 16+ (2%)

ICF/MR 7-15

11%

87%

≤6 Persons
3,213

Other (40%) - 1,301

ICF/MR (2%) - 64

Supported Living (58%) - 1,848

Total: 3,702

PERSONS SERVED BY SETTING

	1990	1991	1992	1993	1994	1995	1996	1997	1998	1999	2000
TOTAL	1,335	1,403	3,259	3,382	3,462	3,543	3,657	3,723	3,753	3,614	3,702
16+ PERSONS	598	517	410	386	347	308	303	272	221	92	99
Nursing Facilities	225	211	164	164	164	164	164	148	133	33	40
State Institutions	308	189	125	113	109	85	80	65	29	0	0
Private ICF/MR	65	117	121	109	74	59	59	59	59	59	59
Other Residential	0	0	0	0	0	0	0	0	0	0	0
7-15 PERSONS	389	503	532	575	612	649	686	486	486	390	390
Public ICF/MR	0	0	0	0	0	0	0	0	0	0	0
Private ICF/MR	271	377	384	390	390	390	390	390	390	390	390
Other Residential	118	126	148	185	222	259	296	96	96	0	0
≤6 PERSONS	348	383	2,317	2,421	2,503	2,586	2,668	2,965	3,046	3,132	3,213
Public ICF/MR	0	0	0	0	0	0	0	0	0	0	0
Private ICF/MR	30	42	43	64	64	64	64	64	64	65	64
Other Residential	318	341	2,274	2,357	2,439	2,522	2,604	2,901	2,982	3,067	3,149

PERSONS SERVED IN PUBLIC AND PRIVATE INSTITUTIONS AND NURSING FACILITIES

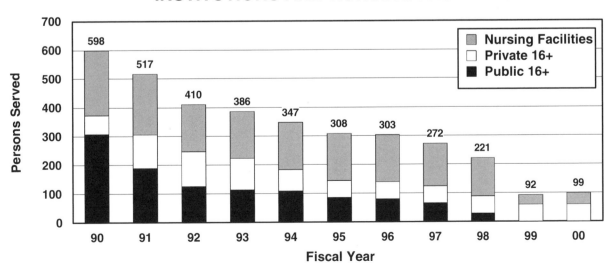

Source: The Coleman Institute and Department of Psychiatry, University of Colorado, 2002.

INDIVIDUAL AND FAMILY SUPPORT

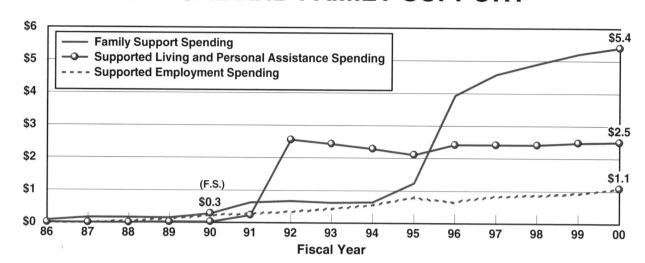

PARTICIPANTS AND SPENDING LEVELS

	1990	1991	1992	1993	1994	1995	1996	1997	1998	1999	2000
TOTAL IFS ($)	386,227	900,835	2,916,779	2,896,466	2,988,205	3,653,942	6,328,523	7,223,226	7,694,456	8,281,231	8,977,175
INDIVIDUAL SUPPORT ($)	171,377	400,835	2,368,529	2,376,466	2,434,086	2,565,337	2,774,783	2,990,226	3,070,120	3,265,977	3,579,980
Supported Employment ($)	150,393	214,340	278,286	342,233	478,283	707,623	592,413	760,460	792,743	876,358	1,078,107
# of Persons	208	273	385	350	273	290	408	425	439	441	390
Supported Living ($)	0	0	0	0	0	0	509,479	707,610	884,512	1,061,400	1,238,300
# of Persons	0	0	0	0	0	0	144	200	250	300	350
Personal Assistance ($)	20,984	186,495	2,090,243	2,034,233	1,955,803	1,857,714	1,672,891	1,522,157	1,392,865	1,328,219	1,263,573
# of Persons	211	1,391	1,872	1,822	1,752	1,664	1,498	1,498	1,498	1,498	1,498
FAMILY SUPPORT ($)	214,850	500,000	548,250	520,000	554,119	1,088,605	3,553,740	4,233,000	4,624,336	5,015,254	5,397,195
Total Families	145	450	n/a	1,082	1,334	1,660	2,140	1,977	2,461	1,870	2,031
Cash Subsidy/Payment ($)	0	0	0	0	0	0	0	0	0	0	0
# of Families	0	0	0	0	0	0	0	0	0	0	0
Other Family Support ($)	214,850	500,000	548,250	520,000	554,119	1,088,605	3,553,740	4,233,000	4,624,336	5,015,254	5,397,195
# of Families	145	450	n/a	1,082	1,334	1,660	2,140	1,977	2,461	1,870	2,031

PARTICIPANTS IN DAY/WORK AND SUPPORTED EMPLOYMENT

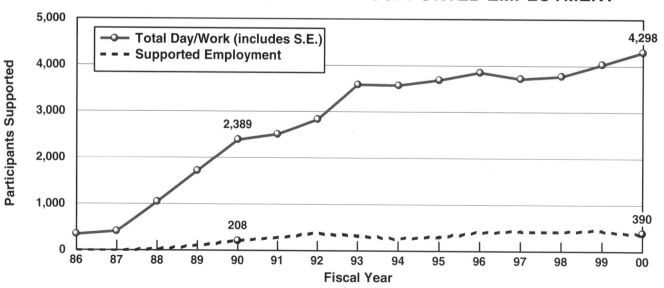

Source: The Coleman Institute and Department of Psychiatry, University of Colorado, 2002.

TRENDS IN SPENDING

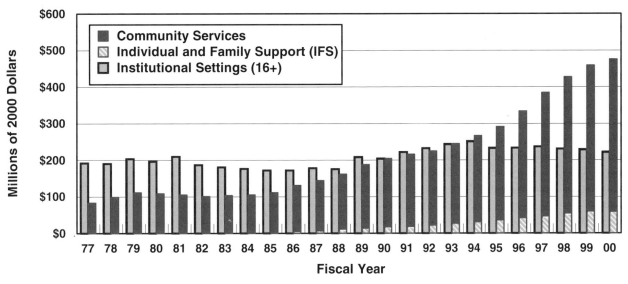

- **Community Services**
- **Individual and Family Support (IFS)**
- **Institutional Settings (16+)**

Millions of 2000 Dollars

Fiscal Year

FISCAL EFFORT

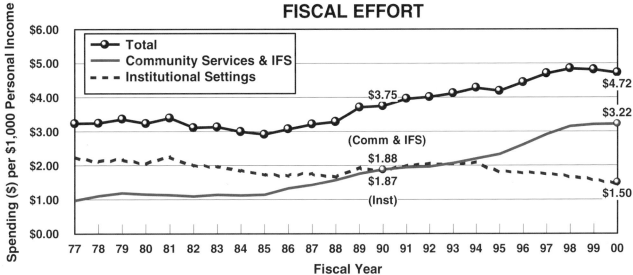

Spending ($) per $1,000 Personal Income

- **Total**
- **Community Services & IFS**
- **Institutional Settings**

$3.75

(Comm & IFS)
$1.88
$1.87
(Inst)

$4.72
$3.22
$1.50

Fiscal Year

TOTAL MR/DD SPENDING AND UNMATCHED STATE/LOCAL FUNDS

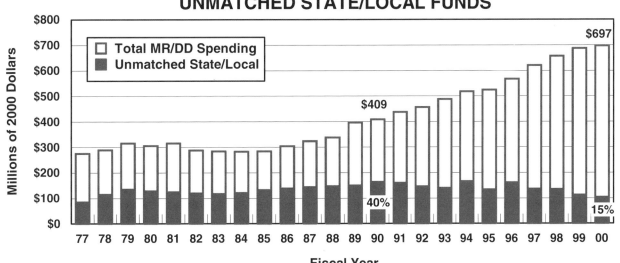

Millions of 2000 Dollars

- ☐ **Total MR/DD Spending**
- ■ **Unmatched State/Local**

$697
$409
40%
15%

Fiscal Year

Source: The Coleman Institute and Department of Psychiatry, University of Colorado, 2002.

TRENDS IN REVENUE

COMMUNITY SERVICES REVENUE IN 2000

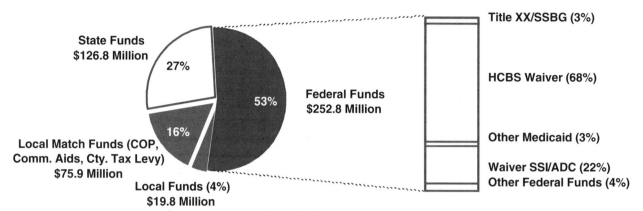

State Funds
$126.8 Million

27%

53%

16%

Federal Funds
$252.8 Million

Local Match Funds (COP,
Comm. Aids, Cty. Tax Levy)
$75.9 Million

Local Funds (4%)
$19.8 Million

Title XX/SSBG (3%)

HCBS Waiver (68%)

Other Medicaid (3%)

Waiver SSI/ADC (22%)
Other Federal Funds (4%)

Total: $475.3 Million

COMPONENTS OF FEDERAL MR/DD MEDICAID REVENUE

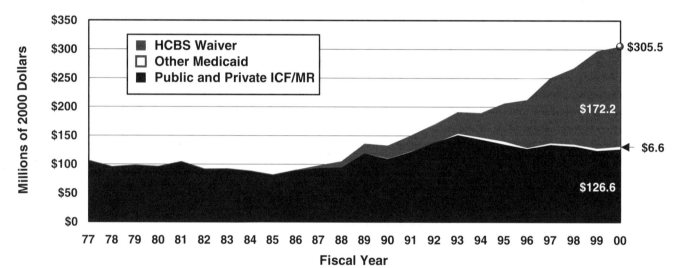

Millions of 2000 Dollars

- HCBS Waiver
- Other Medicaid
- Public and Private ICF/MR

$305.5
$172.2
$6.6
$126.6

Fiscal Year

HCBS WAIVER PARTICIPANTS

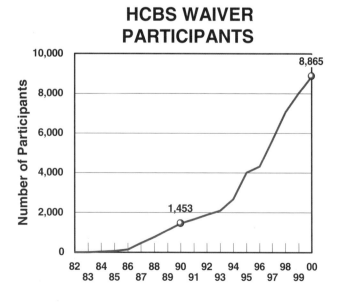

Number of Participants

8,865

1,453

WAIVER SPENDING PER PARTICIPANT

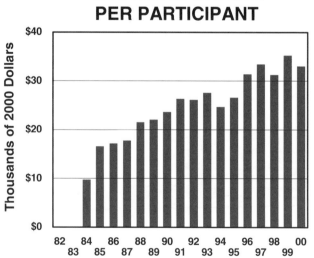

Thousands of 2000 Dollars

Source: The Coleman Institute and Department of Psychiatry, University of Colorado, 2002.

TRENDS IN RESIDENTIAL SERVICES

PERSONS SERVED BY SETTING IN 2000

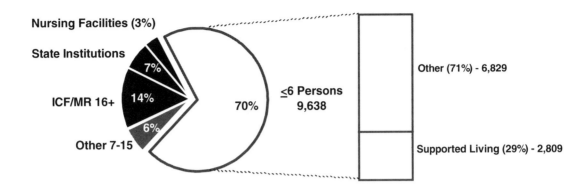

Nursing Facilities (3%)

State Institutions

ICF/MR 16+

Other 7-15

7%

14%

6%

70%

≤6 Persons
9,638

Other (71%) - 6,829

Supported Living (29%) - 2,809

Total: 13,799

PERSONS SERVED BY SETTING

	1990	1991	1992	1993	1994	1995	1996	1997	1998	1999	2000
TOTAL	12,810	12,367	10,899	12,014	12,885	13,622	12,468	13,062	13,278	13,671	13,799
16+ PERSONS	5,660	5,123	4,921	5,009	4,847	4,470	4,171	3,897	3,613	3,479	3,342
Nursing Facilities	1,734	961	857	893	840	748	664	555	496	495	471
State Institutions	1,678	1,640	1,581	1,505	1,492	1,336	1,214	1,219	1,056	968	899
Private ICF/MR	2,181	2,492	2,449	2,566	2,470	2,334	2,241	2,071	2,019	1,982	1,936
Other Residential	67	30	34	45	45	52	52	52	42	34	36
7-15 PERSONS	3,518	3,302	984	914	914	914	896	847	839	825	819
Public ICF/MR	0	0	0	0	0	0	0	0	0	0	0
Private ICF/MR	70	70	70	0	0	0	0	0	0	0	0
Other Residential	3,448	3,232	914	914	914	914	896	847	839	825	819
≤6 PERSONS	3,632	3,942	4,994	6,091	7,124	8,238	7,401	8,318	8,826	9,367	9,638
Public ICF/MR	0	0	0	0	0	0	0	0	0	0	0
Private ICF/MR	0	0	0	0	0	0	0	0	0	0	0
Other Residential	3,632	3,942	4,994	6,091	7,124	8,238	7,401	8,318	8,826	9,367	9,638

PERSONS SERVED IN PUBLIC AND PRIVATE INSTITUTIONS AND NURSING FACILITIES

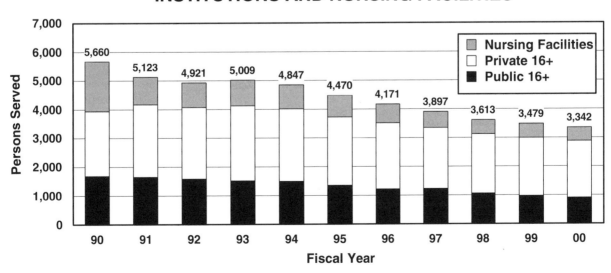

Source: The Coleman Institute and Department of Psychiatry, University of Colorado, 2002.

341

INDIVIDUAL AND FAMILY SUPPORT

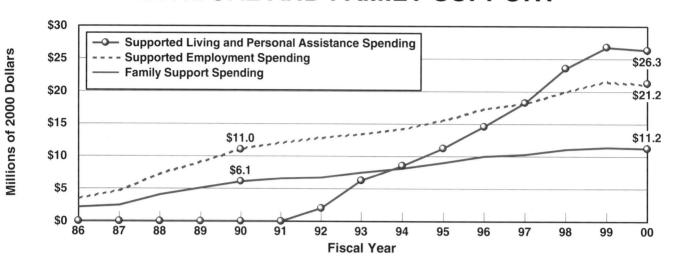

PARTICIPANTS AND SPENDING LEVELS

	1990	1991	1992	1993	1994	1995	1996	1997	1998	1999	2000
TOTAL IFS ($)	13,179,858	14,874,412	17,628,581	22,699,228	26,399,911	31,577,605	37,839,550	43,094,452	51,493,872	57,579,692	58,782,882
INDIVIDUAL SUPPORT ($)	8,489,628	9,576,519	12,123,761	16,429,090	19,401,057	23,595,316	28,777,611	33,546,798	41,029,586	46,578,074	47,545,089
Supported Employment ($)	8,489,628	9,576,519	10,485,943	11,178,251	12,063,638	13,679,964	15,602,231	16,691,993	18,811,817	20,775,701	21,240,405
# of Persons	2,452	2,725	3,091	2,955	3,192	3,346	3,612	3,861	4,031	4,170	4,157
Supported Living ($)	0	0	1,637,818	4,703,953	6,247,990	8,119,832	9,746,735	11,691,784	15,687,561	17,588,770	17,166,801
# of Persons	0	0	159	542	924	1,137	1,275	1,417	1,497	1,549	1,541
Personal Assistance ($)	0	0	0	546,886	1,089,429	1,795,520	3,428,645	5,163,021	6,530,208	8,213,603	9,137,883
# of Persons	0	0	0	83	160	256	474	697	906	1,140	1,268
FAMILY SUPPORT ($)	4,690,230	5,297,893	5,504,820	6,270,138	6,998,854	7,982,289	9,061,939	9,547,654	10,464,286	11,001,618	11,237,793
Total Families	4,255	4,805	5,067	4,907	5,158	5,757	6,098	6,140	6,310	6,760	6,908
Cash Subsidy/Payment ($)	0	0	0	0	0	0	0	0	0	0	0
# of Families	0	0	0	0	0	0	0	0	0	0	0
Other Family Support ($)	4,690,230	5,297,893	5,504,820	6,270,138	6,998,854	7,982,289	9,061,939	9,547,654	10,464,286	11,001,618	11,237,793
# of Families	4,255	4,805	5,067	4,907	5,158	5,757	6,098	6,140	6,310	6,760	6,908

PARTICIPANTS IN DAY/WORK AND SUPPORTED EMPLOYMENT

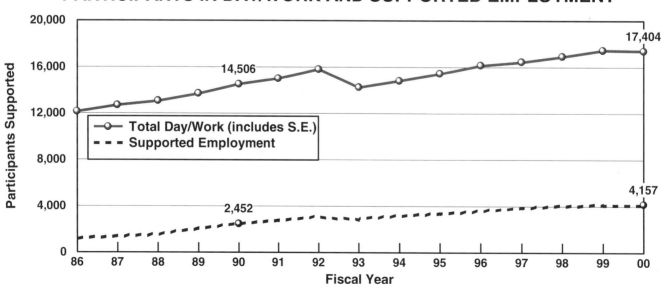

Source: The Coleman Institute and Department of Psychiatry, University of Colorado, 2002.

TRENDS IN SPENDING

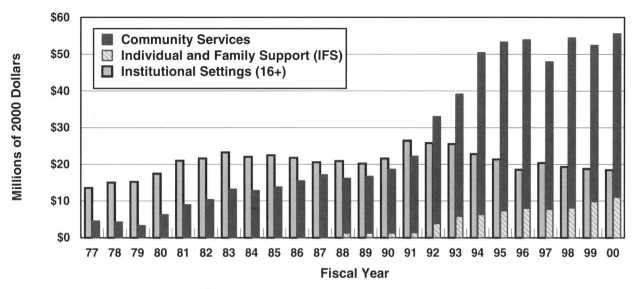

- **Community Services**
- **Individual and Family Support (IFS)**
- **Institutional Settings (16+)**

Millions of 2000 Dollars

Fiscal Year

FISCAL EFFORT

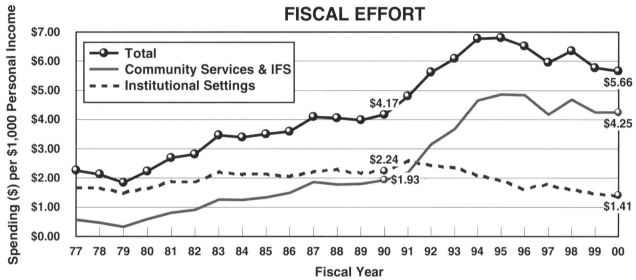

Spending ($) per $1,000 Personal Income

- **Total**
- **Community Services & IFS**
- **Institutional Settings**

$4.17
$5.66
$4.25
$2.24
$1.93
$1.41

Fiscal Year

TOTAL MR/DD SPENDING AND
UNMATCHED STATE/LOCAL FUNDS

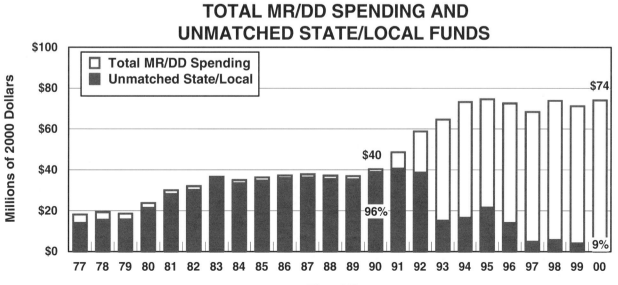

- **Total MR/DD Spending**
- **Unmatched State/Local**

Millions of 2000 Dollars

$40
96%
$74
9%

Fiscal Year

Source: The Coleman Institute and Department of Psychiatry, University of Colorado, 2002.

TRENDS IN REVENUE

COMMUNITY SERVICES REVENUE IN 2000

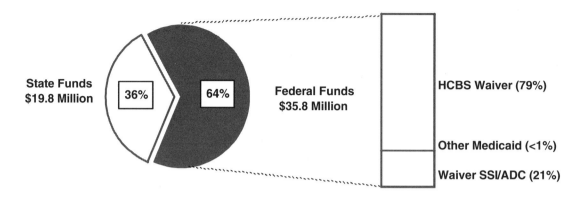

State Funds
$19.8 Million

36%

64%

Federal Funds
$35.8 Million

HCBS Waiver (79%)

Other Medicaid (<1%)

Waiver SSI/ADC (21%)

Total: $55.6 Million

COMPONENTS OF FEDERAL MR/DD MEDICAID REVENUE

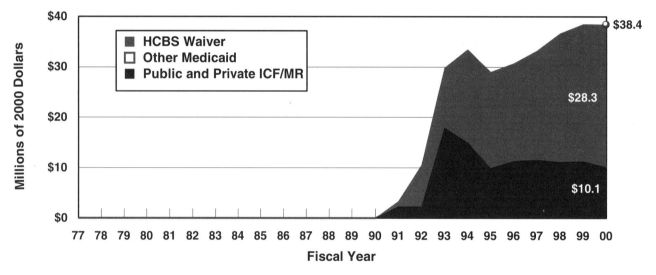

Millions of 2000 Dollars

- ■ HCBS Waiver
- □ Other Medicaid
- ■ Public and Private ICF/MR

$40
$30
$20
$10
$0

$38.4
$28.3
$10.1

77 78 79 80 81 82 83 84 85 86 87 88 89 90 91 92 93 94 95 96 97 98 99 00

Fiscal Year

HCBS WAIVER PARTICIPANTS

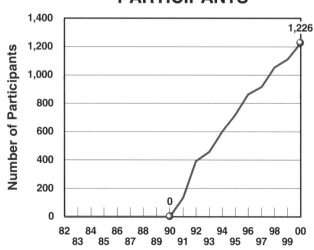

Number of Participants

1,400
1,200
1,000
800
600
400
200
0

1,226

0

82 84 86 88 90 92 94 96 98 00
83 85 87 89 91 93 95 97 99

WAIVER SPENDING PER PARTICIPANT

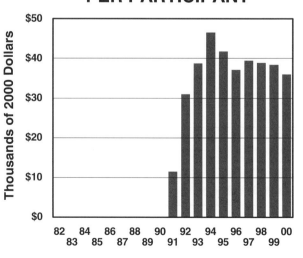

Thousands of 2000 Dollars

$50
$40
$30
$20
$10
$0

82 84 86 88 90 92 94 96 98 00
83 85 87 89 91 93 95 97 99

Source: The Coleman Institute and Department of Psychiatry, University of Colorado, 2002.

TRENDS IN RESIDENTIAL SERVICES

PERSONS SERVED BY SETTING IN 2000

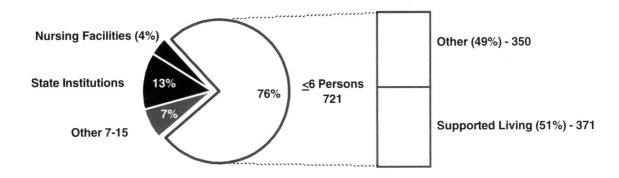

Nursing Facilities (4%)

State Institutions 13%

Other 7-15 7%

76%

≤6 Persons 721

Other (49%) - 350

Supported Living (51%) - 371

Total: 951

PERSONS SERVED BY SETTING

	1990	1991	1992	1993	1994	1995	1996	1997	1998	1999	2000
TOTAL	662	626	753	766	1,043	1,035	1,219	849	982	988	951
16+ PERSONS	352	290	308	243	198	180	188	184	176	173	163
Nursing Facilities	41	21	64	55	42	33	43	41	42	42	40
State Institutions	311	269	244	188	156	147	145	143	134	131	123
Private ICF/MR	0	0	0	0	0	0	0	0	0	0	0
Other Residential	0	0	0	0	0	0	0	0	0	0	0
7-15 PERSONS	170	170	114	111	64	60	75	55	91	87	67
Public ICF/MR	0	0	0	0	0	0	0	0	0	0	0
Private ICF/MR	0	0	0	0	0	0	0	0	0	0	0
Other Residential	170	170	114	111	64	60	75	55	91	87	67
≤6 PERSONS	140	166	331	412	781	795	956	610	715	728	721
Public ICF/MR	0	0	0	0	0	0	0	0	0	0	0
Private ICF/MR	0	0	0	0	0	0	0	0	0	0	0
Other Residential	140	166	331	412	781	795	956	610	715	728	721

PERSONS SERVED IN PUBLIC AND PRIVATE INSTITUTIONS AND NURSING FACILITIES

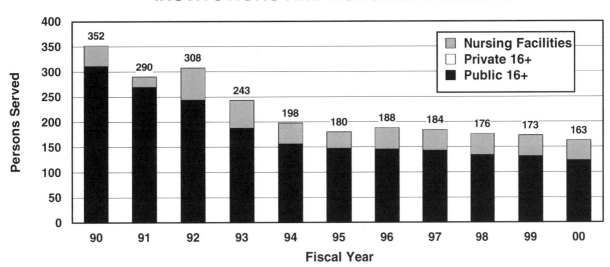

Persons Served

Fiscal Year

- Nursing Facilities
- Private 16+
- Public 16+

Source: The Coleman Institute and Department of Psychiatry, University of Colorado, 2002.

INDIVIDUAL AND FAMILY SUPPORT

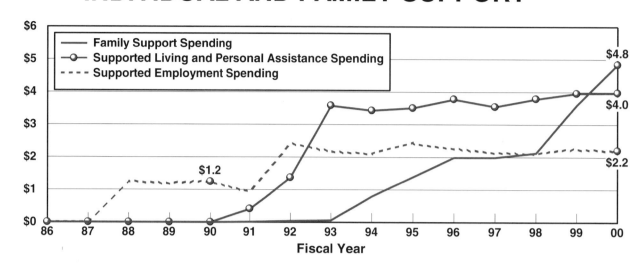

PARTICIPANTS AND SPENDING LEVELS

	1990	1991	1992	1993	1994	1995	1996	1997	1998	1999	2000
TOTAL IFS ($)	960,000	1,093,944	3,149,301	4,878,684	5,435,519	6,468,083	7,265,785	7,105,852	7,600,578	9,463,451	11,018,758
INDIVIDUAL SUPPORT ($)	960,000	1,087,883	3,118,181	4,826,496	4,753,359	5,238,268	5,465,828	5,261,821	5,589,342	5,992,992	6,177,627
Supported Employment ($)	960,000	761,061	1,995,616	1,826,496	1,809,584	2,139,368	2,046,352	1,978,704	2,012,528	2,173,462	2,202,627
# of Persons	120	160	236	216	214	253	242	234	238	305	317
Supported Living ($)	0	326,822	1,122,565	3,000,000	2,943,775	3,098,900	3,419,476	3,283,117	3,576,814	3,819,530	3,975,000
# of Persons	0	23	79	113	218	217	326	313	341	405	371
Personal Assistance ($)	0	0	0	0	0	0	0	0	0	0	0
# of Persons	0	0	0	0	0	0	0	0	0	0	0
FAMILY SUPPORT ($)	0	6,061	31,120	52,188	682,160	1,229,815	1,799,957	1,844,031	2,011,236	3,470,459	4,841,131
Total Families	0	4	13	21	236	321	414	426	512	621	641
Cash Subsidy/Payment ($)	0	0	0	0	0	0	0	0	0	0	0
# of Families	0	0	0	0	0	0	0	0	0	0	0
Other Family Support ($)	0	6,061	31,120	52,188	682,160	1,229,815	1,799,957	1,844,031	2,011,236	3,470,459	4,841,131
# of Families	0	4	13	21	236	321	414	426	512	621	641

PARTICIPANTS IN DAY/WORK AND SUPPORTED EMPLOYMENT

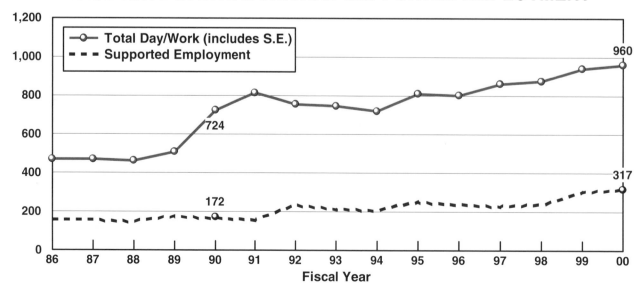

Source: The Coleman Institute and Department of Psychiatry, University of Colorado, 2002.

TRENDS IN SPENDING

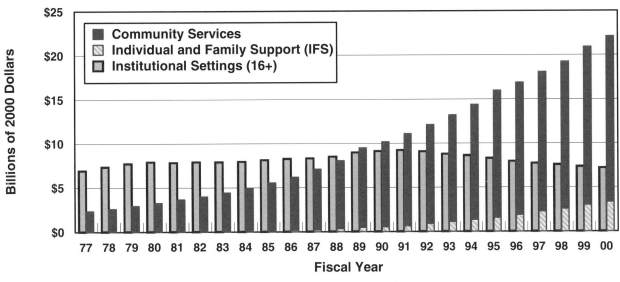

FISCAL EFFORT

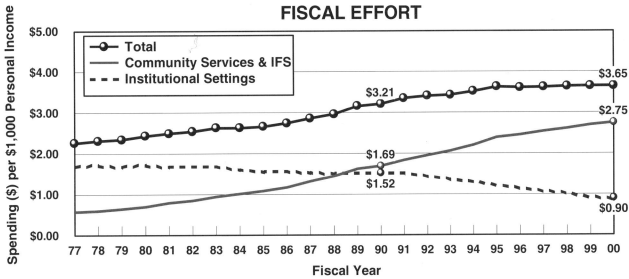

TOTAL MR/DD SPENDING AND
UNMATCHED STATE/LOCAL FUNDS

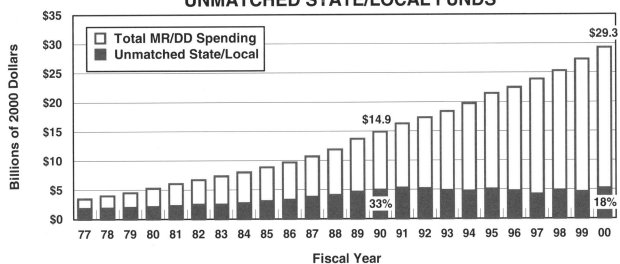

Source: The Coleman Institute and Department of Psychiatry, University of Colorado, 2002.

TRENDS IN REVENUE

COMMUNITY SERVICES REVENUE IN 2000

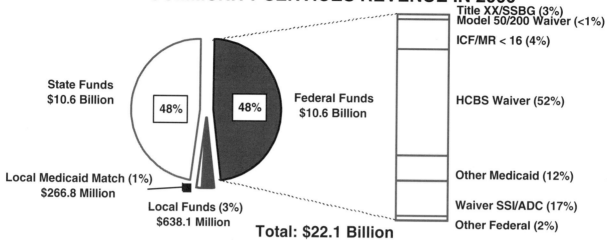

Title XX/SSBG (3%)
Model 50/200 Waiver (<1%)
ICF/MR < 16 (4%)
HCBS Waiver (52%)
Other Medicaid (12%)
Waiver SSI/ADC (17%)
Other Federal (2%)

State Funds
$10.6 Billion — 48%

Federal Funds
$10.6 Billion — 48%

Local Medicaid Match (1%)
$266.8 Million

Local Funds (3%)
$638.1 Million

Total: $22.1 Billion

COMPONENTS OF FEDERAL MR/DD MEDICAID REVENUE

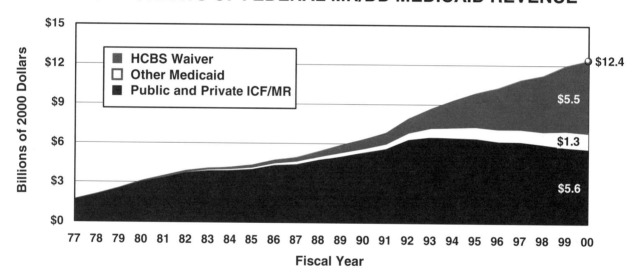

- HCBS Waiver
- Other Medicaid
- Public and Private ICF/MR

$12.4
$5.5
$1.3
$5.6

Billions of 2000 Dollars

Fiscal Year

HCBS WAIVER PARTICIPANTS

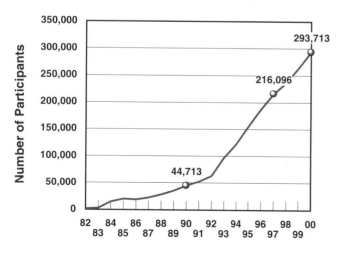

293,713
216,096
44,713

Number of Participants

WAIVER SPENDING PER PARTICIPANT

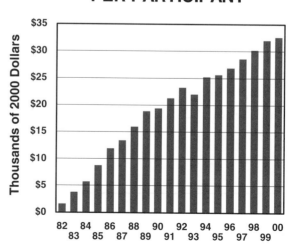

Thousands of 2000 Dollars

Source: The Coleman Institute and Department of Psychiatry, University of Colorado, 2002.

TRENDS IN RESIDENTIAL SERVICES

PERSONS SERVED BY SETTING IN 2000

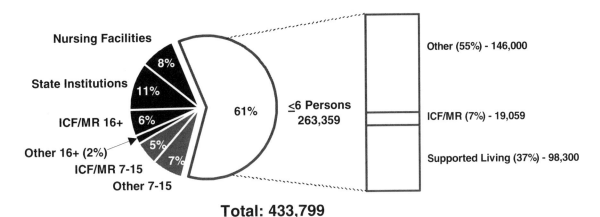

Total: 433,799

PERSONS SERVED BY SETTING

	1990	1991	1992	1993	1994	1995	1996	1997	1998	1999	2000
TOTAL	323,479	328,964	355,868	359,478	368,328	380,721	390,586	401,559	412,785	422,351	433,799
16+ PERSONS	176,037	169,841	168,103	158,288	151,827	145,442	137,618	131,012	125,424	119,022	116,527
Nursing Facilities	44,903	42,696	44,291	41,759	40,752	40,249	38,960	37,229	36,252	35,132	34,743
State Institutions	84,818	81,245	77,600	73,032	68,867	64,187	59,775	56,343	52,754	49,276	47,374
Private ICF/MR	32,926	33,091	33,577	32,222	31,204	30,752	28,777	27,744	27,271	26,218	26,107
Other Residential	13,389	12,809	12,635	11,276	11,004	10,255	10,106	9,696	9,147	8,396	8,303
7-15 PERSONS	78,819	81,072	59,016	55,458	54,883	55,755	54,493	54,399	53,672	53,255	53,913
Public ICF/MR	4,027	4,296	4,450	4,765	4,417	4,434	1,579	1,594	1,431	1,259	1,368
Private ICF/MR	21,008	23,312	23,238	22,343	22,834	23,197	23,443	22,949	22,813	21,818	21,927
Other Residential	53,784	53,464	31,328	28,350	27,632	28,124	29,471	29,856	29,428	30,178	30,618
≤6 PERSONS	68,623	78,052	128,749	145,732	161,618	179,524	198,475	216,148	233,689	250,074	263,359
Public ICF/MR	300	334	461	539	551	775	983	1,275	1,192	1,079	1,137
Private ICF/MR	8,940	10,027	12,450	14,342	15,756	17,303	18,001	19,083	19,269	17,904	17,922
Other Residential	59,383	67,691	115,838	130,851	145,312	161,446	179,491	195,790	213,228	231,091	244,300

PERSONS SERVED IN PUBLIC AND PRIVATE INSTITUTIONS AND NURSING FACILITIES

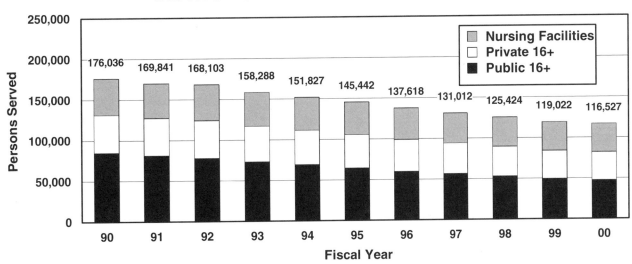

Source: The Coleman Institute and Department of Psychiatry, University of Colorado, 2002.

INDIVIDUAL AND FAMILY SUPPORT

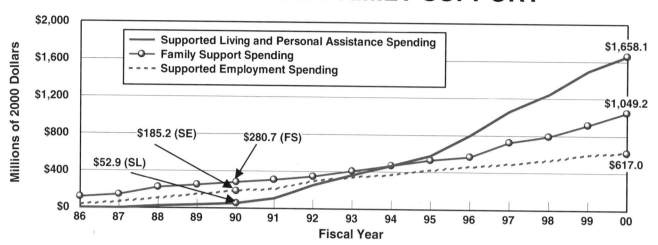

PARTICIPANTS AND SPENDING LEVELS

	1993	1994	1995	1996	1997	1998	1999	2000
TOTAL IFS ($)	926,923,053	1,121,542,547	1,348,405,574	1,657,168,060	2,107,811,126	2,417,993,992	2,890,806,497	3,324,296,279
INDIVIDUAL SUPPORT ($)	586,820,514	718,986,545	879,572,910	1,142,699,926	1,435,854,775	1,670,739,343	2,007,955,946	2,275,126,330
Supported Employment ($)	283,156,149	315,729,596	367,803,723	419,809,751	456,282,986	496,022,163	566,046,793	617,013,500
# of Persons	68,358	72,331	83,289	88,662	87,791	94,106	101,205	108,004
Supported Living ($)	281,000,597	367,377,685	462,568,976	628,921,360	834,365,015	999,694,708	1,272,167,558	1,462,822,420
# of Persons	26,417	30,519	37,052	43,294	52,065	59,319	74,111	79,474
Personal Assistance ($)*	22,663,769	35,879,263	49,200,211	93,968,814	145,206,774	175,022,473	169,741,595	195,290,410
# of Persons*	6,480	8,199	9,581	13,098	16,421	18,250	17,615	18,826
FAMILY SUPPORT ($)	340,102,539	402,556,002	468,832,664	514,468,134	671,956,351	747,254,649	882,850,551	1,049,169,949
Total Families	204,639	230,597	258,508	279,266	311,785	324,678	353,628	385,414
Cash Subsidy/Payment ($)	31,197,028	36,793,661	37,729,756	42,795,628	47,434,456	48,328,570	56,234,062	69,000,749
# of Families	13,024	15,268	15,943	17,495	18,943	20,893	23,313	25,802
Other Family Support ($)	308,905,511	365,762,341	431,102,908	471,672,506	624,521,895	698,926,080	826,616,489	980,159,200
# of Families	194,578	218,482	246,535	267,123	308,162	318,062	333,568	363,089

PARTICIPANTS IN DAY/WORK AND SUPPORTED EMPLOYMENT

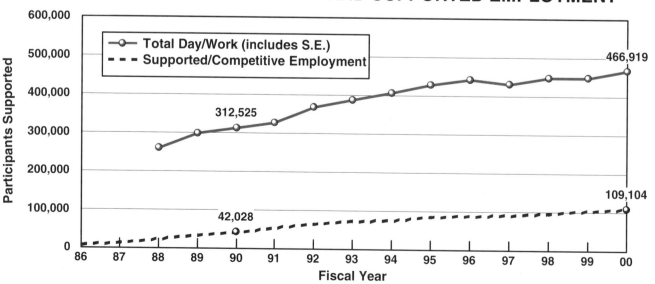

Source: The Coleman Institute and Department of Psychiatry, University of Colorado, 2002.

PART III

Forces Shaping Developmental Disabilities Services in the States: A Comparative Study

Forces Shaping Developmental Disabilities Services in the States: A Comparative Study

Susan L. Parish

INTRODUCTION

Background

Attitudes toward persons with developmental disabilities have undergone profound changes during the past three decades. Society's view that these individuals represented a burden to be segregated and medically treated has largely given way, replaced by notions that people with developmental disabilities are entitled to rights and respect. A philosophical orientation of normalization has gradually edged out segregationist conceptions of the role of people with developmental disabilities in contemporary American society.

Concurrently, the landscape of residential services for persons with developmental disabilities has changed dramatically during the past three decades. Public institutions, the mainstay of state service systems since the 19th century, have increasingly been supplanted by a network of community-based residential programs and supports (Part I, this volume). The magnitude of this transformation is such that since 1967, when the public institutional population peaked at nearly 200,000 persons, the census has declined by more than 140,000 persons. Residential services provided in the community, available to only a negligible number of persons in the 1960s, were received by nearly 400,000 persons with developmental disabilities in 2000. Furthermore, the complete closure of institutional facilities has accelerated. Between 1970 and 1984, Braddock and Heller (1985) identified 20 institutional closures in 12 states. By 2000, 125 facilities had either closed or were targeted for closure, as noted earlier in this volume.

Across the nation, this veritable revolution in the residential service system has occurred alongside many other dramatic changes. Federal legislation was enacted in 1975 that guaranteed children with disabilities the right to a free, appropriate, public education (Pub. L. 94-142, the Education for All Handicapped Children Act). Parent advocacy groups continued the organizing that they had begun in the 1950s, increasingly advocating for developmental disabilities services at the state, local, and national level (Part I, this volume). More than 70 class-action federal lawsuits demanding institutional reform or closure have been litigated (Hayden, 1997). Individuals with developmental disabilities have organized themselves into an advocacy group as well (Dybwad, 1996; *People First of Tennessee v. Arlington Developmental Ctr.,* 1992) with an agenda to close institutions across the nation (Nelis, 1995; Nelis & Ward, 1995). Federal legislation was enacted in 1981 that provided states with the option of funding for individualized services and supports through the Home and Community-Based Services (HCBS) Waiver (Braddock, Hemp, Parish, & Westrich, 1998). There have also been advances in the state of knowledge regarding supporting individuals with behavior problems and emotional disturbances (Braddock, 2001). These developments have contributed to a residential service system that is in tremendous flux.

Statement of the Problem

This picture of the national trend obscures the variability among the states that is a hallmark of our federalist system of government. No national policy mandates how residential services for people with developmental disabilities should be provided (Braddock, 1987). As such, the organization of services is controlled and directed by the individual states. While there are significant federal funding sources available for residential services, the states enjoy substantial latitude in defining the shape and extent of their residential service systems, and the allocation of resources within their borders. By 2000, nine states had closed all of their public institutions for persons with developmental disabilities, and were funding only community-based residential services. However, 10 other states still provided more than 40% of their residential services in institutions in 2000, as noted earlier in this volume. Clearly, not all states have vigorously embraced the transformation of residential service systems that began in the 1970s.

States have pursued deinstitutionalization programs in different ways and to different degrees. For example, New York aggressively depopulated its public developmental disabilities institutions, moving more than 16,000 people into community settings and other private institutional facilities between 1977 and 2000. However, the majority of New York's community-based residential services in 2000 were in settings for 7 to 15 persons, and not the smaller-scale settings preferred by advocates and some researchers (Biklen, 1991; O'Brien & O'Brien, 1991; Racino, 1991; Racino & Taylor, 1993; Taylor, 1991). Vermont, alternatively, eliminated its system of public institutional care in 1993, and provided nearly all residential placements in settings for four or fewer people, the majority in foster care (Braddock et al., 2002). Arkansas and Nevada, by way of contrast, had nearly the same numbers of people living in public institutions in 2000 as had been there in 1977. State variation is the rule in the provision of residential services for persons with developmental disabilities.

Why states vary in their provision of residential care is the chief question that emerges from even the most cursory examination of the status of residential services nationally. Why have states pursued deinstitutionalization and the development of community residential systems in such different ways? What factors contributed to the aggressive pursuit of community services in some states and the retention of institutional models of service delivery in others?

The issue of why states have pursued disparate paths in their provision of residential services is of paramount importance in the United States, for two important reasons. First, the operation of dual systems of community-based and institutional care systems is expensive for states, as economies of scale are less possible. As noted, only nine states had completely made the transition to community services, and closed all of their public institutions; every other state grappled with the issue of how to allocate resources between competing community and institutional programs.

The second important factor is there are large numbers of individuals who need, but do not receive, residential services. The number of people with de-

velopmental disabilities awaiting residential services was estimated to be 87,187 in 1996 (Prouty & Lakin, 1997). This represented 22% of the nation's total residential service system that year. In addition, 17 class-action lawsuits have been filed on behalf of people who are waiting for community residential placements (Smith, 2002). The need for residential services is extraordinary (Braddock, 1999; Davis, 1997). The aging of the nation's population will press the service system even beyond the extent to which it is currently stretched (Braddock, 1999). Ongoing commitments to institutional services make it more difficult for states to expand community services. For these two critical reasons, an investigation of the factors that influenced the differential adoption of community services in the states was pursued. The two states selected for this inquiry, Michigan and Illinois, as will be demonstrated, each represent one end of the spectrum of developing community-based residential services. Michigan led the nation in depopulating its public institutions in the 1970s and 1980s, rapidly developing community-based residences for persons with developmental disabilities. Illinois still lags the national trend to depopulate its public institutions, and has been quite slow to develop a community-based residential service system.

The objective of this investigation was to elucidate the reasons Michigan and Illinois pursued divergent paths in transforming, or not transforming, their institutional service systems to community-based services. The present study is a revised and updated version of the *Comparative study of the development of MR/DD services in two midwestern states: 1970-1990* (Parish, 2001).

LITERATURE REVIEW

The Deinstitutionalization Movement and Related Research

Public institutions began moving out people with developmental disabilities in the 1960s, discharging residents into community settings as well as into other types of institutions, including nursing homes and private institutions (Wolfensberger, 1971). Analyses of the factors related to deinstitutionalization have postulated that the passage of the Intermediate Care Facility for People with Mental Retardation program (ICF/MR), class-action litigation, and advocate pressure culminated in deinstitutionalization and the concurrent development of community-based services (Braddock, Hemp, Parish, Westrich, & Park, 1998; Hayden, 1997; Moss, 1983; Switzky, Dudzinsky, Van Acker, & Gambro, 1988; Topper, 1997). However, results of these analyses have been mixed.

The only systematic investigation of factors related to state-by-state deinstitutionalization efforts was Topper's (1997). She used multivariate regression analysis to identify the predictors of deinstitutionalization, which she operationalized as the percentage of people in a state's total residential service system living in public institutions (Topper, 1997). She found the factors that predicted deinstitutionalization in 1977 included whether or not states funded Supplemental Security Income (SSI), whether or not states received federal ICF/MR funds, and the daily costs of institutional care. However, these variables were no longer predictive in 1995, and the only variable she found to predict deinstitutionalization for that year was whether or not state legislatures were controlled by the Democratic Party. The fact that Topper was not able to find variables that had stable predictive powers over time suggests it would be useful to do more exploratory research into the way developmental disabilities policy is shaped in the states.

The preponderance of existing studies of deinstitutionalization has focused on individual outcomes for formerly institutionalized persons (e.g., Belcher, 1994; Lynch, Kellow, & Wilson, 1997; Spreat, Conroy, & Rice, 1998), on family members' perceptions of institutional versus community placement (e.g., Berry, 1995; Grimes & Vitello, 1990; Spreat, Telles, Conroy, & Feinstein, 1987) and on comparison of the costs of institutional versus community care (e.g., Knobbe, Carey, Rhodes, & Horner, 1995; Schalock & Fredericks, 1990). Another common form of research evaluating deinstitutionalization has been case studies based on single facilities in individual states. These case studies have included examinations of the extent to which formerly institutionalized persons remained in the community (e.g., Smith & Polloway, 1995), comprehensive evaluations of the closure of a single facility (e.g., Heller & Braddock, 1986; Rothman & Rothman, 1984), or a single state's deinstitutionaliza-

tion experience (e.g., Stone, 1990; Zirpoli & Wieck, 1989). A comparatively smaller body of literature has examined the impact of federal policy on community and institutional service systems (e.g., Boggs, Hanley-Maxwell, Lakin, & Bradley, 1988; Braddock, 1987; Smith & Gettings, 1994). These studies have delineated the ways in which federal policy evolved, the forces that shaped federal policy, and how state and federal developmental disabilities policies interact. They have particularly added value to the field by explicating the complexity of federal policy related to people with developmental disabilities, and the impact of this policy on the service system.

Determinants of State Policy

Historically, there have been several leading theories of the predictors or determinants of public policy in the political sciences field. These models are known as the economic, political socioeconomic, and cultural models (Calia, 1996). Economic models presume that economic indicators such as state wealth or slack resources predict the development of public policy (Dye, 1966), and therein wealthier states are expected to have greater levels of spending for social programs. The political socioeconomic model argues that both political and socioeconomic variables, such as wealth and party competition, interact as determinants of the development of policy (Hofferbert, 1966). Finally, the cultural model postulates that certain policy activities, such as state spending, are influenced by the extent to which the state's political culture can be characterized or classified as traditionalistic, moralistic, or individualistic (Elazar, 1984; Gray, 1999). The relationship between these models and the disability policy interest of the proposed investigation is the subject of this discussion.

Holbrook and Percy (1992) examined state variance in civil rights protections for persons with disabilities. They found that a history of positive governance and democratic strength in states with competitive two-party systems were predictors of strong civil rights protections for persons with disabilities. These researchers defined positive governance as "employing governmental powers to tax and regulate in order to achieve social objectives such as aiding disadvantaged groups" (Holbrook & Percy, 1992, p. 210).

Further, they found no support for other traditional political science predictors of social policy, including political ideology or socioeconomic indicators.

Within the field of developmental disabilities, Braddock and Fujiura (1987, 1991) examined the relevance of these political science models to states' spending for community services. They found that traditional predictors of social policy in the states, including state wealth and size, did not predict state spending for community services. In evaluating state spending patterns for developmental disabilities services, Braddock and his colleagues have consistently found that states that spend money for community services cannot be predicted by traditional models of social welfare spending (Braddock, Hemp, Bachelder, & Fujiura, 1995, 1998; Braddock & Fujiura, 1987, 1991). Instead, they found that states' historical commitment to civil rights and advocates' efforts are determinants of state spending for community services. As such, the analysis of state wealth does not provide adequate insight into why some states aggressively pursued deinstitutionalization, while others retained their institutional systems of care.

In light of the lack of clear evidence regarding the development of residential services for people with developmental disabilities in the U.S., this inquiry was conducted to facilitate the identification of all relevant factors, including those from the developmental disabilities literature, and those from the political science literature. The study design, described in greater detail in a subsequent section of the chapter, explains this structure more fully. However, due to the lack of consensus in the literature regarding the impact of an array of different factors, it was important for the present investigation not to preclude the identification of any.

Variables

To understand the complexities of the factors that influenced the development of community services in states that aggressively developed community services and those that did not, it is necessary to examine a broad array of suitable variables. Narrowly focused research can result in the omission of critical, influential factors. The work of previous political scientists and developmental disabilities researchers was used as the basis for identifying variables germane to this

analysis. These variables can be identified within the following categories: leadership, litigation, legislation, and sociopolitical factors. A discussion of these domains follows.

Personal leadership generally plays a pre-eminent role in the establishment of new social policies. Various theories of leadership have been developed, including the role of so-called agenda setters and public entrepreneurs (Kingdon, 1995; Schneider, Teske, & Mintrom, 1995). What is clear from these theories is that leadership is an essential element in the generation of social policy. Leadership in the developmental disabilities field is distributed among three distinct groups: persons with developmental disabilities, professionals, and family members of persons with developmental disabilities. While these categories may seem distinct, some people have membership in more than one group. For instance, President John Kennedy was both an elected official and the brother of a woman with a developmental disability.

The assumption of leadership roles by persons with developmental disabilities has been an important recent advancement in the field. For example, the self-advocacy group People First successfully sued the state of Tennessee and won community placement for many individuals residing in institutions (*People First of Tennessee v. Arlington Developmental Ctr.,* 1992). While national self-advocacy efforts are a relatively recent phenomena (Dybwad, 1996), their leadership in the states goes back to the 1970s, and was examined in this investigation.

Leadership by bureaucrats often occurs at the level of policy implementation. Upper level managers in state agencies may have considerable discretion in executing legislative mandates (Meier, 1989; Neugeboren, 1985). In an analysis of changes to the Texas mental health system, Luke (1975) found that leadership, shared among elected officials and state agency bureaucrats, was critical for the realization of systems change in that state. Bureaucratic leadership was examined as it relates to the development of community-based residential services for people with developmental disabilities.

Elected officials have also been in positions to provide leadership in the developmental disabilities field. At the national level, President John Kennedy's leadership culminated in the federal government's first significant funding for services to people with developmental disabilities (Braddock, 1987). A component of professional leadership, elected leadership was therefore examined in the proposed investigation.

Parents and other family members have been a significant political force in the developmental disabilities field since the 1950s (Allard, Howard, Vorderer, & Wells, 1999; Dybwad, 1996). They have pressed the existing formal service system for expansion of services and fundamental changes in service delivery. In the absence of services altogether, they often worked together to collectively meet their children's needs, establishing schools and day programs for adults in the 1960s. Before the 1975 passage of Pub. L. 94-142, the Education for All Handicapped Children Act, parents often organized schools for their children with developmental disabilities (Lerner, 1972). One exemplar of parental leadership was Elizabeth Boggs, who provided leadership to the field at the national level. She was instrumental in drafting the Developmental Disabilities Act, and worked on developmental disabilities policy at the national level for decades (Scheerenberger, 1983; Spitalnick, 1996). Parental leadership was defined for purposes of this study as those actions taken by parents of persons with developmental disabilities regarding the development of community-based services in the state.

Opposition to the downsizing and closure of institutions has come from some parent groups opposed to the community placement of their (adult) children living in institutions. These parent groups have advocated for the retention of institutional services for people with developmental disabilities (Burke & Hopp, 1999; Burke & Sherman, 1998; Spare, 1997, 1999; Voice of the Retarded, 1999). In a recent Supreme Court case (*Olmstead v. L. C.*, 1999) that decided the right of people with developmental disabilities to live in the community, *amicus curiae* briefs were filed in support of the state agency plaintiffs by more than 74 parent groups. These parents supported the state of Georgia's contention that people with disabilities do not have a right under Title II of the Americans with Disabilities Act to live in community settings (Burke & Hopp, 1999). Parental opposition to the downsizing of institutions is not a recent phenomenon, either. In a relatively early investigation, Frohboese and Sales (1980) found that parents opposed to moving their

children from institutions to community homes represented a significant and growing challenge to community placement and deinstitutionalization across the nation. As such, it was important to examine leadership exerted by parents in opposition to community services as well as that which supported it.

The second domain of variables investigated is litigation. Courts are recognized as having a profound impact on the development of policy. Judicial innovation can have consequences that reach far beyond the decisions made in a single case (Glick, 1999). Chronicling the status and outcomes of more than 70 cases in more than 40 states between 1970 and 1996, Hayden (1997) found that court orders and consent decrees from class-action cases often contained directives to the states that mandated the development of community services for class members. Other researchers have argued that the impact of federal court actions in particular can have far-reaching implications for the entire service system (Grumet, 1985; Moss, 1983, 1985; Sloan & Biloon, 1992). The impact of such cases is often difficult to predict, however. Some states, such as Tennessee, have poured tremendous resources into improving their institutional services in the face of class-action litigation (Braddock, Hemp, Parish, & Westrich, 1998). New Hampshire, West Virginia, New Mexico, Vermont, and Rhode Island, however, closed their public institutions after facing class-action lawsuits (Braddock, Hemp, Parish, Westrich, & Park, 1998; Hayden, 1997). Institutional closures have occurred even when courts did not find a right to community services as in New Hampshire (Covert, MacIntosh, & Shumway, 1994; *Garrity v. Gallen,* 1981). Topper's (1997) multivariate investigation found that the presence or absence of litigation is not predictive of deinstitutionalization. However, the present study examined litigation as more than a dichotomous variable, investigating differences in litigation outcomes and their relationship to the development of community services.

Of great concern to states is the extent to which the courts maintain control of the administrative aspects of the institution and the larger residential service system (Castellani, 1992; Covert et al., 1994). The variable court control was thus defined as the breadth of administrative control exerted by the courts over a state's residential services system. Plaintiffs' attorneys have become concerned that states take extreme steps to delay implementation of court orders, driving up the costs of litigation for plaintiffs and reducing the impact of cases over time (A. Hamlet, Alabama Protection & Advocacy Agency, personal communication, August 27, 1996; S. Kaska, former plaintiffs' attorney, *Conner v. Branstad,* personal communication, August 29, 1996). Therefore, this analysis examined the duration of the case between filing and disposition, and the outcomes of court intervention.

Legislation has also influenced the shape of residential services nationally. The passage of Pub. L. 92-223, which authorized states to obtain federal funding for institutional services through the Medicaid ICF/MR program in 1972, resulted in billions of federal dollars flowing to the states from the federal government for institutional services (Braddock, Hemp, Parish, Westrich, & Park, 1998, Braddock et al., 2002). In order to receive federal funding, the states were compelled to comply with federal ICF/MR regulations, and as such, states had to enhance the quality of care provided in institutional settings. In order to meet minimum square footage standards for residents, many facilities had to depopulate, which is how the ICF/MR program was a catalyst for deinstitutionalization, even as it catalyzed a tremendous influx of resources for institutional improvements (Taylor et al., 1981).

Researchers have found other laws to be important at the state level, and nationally. Passage of the Omnibus Budget Reconciliation Act (OBRA) of 1981 authorized states to receive federal Medicaid funds for individualized community-based services under the auspices of the HCBS Waiver program. As a result of this federal law, millions of federal Medicaid funds flowed to the states for their developmental disabilities service systems.

State and local legislation is also believed to influence developmental disabilities services. Braddock (1986c) has asserted that "the lack of a pre-emptive statewide zoning ordinance [was] perhaps the largest single legal obstacle to the development of community facilities" (p. 10). Given states' discretion in structuring their Medicaid programs, examination of state legislation was particularly important.

Legislation is inadequate in and of itself to understanding the scope of implementation, because policies are often implemented in ways not explicitly delineated by the original legislation (Bardach, 1977; Mazmanian & Sabatier, 1983; Pressman & Wildavsky, 1973). However, legislation is a critical variable in understanding deinstitutionalization and the concomitant development of community services (Hammer & Howse, 1977). The scope and implementation of legislation related to residential services in the comparison states was an important variable for the present investigation.

In the final domain of political socioeconomic factors, the perceived need for prison space was evaluated. Traditional political socioeconomic factors have not been demonstrated to be predictive of developmental disabilities services (Braddock & Fujiura, 1987, 1991; Topper, 1997) or of civil rights for people with disabilities (Holbrook & Percy, 1992). However, researchers have found that one political factor, the need for prison space, was related to states' decisions to close institutions for people with developmental disabilities (Braddock & Heller, 1985). Of the 24 institutional closures Braddock and Heller identified nationally, they found that one third were converted to prisons. A more recent update of Braddock and Heller's analysis indicated the conversion of developmental disabilities institutions to prisons has persisted. By 2000, 17% of the 125 closures were prison conversions (see Part II, this volume).

Conceptual Framework

Even for researchers who are interested in using qualitative strategies, and who expect theory to emerge as a product of their research, the articulation of a conceptual framework is useful. It enables the researcher to bound the limits of the investigation, and to make explicit preconceived relationships between variables (Miles & Huberman, 1994). While this investigation was inductive, and focused on the emergence of a theory that explains the development of community-based residential services, the explication of a conceptual framework was nonetheless important. *Figure 3.1*, on the next page, graphically depicts the initial conceptual framework of this investigation. Variables selected are specifically drawn from the developmental disabilities and political science research fields, as discussed in the preceding section.

The essence of this conceptual framework is that several sets of actors exert influence on, and are influenced by, one another. The arrows in the figure represent the direction in which influence was expected to occur. The boxes represent the different types of actors that exist in the larger sociopolitical arena. As is evident, influence was expected to be shared among groups, and to be dynamic. For instance, in some situations, it was expected that advocate organizations would influence public officials; in other situations, it was expected that public officials would influence advocacy organizations. It was expected that the flow of influence among the actors would be dynamic, and not occur in a linear manner.

The next section delineates the methodology employed to investigate these questions. The study targeted the evolution of residential services in both Michigan and Illinois during the 1970-90 period, which was the time when the deinstitutionalization movement began and expanded across the nation. However, an overview of developments in these two states from 1990-2000 is presented in the final section of the chapter.

METHODS

Overview

A multiple-case study of Michigan and Illinois was utilized to identify the factors that influenced the development of community-based residential services for persons with developmental disabilities.

This section discusses the rationale for the selection of Illinois and Michigan, followed by subsections detailing data collection and analysis procedures. The section concludes with a discussion of the credibility of the findings, and the steps taken to enhance the study's validity and reliability.

Using the criteria of similar demographic characteristics (e.g., population density, per capita wealth, total population), extreme differences in adoption of deinstitutionalization, and being located in the same region of the country, two states emerge that would be ideal for such a comparison, Illinois and Michigan. While histories of residential services in these states have been recorded (Curtis, 1983; Slater, 1986), a comprehensive analysis of the factors that influenced

the development of community services in each state has not been undertaken.

In terms of socioeconomic, political, and demographic variables, Illinois and Michigan are quite similar. Illinois had the sixth largest population in 1996; Michigan ranked eighth. Both states had the same approximate rate of population growth between 1980 and 1997, a factor that has been identified as influencing state policy development (Gray, 1999). Both states exemplify those with significant rural-urban splits in their populations, and both states have similar economies, with strong manufacturing sectors. In terms of the absolute size of each state's economy, Illinois had the fourth largest "gross state product" in the nation, while Michigan's ranked ninth (Gray, 1999). The proportion of each state's population that live below the federal poverty line is similar, although in terms of per capita personal income, Illinois is wealthier than Michigan. Illinois had the seventh highest per capita personal income in 1996; Michigan ranked 16th (Gray, 1999).

Important for the purpose of this investigation, these two states have similar historical patterns of residential services for people with developmental disabilities. Both states were among the earliest to develop public institutional facilities for people with developmental disabilities. Illinois opened its first institution in 1865 at Jacksonville (Curtis, 1983). Michigan's first institution, Lapeer, opened in 1895 (Slater, 1986). Institutions were each state's only significant form of residential care from the turn of the century into the 1950s, by which time a small number of community-based residential programs had been opened in each state (American Association on Mental Deficiency, 1959).

In 1977, Michigan and Illinois still had comparable numbers of people with developmental disabilities living in their public institutions, 6,047 and 6,580, respectively. Each state's spending for community-based services was below the national average, at 17% and 22% of total developmental disabilities spending, respectively. Each state's fiscal effort, or total spending per $1,000 of state personal income, was also below the national average, at $2.00 per $1,000 of state personal income for Michigan, and $2.11 per $1,000 for Illinois (see Part II, this volume). Michigan and Illinois had comparable numbers of institutional

sons. The state's community fiscal effort was similarly low, at 38% below the national. In 2000, Illinois operated nine institutions for people with developmental disabilities, and two for people with developmental disabilities and mental illness. That year, Michigan operated two institutions for people with developmental disabilities, and announced that one of these facilities would close by early 2002.

On nearly every measure, Michigan is one of the strongest states, and Illinois is one of the weakest states, in terms of the provision of community-based residential services. Given their present polarity, their demographic similarities, their regional proximity, and their similar histories of developmental disabilities services, these two states are ideal for the present comparison.

Data Collection Procedures

Data collection consisted of document evaluation and interviews. The general sequence in the collection of documentary evidence was to identify sites where documents are located, obtain permission to review documents, read the relevant documents at the sites, evaluate the documents using a quality control standard, and code the documents for data related to the present inquiry. The procedures for analysis of the content are discussed in the data analysis section of this chapter.

Sample

It is not possible to identify the entire population of documents related to the development of community-based residential services in Illinois and Michigan. As such, documents were obtained from a purposive sample of locations. Sampling for the present inquiry occurred at the level of document location. Seven documentary repositories were selected: the Archives and Library on Disability formerly at the University of Illinois at Chicago's Department of Dis-

Figure 3.1
CONCEPTUAL FRAMEWORK OF THE INVESTIGATION

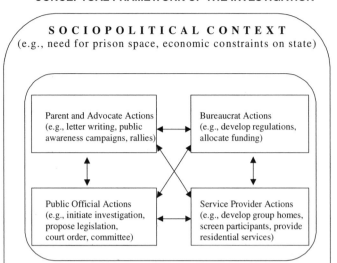

residents per capita (of state general population) as well, at 154 and 137, respectively.

Twenty years later, things have changed considerably. In 2000, Michigan had one of the country's strongest community-based residential systems for persons with developmental disabilities. The State had the fourth highest portion of its entire system of residential services in settings for six or fewer persons. The State spent 95% of all its developmental disabilities resources for community services.

By comparison, Illinois' service system was one of the most institutionally based in the country. In 2000, only Arkansas and Delaware allocated a smaller proportion of their total developmental disabilities resources for community services. Illinois allocated 57% of its resources for community services that year. The national average spending for community services was 75%. Illinois also provided a majority of residential services in institutional settings, and had the fourth lowest rate of utilization of settings for six or fewer per-

ability and Human Development, the Illinois State Archives, Illinois State Library, Michigan State Library, the State Archives of Michigan, the ARC of Illinois and the ARC of Michigan. These sites were selected because of the extraordinary breadth and depth of materials they were expected to contain. Finding aids and published reference guides reviewed for the four public sites, and the Archives and Library on Disability at the University of Illinois at Chicago, indicated each held hundreds of documents that were potentially valuable for the inquiry. The materials of each state's Association for Retarded Citizens was expected to be valuable because it would provide access to documents that offered the perspective of the largest advocacy organizations in the states. Other sites that were considered as well included the public institutions in each state. However, the materials that would have been yielded from these facilities would have been much more limited. Since these were expected to relate mostly to institutional and not community-based residential services, these were rejected as potential sites.

In addition to securing documents from these seven sites, the study employed a systematic strategy of pursuing all possible leads for other relevant documentary evidence. As such, when the documents reviewed at the seven archival sites illuminated other materials that seemed relevant, efforts were made to obtain these materials. In this way, trails were followed that frequently led well beyond the materials at the seven archival sites. The same procedure was followed to obtain documents related to information supplied by interview respondents. When interview respondents disclosed information not known to the investigator, searches were initiated in an attempt to find related materials. These searches included the electronic catalogs of the public university libraries in Illinois and Michigan and internet searches. There were relatively few instances where no documentary sources were located as a result of these secondary searches.

More than half of the Illinois interview respondents reported the importance of politics and the influence of money on the development of the state's developmental disabilities service system. To attempt to "follow the money," as so many respondents suggested was vital, Freedom of Information Act requests were filed to obtain documents from the state's De-

partment of Public Health and Department of Human Services related to the size, cost, and ownership of privately operated facilities. Campaign contributions, submitted on Illinois State Board of Elections' D-2 forms, were obtained for all nursing home and ICF/MR owners with greater than 5% share in any single facility. D-2 forms were also obtained for the nursing home lobby and for The American Federation of State, County, and Municipal Employees (AFSCME), the union that represents most state institutional workers in Illinois. Copies of the "Statement of Financial Interest" for the political party leaders and for all legislators living in a district with a public institution were also obtained. However, the records for the 1970-90 period were not available, as state law does not mandate keeping records for more than a few years. The most current available records were reviewed, to provide the author with a sense of the scope of these issues for the present.

Freedom of Information Act requests were filed to obtain the contracts for garbage removal, pharmacy services, and food at the state institutions in Illinois. However, these contracts were not available for the 1970-90 study period, due to the state's record retention policy. In the mid-1990s, the State changed its contracting procedures, and contracts for all state agencies are centrally negotiated, with a single, combined contract for all facilities, including prisons, psychiatric hospitals, developmental disabilities institutions, and children's institutions.

In Illinois, meeting minutes of the Health Facilities Planning Board were scrutinized, as well as the Department of Public Health's reports on contractor applications submitted to the Health Facilities Planning Board. The Health Facilities Planning Board controls the Certificate of Need process, which is the procedure states use to control development, licensure, and modification of health-care facilities, including ICFs/MR. These documents were obtained and reviewed in order to get a more complete understanding of the current utilization of ICFs/MR in the State, including new development of such facilities.

In Michigan, a less exhaustive effort was mounted to examine the relationship between money and the developmental disabilities service system. Documents were obtained regarding the state's politics, structure of government, and other sociopolitical factors. Documents were also obtained related to the state's campaign finance laws. However, the specific types of inquiries pursued for Illinois were not followed in Michigan for the following reasons: First, no interview respondents reported politics or provider influence as relevant to the development of community-based residential services in the State. Second, Michigan operated only two public institutions for 250 persons in 2000. As such, the institutions are not currently of a sufficient size to influence the state's political process.

Documents related to institutional contracts for the 1970-90 period, as in Illinois, were not available due to Michigan's document retention policies. Related to privately operated facilities, there are a number of structural issues that limited provider power. During much of the 1970-90 period, there was an enforced separation between the provision of services and the ownership of housing. Providers were also restricted in the number of facilities they could operate. As such, their political influence was limited. In addition, Michigan's campaign finance laws severely restrict campaign contributions for state campaigns. The final barrier to obtaining more detailed political or financial information on service providers was related to the structure of the service delivery system itself. The State does not centrally contract with service providers; instead, local Community Mental Health (CMH) boards either provide services directly, or contract with service providers to do so. Therefore, the contracting procedures are diffused among the state's CMH boards and were beyond the scope of the present inquiry.

The final method documents were obtained was directly from some interview respondents, who provided original or copied materials related to the development of community-based residential services in their state. These documents were quite varied, and included personal materials and correspondence, news clippings, and reports not available from other sources.

The general approach taken in obtaining documents for this study was that information obtained from one source (whether documentary or from interview respondents) needed to be corroborated or confirmed by another. While it was not always possible to do this, particularly in the case of sensitive political situations in Illinois, attempts were made to try to track down all significant leads. Criteria were established

for eliminating unsubstantiated data from the analysis. If events were disclosed during interviews that could not be corroborated by any documentary sources, the events were excluded if it was felt that any of the following conditions was met: (a) It was unlikely that the individual was in a position to possess first-hand knowledge of an event or individual's leadership; (b) it was possible or likely the interview respondent was expressing an opinion about a situation that was unduly influenced by animosity or personal conflicts with other policy stakeholders; or (c) data revealed by other sources provided sufficient evidence contradicting the interview respondent's interpretation of the event.

Utilization of these criteria ensured events that could not reliably be confirmed were not included as findings. While this procedure may have led to the exclusion of pertinent or relevant data, it was felt a conservative approach, requiring data to meet minimal standards of credibility, was important. Given the polemical positions taken by many interview respondents on an array of issues, these standards were felt to preserve the integrity of the study's overall findings. The reporting of rumors or events that were engendered from personal conflicts would have contaminated the study's findings.

An overview of the sources of documents included for data collection purposes is indicated in *Table 3.1*, on the next page. While this table provides a document tally, it is important to reiterate that the frequency of author/publisher is provided only to give a general sense of the breadth of materials reviewed, and is not suggestive of the importance of individual documents as related to the study's findings.

Upon close inspection, there are a number of categories in which there were great discrepancies in the proportionate representation of documents across the two states. The largest difference is that of "Other State Agency," with considerably larger collection of documents reviewed in the category in Illinois than in Michigan. This was the case because in Illinois, it was necessary to review documents from other agencies (Department of Public Health, Health Facilities Planning Board, Department of Public Aid) to get a full sense of the operations of the ICF/MR program. Campaign contribution forms and statement of economic interest materials obtained for Illinois are also included in this figure. A larger number of documents from the

Illinois Association for Retarded Citizens was reviewed because the Michigan Association for Retarded Citizens had discarded its historical materials when it moved offices in the early 1990s. Michigan governors generated greater numbers of written documents related to developmental disabilities services than did Illinois governors. This was the case largely because developmental disabilities issues were not often mentioned by Illinois governors in their annual addresses, and the Michigan governors nearly always discussed developmental disabilities issues in some detail. In addition, Governor Milliken of Michigan wrote a number of items related to the Plymouth institution. Generally, the number of documents reviewed within a particular category was not representative of the amount of information that was gathered from the various sources. For example, statements of economic interest were reviewed for more than 20 Illinois legislators, and they yielded almost no information whatsoever.

Document Evaluation

In reviewing pertinent documents to determine their appropriateness as data sources, two standard practices of historical inquiry, relevance and quality, were employed (Brundage, 1989; Shafer, 1980). Attempts were made to use primary sources for the majority of data collected . For documents to be used as data sources for the project, they needed to be pertinent to the study's objectives of illuminating the evolution of residential services, or the larger socio-political context. Therefore, to assess relevance, at least one of the following questions was answered affirmatively for each document that became a data source: (a) Is the document related to the development of residential services for persons with developmental disabilities? (b) is the document related to the developmental disabilities service system in general (e.g., employment services, family support, funding mechanisms, etc.)? (c) does the document provide insight into the state's economic, social, or political context?

The second aspect of the document evaluation process used the quality control criteria of authenticity, credibility, and meaning, as recommended by Scott (1990). Authenticity is related to whether or not documents are genuine, that they are what they purport to be. Credibility is the extent to which documents have

not been distorted and are error-free. Meaning connotes whether or not documents are clear and readily understood. While this standard was adopted prior to data collection, in practice no document was excluded from the study due to concerns related to authenticity, credibility, or meaning. The nature of this study was such that documents were what they appeared to be, and had meanings that were readily apparent. This three-part standard of document quality, however, must be distinguished from an evaluation of a document's intended purpose, or the truth of its claims. Clearly a document can be authentic, and credible, without being perfectly true. For this study, it was more important for documents to be evaluated in the context of what their meaning, intent, and implications were, rather than their authenticity. This evaluative aspect became a part of the data analysis, as will be discussed shortly.

Interview Phase

The general sequence of steps in the interview phase of data collection was to construct a general questionnaire for each state, identify suitable interviewees, contact them, obtain their informed consent to participate in the study, schedule and conduct the interviews by telephone, and iteratively listen and take notes of the tape recorded interviews from the interviews. Thematic content analysis of the interview data was also done, and is discussed in a later section.

In the telephone interview phase of data collection, semi-structured interviews were conducted with individuals identified as experts or participants in the development of residential services in either Illinois or Michigan. These individuals were identified through the documentary data collection process, and were nominated by other interviewees. Telephone interviews afford the greatest combination of fast completion time and high response rates in surveys of experts (Czaja & Blair, 1996; Dillman, 1978). The procedure used for conducting this phase of data collection was based on the recommendations of Dillman (1978).

In addition, telephone interviews were also conducted with four national experts in developmental disabilities residential services policy. These four individuals each had a minimum of 20 years experience in the developmental disabilities field, and were not from Illinois or Michigan. However, their expertise enabled

Table 3.1
DOCUMENTARY SOURCES OF DATA, BY AUTHOR OR PUBLISHER

Author/Publisher	Illinois	Michigan
Governor	16	43
Department of Mental Health	131	149
State/Local ARC	105	57
Newspaper	38	71
State Legislature	54	74
Task Force/Commission	22	18
Court Official/Document	20	15
State Protection & Advocacy	17	23
State DD Planning Council	38	71
Community Mental Health Agencies	1	10
Accrediting Organization	1	0
Health Care Financing Administration	3	0
Journal Article	0	2
Book	14	2
State's Attorney General	0	3
National DD Organization	3	11
U.S. Congress	0	1
University Research Report	12	3
Other State Agency	228	32

them to compare the developments in the two states. These four interviews were conducted in order to verify the validity of the comparisons completed. All four respondents confirmed the study's findings.

Instrument Development

The purpose of the second phase of the study's data collection scheme was to obtain from experts and participants the circumstances, context, and factors associated with the development of community-based services in each state. However, because a measure of the type needed by this investigation does not exist, one was developed by the investigator. An instrument using open-ended questions was developed.

Development of the questions for the instrument was closely based on the literature review of each domain of variables (legislation, leadership, litigation, and sociopolitical context), and the preliminary analysis of the documentary data. The second step in the development of the questions, expert panel review and revision, is also a means of ensuring content validity (Aday, 1996). For this part of the study, the expert

panel consisted of two university researchers, a parent, and a service provider. The university experts had extensive experience in national developmental disabilities policy. The remaining panelists also had extensive experience (at least 10 years) as service providers or parent advocates in the developmental disabilities field. These experts evaluated the congruency of the items with the concepts they were intended to represent, and appropriateness of the questions for respondents. An iterative process of revision and review was adopted, wherein the experts' suggestions were incorporated into a revision of the original draft. Panelists were then asked to review the revised instrument until consensus was reached that content validity had been achieved. This consensus was achieved after the first revision of the draft instrument.

One important distinction of the interviews was that respondents were not asked identical questions. A base instrument was developed and tested, but questions were added for individual respondents, depending on their role and knowledge of the service system. To be able to effectively interview each respondent, information was gathered about the respondents' background and experiences during the 1970-90 period. For many of the respondents, this was easily accomplished by careful scrutiny of documents that had been obtained from the seven archival sites. In situations where interview respondents were nominated by others, and whose background was not known to the interviewer, attempts were made to ascertain the individuals' participation in the development of developmental disabilities policy and services during the 1970-90 period. Respondents were also asked to describe their role in the service system. The gathering of information related to each person's background proved to be crucial, because it facilitated clearer assessments of the data provided by each individual respondent. For instance, a number of interview respondents had played multiple roles during the period, but may have been most visible in one particular role. By uncovering the broader scope of each individual's background, more targeted questions could be asked, and a more systematic attempt was made to utilize the full breadth of knowledge and experience that each respondent possessed.

The individualized nature of each interview was a crucial aspect of this study, as it allowed each individual respondent's area of knowledge and expertise to be fully explored, or at least explored to the extent his or her schedule would permit. Had a single, standardized interview instrument been used, much valuable data would have been lost. Generally, questions asked respondents for their impressions and interpretations of the significance of different events, including state and federal laws, scandals, news media coverage, legislative investigations, lawsuits, and committee or task force work. Respondents were also asked about the contributions made by various groups and leaders in the state, including the directors of the Departments of Mental Health/Developmental Disabilities (DMHDD), the Association for Retarded Citizens, and the Planning Council on Developmental Disabilities, among others.

Sample

Since an existing list of experts in the Illinois and Michigan residential service systems does not exist, a sampling frame was constructed in stages. First, a table of the leadership in each state's MR/DD organizations (Department of Mental Health, Association for Retarded Citizens, Division of Developmental Disabilities, Protection and Advocacy, Governor's Planning Council on Developmental Disabilities) was prepared for each year, 1970-90. Next, individuals who were participants or seemed to have been knowledgeable or influential in the development of community residential services in each state were identified from the documents that had been reviewed. From this leadership table and the review of documents, a core set of individuals was identified for participation in the study. For both states, this core set initially totaled approximately 12 individuals.

In addition to inviting these individuals to participate, the study employed the snowball or chain referral sampling technique. Snowball sampling is the process whereby respondents nominate others who might be eligible to provide information about the topic. Snowball sampling techniques have been found to be effective for use with "hidden" populations (van Meter, 1990) such as these experts. As the universe of experts in each state's residential service system is relatively small, and mostly known to one another, it was expected that a reasonable representation of experts could be obtained.

Thirty-seven individuals with involvement in the Illinois service system were invited to participate in the study. Thirty-one consented, yielding a response rate of 84%. In Illinois, one individual agreed to participate, signed and submitted the consent, and was interviewed. However, three days after the interview, the person contacted the author to rescind the consent that had previously been given. In accordance with the person's wishes, the audiotapes and notes from the interview were immediately destroyed. This individual reported being troubled by aspects of the history in Illinois, and did not want to be a part of the study. While the tape and the notes were destroyed, there was no way to change the fact that this person's insights and answers had contributed to the investigator's thinking on an array of issues. There was obviously no practical way to "purge" this consciousness from the investigator.

Twenty-four individuals with experience in the Michigan service system were invited to participate, and 21 accepted, yielding a response rate of 88%. *Table 3.2* indicates the affiliation of interviewees for both states. This table provides a duplicated count, because some interview respondents, during the course of their careers, had different roles in the residential service system or had dual roles (e.g., parent and professional). In these instances, they are counted twice. To preserve the guarantee of confidentiality afforded to each interviewee, the affiliations are reported together for both states. The distribution was relatively even across states.

Nearly 30% more respondents participated in the interviews related to Illinois than related to Michigan. Greater numbers of Illinois respondents were sought because there was less convergence of agreement among respondents regarding the factors that had influenced the service system. In Michigan, most interview respondents shared a common understanding of what factors had facilitated the development of the state's service system. In Illinois, there was considerable disagreement among respondents over the impact of certain disability groups, most notably the Illinois Association for Retarded Citizens.

Michigan interviews ranged in duration from 50 to 203 minutes, with an average of 109 minutes per interview. All Michigan interviews were conducted as a single, uninterrupted telephone call. The duration of Illinois interviews ranged from 45 to 190 minutes, with an average of 107 minutes per interview. All of the Illinois interviews except three were conducted as a single telephone call. In three instances, the interviews took place as two phone calls. One of the interviews was interrupted for an hour due to equipment failure; the other two were held in two sessions due to time constraints.

Data Analysis

In qualitative research, there is considerable overlap between data collection and data analysis techniques. Analysis is posited as an iterative process, whereby when a "theme, hypothesis, or pattern is identified inductively, the researcher then moves into a verification mode, trying to confirm or qualify the finding" (Huberman & Miles, 1994, p. 431).

For this investigation, as suggested by Huberman and Miles (1994), a strategy of interim analysis and final analysis procedures was employed. The interim analysis consisted of the constant comparison of the data to the conceptual framework articulated in the previous section. In addition, analytical memos were periodically generated, with the explicit purpose of assessing the fit of the data to this conceptual framework. In this way, memos provided an overview of the ways in which the conceptual framework was, and was not, supported by the data. Analytical memos were also used to identify emerging themes and patterns. Such memos are considered integral to qualitative data analysis, facilitating an ongoing assessment of the fit of the data to the conceptual framework (Marshall & Rossman, 1999; Miles & Huberman, 1994;

Table 3.2
AFFILIATION OF INTERVIEWEES

Affiliation	Total
Dept. of Mental Health/Developmental Disabilities	22
Association for Retarded Citizens/ARC	16
Residential Service Provider	12
Other State Agency	7
Parent	6
Lawyer	4
Governor's Staff	5
Protection & Advocacy Organization	3
Planning Council on Developmental Disabilities	3
Legislator or Legislative Staff	4
Court Official	3
United Cerebral Palsy/UCP	2
University Researcher	2
County Mental Health organization	2
Lobbyist	2
Labor Union	1
Self-Advocate	1

Wolcott, 1994).

For the final analysis, the four techniques of coding, thematic-content analysis, pattern matching, and chronological event analysis were employed to build upon the interim analysis. Coding is an analytical technique commonly used in qualitative research methods (Tesch, 1990). Thematic-content analysis is a technique common to qualitative research (Miles & Huberman, 1994). Pattern matching and chronological event analysis are analytical techniques employed frequently in case study research, and are considered superior to other alternatives such as descriptive analysis (Grosshans & Chelimsky, 1990; Yin, 1994). Using these four analytical strategies strengthens confidence in the study's findings, essentially triangulating the analysis. Following completion of data analysis, written summaries of each case were developed. Subsequent to the development of individual case study summaries, a cross-case analysis was crafted. This two-phase procedure of within-case and cross-case analysis is the preferred analysis method for multiple-case study research (Merriam, 1997; Yin, 1994).

Credibility of Findings

Rigor in scientific experiments results from the investigator's controlled design and execution of the entire environment in which phenomenon in question occur, as well as all aspects of measurement of the phenomenon (Cook & Campbell, 1979). In qualitative research, by contrast, the empirical process is engaged to coax theory to emerge, and the role of validity and reliability has been the subject of great debate. Some researchers have argued that validity and reliability are completely inappropriate concepts for qualitative research (Merriam, 1997). This rejection has frequently been predicated on beliefs that the goals of verifying knowledge, most often operationalized as estimates of validity and reliability, are inappropriate because of their association with positivist concepts of singular truths (Kvale, 1996). Other researchers have called for qualitative research that is verifiable (Kvale, 1996). Some have argued that validity and reliability are important to qualitative research because they strengthen the contributions of such research to the body of knowledge by providing replicable and Keohane, & Verba, 1994).

In spite of this debate, it is this investigator's standpoint that the need for results that are reliable and valid, and represent a credible picture of the evolution of residential services in each state, is imperative. As such, this section will provide a brief discussion of validity and reliability, describe the main threats to the validity and reliability of this investigation, and explain the steps taken to reduce these threats. The section also delineates the basis of the overall credibility of the study's findings.

Internal Validity

Threats to the internal validity of the study included maturation bias, test effects, and recall bias. Maturation bias is the extent to which respondents' accounts of the events that transpired are influenced by changes in their perceptions and perspectives over time. Three decades have passed since the outset of the 1970-1990 study period. There have been profound changes in the philosophical underpinnings of the developmental disabilities field, including notable advances in human rights expectations by and for people with developmental disabilities. Institutionalization is a concept that has lost favor with much of the developmental disabilities field. The development of community services for persons with developmental disabilities in both states was (and is, in Illinois) an extremely charged, controversial issue. Society's thinking about the role of persons with developmental disabilities has changed considerably over the years, and it is quite likely this evolution in philosophy shaped the responses some interviewees provided. It was the clear perception of the interviewer that "political correctness" shaped many interviewees' responses. In this way, it is difficult to know what the actual thinking was at the time events were unfolding. To address this issue, the interviewer challenged respondents with evidence from other sources, and probed for examples and details. By seeking deeper and richer explanations and assessments from respondents, it was hoped respondents would move beyond superficial generalizations that echo a politically correct standpoint.

Test effects are a threat to validity related to the possibility that respondents provided information that was altered as a result of their participation in the study. These test effects may have arisen because of the way questions were asked, or respondents' perceptions of the goals of the research. To address test effects arising from the interview instrument, questions were framed to be as value-neutral as possible. In addition, extensive probing was done with respondents, in a systematic attempt to delve beneath the surface of answers. By probing carefully, seeking clarification, and requesting extensive details, the investigator attempted to obtain data that reflected respondents' actual insights into issues and not a statement that was unduly influenced by the interview process itself. There was considerable evidence these procedures were successful. Numerous interview respondents offered detailed explanations of the ways in which they disagreed with data reported by other respondents.

The other way these threats to the study's internal validity were addressed was the use of the documentary data itself. A great strength of using archival records is their nonreactivity (Webb, Campbell, Schwartz, & Sechrest, 2000). In this way, the documents complemented the interview data, which was generated from respondents who could have altered their responses due to their participation in the study. The data collected from documentary sources are not subject to effects arising from participation in the research project. The documents provided a valuable record of events that had transpired, as well as some insight into the official or public thinking related to the service system for persons with developmental disabilities.

Recall bias in the study is related to the burden placed on respondents in accurately remembering events that took place as much as three decades ago. It is likely that individuals have forgotten information related to the period and the service system at the time. To assist respondents in this regard, the interviewer provided as much detail of substantiated events (e.g., passage of legislation, filing of court cases, change in departmental leadership) as was practicable. During interviews, recounting specific details of an event for respondents was frequently helpful in assisting with recall of events. It was possible that relaying event details to respondents biased them toward identifying such events as important. However, because of the number of years that passed, and the serious concerns with memory limitations over time, it was decided that the latter represented more of a problem than the

former. It was also expected that because respondents were experts, they were likely to have strong opinions regarding the impact of different factors, and would not be likely to be influenced by the interviewer. This generally proved to be true; most respondents seemed to provide a considered judgment of the importance of particular events, investigations, task forces, and even people. In numerous instances respondents indicated that situations or people had or had not influenced the development of policy. Most respondents volunteered situations or events not known to the investigator as illustrations of their perceptions. It was therefore concluded that the procedure of providing respondents with situation reminders did not appear to bias their judgments.

Attempts to maximize the internal validity of research are intended to exclude alternative explanations for the phenomena in question. For the present study, the comprehensiveness of the variables explored increased the study's internal validity. The variables that were examined were drawn from both the developmental disabilities and political science research literature, and included sociopolitical factors like state economic conditions as well as leadership, litigation, and legislation, which are traditional developmental disabilities policy variables. The breadth of variables covered does not obviate the possibility that influential factors were omitted. To address this issue, however, all interview respondents were asked if they felt any other issues were germane to understanding the development of community residences. The design of the investigation, which was explicitly open to letting unanticipated variables emerge, helped assuage the possibility that some relevant variables were overlooked.

External Validity

External validity is the extent to which study findings can be generalized to other settings, people, and times (Cook & Campbell, 1979). Case studies are not usually intended to generate findings that can be generalized to other cases, for our purposes, American states. The generalizability sought in this investigation, therefore, was the entire state experience, or, the universe of people, events, and situations that led to the particular development of each state's residential service system. Generalizing to other settings with external validity is partly dependent on representative sampling, which does not occur at the level of sampling of cases. In case study research, cases are selected on the basis of theoretical concerns, and not representativeness. In this example, the two cases were drawn due to the polarity of their adoption of the innovation of institutional depopulation and the development of community-based residential services. As such, no claims are made that the results from these two states are representative of any other states.

The primary threats to the study's external validity were sampling bias and selection bias. Sampling bias is possible if data elements are obtained from sources that differ in systematic ways from the population or universe of sources. Selection bias occurs when interview respondents who participate in a study differ from those who do not participate.

Sampling bias may have occurred in this study because the documents available for review may not reflect the population of all relevant documents, and they may have been materially different from those that were unavailable. Archival sites have specific rules governing the materials they accept into their collections (Bailey & Evans, 1996). The official sites for each state contained substantial holdings of official materials, but were expected to have limited collections of documents related to the political process that were not intended for public consumption.

To address this potential problem, a wider net of sites for document retrieval was cast than the official sites run by the states. The inclusion of the ARC collections, documents obtained from interview respondents, documents obtained via Freedom of Information Act requests, the Illinois Secretary of State and from the Illinois State Board of Elections, and, most important, from the Archives and Library on Disability, ensured the documents used in the study were not only those that represented the official state positions. As mentioned previously, Department of Mental Health materials at the Michigan State Archives were not accessible to the public. It is impossible to know what was contained in these documents that might have been informative to the study. However, the collection of the Archives and Library on Disability included a substantial set of materials (42 boxes) from a former high level staff person at the Michigan Department of Mental Health. As such, access was gained to interoffice memoranda and other documents that proved important, and filled this gap.

Selection bias was a limitation of the study, since everyone who played a role in the development of the service system did not participate in the study. Individuals who declined to participate in Illinois included people who were expected to have considerable "insider" information on the ways politics influenced the development of developmental disabilities policy. It is unclear how these individuals' lack of participation affected the study results. It is likely, however, that the data that could have been provided by these people would have been valuable.

Related to this selection bias is the fact that some of the leaders in both states from the early 1970s are deceased, particularly the directors of the Departments of Mental Health and the Illinois Division of Developmental Disabilities. Many of these deceased individuals became professionals in a much earlier and, frankly, harsher time for the field. Their perspectives might have been markedly different than the younger people who survived to be interviewed. Whereas other interview respondents had the ability to provide commentary to accompany the documents by which their roles were assessed, this group of leaders had to be assessed by virtue of the extant documents and the perspectives of other interviewees. There was no way to address this issue in the study, but it is likely that some form of bias was probably introduced due to the inability to interview the most powerful officials of the late 1960s and early 1970s.

Reliability

Inter-rater reliability was within acceptable limits on both analyses. Test-retest reliability was also conducted by the principal investigator for the thematic-content analysis and the coding of documentary data. The results of these reliability tests were within acceptable limits as well.

Threats to the study's reliability were also related to decisions about the inclusion of documents as data sources and decisions about what data should be excluded from the analysis. To consistently identify relevant documents as data sources, a systematic evaluative criteria was employed, as described previously. This criteria minimized some of the reliability threats to which the study was exposed. Also described previously was the criteria for excluding evidence from the analysis and subsequent findings. This most frequently occurred with interview data, for which a conservative standard of corroborating evidence was employed.

Study Strengths

The credibility of this study rests on three interrelated methodological components: triangulation, member checks, and national expert interviews. Triangulation refers to the use of multiple strategies that, one hopes, converge toward one outcome. Member checks are commonly employed in qualitative research, and comprise a process of reviewing findings with interview respondents in order to get their feedback. Finally, study findings were shared with national experts, who were invited to critique and assess them.

By employing triangulation, the shortcomings of one method were addressed by employing another. Triangulation was employed in multiple levels in this study, and occurred during data collection and data analysis. Data collection was triangulated by relying on different sources of data (documents and interviews). Triangulation occurred within the two phases of data collection as well. Interview respondents were drawn from different arenas (advocacy organizations, professionals, public officials) in order to obtain divergent perspectives on the evolution of the residential service system. In the documentary phase of data collection, an array of document types provided data for the study (e.g., official reports, newspaper articles, meeting minutes, testimony, court records, legislative records, laws). In addition, documents were used from varied sites, and had been created by diverse authors. The use of seven document repositories ensured that an array of perspectives was represented. The use of different document types ensured that if certain documents possessed systematic errors, other documents might provide counterbalancing perspectives.

Member checks and national expert interviews were also conducted to verify the study findings. Five interview respondents were randomly drawn from each pool of respondents who had participated for Illinois and Michigan. These individuals were contacted by telephone, and the principal investigator reviewed the study findings with them. These individuals largely supported the study's conclusions about the factors that influenced the development of the service system in each state. There was some disagreement in Illinois related to the ARC's role, however. Individuals who had been part of the ARC generally (although not always) felt that their advocacy efforts were not compromised becase of their dual role as service provider and as advocate. In Michigan, there was widespread support expressed for the accuracy of the study's findings.

Finally, interviews were conducted with four national experts in state residential service systems. Given their situation as experts in state policy development, they were the only interview respondents who were positioned to compare Michigan and Illinois. All four supported the study's conclusions as well.

One of the most important strengths of this study was the way in which each of the phases of data collection helped frame interpretation of data collected by the other phase. In this way, the two forms of data collection complemented each other, and provided data not available from each other form. Documents complemented interviews because they often could be used to examine contradictions among and between respondents' recollections and assessments. Interviews often complemented the documents because they provided background and context that was frequently missing from the documents. In building coalitions of disability advocates, individual personalities proved to be important. The ability of coalition members to "speak with one voice" was frequently cited by Michigan advocates as a significant element of their success. This type of nuance was nowhere reflected in the documents related to Michigan, but it helped to understand the dynamics of what had occurred.

MICHIGAN CASE STUDY

This section will present the case study related to the development of residential services from 1970-90 in Michigan. To facilitate understanding of a complex interplay of factors and forces, this section is organized as follows: trends in residential services, which provides a brief description of the development of residential services; and administrative structure, which delineates the organizational aspects of funding and providing residential services. A discussion of the role of public scandals in shaping Michigan's service system is then presented. Subsequent sections describe and discuss the role politics, federal influences, the governors, the legislature, the judiciary, the Department of Mental Health, and advocacy groups played in the development of community-based residential services.

Trends and Developments in Residential Services

The residential service systems of Michigan and Illinois shared remarkable similarities in the 1960s. Public institutions were the dominant form of residential care available at the time, with just a small handful of private residential alternatives available to those who could afford them (Michigan Departments of Public Health and Mental Health, 1966). The states' facilities were severely overcrowded, and conditions were brutal. A parent of an individual living in a public institution in one of the states in the 1960s recounted this experience:

> The house manager told me I couldn't go down into the basement. I told her that I was going anyway unless they threw me out bodily. Then she went into the office--I'm sure to call security. I went downstairs. And the sight that I saw made me so damn mad that I really thought I was going to kill someone. They had three attendants sitting on three chairs. And in front of each attendant was a regular scrubbing bucket of soap and water. And then in front of each one was this line of naked boys. Three lines of naked boys. One attendant washed hands and faces using the same water for every boy. And then they went to the next row and they washed the bodies. And the next row, they washed the feet. Then they sent them through the adjoining shower room and they hosed them down.

In spite of these poor conditions, waiting lists for the public institutions were long, exceeding 1,500 persons in 1962 (Michigan Department of Mental Health [hereafter, DMH], 1962). To relieve overcrowding and address the waiting list, Michigan opened a number of

public institutions in the 1960s. The newly constructed Plymouth Center opened in 1960, and Howell (later Hillcrest), a former tuberculosis sanatorium, was converted to become an institution for people with developmental disabilities in 1961. In 1963, the Gaylord State Home (later Alpine) opened, and, in 1969, a newly constructed facility opened in Muskegon (Michigan Departments of Public Health and Mental Health, 1966). In 1965, the population of people with developmental disabilities in the public institutions exceeded 12,500. In the 1960s, the majority of available community services were sheltered workshops and adult daycare programs (Michigan Departments of Public Health and Mental Health, 1966).

Funding for public institutions in Michigan was limited during this period. Like many states, Michigan relied upon the work provided by patients in its state institutions. DMH (1967) reported that a total of nearly 2,700 patients were working in six of its eight developmental disabilities institutions. By the author's calculations, the combined efforts of these individuals yielded an estimated 1,929 full-time equivalent positions. Given there were fewer than 5,000 staff in the facilities, the contribution of the patients was substantial. These patients were not compensated for their work and therefore they represented a cost savings to the State and the ongoing operations of the institutions.

In 1966, Congress amended the Fair Labor Standards Act to cover patients in mental facilities and mandated they be paid for the work they provided. Policy briefs were subsequently issued stating the new law "provided for application of the Act to hospitals and institutions primarily engaged in the care of the sick, the aged, the mentally ill or defective. Workshops and other programs operated by hospitals and institutions are considered to be within the coverage of the act" (U.S. Department of Labor, 1968, p. 1). In spite of the promulgation of these guidelines, it took Michigan a number of years to address it. Peonage or unpaid work by mental patients had been a practice in the state of Michigan for decades. The state's long-term patient labor law stated that patients in mental facilities were to be furnished with "every proper means" of employment, and were not to receive compensation for doing so (Pub. Act 151 of 1923). This longstanding practice of peonage and the reliance on patients to assist in the financing of their care continued for a number of years after the federal regulations were promulgated.

Discussions within the House Mental Health Committee in 1970 concerned passage of new laws related to patient employment. However, it was not until the mid-1970s that Michigan finally abolished the practice of peonage and mandated the compensation of residents' labor contributing to the facility operations (Pub. Act 117 of 1975). This legislation authorized the institutions to keep half of a resident worker's compensation as payment for room and board.

Although the decade of the 1970s ushered in a period of considerable change in Michigan's residential service system for people with developmental disabilities, at its outset, institutional services were the mainstay of care in the State. *Figure 3.2*, below, shows the construction and closure of Michigan's public developmental disabilities institutions from 1960-90.

In 1970, the State was beset with a severe recession and the governor cut $108 million from the state's total budget for fiscal year 1971, including a 3% reduction in DMH allocations (Milliken, 1970a). Partly in response to the budget difficulties confronting the State and partly due to the rising costs of maintaining an aging and dilapidated facility, the governor proposed the closure of the Ft. Custer Developmental Center. This facility had been leased from the United States Army since 1956.

The impending closure of Custer was not an opportunity to implement community services in the State.

Indeed, all 331 residents at the facility were intended to be transferred to other state institutions. In response to the governor's announcement, Representative Groat introduced a resolution to prohibit the transfer of patients to stop closure of the facility.

> Resolved, that it is being the intent of the House of Representatives, that any action to transfer patients from the Ft. Custer State Home to terminate the employment of any of their employees be delayed until this legislative body conducts a full investigation of the contemplated action to transfer patients and terminate employment of the employees at the Ft. Custer State Home. (Michigan House of Representatives, 1972, p. 2)

While the resolution was subsequently passed by the House, it was not successful in preventing the facility's closure, which occurred in 1972 over the legislators' objections. However, the passage of this resolution is instructive of the legislative support for the employees in the facility. The resolution noted that 150 employees would lose their jobs due to the closure of the facility.

In his 1970 address to the legislature, Governor Milliken reported there had been an ongoing decline in the population of facilities for people with developmental disabilities. He explained that the total capacity of state institutions for people with developmental disabilities had expanded by 1,000 persons between

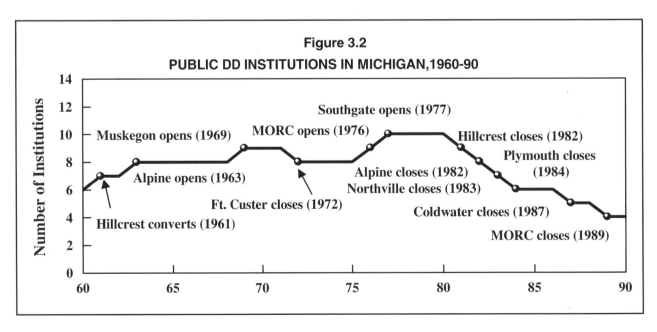

Figure 3.2
PUBLIC DD INSTITUTIONS IN MICHIGAN, 1960-90

1963 and 1970. He also noted that people waiting for admission to state DD institutions had been reduced by more than 400 since 1962, and an additional 895 were deferred (Milliken, 1970b). Deferral was a process whereby an individual received some form of community service, possibly adult day care, sheltered workshop, or other ancillary service and waited to be admitted to a state institution. The population in Michigan's developmental disabilities institutions peaked in 1967 at 12,700. Like many states across the country, Michigan began moving people out of state facilities in the late 1960s, a trend that continued into the 1970s (DMH, 1966, 1981b).

As Custer closed, its residents moved into one of three types of facilities: nursing homes, homes for the aged, which were boarding homes, and adult foster care. Adult foster care was a form of board and care with some minimal supervision open to individuals with developmental disabilities, mental illness, and the aged (Office of Health and Medical Affairs, 1974).

There were numerous problems in the early stages of Michigan's community placement program. In a study issued in 1974, the Office of Health and Medical Affairs concluded that patients transferred from the state institutions often went into facilities that were not subject to adequate inspection, licensing, or regulation. The Department of Public Health frequently found substantial noncompliance with the existing licensing standards. Providers or facility operators were concerned with what they termed to be inadequate rates of reimbursement, and after an individual was placed, there was often a lack of supervision and care that was termed "inadequate by any reasonable criteria" (Office of Health and Medical Affairs, 1974, p. 3). Problems with oversight of facility operators and quality assurance existed in Michigan for a number of years.

One of the state's first initiatives to develop community-based residential services for people with developmental disabilities came about due to an agreement between the DMH, Social Services, and the Michigan State Housing Development Authority (MSHDA). This prototype program was instituted to create 10 community-based facilities for adults with developmental disabilities; in 1974, it was expanded to provide for 24 facilities (Michigan Department of Social Services et al., 1976). These early group homes designed for 16 persons with developmental disabili-

ties, were regarded as progressive. But, by the time the facilities were completed, the philosophy had changed and 16 person homes were no longer considered appropriate or in accordance with the normalization principles taking hold in the State. When it became apparent that these facilities were inappropriate due to their large size, they were discontinued. However, according to later analyses MSHDA was unable to build facilities for fewer than 16 that were economically feasible, so capital development became more difficult (Human Services Research Institute, 1978).

Another of the state's early deinstitutionalization initiatives implemented between 1970-75 was to build specialized nursing homes for people with developmental disabilities. By 1973, plans were underway to build 10 of these new nursing homes intended to serve up to 150 people per facility by the end of 1974 (DMH, 1973; Harris, 1974; Harris & Miller, 1974).

In a project funded under the Developmental Disabilities Act, the ARC conducted a comprehensive evaluation of Michigan's service system and developed a plan to improve services to people with developmental disabilities (Harris & Miller, 1974). The report stated that nursing homes for people with developmental disabilities lacked individualized programming and were inappropriate for individuals who did not need 24-hour nursing care. In spite of these weaknesses, the report called for the development of more nursing facilities because they provide a better opportunity for individuals to return to community functioning than institutions. "Nursing homes are new and modern with semi-private rooms with baths and other special structural accommodations to meet Medicaid standards." (Harris & Miller, 1974, p. 73)

By 1974, there were 1,048 individuals with developmental disabilities residing in nursing homes (Harris & Miller, 1974). One interview respondent indicated that the incremental changes that occurred in the State were considered to be advances, whether or not they truly were. Related to the development of nursing homes, he stated:

> All of us tend to take success as something that is better than what we did yesterday. If you think in the history of care for people, the state institutions were better than what was provided before them, in people's mind

at the time. Then it became unacceptable. We took the same people, and put them in these nursing homes, which was better than what we took them from, but they became hell holes. We took people out of state institutions and we put them in adult foster care, a number of which were high quality, delivering services, a lot of them were prisons and worse, torture chambers, and we slapped ourselves on the back and gave ourselves high fives.

One event from the early 1970s had important implications for the residential service system in the State. In 1972, Michigan enacted legislation calling for the construction of the Macomb-Oakland Regional Center (MORC). This legislation authorized the allocation of funds to construct a 650-bed facility located on a single campus consisting of 54 duplex homes. In addition, the center was to include a 26-bed medical unit and six 16-bed nursing care units. David Rosen was hired as the facility's superintendent, and he recruited Gerald Provencal and Ben Censoni as part of the new facility's administrative team. Immediately, MORC staff began developing plans for the individuals who were intended for the new facility including those living in other state institutions. In the summer of 1972, staff began planning for the facility's physical plant and, without even having broken ground, began to aggressively develop a significant community services program. In the beginning, these community placements were not specifically intended to replace the targeted number of residents that the facility would eventually serve. However, as the years passed, the number of residents that the institution was intended to serve was continually reduced. In the first year alone, 236 people with developmental disabilities were moved from "inappropriate" community settings or out of existing public institutions (DMH, 1973).

Group homes for 77 people were developed and family care home programs served 17 children the first year. Family care homes were situations in which children were placed with a foster family. A family training home program, which was a program whereby foster parents were heavily involved in daily training programs, was also established and served 92 people in its first year of operation. MORC was also respon-

sible for planning the development of 10 new specialty nursing homes for approximately 150 persons, which were intended only to serve persons with developmental disabilities (DMH, 1973).

In 1973, MORC received a grant from the federal Department of Health, Education, and Welfare for nearly $400,000 over three years with the goal of placing and fully serving 100 new residents in community-based residences per year. This grant, "deinstitutionalization of the hard-to-place retarded," was intended to serve individuals whose disabilities or medical needs were so severe that they would have normally have been precluded from being considered community placement candidates (DMH, 1973).

An important contribution MORC made to the Michigan residential service system was its commitment to community placement for individuals who were classified in the severe or profound level of developmental disabilities. By 1978, approximately 54% of individuals whom MORC had placed into community settings were classified as having severe or profound mental retardation. Put into the context of the time nationally, individuals labeled with severe or profound mental retardation were generally not considered to be appropriate for living in community residences at all (DMH, 1978).

Nearly all of the interview respondents who had worked in the State during this period indicated that Gerry Provencal and Ben Censoni were "absolute visionaries." These men were able to inspire an appreciation for how community placement was the necessary home for individuals with developmental disabilities. While institutional superintendents reportedly were opposed to the community residential development MORC orchestrated, this opposition was not well organized and did little to slow its progress. Early on, MORC staff regarded their mission to be the implementation of the normalization philosophy which was popularized by Nirje (1976) and Wolfensberger (1972). Macomb-Oakland Regional Center staff were perceived as mavericks by others in the state, but what gave the organization credibility and legitimacy at the state level was its direction by superintendent David Rosen.

Rosen was the president of the American Association on Mental Deficiency and had been an institutional superintendent both in New Jersey and in Washington State before he was recruited to head the MORC. Rosen shared the vision of community placement and the development of community services and a sense of creativity but he also provided legitimacy and credibility to the new undertaking.

A number of the ways in which the Macomb-Oakland Regional Center was developed, in retrospect, have been important to the success of the development of community services. While it was to be a hotbed of innovation in the State for a number of years, MORC was part of the Department of Mental Health. As such, the DMH had considerable discretion in the way MORC was organized and how it was able to work with other institutions to pursue deinstitutionalization. From the outset, the fact that service providers did not control the housing would prove to be important. In many states, when a group home was developed, the entity providing the services, training, and supervision typically owned and therefore controlled the mortgage or lease. Within this structure, two important things emerge. If an individual's behavior or medical needs become challenging, it is a simple matter for the service provider to discharge the resident and fill his or her place with someone else, because the provider has complete control over where the person lives and what services the individual receives. Many advocates have argued that this creates an inherent imbalance whereby providers have a stranglehold on the service system. The second important issue that emerges when the service provider controls the housing is that service providers then have an additional source of income from the housing, which can be considerable. When the provider owns the group home, the rental or mortgage costs can be charged to the contract and wealth can be accumulated.

In some states, this has led facility operators to accumulate considerable wealth, again, adding to an imbalance in the system among service providers, the state, and individuals receiving services. In Michigan, this did not happen to as large an extent because housing was controlled by the State and service providers had contracts only to provide services. In this kind of a situation, an individual could not be discharged from his or her placement as readily for failing to conform to the standards of the service provider.

The Macomb-Oakland Regional Center made another important contribution to the Michigan service system: As it developed group homes, it fought local zoning battles (Joint Mental Health Oversight Committee, 1980; Michigan Mental Health Advisory Council, 1982). This was important from the standpoint that the agency, as part of the state's DMH, had sufficient resources to employ attorneys who in turn developed considerable zoning litigation experience over time. These attorneys were quite successful in winning zoning challenges that might have precluded the development of group homes in other situations.

The services developed by the MORC gained the respect and admiration of professionals from other states and indeed even from other countries. Visits to MORC facilities took place as dignitaries and other individuals visited from around the world. This attention also served to enhance the credibility of what the organization was doing. The Department of Mental Health and the governor must have been pleased with the positive press received by MORC. And while there was dissent in the State over the development of community residences, it might have been difficult politically to walk away from the positive press that MORC and DMH were receiving from Macomb-Oakland Regional Center's activities.

The Macomb-Oakland Regional Center offered the State an exciting opportunity whereby innovations could be piloted in a way that was still relatively easy for the State to control. The development of innovations became an important function of the agency over time. Smaller scale group homes were initially developed at MORC and then spun out to the rest of the State. The same was true of small-scale foster care placements whereby children were placed with families. Family support was similarly piloted at the Macomb-Oakland Regional Center. In 1976, when the State embarked upon its plan to develop community-based ICFs/MR, they began with MORC (DMH, 1977, 1980).

Another important event in the history of residential services in Michigan occurred in 1971, when Congress amended the Social Security Act (Pub. L. 91-517) and authorized the Intermediate Care Facilities for the Mentally Retarded (ICF/MR) program as an option under the Medicaid program. This new program enabled states to obtain federal Medicaid reimbursement for facilities certified as ICF/MR by meeting an extensive array of conditions and regulations. In return for meeting the conditions or the standards, states received federal reimbursement based on their wealth in amounts ranging from 50% to approximately 80% of their institutional service costs (Braddock, Hemp, Parish, & Westrich, 1998).

Michigan embarked upon a plan to comply with the federal regulations and thus obtain what eventually resulted in millions of dollars in federal reimbursements over time. Steps taken to comply with the federal regulations resulted in reducing the number of people living in institutions because of strict standards of minimum square footage per person (Joint Mental Health Oversight Committee, 1980).

The Michigan plan set a goal of establishing a state institutional population of fewer than 4,000 persons by 1980. The plan also included the construction of Alternative Intermediate Services for the Mentally Retarded (AIS/MR) homes, which were privately operated ICFs/MR. In Michigan, 1000 people were to be transferred from the state institutions into the AIS/MR homes. Per the planners' agenda, these AIS/MR homes fulfilled the need for one part of a continuum of residential services ranging from independent living at the one end to institutional placement at the other. The AIS/MR homes, designed for eight or fewer persons, were to be slightly less restrictive than the traditional state institutions. Their development was seen as a way the State could place individuals with severe impairments or behavioral challenges in the community and still engage in the institutional depopulation plan that was mandated by the federal regulations. The incentive to the State to participate in the ICF/MR program was considerable. Between fiscal years 1977 and 1987, federal ICF/MR reimbursement to the state of Michigan totaled nearly $826 million (Braddock, Hemp, Parish, & Westrich, 1998). At the time Michigan developed its ICF/MR compliance plan, their were no formal goals to close any of the state's public institutions (DMH, 1977).

The submission of Michigan's ICF/MR compliance plan marked the beginning of an aggressive depopulation strategy that had a federal incentive attached to it. Prior to the enactment of ICF/MR legislation, depopulation of the state's public institutions had not had the sense of urgency that it received when it negotiated its compliance plan with the federal government. Failure to meet the plan's objectives and institutional

improvement targets could result in the loss of millions of federal ICF/MR dollars to the State.

Passage of several zoning acts occurred in 1976 (Pub. Acts 394-398). These new statutes established a statewide standard that if a community residence was licensed to serve six or fewer people, municipalities could not impose any zoning restrictions on them. These laws were unsuccessfully challenged by neighborhood groups and towns more than a hundred times between 1976 and 1985. Thus the laws proved to be an important factor that facilitated the ongoing development of the state's community residential programs.

Because the zoning statutes established a standard that homes for six or fewer individuals did not need a town's permission to open, most homes developed after 1976 were for six or fewer individuals and therfore avoided entanglements with local municipalities. Partly as a result of this law, Michigan avoided the development of larger private facilities.

Legislation was enacted in 1977 to prohibit the close development of community residences (Pub. Acts 28-30 of 1977), and mandated that facilities could not be developed within 1,500 feet of one another, or within 3,000 feet of one another in Detroit. The Department of Social Services was also mandated to conduct public notification of pending group home development for neighbors in close proximity to the proposed site. Such notification provisions were intended to give residents the opportunity to air their concerns, and for the DMH and Social Services to explain the community placement program to the new neighbors. While such notification was mandated, the hearings did not allow neighbors to block the development of the programs, and most interview respondents indicated that these laws did not have a major impact on the continuing operation of the community placement program. Finally, the Department of Social Services was required not to license facilities when doing so would contribute to "excessive concentration" in a neighborhood. However, the statute did not specify what excessive concentration was, and the Department of Social Services was directed to develop its own standards. The Department of Social Services subsequently used the distance criteria stipulated in the law as its measure of excessive concentration, and did not impose further restrictions on the community placement program (Michigan Department of Social Services, 1980).

In February 1978, the *Detroit Free Press* broke a sensational and horrific story, reporting rampant abuse of residents occurring, and being covered up, at the Plymouth Center for Human Development, which was one of the state's largest developmental disabilities institutions. In their series of 10 articles, replete with shocking and gruesome photographs, Paul Magnusson and Susan Watson opened the door to what became another watershed in the evolution of Michigan's residential service system.

The exposé published by the *Detroit Free Press* was not unlike others around the country. The pictures are alarmingly similar to Geraldo Rivera's televised footage of the Willowbrook State School in New York several years earlier. Like the Willowbrook exposé, the Plymouth scandal catalyzed the filing of a class-action lawsuit by the state Association for Retarded Citizens. The case was filed against DMH in federal court on February 21, 1978, on behalf of the Center's 830 residents. The attorneys representing the ARC and the Plymouth residents were from the Michigan Protection and Advocacy Service. On March 4, the courts recognized the plaintiffs as a class and the suit henceforth represented all of Plymouth's residents (*Michigan ARC v. Smith,* 1979; Michigan Protection and Advocacy, 1979).

On February 24, 1978, in response to the scandal, Governor Milliken outlined a 13-step plan designed to address and eliminate abuse in state mental health facilities. The governor directed DMH to take a number of steps to address abuse. Administrative changes ordered by the governor included improvement in the system of reporting and filing abuse injuries and medical treatment reports, development and submission of a plan to safeguard patients' rights, involvement of parent groups in the recipient rights process, expansion of parental and community involvement in state institutions, the development and distribution of instructional materials defining abuse, and wide dissemination of DMH's agreement with the Department of Social Services regarding their respective responsibilities related to the abuse investigations (Milliken, 1978a, 1978b).

The governor's plan also called for changes in staff management and supervision practices, including strengthening and standardizing new employee orien-

tation, establishment of a career ladder for institutional employees, development of new in-service training programs, reviewing civil service job descriptions, and review of the existing discipline procedures with the goal of eliminating barriers to the speedy resolution of disciplinary cases. The governor called for an immediate reassessment of the resources needed by the institutions, which was to be completed in conjunction with the Department of Management and Budget. He also directed the Department of Mental Health to ensure all abuse and neglect allegations were promptly investigated and the disposition of the investigation be reported to the person who initiated the complaint (Milliken, 1978a, 1978b).

On March 9, 1978, Governor Milliken appointed the Task Force on Prevention and Investigation of Abuse in State Institutions, chaired by Wilbur Cohen, who was then the dean of the University of Michigan's School of Education. Cohen headed the federal Department of Health, Education, and Welfare for many years and was one of the principal architects of the Social Security Act (Berkowitz, 1995).

In a special report to the legislature issued a few weeks after the establishment of his 13-step plan, the governor reported that the Cohen Task Force had been directed to:

> ascertain the facts and disposition of incidents and allegations of abuse and neglect at Plymouth, review administrative response to allegations, assist present Plymouth Center administration in pursuing any new allegations of abuse and neglect and undertake the broader role of reviewing the method by which abuse cases are addressed in other state institutions that provide live-in care and treatment programs. (Milliken, 1978b, p. 1)

While the governor's charge to the Cohen Task Force was largely restricted to abuse and neglect at the Plymouth Center and other state institutions, the Task Force interpreted its mandate much more broadly. Its interim and final reports, issued in May and July, respectively, of 1978, offered far-reaching recommendations related to all of the state's institutions, presenting the solution to abuse as the development of community-based residences:

We believe that the policy of placing each mentally retarded person in the least restrictive environment is sound and should be pursued vigorously and effectively. Full implementation of this policy will require substantial additional funds and cooperation among the parents, the staff and the community. The Task Force believes the involvement of the community is essential in the development of such facilities and the subsequent placement of residents. We favor the allocation of special project grants or contracts to develop pilot demonstrations of how such cooperation can be carried out. (Governor's Task Force on Prevention and Investigation of Abuse in State Institutions, 1978, pp. 9-10)

These recommendations related to community services clearly exceeded the governor's directions to the Task Force. Because the Task Force concluded that the atmosphere at Plymouth was supportive of abuse, Task Force members felt it was important to address the need for expanded community-based residential services and the dismantling of state institutional facilities.

Most interview respondents were only vaguely aware of the Task Force's report and were unconvinced it had been important in influencing public policy in Michigan. However, the report's impact on Governor Milliken, who certainly did influence public policy, is less clear. Cohen's long-standing tenure at the federal Department of Health, Education, and Welfare and his widely respected leadership on social services issues, must have offered the Task Force considerable credibility in the eyes of the governor. Given the immense problems confronting the DMH at the time, and the lack of effective leadership of the DMH, such credibility may have been vital to the governor. One interviewee suggested Cohen might have been selected to chair the Task Force because the governor knew in advance the kinds of recommendations that could be expected to emerge from an enterprise that Cohen headed.

What is meaningful for our purposes is that the Task Force's reports provided additional support to the nascent community services movement. By defin-

ing large institutions as fundamentally conducive to abuse, the Task Force suggested that the community was the only appropriate route the State could take in developing its residential service system.

Coincident with the administration's investigation into the Plymouth Center, the legislature conducted its own inquiry into the situation at Plymouth. The Joint Legislative Committee to Study Abuse in State Mental Health Facilities was cochaired by Sen. Jerome Hart and Rep. David Hollister. This committee reviewed recommendations of other groups, held its own hearings, and monitored the administration's activities. Wilbur Cohen testified before the Joint Committee in September 1978 and conveyed his recommendations in terms of abuse and neglect, as well as the costs of maintaining institutional facilities. Related to abuse and neglect, he stated:

> My own personal belief is that in the limited time our Task Force had at its disposal to make its report, we were only able to discover the tip of the iceberg of abuse and neglect that exists. It seems clear to me from letters and telephone calls which I received that there is more abuse than generally realized. I believe that there probably exists a substantial amount of neglect with respect to many children in the state and with respect to many older persons in nursing homes. I urge you to give special attention to these two areas. (Cohen, 1978, p. 3)

His convictions that abuse and neglect were common in state institutions, and his understanding of the considerable cost savings that community-based services represented to the State, led him to conclude for the committee that:

> It is essential that the state prepare and obtain agreement on a long-range plan for accelerating the process of reducing the size of state institutions, accelerating community placement and improving that quality of life for the vulnerable individuals for whom the state has assumed responsibility. (Cohen, 1978, p. 5)

By September 1978, the Joint Legislative Committee had produced its final report. Its recommendations included short-term improvements to quickly improve the quality of institutional care for people with mental disabilities. However, the report also took a firm stand on the state's long-term approach to institutions stating that:

> [I]n the long run, the state must phase out the large institution approach to mental health care and replace it with a comprehensive community-based system of care and treatment… the present community network of residential and treatment services for the mentally disabled must be broadened, strengthened and effectively coordinated…funds for care and treatment must precede the patient into the community from the institution. Public attitudes toward and community acceptance of mentally disabled persons must be improved. A meaningful, useful role in society is inherently rehabilitative and must be promoted. (Hart & Hollister, 1978, p. 2)

In the meantime, the lawsuit related to conditions at the Plymouth Center brought by the Michigan ARC against the DMH was proceeding. By the following year, the parties reached agreement on the shape of a consent decree which was signed by Judge Joiner on August 30, 1979. The following month, Joiner appointed David Rosen to be the master responsible for oversight of consent decree implementation. In November, DMH finalized its plan to implement the decree (*Michigan ARC v. Smith,* 1979).

The consent decree ordered DMH to develop community placements for all Plymouth residents and residential services were to be provided in facilities that served no more than eight persons. In October 1979, DMH Director Frank Ochberg appointed Ben Censoni to be the director of a new unit with the sole responsibility of implementing the consent decree (Ochberg, 1979). Censoni had been with the MORC and was a visionary in the development of Michigan's community-based residential services system.

The lawsuit eventually resulted in the placement of Plymouth residents into community homes and the

facility's closure in 1984. Most interview respondents felt the Plymouth Center played a central role in shaping the development of community services in Michigan. While documentary evidence indicates community residences had begun to develop in earnest before the Plymouth lawsuit, interview respondents agree the lawsuit accelerated the development of community-based residences.

At the end of the 1970s, as the development of community-based residential services accelerated, so did the opposition by neighborhoods of the placement of such facilities within their midst. Many municipalities across the State filed legal challenges to the state's zoning laws with the hope that the Michigan courts would undo the work of the legislature. Governor Milliken, in his annual State of the State message, characterized the problems in the community placement program as follows:

> Now we must address the other half to the equation. It is no secret that some communities in this state discriminate against the mentally ill and the mentally retarded through restrictive zoning ordinances. It is time to stop that discrimination. (Milliken, 1976, p. 64)

His commitment to the community placement program, in the face of ongoing community opposition, was clearly articulated again in his 1980 message to the State:

> [In spite of local community resistance to community placement] I remain determined to strengthen and build our community placement program in Michigan. I believe that a successful community placement program enriches the quality of life for all concerned. My budget recommendation to the Legislature will include a substantial increase in the budget for community placement services. (Milliken, 1980, p. 69)

In 1979, the Michigan Supreme Court refused to hear a case involving a group home for six children challenged by Avon Township, the Bellarmine case (DMH, 1979). By refusing to hear the case, the Michigan Supreme Court let stand the Court of Appeals' ruling that the group home had the right to exist in the local community. The following year, the Court of Appeals issued a ruling in a case involving five women with developmental disabilities who lived in a group home in St. Clair Shores. The Court of Appeals decided in favor of the women, ruling that they were living together as a family and again holding that the state's zoning ordinances were constitutional (*Malcolm v. Shamie,* 1980). Communities, however, continued to oppose the development of group homes.

In an effort to address heightened community opposition to group home development, legislation was passed which compelled DMH to issue a community notification policy whereby neighbors in close proximity to a proposed group home were told of its pending development (Pub. Act 423 of 1980). This was an expansion of the previous policy that mandated the Department of Social Services conduct such notifications.

In spite of the passage of this law, a number of legislators continued to be concerned with the development of group homes in the State. Several legislators called for a moratorium on further placements until the community placement program could be fully investigated. At the request of House Speaker Gary Owen, the Auditor General evaluated the state's community placement program, and released its preliminary analysis of group home leases in June 1981. This report leveled serious accusations of mismanagement against DMH, noting instances where DMH staff were running foster care homes or were married to foster care operators, and where there were notable differences in reimbursement rates and differences in lease agreements across substantively identical facilities. The auditors asserted that waste in the community placement program totaled more than $30 million (Michigan Office of the Auditor General, 1981).

House Speaker Gary Owen seized the opportunity presented by the report, and initiated his own inquiry into its findings. DMH Director Ochberg was unable to satisfy the legislature that DMH did, in fact, have a community placement system that was functioning and effective (Joint Capital Outlay Subcommittee, 1981). A number of legislators used the Office of the Auditor General's report as a springboard from which to introduce legislation intended to restrict or curtail the further development of community homes

by DMH.

Several members of the Joint Capital Outlay Subcommittee wanted the community placement program to be stopped until the problems were fixed and the subcommittee voted unanimously to refer the findings of the auditor general to the attorney general and the state police for investigation and possible prosecution. The State Department of Management and Budget subsequently requested an investigation by the attorney general and the state police into an insurance agency in Wayne County that had received a seemingly excessive amount of DMH insurance business for community group homes (Miller, 1981).

In response to the Joint Capital Outlay Subcommittee's activities, the Michigan ARC held a press conference attacking the Subcommittee and its proceedings. Coverage in the *Detroit Free Press* and the *Lansing Journal* was similar; both papers gave airtime to the notion that the Subcommittee had political motives in pressing for the termination of the community placement program.

> "The questions and innuendoes raised by the committee give the public a bad image of the entire program," said Beth Ferguson, acting director of the Michigan State Planning Council for Developmental Disabilities [Michigan Association for Retarded Citizens Executive Director Harvey] Zuckerberg said "unfair treatment of the program was partly due to lawmaker's displeasure with the way former Mental Health Director Dr. Frank Ochberg ran the department. Ochberg had been a strong proponent of the program." (Benac, 1981, p. 3A)

In response to the legislature's concerns, Governor Milliken established the Interagency Community Placement Coordinating Council to investigate and address the issues. This council was composed of the directors of the Departments of Social Services, Mental Health, Public Health, Labor, Corrections, and Management and Budget, and the Superintendent of Public Instruction. At its first meeting in June 1981, the Council agreed that the major crisis facing the community placement program was in fact a crisis of "credibility" (Governor's Interagency Community Placement

Coordinating Council, 1981).

Each department addressed by the auditor general's report participated in a response coordinated by the Council. In its response, DMH largely disagreed with the interpretation of the facts by the auditor general. In its defense, the DMH noted that considerable corrective action was already underway, including the implementation of new policies, and cooperation with the Department of Management and Budget on leasing issues (Governor's Interagency Community Placement Coordinating Council, 1981).

In 1980 and 1981, in reaction to concerns about the community placement program, the legislature enacted measures that directed DMH to provide greater oversight to the program (Pub. Act 39 of 1981; Pub. Act 360 of 1980). In response to these legislative directives, Ben Censoni was appointed director of the Office of Community Placement Coordination in June 1981. This office was established to provide a single, cohesive administrative structure for the ongoing community placement program (Ochberg, 1981).

DMH Director Ochberg subsequently resigned in response to persistent criticisms of the community placement process and other concerns about his leadership. Governor Milliken replaced him with C. Patrick Babcock, who had formerly been director of the Department of Labor, and had served the governor and the legislature in a number of different capacities (Babcock, 1982a; DMH, 1981a). Babcock's appointment represented a turning point for the Department. By all accounts, he was the first director to truly champion the cause of community placement for persons with developmental disabilities, and to provide effective leadership in doing so. He was also the first director in more than a decade to be widely respected by the governor, the legislature, and the advocacy community. Babcock's appointment represented a transition in departmental leadership for the community placement movement. Prior to his appointment, the Department's leadership in community placement issues had come from the MORC; after Babcock became director, departmental leadership was shared between the central office staff and MORC.

The opposition to the development of community homes continued to be a problem into the mid-1980s. Opposition took the form of legislation introduced to slow or stop community homes from being developed, lawsuits against proposed homes, and violence from neighbors.

New legislation mandated establishment of new neighborhood notification policies had the direct effect of slowing group home development, as did the new leasing policies that resulted from the auditor general's investigation and subsequent report. In 1981, the Plymouth master wrote to the Michigan ARC, indicating that DMH was not meeting its placement objectives for the Plymouth class because of the imposition of these new policies, and because of continued opposition from neighbors.

The Department of Mental Health's inability to meet the census reduction schedule delineated in the Stipulation for Modification of the Court's Order of August 30, 1979, has in part been related to the... recently developed procedures regarding the negotiation and renegotiation of leases with investors. This Office is aware that up to twenty-five six-bed group homes were lost by the Department of Mental Health... as a direct result of restrictions in the letting of leases as related to determining rental amounts. Furthermore, there are a number of group homes currently in operation containing both Class and non-class members which are in jeopardy of closing because the leases are being renegotiated for substantially lower rental amount than would justify their continuance. The loss of these homes may result in the return of the clients to institutions. The impact of the policies and procedures now being implemented by DMH and [the Department of Management and the Budget] at the behest of the Legislature has resulted in the deceleration of community placement and will prolong the process of developing new homes and may result in the loss of existing homes. Our concern regarding the impact of these measures encompasses all of Michigan's developmentally disabled citizens who are in need of community placement, not only members of the Class. The cutbacks in institutional staffing and services have caused more persons to turn with hope toward the community. The gains which have been made over recent years in the community placement arena are in danger of being lost unless a coordinated, intensive effort is made to reactivate the community placement momentum which has been stalled by recent actions generated by individuals and groups opposed to community placement. (Rosen, 1981, pp. 1-2)

Neighborhood opposition to group homes became violent in 1982. In April and May, two group homes under construction were firebombed in Livonia and Pleasant Ridge, respectively (Flanigan, 1982). In 1985, three legislators introduced a measure that would have instituted quotas on the number of facilities that could be located in a municipality. These legislators claimed some towns were forced to bear a disproportionate share of the number of homes being developed, while other towns did not experience the development of any (Goldberg, 1985). Most interview respondents felt that the notion of "overconcentration," as it was termed, or locating too many facilities in one place, was a cover for legislative attempts to block further community placement entirely. This measure was not enacted, but it is indicative of the ways in which some legislators sought to curb the community placement program.

In spite of the opposition and problems raised related to the development of community-based residences, their growth continued. In 1980, there were 27 AIS/MR homes under construction, and an additional 47 homes had been completed (DMH, 1980). By 1984, there were 157 AIS/MR homes operating in the State (Michigan Department of Public Health, 1984). By 1988, the number of facilities had expanded to exceed 350 (DMH, 1988a).

In 1985, the Michigan Supreme Court issued a ruling in the first zoning challenge that it heard. Arguments before the Court took place in 1984, in a combined case involving persons with developmental disabilities and persons with mental illness. The Court ruled that the 1976 zoning laws did not violate the state's Constitution, and community residences for six or fewer persons were not subject to local zoning restrictions (*City of Livonia v. Department of Social Services, Greentrees Civic Association Inc. v.*

Pignatiello, 1985).

The early 1980s were also marked by severe fiscal conditions in Michigan. The State was clearly affected by the national recession and tax cuts enacted in the 1970s made the State budget situation even worse (Brazer, 1982). The state's economic problems resulted in deep budget cuts to all departments, particularly in fiscal years 1981-83. The gravity of the situation was explained by this memo to all of the state's departments from the director of the Department of Management:

Having begun the fiscal year with the largest Executive Order [reducing the budget] in the state's history, many of you may still be adjusting your program plans to accommodate a lower than expected level of spending. As you proceed with the difficult task of balancing a constant, or increasing, demand with diminished resources, I must ask that you also keep in mind the precarious nature of our financial stability... As you continue the strong management controls that have been used over the past year, it would be prudent and sound to establish a goal of lapsing at least 4 percent of your net general fund/general purpose appropriate, after the Executive Order. You should regard these steps as necessary and minimal actions for dealing with the most difficult year which lies ahead of us. (Miller, 1981, p. 1)

In addition to having sustained serious cuts, departments were also expected to ensure they spent only 96% of the portion of their budget derived from state funds (as opposed to federal) sources. In the face of these budget cuts, and the ones that followed in subsequent years, public institutional staff were cut, and accreditation of a number of facilities was lost. In 1979, nine of the state's public institutions had been accredited. By November 1983, only Coldwater, Mt. Pleasant, and Muskegon were accredited (DMH, 1983). Efforts to regain accreditation resulted in all facilities except Northville achieving accreditation by fiscal year 1986 (Babcock, 1985).

In his 1982 message to the State, Governor Milliken noted that the Alpine Center had closed, and the State planned to close the Hillcrest, Plymouth, and Northville Centers. Alpine was closed as a result of transferring all residents to community-based homes (Milliken, 1982). In December 1982 Governor Blanchard was elected, and, he carried on with the institutional closure program begun under Governor Milliken. Hillcrest was closed in 1982, Northville in 1983, and Plymouth in 1984 (Angelotti, 1997). By the end of Blanchard's tenure as governor, Coldwater, the Macomb-Oakland Regional Center, and Oakdale (formerly Lapeer) were closed as well, in 1987, 1989, and 1991, respectively (Braddock, Hemp, Parish, Westrich, & Park, 1998).

Babcock had so impressed the advocacy community that the Mental Health Coalition, a nonprofit advocacy group, petitioned governor-elect Blanchard to keep Babcock on as DMH director (Rave, 1982), which he subsequently did.

> One of your early decisions must be the choice of a director for the Department of Mental Health. Pat Babcock has enormously strengthened the department in the relatively short time he has served as its director. His management ability, decisiveness, leadership, skill with the Legislature, and open, consultative style have earned him nearly universal respect.... The Department of Mental Health is one of the potential trouble areas for your administration. It has suffered scandal, severe budget cuts, and frequent changes in leadership during a period when the basic philosophy for delivery of mental health services is changing. At current budget levels, the safety of staff and clients is in jeopardy. We urge you to select the director of this sensitive department with the utmost care. (Rave, 1982, p. 1)

In 1983, the State took another major step in the development of its community service system. In December, championed by Rep. Debbie Stabenow, the State passed the Family Support Subsidy Act, which authorized payments to the families of children with severe disabilities (Pub. Act 249 of 1983). Stabenow had worked tirelessly to campaign for passage of the bill, which was pushed as a major cost-saving measure for the State. By paying families a monthly stipend for caring for their disabled child, the State could avoid the more expensive alternative of residential placement (House Committee on Mental Health, 1983; Stabenow, 1983a, 1983b). This program was very successful, both in terms of the families' satisfaction with it, and its utility in preventing institutional placement. Preventive impact was assessed by counting the number of families that sought residential placements for their children, and then rescinded their requests after receiving family support subsidies (DMH, 1988b).

The 1980s also witnessed extensive problems with the state's system of nursing home care for persons with developmental disabilities. In 1983, the eight existing specialized nursing homes were phased into five such facilities. The Warren Manor home, which was not a specialized nursing home, but a facility with a considerable population of children with developmental disabilities, was closed in 1986. This facility's closure was prompted by concerns related to care that were uncovered by the state's Protection and Advocacy organization. By 1988, the census of the specialized nursing homes totaled 496 persons (DMH, 1988a). That year, Michigan submitted an application for OBRA-87 Waiver funds. These funds were made available by the federal government with passage of the Omnibus Budget Reconciliation Act (OBRA) of 1987, which contained federal nursing home reform standards. Under this new legislation, states were required to assess individuals with developmental disabilities living in nursing homes, and provide them with active treatment as needed. As part of its plan of compliance with the new federal law, Michigan proposed to close three of its specialized nursing homes by 1990.

Advocates had been raising concerns about conditions in the specialized nursing homes throughout the 1980s, and particularly at the Wayne Total Living Center. In February 1988, before the December 1988 finalization of the state's OBRA-87 compliance plan, advocates filed a lawsuit on behalf of all persons with developmental disabilities living in nursing homes (*Kope v. Watkins,* 1988). This lawsuit eventually resulted in the closure of all the specialized nursing homes.

At the end of the 1980s, Michigan's residential service system for persons with developmental disabilities had grown considerably, and looked very little like it had in the early 1970s. Institutions had been displaced as the major service type, and small community residences were the norm. *Figure 3.3* depicts the state's residential service system for persons with developmental disabilities in 1977 and in 1990. As is evident from the figure, the greatest growth in Michigan's residential service system between 1977 and 1990, in terms of the number of residents, occurred in settings for six or fewer persons. Reliable pre-1977 data could not be located for the number of persons with developmental disabilities in private residential settings, which is why the later point of 1977 was selected.

Administrative Overview

This section will explain, in general terms, how residential services for persons with developmental disabilities in Michigan were organized and provided during the 1970-90 study period. Also, the ways in which this administrative structure affected the evolution of the service system will be discussed.

The role of the MORC within DMH has been discussed previously. Its role was an important way in which the state's administrative structure facilitated the development of community-based residential services. As noted, the Department's authority over the main

innovator in Michigan provided opportunities to pilot new initiatives in a controlled fashion. By the same token, MORC had the latitude and support of the DMH in depopulating other state institutions.

The second important aspect of the structure of the service delivery system was that DMH and the Community Mental Health (CMH) Boards jointly shared responsibility for the provision of developmental disabilities services. In 1974, Michigan enacted major changes to its Mental Health Code. The most important achievement of the new Code was that it established a structure for the provision of community-based services. The Act stated:

> It shall be the objective of the Department to shift from the state to a county, the primary responsibility for the direct delivery of public mental health services, whenever such county shall have demonstrated a willingness and capacity to provide an adequate and appropriate system of mental health services for the citizens of such county. (Pub. Act 258 of 1974)

Under this new structure, counties were allowed to provide services as they developed the ability to do so. Three levels of CMH Board control over services

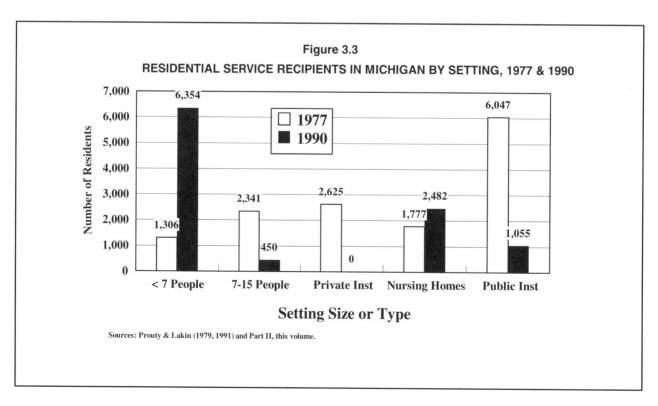

Figure 3.3
RESIDENTIAL SERVICE RECIPIENTS IN MICHIGAN BY SETTING, 1977 & 1990

Sources: Prouty & Lakin (1979, 1991) and Part II, this volume.

were established: full management, where the CMH had the total responsibility for contracting for or providing services; shared management, where DMH and CMH together contracted for the services, and DMH management, where the DMH controlled the service system. Counties were allowed to gradually transition to greater levels of authority, ensuring the transition to CMH control was smooth. Concurrent with this development was the implementation of the governor's priority of establishing a unified system of delivering mental health and developmental disabilities services.

The financing structure was such that 90% of the resources allocated within counties for mental health and developmental disabilities services came from DMH, and 10% was derived from the county (Pub. Act 258 of 1974). The decentralization of the development of community-based services was identified by many interview respondents as one of the hallmarks of success in the Michigan service system. This structure put in place a specific and concrete mechanism for the widespread development of community services across the State. The language of the statute mandated county participation only to the extent that a county was willing and able to provide it; DMH remained the safety net until such capacity was developed, and therefore, community mental health programs developed slowly and took over responsibilities from the Department as they were able to do so.

Another aspect of the administration of services in Michigan helped facilitate the development of community-based residential services: From the outset, there was a separation between service provision and housing ownership. As noted previously, in Michigan separate financing arrangements were made to pay for the capital development of new group homes and the provision of services. This structure allowed DMH to better control services. Service providers did not become overly powerful because they did not have access to considerable sums of money available by owning housing. In this way, the concentration of power was not vested solely with one constituency group. Related to this balance of power was the fact that the Department initially limited the number of homes service providers could operate. Generally, service providers were limited to operating 10 homes, which provided another check on their development of power.

Another important structural or administrative aspect of the development of community services was that when the State embarked upon its plan to develop AIS/MR homes, the Departments of Mental Health and Social Services agreed that DMH would have sole responsibility for these homes. As the state's Medicaid agency in Michigan, the Department of Social Services would otherwise have been required to run the new AIS/MR homes. However, according to the memorandum of understanding between the two departments, DMH had total control over its community-based AIS/MR program, and, more important, over its ICF/MR budget. This ensured DMH received the federal revenues it generated by quickly developing the AIS/MR homes. In many other states, when a state receives federal Medicaid reimbursement, the revenues go back to the general treasury; the budget process does not return these funds to the state's developmental disabilities agency (R. Gettings, personal communication, July 2001). In Michigan, however, due to this early agreement, DMH was able to use the revenues it generated by expanding its ICF/MR program, another incentive to develop community residential services.

It is clear the state's administrative structure played a supporting role in the evolution of the developmental disabilities residential service system. Most important, the latitude DMH gave the MORC for innovation provided a foundation for the rest of the State. MORC also proved that people with severe impairments could be successfully supported in community services, which established the state's capacity to serve everyone in the community. The planned and careful transition to locally controlled and administered services provided a framework within which group homes could be developed. The Department's control over the ICF/MR program gave it resources that were an incentive to continue the expansion of community services. The division between service provision and control of housing prevented service providers from becoming all-powerful. All of these factors worked together to provide a capacity for the innovations that the State pursued, and a foundation from which the State could expand its community-based service system.

Scandals

This section will discuss some of the scandals that

have beset the Michigan residential services system during the 1970-90 period, with a particular emphasis on their implications for public policy. One interview respondent stated, "scandals are only useful if the media hangs onto them and there are people in leadership positions who take actions to address them." This respondent's characterization of the role scandals play in shaping public policy seems to be a fairly accurate representation of what occurred in Michigan.

In situations where the media "held" a story, and the state's leadership, whether advocates or state officials, exploited the notoriety, public policy was shifted. A requirement for public policy to be changed was the capacity within the system to do so. In instances where these forces did not coincide, public policy remained relatively unaffected.

The exposé that the *Detroit Free Press* published, which uncovered conditions at the Plymouth Center, led to the filing of a class-action lawsuit that resulted in the facility's closure, and an accelerated program of community-based residential expansion. The Plymouth scandal was clearly the one that made the greatest impact on the evolution of the state's developmental disabilities service system.

It seems that in order to shape policy, scandals must also occur at a timely moment. When the *Detroit Free Press* broke the Plymouth story, the MORC had been developing community-based residential services for a number of years (DMH, 1979). As such, MORC provided the State with the capacity or foundation from which it could structure changes to its residential service systems. The Plymouth scandal also occurred as the depopulation of public developmental disabilities institutions and the development of community services was increasingly recognized as a civil rights movement. In one final way, the timing of the scandal was propitious. The scandal occurred at a time when the state's elected leadership, both the legislature and the governor, was receptive to, and supportive of, changing the service system (Hart & Hollister, 1978; Milliken, 1978b).

The ARC also seized the opportunity offered by the *Detroit Free Press*, and immediately filed the class-action lawsuit (*Michigan ARC v. Smith,* 1978). The Association for Retarded Citizens was able to do so because it had established credibility and sufficient organizational resources that positioned it to continue to be a leader in the State and to make such a bold move.

The *Detroit Free Press* ran 10 stories on the Plymouth Center and made coverage of Plymouth a centerpiece of its news reporting. Their attention to this issue was important to the unfolding of the Plymouth crisis because in addition to revealing the horrors of life in the institution for the residents, they continued to hold the governor and DMH accountable.

These were all important aspects of the way in which Plymouth became an important catalyst for the growth of community-based residential services. The Plymouth scandal was by no means the state's first developmental disabilities scandal. The 1970s saw a series of deaths of adult foster care residents. In one particularly gruesome beating death of a man with disabilities in such a facility, Department of Social Services Director John Dempsey (1977) called for a complete investigation into the overall operation of the residential program. He wrote a personal memo to all field workers reminding them of the importance of investigating and attempting to prevent abuse in such facilities.

However, most respondents reported these types of situations, which were not uncommon in the 1970s, did not capture the media's attention the way Plymouth did and were not a means by which major changes in public policy occurred. One respondent spoke for many, stating that these incidents "might have facilitated an emergency response to that moment in time. But the movement in Michigan was driven far more by bigger public policy perspectives than a single incident."

In 1979, eighteen months after the Plymouth story broke, there were 11 deaths at the state's Hillcrest Center, another public institution for people with developmental disabilities (Pomeroy, 1980). These deaths also attracted media attention, and were subsequently investigated by the state police. The Department of Mental Health conducted its own inquiry and, like the state police, concluded that the deaths had not occurred because of abuse or neglect. However, the DMH did conclude that numerous policies were not followed, and the lack of adherence to some policies may have contributed to the deaths. In reviewing the Department's inquiry, it appeared there were considerable problems with staff supervision that were related to the deaths (Pomeroy, 1980). The Hillcrest Center incidents, however, did not precipitate major changes in the residential service system.

In the 1980s, nursing homes became a target for investigations. In 1986, Warren Village, which had been a nursing home for 150 children with developmental disabilities, was closed after serious questions about care were raised by the Protection and Advocacy organization. Two years later, this organization joined forces with advocates from across the State. This group wrote to Governor Blanchard protesting conditions for people with disabilities who were living at the Wayne Total Living Center, another specialized nursing home (Bauer et al., 1988). Protection and Advocacy subsequently filed a lawsuit on behalf of 535 nursing home residents with developmental disabilities, all of whom had been transferred from the state's public institutions (*Kope v. Watkins*, 1988). This lawsuit was eventually settled in the 1990s and all of Michigan's specialized nursing homes for people with developmental disabilities were closed.

In evaluating the role scandals played in the development of Michigan's residential service system, the incidents at the Plymouth Center did the most to accelerate the expansion of community-based residential services. While several interview respondents felt the community-based residential service system really began with Plymouth, there is considerable evidence this residential transformation actually began with the activities of the MORC much earlier in the decade. There is no doubt, however, that Plymouth accelerated the state's expansion of services. The fact that the State was under court orders to develop community placement for Plymouth class members during its period of most financial difficulty was also a helpful aspect of the transformation of the state's residential service system. But scandals have had a limited impact by themselves. It seems the scandal must be seized as an opportunity by advocates to press for change. It is also possible that a scandal needs to receive considerable media attention before it can become an important catalyst.

Politics

Politics played a much smaller role in shaping the residential service system in Michigan than it did in Illinois. In fact, when asked the main contributing factors to the emergence of community-based residences, no Michigan respondent directly identified politics. This is not to say that politics did not play a role, but it was more subtle than what occurred in Illinois.

The structure of Michigan politics did more to facilitate the development of community residential services than to bar such development, and this was the case for a number of reasons. The first was that under the structure of the legislature "Power is shared extensively; it's like fine old wine, nobody gets much" (Browne & Verburg, 1995, pp. 114-15). The dispersion of power among legislators means there was a need for cooperation across party lines and among different regional representatives. There was considerable regional fragmentation in Michigan, and the party leadership was often unable to keep members in line (Browne & Verburg, 1995). Minority views in such a system appear to have a greater chance at effecting change because individual legislators had considerable independence, and power was not consolidated. As such, protection of the status quo was not necessarily an implicit goal of politics in the State.

In contrast with Illinois, patronage never emerged as a major part of State government in Michigan, largely due to so-called "outstate" (non-Detroit) control. Prior to the U.S. Supreme Court-order redistricting for the 1964 election, it was possible for the rural counties, even though they were in a minority of the population, to elect Republican governors (Browne & Verburg, 1995). Prior to redistricting, legislative districts were constructed along disproportionate county lines. The Supreme Court mandated redistricting that was proportionate to the population, and established a one-person-one-vote election system. But due to the long-standing power of the outstate counties, patronage did not emerge as a major component of the state's political system (Browne & Verburg, 1995). The lack of patronage in Michigan meant that state jobs, particularly those in public institutions, were not widely used as rewards for political loyalty or service. This is not to imply, however, that Michigan legislators were immune to concerns over the employment of institutional workers in their districts. There is considerable evidence that legislators viewed institutions as major sources of employment for their constituents, particularly in rural areas (e.g., Michigan House of Representatives, 1972).

Several interview respondents argued that the influence of politics was probably most evident in the closure of the state's public institutions. The first three public institutions to close were Alpine, Hillcrest, and Northville, which closed in the early 1980s, during Governor Milliken's administration. These facilities were among the state's smallest, which several interview respondents felt was undoubtedly a concession to the unions that represented institutional workers. During Governor Blanchard's administration, DMH closed the Coldwater and Macomb-Oakland facilities voluntarily, and Plymouth closed under court order. Some interview respondents felt that Blanchard did not aggressively pursue closure because of the connections between the Democratic Party and the powerful labor unions in the State. As is the case with much of politics, which often occurs in ways that are not recorded, these claims could not be verified or refuted by review of the documentary evidence.

Federal Influences

Congressional passage of the ICF/MR law in 1971 offered the same impetus for Michigan to depopulate its state institutions that it offered the rest of the country. States that met the federal ICF/MR standards were eligible to receive federal reimbursement for their programs, ranging from 50% to approximately 80% of the costs. However, by federal standards, Michigan's institutions were woefully overcrowded, staffing ratios were inadequate, and the level of care provided was substandard.

To capture the available federal funds, Michigan embarked upon a major program of institutional depopulation and facility renovation to achieve compliance. The plan that the State developed to comply with the federal ICF/MR regulations initially called for reducing the State institutional population by 1,200 persons by 1980 (DMH, 1977).

As discussed previously, another notable aspect of Michigan's compliance plan was the construction of AIS/MR homes, which were intended to complete the continuum of residential care for persons with developmental disabilities in Michigan. These facilities were located in the community and were the size of other group homes, but they received federal ICF/ MR funds. They were intended to serve individuals whose needs ostensibly did not require ongoing institutional placement, but whose needs were considerable enough that the individuals were not considered to be "appropriate" for regular group homes or foster care.

These facilities represented the opportunity to obtain federal Medicaid reimbursement for a form of community services. By 1984, there were 157 operating AIS/MR homes for more than 1,000 people, located in 56 of Michigan's 83 counties (DMH, 1985). Using these AIS/MR homes netted Michigan considerable federal revenue into its developmental disabilities service system. From the program's inception in 1977 to 1990, federal ICF/MR reimbursement that resulted from the AIS/MR program totaled $1.2 billion (Braddock, Hemp, Parish, & Westrich, 1998)

Several interview respondents indicated there was nothing particularly innovative in Michigan's approach to using federal ICF/MR funds to create community-based AIS/MR homes. Many states across the country embarked upon similar plans during the time period. What is important to our understanding of the evolution of the service system, however, is that Michigan did pursue the development of these AIS/MR homes aggressively, and their development helped the State to depopulate its large public facilities more quickly than might otherwise have been possible. The incentive offered by federal Medicaid funds was considerable. *Figure 3.4* depicts the annual level of federal ICF/MR funding Michigan received from 1977-90. The figure also includes all other sources of funding for developmental disabilities services, in order to represent the relative importance of federal ICF/MR revenues to the state's total budget. Michigan first received federal ICF/MR reimbursement in 1977. ICF/ MR revenues are shown for the state's institutions and for the AIS/MR homes.

Also important, however, was that the size of these facilities was strictly limited. Unlike its neighboring state of Illinois, which did not initially impose size limits on privately operated ICFs/MR, AIS/MR homes in Michigan were generally for six to eight people. This was relatively constant across the State as well. By 1984, six of the 157 operating AIS/MR homes in the State were for eight people, and none of the remainder served more than six people.

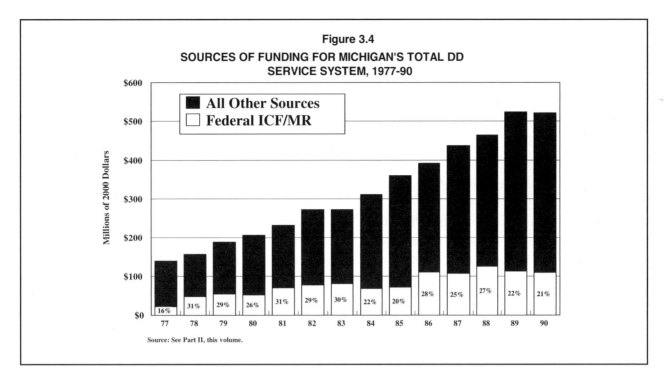

Figure 3.4
SOURCES OF FUNDING FOR MICHIGAN'S TOTAL DD
SERVICE SYSTEM, 1977-90

Source: See Part II, this volume.

The state's problems with the community placement program that began in the late 1970s were understood to represent a threat to the potential to obtain federal ICF/MR revenues. If the State didn't continue to develop group homes, it wouldn't meet its institutional depopulation targets. The Joint Mental Health Oversight Committee, chaired by Rep. David Hollister and Sen. Jerome Hart characterized its importance as follows:

> Michigan's entry into the Federal ICF/MR Medicaid program has resulted in the state receiving Federal reimbursement for 50% of the costs of care for mentally retarded persons in certified programs. Reimbursements were first received in 1977 and have continued to date, because Michigan has met annual goals toward achieving full compliance with ICF/MR plan requirements by July, 1982. To date, the state has received $126 million under this program, and projects receiving an average of $70 million per year for each of the next three fiscal years, through FY 1981-82. This would be an additional amount of $210 million. However, if the state is found to be out of compliance with its plan, because institutional populations didn't meet the planned levels and were too high, then

the state could stop receiving reimbursements, or even be required to return some funds received in previous years. A slowdown or moratorium on the AIS/MR program development, or on the other community placement alternatives would most certainly impact the progress toward compliance. (Joint Mental Health Oversight Committee, 1980, p. 64)

In 1981, the federal government passed the Omnibus Budget Reconciliation Act of 1981 (Pub. L. 97-35), which authorized states to receive federal Medicaid funds for community-based services. This legislation established the Home and Community Based Services (HCBS) Waiver. States with Waivers were allowed to obtain federal Medicaid reimbursement for approved services, including family support, day programs, and residential programs. Participation in the Waiver was attractive to states for the same reasons that the ICF/MR program was. The Waiver offered the opportunity to obtain considerable federal Medicaid funds for community-based services.

Michigan was not an early participant in the Waiver program. Its initial application was approved beginning October 1987 with a targeted number of service participants of 2,618 people for its first three years (DMH, 1987). Michigan's earliest years in the

Waiver did not reach the targeted population for which it had applied. By 1990, 1,647 participants had been served, with spending at an average of $26,300 per participant (Braddock et al., 2002). The ICF/MR program and the HCBS Waiver allowed Michigan to infuse its service system with federal funds at a time when its financial condition was dismal. Federal resources were a significant part of Michigan's spending for developmental disabilities services in the 1970s and 1980s. *Figure 3.5* shows the levels of combined state-federal HCBS Waiver, ICF/MR, and other funds for Michigan's community-based services spending from 1977-90. Community-based services here include day and employment programs, case management, residential programs in settings for 15 or fewer person, and family support services.

The final way in which federal activities influenced Michigan's service system is related to actions of the federal government that stimulate the formation of advocacy groups or task forces. Federal action, in addition to providing financial resources, catalyzed the advocacy groups and coalitions in Michigan that formed to address changes in national policy. A few examples will be used to illustrate this phenomenon.

When President Reagan took office in 1981, one of his priorities was to reduce the Social Security Administration's payouts that were being made to persons with disabilities. The Reagan Administration targeted Disability Insurance (DI) and Supplemental Security Income (SSI) for cuts, and $200 million was anticipated in savings during the first full year of administrative reinterpretation of entitlement rules (Dilley, 1987). To cut the program, the Social Security Administration accelerated its review of disability determinations; it re-evaluated individuals who had previously been found eligible to receive benefits, and instituted tougher standards for new applicants. As a consequence of these eligibility determinations, the approval rate for new applicants declined from 40% in 1979 to 29% in 1981. Reviews leading to the termination of beneficiaries had been anticipated to be 20%, but instead rose to 47% (Chambers, 1985). People with mental disabilities were heavily affected by the Administration's policy retrenchment; one fourth of all terminations were persons with mental impairments, even though they represented only one ninth of all beneficiaries (Goldman & Gattozzi, 1988). Public outcry about the cuts was substantial, and the U.S. House Select Committee on Aging accused the U.S. Social Security Administration of "deceptive practices" in its attempts to cut disability expenditures.

The cuts to Social Security for individuals with

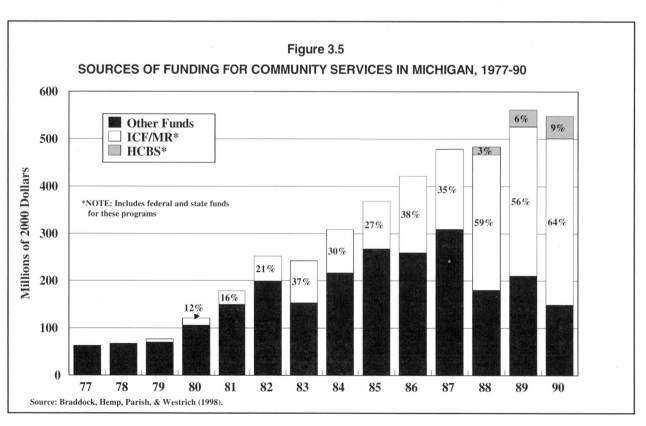

Figure 3.5

SOURCES OF FUNDING FOR COMMUNITY SERVICES IN MICHIGAN, 1977-90

Source: Braddock, Hemp, Parish, & Westrich (1998).

disabilities in Michigan were devastating. One of the important implications of these cuts is the burden of caring for people who were poor shifted from the federal government, which paid for Social Security programs like SSI and DI, to the states, which funded general assistance or poverty payments. Individuals with disabilities who were cut from SSI then sought support from the State through its general assistance (poverty) program. As a result, while Michigan was experiencing its most severe levels of unemployment in decades, the federal government cut its assistance to persons with disabilities.

To address these cuts, the governor created the Michigan Interagency Task Force on Disability (MITF/D). The Interagency Task Force comprised all of the state departments affected by the Social Security cuts including the Departments of Management and Budget, Mental Health, Social Services, Labor, and others. Participants also included advocacy groups, including staff from the DD Planning Council and Protection and Advocacy Services (Babcock, 1983; Michigan State Planning Council on Developmental Disabilities, 1984). The Task Force brought together individuals representing different programs and interests, including professionals and advocacy groups, and a full-scale attack on the Social Security Administration cuts was launched. Actions taken included training Social Security Administration field staff to properly authorize persons with disabilities to receive benefits, thus preventing them from being cut from the programs. The Task Force also educated Michigan's Congressional delegation about the importance of restoring Social Security benefits to individuals with disabilities. Later Congressional action led by Michigan's Senator Levin included passage of legislation that ordered the Social Security Administration to revise its disability determination policies.

The Task Force was not a coalition specifically targeting the needs of individuals with developmental disabilities. However, the Task Force's work served to put disability concerns on the agenda of decision makers at many levels and from many organizations. It also fostered a network of advocates who attempted to influence public policy at the national level. Important for the developmental disabilities movement, the Task Force offered another opportunity for advocates to join forces toward a common purpose. By including such diverse representatives as the Departments of Labor and Management and Budget, the Task Force must have engendered greater understanding of disability issues among groups that were not intimately familiar with them. These kinds of advocacy "occasions," where a single issue was addressed by a broad-based spectrum of advocates and organizations offered opportunities for public policy success to be realized. These activities strengthened the advocacy community and gave it momentum, thus positioning it to address subsequent issues.

Another example of federal action that catalyzed this type of a coalition response was reauthorization of the Developmental Disabilities Act in 1984. The Act identified the development of supported employment as a major priority. Subsequent to the Act's reauthorization, a number of different groups in Michigan worked together to obtain federal grant funds to develop and expand supported employment for people with developmental disabilities. This coalition was led by the state's Division of Rehabilitation Services, which was housed in the Department of Education. Participants, however, included people from the Michigan ARC, the Governor's Planning Council on Developmental Disabilities, DMH, Department of Social Services, and others (Griswold & Walden, 1986). While the Developmental Disabilities Act was a much more positive change in national policy than the Social Security cuts, the situation again created an opportunity for advocates and department officials to work together to meet a common goal, in this case, gaining access to federal funds for a new initiative for persons with developmental disabilities. When the State was successful in getting funding for its supportive employment initiative, bonds among advocates and different state departments were again strengthened.

In reflecting on different advocacy activities that occurred throughout the decades in question, one interview respondent reported that these kinds of single-issue coalitions were important to the developmental disabilities movement in the State. Another interview respondent described the importance of this means of working together as follows:

> We do work a lot in coalition in this state. That's a very valued way of working in this state. It's not perfect, of course. But we form

coalitions around single objectives or single purposes. When they expand beyond that, they usually fall apart. The mental health coalition was made up of groups as disparate as NAMI [National Alliance for the Mentally Ill], psychiatric survivors groups, People First, and the Association for Retarded Citizens. We were very effective when we went to the legislature and said, we want more money. When we fell apart was when we said we want more money for what. NAMI wanted more hospitals and psychiatric survivors wanted no hospitals. But that group was very effective in keeping up the drumbeat of "we want more money" during the state's major budget crises. Working in coalition is a major initiative here.... This has fostered understanding and it allowed for some progress. It all comes down to people.

Another interview respondent supported this individual's claims, stating: "advocacy groups are never so successful as when they are able to move from the momentum of one success."

In evaluating the relative importance of the contribution made by federal policies to the development of community services in Michigan during the 1970s and 1980s, it is clear that the impact was significant. Federal funds provided an important resource to begin and continue the state's deinstitutionalization efforts. The federal ICF/MR program was seized by Michigan leaders to develop small group homes and continue the momentum of community placement during difficult economic times. The state's use of the HCBS Waiver during the 1980s was less of a factor; little growth was evident during the decade. Finally, federal budget cuts and retrenchment provided a vehicle for Michigan advocates to coalesce against a common foe, thus strengthening them for further battles.

Public Officials and Bureaucratic Leadership

In Michigan, public officials and the state's developmental disabilities bureaucracy were an important part of the transformation of the state's residential service system. This section will consider the role and

contributions of the governors, the Legislature, the courts, and the Department of Mental Health.

The Governors

During the 1970-90 study period, Michigan was led by two governors, William Milliken (1967-83) and James Blanchard (1983-91). This section discusses the contributions of these men in succession.

Governor Milliken was a moderate Republican who was widely respected by developmental disabilities advocates. Many interview respondents used the same language to describe Milliken; calling him a kind and decent man who had a genuine concern for people with developmental disabilities. Given the state's considerable economic woes during much of his administration, it is perhaps not surprising that mental health issues were not his primary focus or his main priority. In spite of this, he made ongoing commitments to continue to depopulate the state's public institutions and was completely supportive of community placements for individuals with developmental disabilities. His State of the State messages indicated some level of commitment toward improving services for people with developmental disabilities, and his later messages supported community placement even in the face of considerable opposition from neighborhoods and some legislators (Milliken, 1975, 1976, 1977, 1978d, 1979, 1980).

Most interview respondents acknowledged that Milliken was not a major champion of services for people with developmental disabilities, but the fact that he was so decent led him to seriously work toward improving the service system. When the conditions at Plymouth were uncovered by the *Detroit Free Press*, the governor immediately took action to appoint a task force and address the problems that were rampant at the facility. His directives in response to the scandal were immediate and far-reaching. He did not confine his response to combating abuse and neglect, but instead used the opening provided by the scandal as a mechanism to evaluate the facility as a whole. The solution that was prescribed for Plymouth seemed to be reflective of a governor who was not just interested in a quick patch to get beyond the media attention (Milliken, 1978b).

One other illustration of the governor's commitment to the ongoing development of community-based residential services may be helpful. In response to the introduction of legislation that would have established a moratorium on the community placement program, a rally was held on the steps of the Capitol in Lansing. This had been organized by the Michigan ARC, MORC staff, and other advocates. The governor joined them on the steps. Addressing the crowd, he insisted that the community placement program was going to continue (Shapiro, 1980).

Democratic Governor Blanchard's impact on public policy for persons with developmental disabilities in Michigan is more difficult to evaluate. Many interview respondents were extremely critical of his leadership; many flatly stated he had absolutely no interest in persons with developmental disabilities whatsoever. However, two interview respondents were quick to indicate that under Blanchard, terrific things occurred, including the continuation of Patrick Babcock as the DMH director, the subsequent appointment of Thomas Watkins as director, passage of the Family Support Subsidy Act in 1983, and the closure of three of the state's public institutions.

Other interview respondents countered that the continued depopulation of institutions while Blanchard was Governor had nothing to do with his leadership. The decline in population persisted only because of the constant pressure to do so by advocates, the state's economy, and the commitment of DMH leadership, particularly Ben Censoni and Patrick Babcock.

One interview respondent explained the differences between Milliken and Blanchard as follows:

> Milliken was so humane, he supported developing a continuum, he was thoughtful… he wasn't advocating closing institutions for the institution's sake. He wanted to put together this thoughtful process. Milliken was very much a humanitarian…Blanchard saw mental health issues as a budget issue. Given the big recession, Blanchard was much more of a pragmatic politician who would be somewhat sympathetic because it was the Democratic liberal thing to do, but not really believe it on a personal level. When the big recession hit, we had an economic factor driving the policies, not just good govern-

ment. Now suddenly, the governor embraces the policy primarily so he can close the institutions. So now we see something else happening, it's called dumping. Instead of a thoughtful, progressive, gradual phasing out of the institutions, and the concurrent development of a continuum of care in each community, uniform across the state, the budget crisis became a rationale for closing institutions fairly rapidly. People were simply dumped.

In 1988, a number of advocates, including Protection and Advocacy Services, the Planning Council on Developmetnal Disabilities, ARC, United Cerebral Palsy, the University Affiliated Program, Epilepsy Foundation, and others, wrote to Governor Blanchard telling him of appalling conditions in a nursing home for persons with developmental disabilities reported in 1987. In this letter they recounted horrors that hearkened back to the series of articles the *Detroit Free Press* had printed about Plymouth (Bauer et al., 1988). The governor's response here, however, is quite different from his predecessor's response to the Plymouth crisis:

> I wish to assure you of my continuing commitment that state government does everything possible to provide services to all individuals in a humane and dignified fashion. While resources are not always available to fully or immediately provide for all needs within the state, much has and will continue to be done to direct available funds to the most urgent needs… I have directed that a number of actions be initiated to expedite improvements in current services and the orderly placement of individuals into appropriate community homes…To further my long-standing policy of avoiding institutionalization of children with developmental disabilities, developing appropriate community-based systems for all persons with developmental disabilities, and recent changes in federal law governing use of nursing homes, I have also directed the Departments of Mental Health, Social Services, and Public Health

to provide me with recommendations regarding appropriate services for all persons in nursing homes with mental health needs by June 3, 1988. Further actions will be taken as a result of these recommendations…New funding is not available to the extent preferred. (Blanchard, 1988, pp. 1-2)

This seemed to be a troubling and bureaucratic reaction to the chilling set of abuses and neglect revealed in this facility. In light of this reaction, and what advocates felt was a limited response of DMH, a lawsuit was filed against the State seeking appropriate community placements for nursing home residents with developmental disabilities. This lawsuit (*Kope v. Watkins,* 1988) would not be settled until the 1990s and eventually resulted in the closure of nursing homes for people with developmental disabilities in the State.

However, most of the same respondents who disclaimed that the governor had been a positive force in the State gave high marks to the team that he empowered to handle mental health, particularly under Patrick Babcock and subsequently under Tom Watkins. It is possible that positive public policy changes can come about if a governor lacks the leadership or commitment toward an issue, but allows his administration the latitude to implement changes as they see fit. In the case of Governor Blanchard, this is the most likely explanation for what transpired during his terms in office.

In evaluating the relative contributions of Governors Milliken and Blanchard during the 1970s and 1980s, there is little doubt that Milliken's support facilitated the development of community services. His widely held respect, and his commitment to the role of state government to provide for people with developmental disabilities, proved to be an important ingredient in the ongoing evolution of the service system. Blanchard, as has been discussed, was far from a champion of services for people with developmental disabilities. He clearly lacked Governor Milliken's presence in the movement, and he was not inclined to take controversial positions in support of community homes. However, the individuals he empowered to lead the Department were given the latitude to continue the development of community services begun in the 1970s.

The Legislature

A number of state legislators asserted themselves as champions of the community residential movement. These individuals were both conservatives and liberals, and initially exhibited their leadership during the 1970-90 period with the passage of the state's mandatory special education law in 1971. Later important legislation that was passed related to zoning, licensing regulations, and enactment of the state's Mental Health Code itself (Pub. Act 258 of 1974).

As discussed previously, the Mental Health Code of 1974 established a structure for the provision of community developmental disabilities and mental health services. Under this structure, Community Mental Health Boards were allowed to assume full management of services, or share responsibility with DMH. The new Code also provided for the protection of recipient rights. Individuals who were receiving mental health and developmental disabilities services had a due process protection established in law. In addition, the Code contained language stating that individuals receiving mental health (here includes those with developmental disabilities) services must be placed in the least restrictive environment (Pub. Act 258 of 1974).

In response to community opposition to group home development, the Legislature passed Pub. Acts 394-398 of 1976. The legislation stipulated that for purposes of zoning, six unrelated persons with disabilities living together constituted a family. As such, municipalities could not enact or enforce local laws that barred group homes for six or fewer people. One interview respondent described the way in which this legislation passed as follows:

The person that introduced the legislation on the definition of family for purposes of zoning was Peter Kok, a Republican from Holland, Michigan. He'd been trying to get it through for years…Then the chairman of the Towns & Counties Committee, Tom Brown, who was a very powerful legislator, it was in his committee, and he decided to put it in the hands of David Hollister. And once he did, David picked up the ball and ran and got it through. It was a combination of probably, Tom Brown, for some reason, gave Hollister the go ahead. "If you can do it, young man, then go ahead and do it." And David was resilient and brilliant, and he did it along with Peter Kok. So you had a very liberal Democrat from Lansing and a very conservative Republican from Holland. And the two of them were just what it took. But I think Tom Brown gets some credit here too…It was nearly unanimously passed. Tom Brown was an exceedingly powerful person at this time. I guess once he gave his go ahead that's all that was needed. Peter Kok did it because he was an honorable man and he clearly perceived that it was the right thing to do.

The following year, laws were passed that stipulated group homes could not be placed within 1,500 feet of one another, or within 3,000 feet of one another in Detroit (Pub. Acts 28-30 of 1977). One interview respondent noted that the specific objective of this law had been to address the development of "mental health ghettos," which occurred when less resistant neighborhoods had many group homes, and resistant neighborhoods, none.

> …to avoid dumping them all in one neighborhood, we added concentric zones, and they couldn't be within 1,500 feet of one another. The tendency had been to dump them all in one block. We wanted to balance off the mental health ghettos.

Other legislation also had an important impact on the residential service system for people with developmental disabilities. The Public Health Act (1978) contained nursing home reform provisions and prohibited admission of persons with developmental disabilities who needed active treatment. Nursing homes were required to establish agreements with their local community mental health systems for assistance and training to meet the special needs of patients with developmental disabilities.

In response to concerns about the quality of some of the group homes that were developing, the Adult Foster Care Facility Licensing Act was passed (Pub.

Act 281 of 1979; Michigan Department of Social Services, 1980). This licensing act directed the Department of Social Services, which was the state's licensing authority, to develop minimal standards and establish a protocol for ensuring quality assurance in facilities that served people with developmental disabilities.

It is difficult not to see the clear and consistent progression of laws that passed in the 1970s to facilitate the development of community-based residential services. One respondent characterized it as follows:

> There was a drumbeat. There was a deliberate march to the community. The problems that were identified as we went, the legislature responded. As people moved to the community, we saw the need for regulation and inspection, so the Adult Foster Care Licensing Act was passed. Then there was horrendous opposition to these homes. They burned them down, they shot them up. Neighbors did all kinds of horrible things. And the legislators tried to respond to the neighbors by notifying them. But there was an administrative plan to move to community, and legislative response to create the kinds of supports and protections or door-openers. It was a collaborative effort. That's the best way we worked in those years.

Not every legislator was a champion, though, and a number opposed the development of community services. To placate neighborhoods that were furious about community placement, the legislature passed community notification policies (Pub. Acts 28-30 of 1977). In addition, several legislators introduced bills to halt community placement altogether, or establish population-based limits on community placement. However, the latter two measures were not enacted.

A number of legislators were committed collaborators, who worked closely with advocates and DMH staff in their monitoring role. Rep. David Hollister and DMH Director Patrick Babcock conducted surprise visits to DMH institutions in the middle of the night. Collaboration with the MORC and the Michigan ARC was an important aspect of the leadership that Sen. Joseph Snyder provided as well. He was a tireless champion of developing community services and a staunch supporter of MORC and the ARC. In the early 1980s, Rep. Debbie Stabenow worked closely with the ARC and the Planning Council on Developmental Disabilities to enact the Family Support Subsidy Act. This law was passed in 1983 and is still a model for the nation (Braddock, Hemp, Parish, & Westrich, 1998).

The legislature also fulfilled a watchdog role, providing oversight and monitoring of state programs. In this capacity, it also investigated situations and incidents that were brought to its attention. An example of leadership that the legislature demonstrated in its watchdog capacity is evident in the Joint Committee to Study Abuse in State Mental Health facilities. This Committee was established in response to the publication of abusive and neglectful conditions at the Plymouth Development Center in February 1978 in the *Detroit Free Press*. The Committee was chaired by Rep. David Hollister and Sen. Jerome Hart. The Committee's response to the conditions at Plymouth and in other facilities was that the State had to improve its institutions, but more importantly "in the long run, the state must phase out the large institution approach to mental health care and replace it with a comprehensive community-based system of care and treatment" (Hart & Hollister, 1978, p. 2).

Their recommendations went on to suggest that "funds for care and treatment must precede the patient into the community from the institution [and]... Public attitudes toward and public acceptance of mentally disabled persons must be improved, a meaningful, useful role in society is inherently rehabilitative and must be promoted" (Hart & Hollister, 1978, p. 2). One of the most striking findings of the review of documents related to the development of the residential service system in Michigan during the 1970-90 period was that everywhere one looked there were individuals who were carrying the torch for development of community-based residential services for people with developmental disabilities.

In 1979, the Joint Mental Health Oversight Committee was established, with the express purpose of conducting an extensive review of the entire community placement issue and its related problems. The Committee was co-chaired by the same team that had led the Plymouth investigating committee, Sen. Jerome

Hart and Rep. David Hollister. Hearings were held and the Committee subsequently issued an extraordinarily detailed report. Inasmuch as the Committee was co-chaired by Hollister, who was a clear leader in the State in support of the development of community services, the outcome of the Committee's work was probably quite evident from the outset.

The Committee recommended that steps be taken to establish a comprehensive continuum of care, a statewide network designed to meet people's needs in the community. The range of the Committee's recommendations reached far. Quality assurance was addressed, along with scheduled rates of institutional depopulation, the potential loss to Michigan in federal funds if the community placement process was slowed, and a host of other related issues (Joint Mental Health Oversight Committee, 1980). What is further evident from this report is that at least some legislators had a sophisticated understanding of the issues surrounding community placement, including the nuances of federal ICF/MR regulations and Medicaid law, the standards by which DMH and the Departments of Social Services and Public Health operated, and the range of judicial rulings related to community placement. The breadth of this report is indicative of the level of commitment some of the legislators had to the ongoing development of community-based residential services for persons with developmental disabilities.

Perhaps the best way to understand many of the legislators during the 1970-90 period is simply explained by one interview respondent:

> DMH funds weren't cut as badly as funds in other departments because of the commitment of the appropriations chairs. Joe Young, Sr., was absolutely, 100% committed to public mental health services. These legislators valued men and women with developmental disabilities. We had Joe Snyder in the Senate, Joe Young, Sr., in the House, Dave Hollister in the House. Peter Kok. There were so many. The legislature was just a legion of champions.

The Judiciary

The courts in Michigan had two primary functions as related to the development of community-based residential services for persons with developmental disabilities during the 1970-90 period: class-action litigation and zoning litigation. State courts were involved in zoning litigation, as neighborhoods and towns sued to stop community placement. The federal court was involved in the Plymouth case. As has been noted, neighborhoods were relentless in filing more than 120 challenges to the state's zoning laws, passed in 1976. However, the state courts were nearly as relentless in upholding the laws.

According to one interview respondent, only two zoning cases were lost at the trial court level, and both were subsequently overturned on appeal. These cases largely came to an end with the issuance of the Michigan Supreme Court ruling in 1985. That year, the Court issued its opinion in *City of Livonia v. Department of Social Services and Green Trees Civic Association v. Pignatiello*. The Court addressed zoning and ruled that "the operation of adult foster care small group homes in the cases affected by this decision does not violate building in-use restrictions in the deeds of the homeowners." The Court upheld the right of men and women with disabilities to live in group homes, and permanently closed the door on further challenges to the state's zoning laws.

The other case that became important at the state court level was *Kope v. Watkins*, discussed previously. This case was filed in 1988 on behalf of nursing home residents with developmental disabilities. In the 1990s, it resulted in community placement for these residents and the closure of Michigan's system of specialized nursing homes for persons with developmental disabilities.

The Plymouth case was played out in federal court, as mentioned earlier. In this way, the federal courts played an important role in shaping the ongoing development of Michigan's service system. When he signed the Plymouth consent decree, federal District Court Judge Charles Joiner explained the role of the institutions and community residences for persons with developmental disabilities as follows: "All mentally retarded individuals can and should live in the more normalized environment of the community and do not require institutionalization, given the development of necessary habilitation and support services in the community" (cited in Leismer, 1983, p. 3).

One must conclude that the Plymouth case proved to be an extremely important catalyst for the development of community homes in Michigan. The case provided a mechanism for advocates to use the court's power to compel the DMH to make progress, even in difficult economic times.

The Department of Mental Health

Michigan's Department of Mental Health provided leadership to the community services movement in two distinct phases. In the first phase, the 1970s, leadership was provided by the Macomb-Oakland Regional Center. In the second phase, beginning with Patrick Babcock's appointment to the directorship of the DMH, the central office in Lansing provided leadership as well. This section will review these developments.

In 1972, when Michigan enacted legislation calling for construction of the MORC, it was designed to be a 650- to 750-bed complex located on a 40-acre campus, including a hospital and nursing care units. DMH hired David Rosen to be the superintendent of this facility, with responsibility to oversee facility construction and development. Under Rosen's leadership, while beginning to plan for the facility's construction, the MORC immediately began placing individuals in community homes and in nursing homes. The Macomb-Oakland Regional Center did not wait for the facility to be constructed to start to serve people. By the time the facility was actually built in 1976, hundreds of people had already been placed in community homes by MORC staff (DMH, 1977, 1981b).

Many of the interview respondents indicated that the leadership at the Macomb-Oakland Regional Center, particularly that provided by Gerry Provencal and Ben Censoni, was visionary. MORC became a hotbed for innovation as new and creative programs were piloted here which would later be replicated in other parts of the state and nation.

There are many important aspects of the unique position of the Macomb-Oakland Regional Center in Michigan. It was part of the Department of Mental Health; its employees were state employees; DMH was able to control the financing of the development of community homes and service delivery. This led to the State developing considerable expertise in the development and operation of small-scale community-based homes.

The synergy of leadership between Rosen, Provencal, and Censoni was important to the development and successes enjoyed by MORC. Provencal and Censoni were the radicals with the idea of placing everyone in the community and closing the institutions. Rosen was the one who offered credibility and legitimacy, having been an institutional superintendent in New Jersey and Washington, as well as president of the American Association on Mental Deficiency. The credibility offered Provencal and Censoni the cover under which they could do truly innovative things.

The combined leadership of these men in MORC's early days facilitated a community development program that excelled at placing everyone in community residences, even individuals with severe disabilities who were not widely believed to be "appropriate" for the community.

During the 1970s, DMH was led by three directors, Gordon Yudashkin (1970-74), Donald Smith (1974-78), and Frank Ochberg (1979-81). All three were psychiatrists and all of them had considerable difficulty leading the DMH. All three came under considerable fire for an array of different aspects of the DMH's administration and none were leaders in developing community residences for people with developmental disabilities. However, they each played a different and in some ways instrumental role in what transpired in developmental disabilities services.

Gordon Yudashkin enjoyed a good working relationship with David Rosen, the superintendent of the MORC. Yudashkin gave Rosen considerable latitude in implementing programs and services and in pursuing his community placement objectives at MORC. A number of respondents from that period have suggested that Yudashkin, while not a champion of community placement, provided staff with the latitude to bring about changes in the service system.

Donald Smith took over the DMH's leadership after Yudashkin resigned under fire. Smith was subsequently fired for having known about the conditions at the Plymouth Center and for his lack of ability to lead the DMH and provide it with an effective administrative structure. Smith was widely acknowledged by nearly every interview respondent as not having had any impact on the community services program. The

joint legislative committee that investigated Plymouth concluded, "Perhaps the most crucial element the Michigan mental health system has lacked for a number of years is effective leadership" (Joint Committee to Study Abuse in State Mental Health Facilities, 1978, p. 8).

Smith was replaced by Frank Ochberg, whose immediate mandate from Governor Milliken was to get the situation at Plymouth under control and to end the abusive and neglectful conditions at the facility. Review of Director Ochberg's documents related to Plymouth indicate he was supportive of community placement and he intended to fix the problems there and elsewhere in the DMH and restore the DMH's credibility.

However, Ochberg was unable to work effectively with the legislature. According to numerous interview respondents, at one point he was thrown out of the House chamber, because he did not have permission to be present. Ochberg was also at the helm when the auditor general, at House Speaker Gary Owen's request, conducted an inquiry into DMH's leasing practices and otherwise evaluated the community placement program. The furor caused by this report led a number of legislators to call for a moratorium on further community placement. Ochberg resigned and was subsequently replaced by Patrick Babcock (1981-86). Babcock ushered in a new era for DMH.

Babcock had worked under Governor Milliken for a number of years, and had previously been a legislative liaison. He enjoyed widespread respect for both his administrative skills and for his ability to work effectively with the legislature. He proved to be just what the ailing DMH needed. He was able to gain control over the community placement program and construct effective agreements with the Department of Leasing and Budget over leasing issues. He gave the DMH credibility. He was also a strong champion of the community placement process, characterizing it as a civil rights movement in one interview conducted while he was director.

Babcock's assumption of the leadership of the DMH initiated a transition at the Department, whereby the MORC was no longer the only entity interested in aggressively pursuing community placement. It is important to note that Babcock took over after the Plymouth case, and after the MORC had been operating for a number of years. Although he was not the person who initiated the major changes in the DMH, he was able to usher the Department through a period of continued growth in community placements. The consent decree objectives of the Plymouth Center were eventually met, and a number of facilities closed while he was director. Another important part of the DMH leadership was Ben Censoni. Universally acknowledged to have been a visionary, Censoni was hired by David Rosen to work on community placement for the MORC. In 1976, he moved from his position at the MORC to the DMH office in Lansing. There he would wear a number of different hats and oversee different aspects of the state's community placement program, including its compliance with the stipulations of the Plymouth consent decree. Censoni spearheaded the development of the state's AIS/MR program and worked assiduously to ensure that community placement took place across the State (DMH, 1976, 1977, 1980; Ochberg, 1979).

DMH is best characterized as being an agency that was beset with problems in its administration during the 1970s, and in the opposition to its community placement program in the late-1970s well into the 1980s. In spite of having many problems, there were significant strengths in some of the leaders who facilitated innovation. The Department's capacity for innovation prevailed in spite of the difficulties that it encountered.

Advocacy Groups

A number of different advocacy groups played a role in the development of community-based residential services in Michigan during the 1970-90 study period. The most important of these was, as has been mentioned, the Michigan Association for Retarded Citizens and its local chapters. This section will describe the ways in which the ARC made an impact on services in the State. It will also discuss the contributions of the Protection and Advocacy organization, and the Governor's Planning Council on Developmental Disabilities and their implications for the service system.

The Association for Retarded Citizens in 1970 was the single largest advocacy group on develop-

mental disabilities issues in Michigan, and was interested in securing passage of a mandatory special education law. The ARC secured passage of the legislation basically by hitting the streets and having all of its volunteers and advocates gather signatures to put a referendum on the Michigan ballot to enact this legislation. It then successfully maneuvered the legislature into passing legislation instead of having the measure go before the population on the ballot. At this time, the legislature was opposed to having the people do the business of enacting legislation, and the ARC was able to essentially gather enough signatures to compel the legislature into passing the law or sitting put while the State passed it over the legislators' objections, via the referendum.

The passage of the mandatory special education law in 1971 was an enormous success for the ARC. It was passed four years before the federal Education of All Handicapped Children Act in 1975. In addition to being passed well in advance of the national law, the state's law was more comprehensive and far-reaching, mandating education for children until the age of 26, and establishing a standard of educational services designed to maximize the individual's potential. This was revolutionary language for the time in which it was passed.

Securing passage of this legislation confirmed the power and importance of the ARC as a central advocate and champion in Michigan. Two years later, when the mandatory special education law was supposed to be implemented, the ARC brought suit to enforce the provisions of the law in the state's public institutions. While this lawsuit was not widely known, it enabled the ARC to again precipitate a major change in state public policy and it secured the position of the ARC as the voice on developmental disabilities in the State.

When the Developmental Disabilities Act was amended in 1975, it authorized states to establish Protection and Advocacy organizations for persons with developmental disabilities. When this federal funding came through, most states created their Protection and Advocacy organizations as operating units of their larger developmental disabilities divisions or departments. However, in Michigan, Governor Milliken appointed the ARC as the coordinating agency from which the Protection and Advocacy service was operated. The leadership of the ARC shaped the creation of the Protection and Advocacy organization, and the foundation for a close working relationship was established. When the Protection and Advocacy organization was spun off to be an independent entity five years after its creation in 1976, the ARC maintained its ties with Protection and Advocacy and subsequently joined forces with the Protection and Advocacy in the Plymouth lawsuit.

Several years later, when the *Detroit Free Press* published a series of articles exposing abusive conditions at the Plymouth State School, the ARC filed what came to be known as *Michigan ARC v. Smith* (1979). This lawsuit further catalyzed the development of community residential homes in the State. Family members active in the ARC at the time and other members of ARC leadership acknowledged that they knew from the outset of filing the Plymouth case that they were seeking closure of this facility. There was widespread recognition by this group that individuals with developmental disabilities could not be properly supported or cared for in public institutions.

By the time that the Plymouth lawsuit was filed in February 1978, the ARC had established its credibility as an important political force in the state's mental disabilities arena. One indication of this was Governor Milliken's specific invitation to the ARC to witness and participate in the Plymouth Task Force chaired by Wilbur Cohen (Milliken, 1978c). Minutes from the House Committee on Mental Health throughout the 1970s and 1980s also provide important evidence as to the stature and involvement of the ARC during this time. The ARC was a nearly constant presence during these meetings and legislators therefore had the opportunity to get to know the ARC and to understand its issues in considerable detail. While other advocacy organizations also attended House Mental Health Committee meetings, their attendance was more sporadic and was frequently in response to single issues. In contrast, the ARC made it a priority to maintain a presence at these meetings.

Nearly all interview respondents agreed that the ARC played a pivotal role in shaping the development of the state's community-based residential services system. However, concern was expressed by some interview respondents that the ARC had not always acted as radically or aggressively as it could have.

Because it was a parents' organization, it did not always support the independence of individuals with developmental disabilities. Two interview respondents recounted an example of this related to the Plymouth case, explaining that the lawyers and ARC leadership strategy discussions related to Plymouth sometimes took inappropriate turns. These two interview respondents felt that the lawyers' responsibility was to represent the best interests of the Plymouth residents and not the ARC. In spite of this claim, however, the centrality of the ARC in catalyzing and accelerating the changes that were wrought to the Michigan residential service system should not be understated.

The second advocacy organization that played a role in Michigan was the Protection and Advocacy Services. Protection and Advocacy is one of three programs funded in every state by the Developmental Disabilities Act. The other two were the Planning Councils on Developmental Disabilities and the University Affiliated Programs in Mental Retardation (now University Centers for Excellence). Protection and Advocacy organizations are mandated by federal law to develop a cohesive program of securing the rights of people with mental disabilities. As discussed previously, in Michigan, the Protection and Advocacy organization was initially created within the authority of the ARC; five years later it was spun off and became its own independent entity. Michigan's Protection and Advocacy was also unique in that it received state funding in addition to federal funding.

The most important contribution of Michigan's Protection and Advocacy organization to the service system was two-fold: (a) its role in providing legal representation for the plaintiffs in the Plymouth case and (b) the personal leadership of Elizabeth Bauer, the agency's executive director. Most interview respondents stated that Protection and Advocacy was less instrumental in shaping public policy. However, the same interview respondents indicated that Bauer commanded considerable respect in the State and personally had been a persuasive and respected supporter of the ongoing development of community-based residential services.

The final advocacy group to be considered is the Governor's Planning Council on Developmental Disabilities (the Council), which was also authorized by the federal Developmental Disabilities Act and received federal funds to complete its mission. Its mandate was to coordinate planning for services and provide advice to the governor and legislature on the best practices for people with developmental disabilities. This coordination function came out of recommendations made by President Kennedy's Panel on Mental Retardation in the 1960s. One of the most important issues this panel identified was the need for cohesive and coordinated planning because, in most states, a number of agencies share responsibility for services for people with developmental disabilities, including the Department of Education, the Department of Mental Health, the Department of Social Services, and sometimes even the Department of Public Health. The Council served as the single entity that coordinated the planning function for the State. Most interview respondents indicated that the Council did not play a major role in the development of community-based residential services in Michigan. However, the review of documents indicated that the Council worked behind the scenes and may not have been as visible as the leadership demonstrated by the parent advocates.

Considerable documentary evidence indicates that one of the Council's first major achievements was its support of and assistance provided to Rep. Debbie Stabenow in her drive to pass family support subsidy legislation. For much of the 1970s, the Council conducted an array of needs assessments and attempted to identify the relevant planning issues that it should tackle. The Council developed its own operating structure and worked out the details of what its role and functions would and should be. However, when Representative Stabenow appointed her Ad Hoc Citizens Committee on Family Support in 1982, the Council provided technical assistance and helped coordinate the meetings.

Council staff were involved in other efforts including, as discussed previously, advocacy in Michigan to address the cuts to Social Security that occurred under President Reagan. The Council was also involved in the development of Michigan's application and subsequent implementation of a federal grant on supported employment.

During the 1980s, the Council provided seed grants to an array of organizations across the State, which then implemented innovative or pilot projects. In this way, it had a role similar to the MORC in pilot-

ing initiatives, but to a much lesser extent. One example of an innovative Council-funded project was a family support pilot project.

The Council worked behind the scenes in yet another way: In 1982 when DMH faced one of its most severe budget cuts, it was forced to terminate funding for a family support subsidy pilot program. DMH turned to the Council inviting it to pick up the funding for this program, which was seen as critical to the families who were receiving the subsidy. In return for doing so, the DMH agreed that it would reinstate funding for the program as soon as resources made that possible. The Council used its federal funds to essentially bridge the imminent gap for these families. The following excerpt from Patrick Babcock, DMH director, to Howard Shapiro, Council president, sought the Council's assistance:

As you know, the Department of Mental Health will be still further affected by severe budget cuts in its anticipated 1982-83 budget. CMH programs will have to take a 10% reduction in existing programs. Central Office accounts are also being drastically affected. Among the items eliminated for 1982-83 is funding for any new continuation demonstration and evaluation projects…Withdrawing DMH support for these projects will mean the complete loss of family support services for 80 families in western Wayne, Washtenaw, and Macomb counties…Should the DD Council be able to support the continuation of these family support Projects for an interim period, the Department will commit itself to providing funding for them as soon as any expansion CMH funds are available. DMH policy requiring continuation support of successful demonstration projects is under development and will be incorporated into the Administrative Manual during this fiscal year. (Babcock, 1982b, pp. 1-2)

Self-advocates, or individuals with developmental disabilities championing their own needs, were not a critical force for change during the 1970-90 study period. One individual, Richard Prangley, a former

401

resident of the Coldwater institution, did provide some leadership and participation on task forces and other coalitions. However, he and other self-advocates were not political players in the sense that they facilitated change. A biography was written about Prangley and the considerable hurdles he overcame in order to leave Coldwater and create a life for himself in the community (Schneider, 1998). Numerous interview respondents recommended the book as a way to help understand the difficult lives formerly institutionalized persons with developmental disabilities have had. A number of respondents reported that Prangley had been a source of inspiration to them, as were many other individuals who blossomed once they left the institutions. Self-advocates during the 1970-90 period had their greatest impact on the service system by inspiring leaders with their achievements in the face of great difficulty, and not by directly influencing the service system.

In evaluating the contributions of advocacy groups to the evolution of Michigan's service system during the 1970-90 study period, the most important leadership roles were played by the ARC. The ARC had established its credential as an important political player by the early 1970s, and had the capacity to advocate for significant change in Michigan. The ARC seized the opportunity presented by news stories of horrific conditions at Plymouth, and filed a lawsuit that ultimately expanded the scope of services that were available across the State. The ARC's partnerships with elected officials and DMH bureaucrats were very important as well.

Conclusions

In Michigan, a number of factors effectively transformed the service system from an institutional-based to a community-based network. This conclusion will briefly review the factors and the interrelationships among them, answering the study's fifth research question: What were the relationships among influential factors in Michigan?

The most important factor that influenced the transformation of the state's residential service system was the convergence of leadership among the ARC, a number of legislators, and the DMH. Department of Mental Health leaders came from the MORC beginning in

the 1970s and from DMH's central offices in Lansing beginning in the early 1980s.

Other factors facilitated the development of community services in the State as well. These included support from the governor and other advocacy groups, success in the courts on zoning, passage of a series of laws that provided a shape for the community system, and to a much lesser degree, even the state's recession.

Perhaps the best way to characterize the ways in which the different factors related to one another is to delineate what each contributed to the process. In some sense, each of the players or organizations brought unique attributes to the service system, and each contributed in ways that complemented the others. *Table 3.3* provides a more succinct overview of the resources and contributions of the different influential organizations and leaders. The table lists major and other facilitative influences to the development of community-based residences in Michigan.

Beginning in the early 1970s, MORC established competence and expertise in two critical areas: quickly developing community residences and serving people with severe impairments. Both of these were innovations that laid a foundation of expertise that could later serve the entire State, as programs piloted in Macomb and Oakland Counties were established in other localities. MORC's vision of services and determination to overcome community opposition was very important as well; they made transformation of the service system a possibility by developing the technical capacity.

The ARC provided a set of leaders who were widely respected, and who were unencumbered by commitments to the needs of service providers. The ARC's monitoring and advocacy role was codified by Governor Milliken when he opted to pilot the Protection and Advocacy under the direction of the ARC. While the ARC was agitating for improved services, it was able to point to the programs in operation at the MORC and demand similar quality for other people with developmental disabilities. The ARC also worked hard to be a presence in the legislature, and developed partnerships with legislators, the governor, and DMH leadership. Their willingness and capacity to work with the leadership, but still demand quality services, provided a synergy that was important to the

Table 3.3
RESOURCES AND CONTRIBUTIONS OF INFLUENTIAL FACTORS IN MICHIGAN

Other Facilitators	Resources	Contributions
Macomb-Oakland Regional Center (1970s & 1980s)	Latitude from central DMH office to innovate; finances to pursue innovation; vision to pursue innovation; finances & staff commitment/determination to fight neighbors' opposition lawsuits; civil rights perspective	Created community homes; developed expertise in serving people with severe impairments; controlled innovative test pilots for the State; acclaim for community services; positive press for state leaders
ARC (1970s & 1980s)	Recognized and respected political clout; commitment/determination; advocacy capacity; successful partnerships with elected officials and DMH bureaucracy; not financed by service providers; education of institutional parents	Filed and fought Plymouth lawsuit; advocacy for changes in the service system; monitoring functions; systems change leadership
DMH leadership (1980s)	Ability to work with legislature; civil rights perspective; finances to build group homes; power of the State	Financing; fought zoning litigation; fought community opposition
Legislators (1970s & 1980s)	Power of the State; finances to monitor services; commitment to State role in serving people with developmental disabilities; respected leadership	Monitoring function; passed legislation that structure service system; fought community opposition; civil rights perspective
Other Facilitators	Resources	Contributions
Protection and Advocacy	Finances; legal capacity; respected leadership	Lawyers for Plymouth; coalition participants; monitoring functions; advocacy for systems change
DD Planning Council	Finances	Funded pilot projects; coalition participation; technical assistant to legislators
Governor Milliken	State power; respected leadership	Philosophical and financial support; leadership
Other Advocates	Varied	Coalition participation
Recession	N/A	Justification for cutting institutional jobs & developing cheaper community homes
CMH organizations	Finances; local control of services; financial incentive to develop group homes	Cohesive structure for service development; expanded constituency of support

movement.

A number of legislators complete the triangle of leadership so critical to the development of the state's community-based residential system. These legislators were committed to the provision of quality services and believed the State had a significant role to play in supporting people with developmental disabilities. These legislators passed laws that established a codified structure within which the service system could evolve. These laws included prohibitions against zoning discrimination, prohibitions against mental health ghettos, and quality assurance statutes. As problems arose in the development of group homes, the legislature responded with an agenda intended to solve the problems.

Finally, in the 1980s, leadership from central DMH emerged as well. Ben Censoni, Patrick Babcock, and later Tom Watkins all provided support for community services that facilitated continuing the momentum while the state's economy faltered. DMH resources were particularly critical in fighting the numerous zoning suits that neighborhoods brought and forcing communities to accept group homes in their midst.

Other facilitative factors included Governor Milliken's support, other advocacy groups, and, to a point, the state's recession itself. The CMH structure, whereby local authority for delivering services was established, also facilitated the development of community services.

Figure 3.6 depicts the ways in which influence flowed in the State. Crucial coalitions existed among and between organizations and groups. The partnership among the ARC, some legislators, and some MORC and DMH staff is indicated by collocating them within a circle. Arrows are used to indicate direction of influence that most commonly flowed from one entity to another. What cannot be represented here, of course, is the dynamic nature of these coalitions and partnerships. On a particular issue, different entities emerged as the strongest leaders.

What is most compelling about the

Michigan story is the way in which each of these entities brought its resources to the arena, and worked collaboratively to transform the state's residential service system. The leadership of different groups, the partnerships, and coalitions that struggled to change the system were tremendously effective, as has been described.

ILLINOIS CASE STUDY

This section will present the case study related to the development of residential services from 1970-90 in Illinois. To facilitate understanding a complex interplay of factors and forces, this section is organized as follows: trends in residential services, which provides a brief description of the development of residential services; administrative structure, which delineates the organizational aspects of funding and providing residential services. A discussion of the role of public scandals in shaping Illinois' service system is then presented. Subsequent sections describe and discuss the role

Figure 3.6
CONCEPTUAL FRAMEWORK OF INFLUENCE IN MICHIGAN, 1970-90

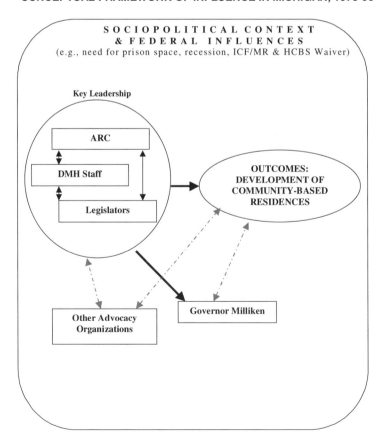

played in the development of community-based residential services of: politics, federal influences, the governors, the legislature, the Department of Mental Health, and advocacy groups.

Trends and Developments in Residential Services

The foundation for Illinois' development of residential services during 1970-90 rests squarely in the 1960s. In 1960, there were two options for residential services in Illinois: placement at the Lincoln or Dixon State Schools, with the cost borne largely by the State, or placement in a private facility with the cost entirely borne by the family. The two state schools in the towns of Lincoln and Dixon were mammoth facilities, among the largest in the nation. The population at Lincoln, which opened in 1877, was 5,381 persons in 1958. Dixon, opened in 1917, peaked in 1954 at 4,920 persons. These facilities were widely acknowledged to be little more than warehouses, and incapable of providing the rudiments of decent care (Commission on Mental Health, 1965; State Advisory Council on Mental Retardation, 1965).

One report (State Advisory Council on Mental Retardation, 1965) from this period stated that the most pressing concerns related to Illinois' residential service system were the waiting lists and the overcrowding at Lincoln and Dixon. The number of people living in the facilities exceeded the licensed capacity by 28% at Lincoln and by 43% at Dixon. This report noted that "on many shifts there is only one employee to care for a cottage housing 160 severely retarded persons" (State Advisory Council on Mental Retardation, 1965, p. 67). This report concluded that in order to address the needs of persons waiting for residential services, and to relieve overcrowding, "Illinois right now, has an urgent need for additional residential facilities for 4,645 mentally retarded persons" (State Advisory Council on Mental Retardation, 1965, p. 73). This number represented nearly 50% of the existing public institutional population at the time.

In Illinois, the Department of Mental Health's residential service-related goals in the 1960s were to relieve overcrowding in these two facilities. Construction of new facilities was part of this strategy, and the Murray and Fox Centers opened in 1964 and 1965,

respectively, in Centralia and Dwight. In 1966, the Bowen Center opened in Harrisburg (Scheerenberger & Wagner, 1968; Interdepartmental Committee on Mental Retardation and Illinois Association for the Mentally Retarded, 1968). Another aspect of the Department's attempts to relieve overcrowding at Lincoln and Dixon was by preventing institutionalization itself. The development of services outside institutions was part of this strategy. In response to the federal stimulus of funds authorized by the Maternal and Child Health and Mental Retardation Planning Act (Pub. L. 88-156), beginning in the mid-1960s, Illinois targeted the development of community services as a priority. Community services, however, were essentially limited to ancillary services: day programs or sheltered workshops, adult daycare programs, clinics and schools. These community services were frequently operated by local chapters of the Association for Retarded Citizens (ARC). Such services were seen as important mechanisms by which the waiting list for residential placement could be reduced (Illinois Department of Mental Health, 1969; Scheerenberger, 1968; Visotsky, 1968).

Private residential facilities were not widely available, and state funds did not flow to these facilities. Families that sought placement for their children bore the entire cost of such services until 1961, when the Department of Mental Health (DMH) enacted its interim care program. This program provided financial assistance to families that had placed their children in private facilities and were on the waiting list for placement in one of the state's public institutions (Committee on Mental Retardation, 1970, 1973; Illinois Mental Health Planning Board, 1968). By 1965, there were 500 families receiving interim care grants of $175 per month. Under the interim care grant program, a family would continue to receive funds until a placement became available in one of the state-operated facilities, at which time the family was expected to place the child in the public facility or risk losing the state's financial assistance with the private placement. In reality, the waiting list was considerable (2,163 persons in 1965) and the DMH did not terminate grants if a family preferred to keep the child in the private facility (Committee on Mental Retardation, 1970, 1973; Developmental Disabilities Study Committee of the House of Representatives, 1973).

The other mechanism used to depopulate the large facilities was what the DMH termed "community placement," which entailed the transfer of individuals from Dixon and Lincoln into facilities that were not operated by the State. These consisted of nursing homes (long-term care facilities) or sheltered care facilities. Nursing homes were generally skilled nursing facilities, and theoretically were able to provide ongoing nursing care to individuals who needed it. Sheltered care facilities provided room and board and minimal levels of supervision. Both nursing homes and sheltered care facilities received small amounts of federal funds, in addition to state funds. While the DMH characterized all placements out of public institutions as "community placement," most facilities into which people were discharged were, in fact, large, privately operated institutions (Committee on Mental Retardation, 1970, 1971c, 1973; Developmental Disabilities Study Committee of the House of Representatives, 1973; Illinois Department of Mental Health, 1972; Ragan, 1974).

The wholesale placement of persons with developmental disabilities into nursing homes and sheltered care resulted in a total of 1,450 persons in such facilities by 1967, and the Department later conceded that the practice of "dumping" had gone on in order to depopulate the large facilities (Ragan, 1974). There was limited aftercare or oversight of the community facilities. In the 1970s, the DMH was beset with numerous scandals investigated by the legislature, which found, among other things, that the DMH failed to adequately monitor its community placement program. Between 1965 and 1968, the population at Lincoln alone declined by nearly 1,000 persons, or 20% of the facility's total. At Dixon, the downsizing during this period was 831 persons, or 17% of the facility's 1965 total population (Commission on Mental Health, 1969; Scheerenberger, 1969).

In spite of the dramatic population declines at Dixon and Lincoln, conditions at the facilities remained notoriously poor. One interview respondent who visited Dixon in the late 1960s reported that:

it was a repulsive scene out of Bedlam. Overwhelming smell of feces and urine. [The superintendent] wanted to shock me into an understanding or an awareness of the con-

ditions in which the children live. It was a scene that I couldn't believe.

Life was grim for the residents. The poor conditions were admitted by Governor Ogilvie at the 1970 groundbreaking ceremony for the Ludeman Developmental Center. In response to suggestions to improve Dixon and Lincoln, the governor stated, "I will have no part of such a plan, for it would only serve to perpetuate the dehumanized conditions which have made those oversized facilities the shame of our state mental health system" (Illinois Information Service, 1970, p. 3).

In answer to charges that the large facilities were inadequate and overcrowded, the construction of more developmental disabilities facilities was sought. In 1967, the State passed Senate Bill 950, and authorized the construction of six new developmental centers near Chicago. The five existing developmental disabilities centers, in Centralia, Dixon, Lincoln, Harrisburg, and Dwight, were all at considerable distance from the state's population center in Chicago. It was felt that building facilities near the city would enable families to remain in closer contact with their institutionalized family members (Commission on Mental Health, 1969; Scheerenberger & Wagner, 1968). As a result of this legislation, funds were eventually released by Governors Ogilvie and Walker for the construction of Ludeman in Park Forest, which opened in 1972; Howe in Tinley Park; and the Kiley Developmental Center in Waukegan, both of which opened in 1975. All three of these facilities were planned to have neighborhoods of eight-person cottages clustered on a single campus (Illinois Department of Mental Health and Developmental Disabilities [hereafter, DMHDD], 1976). *Figure 3.7* depicts the number of public developmental disabilities institutions in Illinois during the 1960-90 period.

Units in psychiatric hospitals are not shown in the figure. Shapiro and Jacksonville, which were converted from psychiatric hospitals to developmental disabilities institutions in 1973 and 1974, respectively, are indicated as opening on those dates.

Another major residential trend that began in the late 1960s was the conversion of portions of state psychiatric hospitals to developmental disabilities units. The population of the state's psychiatric hospitals had been declining since the 1950s, and as this occurred, the patients with mental illness were replaced by people with developmental disabilities.

In 1969, the state's psychiatric hospital in Anna developed a developmental disabilities unit for 200 residents, made up of 83 individuals who had already been living at the facility, and transfers from Dixon and Lincoln. By 1970, similar units had also been developed at the state's Galesburg, Peoria, Kankakee, Alton, Elgin, and Jacksonville psychiatric hospitals (Scheerenberger, 1970). This pattern of transferring people among institutional facilities would become a hallmark of the ongoing development of residential services in Illinois well into the 1980s. In 1973, the Kankakee State Hospital was completely converted into a developmental center for persons with developmental disabilities (Illinois Department of Mental Health, 1973a). The following year, this conversion was repeated at the Jacksonville State Hospital. The depletion of the population of persons with mental illness in state hospitals presented ongoing opportunities for expanding institutional care for persons with developmental disabilities in Illinois.

In June 1972, the General Assembly passed House Resolution 668, which established a study commission on the state's developmental disabilities service system (Developmental Disabilities Study Committee of the House of Representatives, 1973). A private consultant was brought in to assess the status of the DMH's developmental disabilities service system. The resulting report indicated that there were extensive, systemic problems with the administration of the state's services for persons with developmental disabilities. In addition, the report concluded that there had been an excessive reliance on state institutions, and families were largely not interested in this form of care for their children. The report stated:

[There is a clear] need for review of the state's policy of construction and operation of residential institutions. For many years, the State of Illinois has attempted to meet the needs of the retarded by building and operating state institutions. The findings of the survey of families-- presented in Part II of this report-- show that only 7.3% of 1,031 families who responded to the Committee's questionnaire desired care for their children in state institutions. In contrast, 38.3% requested care in private institutions while 41.2% of the respondents desire help to care for their children at home. In view of these findings, and because there is a lack of cost/ benefit evaluation data to provide firm justi-

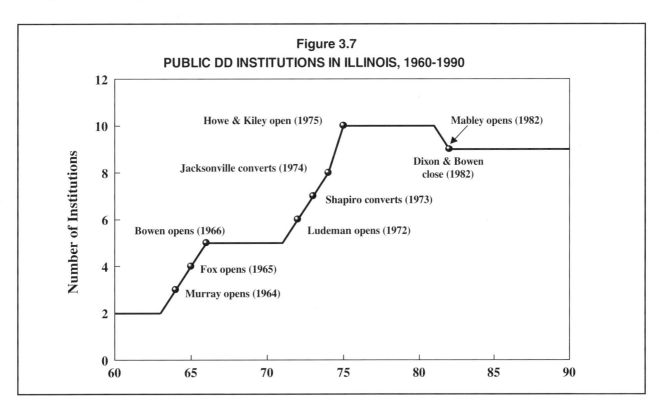

Figure 3.7
PUBLIC DD INSTITUTIONS IN ILLINOIS, 1960-1990

fication for large, capital outlay expenditures on permanent state residential care facility, and because the new community service system proposed herein should reduce the total requirements for state institutions, it is recommended that the further development of any major state residential facilities be held in abeyance. (pp. 14-15)

Alternatives to institutional services began to slowly emerge in Illinois in the early 1970s. The most prevalent institutional alternative in the 1960s and early 1970s was the nursing home (Ragan, 1974). These facilities were often converted from boarding homes, in order to obtain federal funding. According to a number of interviewees, nursing homes had been used for the "dumping" of institutional residents. As noted previously, the Department of Mental Health even publicly acknowledged that this had been the case (Ragan, 1974).

To meet its depopulation objectives, the DMH also sought to support new private residential alternatives. In 1970, it contracted with Unicare, a company which purchased the former North Aurora Hilton Hotel. The property was remodeled to accommodate 500 residents from Lincoln and Dixon. By 1971, 370 former public institutional residents were living at the North Aurora facility (Committee on Mental Retardation, 1971b).

Illinois' first new community-based residential program began with the 1970 application for licensure of a community living facility (CLF) by Aid to the Retarded Children in Springfield, which was a local chapter of the state Association for Retarded Citizens (Scheerenberger, 1970). These facilities were new in the sense that they represented a new service type, as opposed to the use of nursing homes or sheltered care. Community living facilities generally comprised 10 apartments under one roof, and served approximately 20 individuals with developmental disabilities. By 1977, there were 414 people with developmental disabilities living in such facilities across the State. However, these facilities represented a small proportion of the state's entire residential service system, which served thousands of individuals (DMHDD, 1983).

Another important event in the history of residential services in Illinois occurred in 1971, when Con-

gress amended the Social Security Act (Pub. L. 91-517) and authorized the Intermediate Care Facilities for the Mentally Retarded (ICF/MR) program as an option under the Medicaid program. This new program enabled states to obtain federal Medicaid reimbursement for facilities that were certified as ICF/MR, meeting an extensive array of conditions and regulations in order to participate. According to many interview respondents, in order to capture this new stream of funding, the Department of Mental Health offered nursing home operators rate incentives to convert. These new facilities were termed Intermediate Care Facilities/Developmentally Disabled (ICF/DD). These "add-ons" enhanced the reimbursement rates the nursing home operators were receiving. One interviewee reported:

In the beginning, the development of private ICF/MR was really a transition of licensure. These mentally retarded individuals were already in nursing homes and many of the nursing homes had large numbers of mentally retarded people because there was no prohibition on mentally retarded people going into nursing homes. There was a pretty aggressive effort to deflect people from going into the state institutions. There was no room in the institutions. It wasn't done for altruistic reasons. So they discharged or deflected people into nursing homes. When the ICF/MR program came into existence, the nursing homes had a choice to specialize in MR and if there were elderly people living there, they had to move them out, make changes in their operations, and then re-license to specialize with the MR population. They weren't built as ICFs/MR.

The incentives offered to providers worked. By 1978, there were 2,550 persons with developmental disabilities living in privately operated ICFs/DD in the State, many of whom had previously been in nursing homes. Extensive utilization of ICFs/DD in Illinois was an enduring trend throughout the 1980s (DMHDD, 1983).

Another community residential program that developed in the 1970s was the Specialized Living Center. These centers were constructed by the State with capital development grant money, as part of a new economic stimulus program. In a special message to the General Assembly, Governor Walker (1975) noted that the State faced its worst economic conditions since World War II, and proposed a $4.1 billion construction package to stimulate the faltering economy. He noted that most of the projects were necessary and already in the planning stages, and included $15 million to construct new community facilities and earmarked $12 million for capital improvements at state mental facilities. A year earlier, the General Assembly had voted down a similar proposal; in 1975, the measure passed (Illinois Commission on Mental Health and Developmental Disabilities, 1977; Walker, 1976).

As part of this program, six specialized living centers were eventually constructed around the State. They were initially intended for 150 people per facility. One new aspect of these facilities was that their construction was financed by the State, and they were subsequently turned over to private providers to own and operate. In most other residential developments in Illinois, providers were required to finance the building of projects themselves.

In 1981, new laws mandated the licensure of community living facilities (Pub. Act 82-567) and community residential alternatives (Pub. Act 82-584) by the Department of Public Health. The latter facilitated the development of smaller group homes for no more than eight individuals. This ushered in the development of residential facilities that were considerably smaller than the existing ICFs/DD, community living facilities, and specialized living centers. Development of these proceeded slowly, however. By 1985, there were fewer than 500 persons residing in community residential alternatives, as compared to over 650 living in community living facilities and approximately 5,000 people in privately operated ICFs/DD (DMHDD, 1985).

In response to the national recession that was gripping Illinois, Governor Thompson in 1982 announced the closure of the Dixon Developmental Center. At the time of his announcement, the facility's population was 823 persons, all of whom would be transferred to other state facilities. Six days after the governor's announcement, the Dixon Association for Retarded Citizens, representing the families of Dixon

residents, filed a lawsuit in state court to prevent the facility's closure. The Circuit Court found in favor of the families and issued an order halting further transfers of the residents. On appeal, the Illinois Supreme Court upheld the governor's right to close the facility (*Dixon Association for Retarded Citizens v. Thompson,* 1982). On a delayed schedule, the Dixon residents were transferred to facilities across the State. The expansion of community-based residential services was not an outcome of the facility closure.

However, the closure did not result in the complete termination of institutional services at the site. As a concession to the families, the governor agreed to construct a new, smaller institution for individuals with deafness, blindness, and mental retardation. This facility was built on the grounds for 100 residents and named the Mabley Developmental Center. By 1982, the Department of Mental Health and Developmental Disabilities (DMHDD) was leasing two buildings of the former Dixon Developmental Center to Kreider Services, which operated two group homes for 12 and 10 persons on the former Dixon campus (Health Facilities Planning Board, 1985). The remainder of Dixon was converted to a prison.

Dixon was not the state's first conversion of a state developmental disabilities institution into a prison. In 1977, part of the Lincoln Developmental Center known as the Annex was turned over to the Department of Corrections and converted into a prison (DMHDD, 1980). In 1982, the Bowen Developmental Center was also converted to a prison, with most residents being transferred to the Anna Psychiatric Hospital, and a small number placed in privately operated facilities (DMHDD, 1984). During his term as governor, Thompson converted three psychiatric hospitals to prisons as well. Most of the state's psychiatric hospitals were perceived to be seriously underutilized (House Democratic Staff, 1980; Illinois Office of the Auditor General, 1978). The auditor general reported that there were 74 vacant buildings at seven DMHDD psychiatric and developmental disabilities institutions.

By the early 1980s, community residential services in Illinois meant facilities that were not operated by the State, but certainly did not connote small-scale homes for persons with developmental disabilities. In an inventory of residential facilities licensed by the Department of Public Health for adults with developmental disabilities, the Health Facilities Planning Board (1982) identified 54 facilities with 20 or more individuals per setting, and just 10 for fewer than 20 persons. The largest private facilities in the State, Beverly Farms and St. Mary's Square, had 390 and 227 beds, respectively. Furthermore, a number of facilities operated general long-term care beds in the same facility with beds for persons with developmental disabilities, so facilities in these cases were considerably larger than is readily apparent. For example, Somerset House in Chicago operated 80 ICF/DD beds and 370 general long-term care beds at the same location. Mattingly Health Care in the town of Energy operated 73 beds for persons with developmental disabilities and 86 general long-term care beds in the same facility (Health Facilities Planning Board, 1982).

General long-term care beds were for "regular" nursing home patients. Numerous facilities provided services to a mixed clientele, and transitions in licensure were extremely common. Beds were frequently converted from community living facility to ICF/DD in order to secure higher reimbursement rates. Facilities also commonly terminated their community living facility or ICF/DD beds, converting them back to general long-term care beds (Health Facilities Planning Board, 1982), possibly in response to the threat of decertification by the Department of Public Health for failure to comply with ICF/DD certification standards. What is clear from this report is that in 1982, a cohesive plan to provide residential services to persons with developmental disabilities was not in place. Facilities were able to apply to the Health Facilities Planning Board to change their operating status, and DMHDD did not directly control the process. Several interview respondents indicated that the political nature of the Health Facilities Planning Board facilitated the development of large, private institutional facilities for persons with developmental disabilities.

Illinois was among the earliest states to apply to the Health Care Financing Administration (HCFA) to participate in the new Waiver program. Illinois' first Waiver application was approved by HCFA to begin November 30, 1983, and was approved to serve 770 persons in its first year (DMHDD, 1984). Illinois' Waiver application intended to target services to three primary groups: public institutional residents, individuals living in private ICFs/DD, and finally, individuals

living in the community. Illinois structured its Waiver to provide services including day programs, supported employment, residential services, and behavioral interventions (DMHDD, 1984). In 1982, Illinois enacted legislation mandating inter-departmental cooperation in the development of Waiver services (Pub. Act 82-921 of 1982).

The state's implementation of the Waiver was quite anemic during the 1980s. While approved to serve 1,497 persons by its third year of operation, the State in fact served only 720 persons through the Waiver by 1990. Six years after implementation, the Illinois Waiver served fewer people than had been approved for the first year of the operation (Braddock, Hemp, Parish, & Westrich, 1998). The lack of expansion of the HCBS Waiver was commonly attributed to a lack of funds to expand it.

Throughout the 1980s, growth in the state's residential service system largely occurred in either nursing home placements or private ICFs/DD placements. While a number of new initiatives were piloted and implemented in the 1980s, few expanded to become large-scale aspects of the state's residential service delivery system. For instance, in 1982, the Home/Individual Program (H/IP) was initially piloted in one region of the State. This new initiative funded the care and training of one or two person(s) living with house parents (DMHDD, 1984). While the program subsequently moved beyond the pilot level and was implemented in other locations, it never became a large component of the state's service delivery system. By 1996, there were only 120 individuals in H/IP programs around the State (Braddock, Hemp, Parish, & Westrich, 1998).

In 1983, a decade after the DMHDD had acknowledged dumping individuals with developmental disabilities into nursing homes to downsize its public institutions, the federal Health Care Financing Administration identified more than 3,000 persons with developmental disabilities living in Illinois nursing homes. The HCFA report found serious problems with the placements; individuals were not receiving adequate care, treatment was not being provided, individuals were placed in nursing homes without adequate facility preparation, in addition to a host of other problems (DMHDD, 1985). The publication of this report indicated that attempts to address the problems in Illinois nursing homes, which had been uncovered by a number of scandals in the 1970s, had not been adequate or successful. Nursing homes continued to be a dominant part of the residential service system for people with developmental disabilities throughout the 1980s (Braddock, Hemp, Parish, & Westrich, 1998; DMHDD, 1990).

In the 1970s and 1980s, operation of the ICF/MR program in Illinois was coordinated by three separate state agencies. The Department of Mental Health and Developmental Disabilities was responsible for operating the facilities according to ICF/MR regulations. The Department of Public Health (DPH) was responsible for inspecting facilities and certifying them for continued participation in the ICF/MR program and the Department of Public Aid (IDPA) was responsible for Medicaid financing. A facility found to be out of compliance during one of DPH's inspections would receive a statement of deficiencies and was required to submit a plan of correction. If the plan of correction was approved by the DPH, no further measures would be taken to address the deficiencies. However, if the deficiencies were sufficiently significant, or the operating agency was felt not to be able to implement the plan of correction quickly enough, DPH was empowered by state law to recommend termination of a facility's ICF/MR participation. In these cases, the termination recommendation would be submitted to the IDPA, which, as the state's Medicaid agency, paid for the ICF/MR program. Once the IDPA terminated the facility from the ICF/MR program, federal reimbursement for the program stopped. In Illinois, all Medicaid programs, including the ICFs/DD, have always been reimbursed 50% by the federal government. As such, when a facility was terminated from the federal ICF/MR program, the federal reimbursement of 50% of the operating costs were lost to the State; in essence, the state's actual operating costs doubled when federal participation ceased (Citizens Council on Mental Health and Developmental Disabilities, 1986).

Maintaining compliance with federal ICF/MR certification standards became a serious problem for the State in the mid-1980s (Citizens Council on Mental Health and Developmental Disabilities, 1986). In order to obtain federal Medicaid funding for its state institutions, the DMHDD had submitted to HCFA a comprehensive plan to bring the state facilities into compliance with federal ICF/MR regulations. This plan was submitted and subsequently revised in the 1970s. It called for the continued downsizing of the state's public institutions, improvement of institutional living conditions, and, perhaps most important, enhanced staffing levels. These objectives needed to be met in order to conform to ICF/MR regulations related to minimum staffing, minimum square footage, and minimal living conditions for institutional residents. The consequences of failing to comply with ICF/MR regulations was the potential loss of millions of federal Medicaid funds.

Illinois submitted an amended plan to the HCFA in 1980, and sought a 24-month extension to improve conditions at Shapiro, Dixon, Lincoln, Murray, and Bowen. Dixon and Bowen subsequently closed in 1982, and the compliance project plans were completed for Shapiro, Lincoln, and Murray in 1983. As part of this plan, 707 residents were transferred to other facilities and 19 buildings were renovated (DMHDD, 1984). However, conditions were still unacceptable in many of the state facilities in the mid-1980s. In 1982, prior to the facility's closure, DMHDD received notification from HCFA that the Dixon Developmental Center would be terminated from the ICF/MR program if it was unable to meet certification standards within two months (Wells, 1982). In 1984, the DPH, which, by state statute was the licensing and certification authority for the ICF/MR program in Illinois, issued a short-term agreement and a cancellation clause related to the Howe Developmental Center. This stipulated that if Howe could not be brought up to standards immediately, DPH would recommend final termination of the ICF/MR participation of this facility to the Department of Public Aid (Citizens Council on Mental Health and Developmental Disabilities, 1986).

On August 6, 1986, the DPH recommended final termination of Howe from the ICF/MR program to the Department of Public Aid. In response to this, DMHDD Director Michael Belletire voluntarily withdrew the facility from the program, ostensibly to salvage a politically embarrassing situation. The financial loss to the State due to Howe's withdrawal from the ICF/MR program was considerable, exceeding $11 million in federal Medicaid funds (Citizens Council on

Mental Health and Developmental Disabilities, 1986). Several interview respondents indicated that this was a poor decision and a clear miscalculation of the length of time it would take to return the facility to ICF/MR compliance.

Although Howe was the only state institution terminated from the ICF/MR program, a number of other facilities had serious difficulties. A survey conducted in 1985 by federal HCFA auditors at the Ludeman Center resulted in a notification of termination of the facility's participation in the ICF/MR program. Five months later, improvements at Ludeman resulted in the rescinding of termination proceedings by the HCFA; no federal funds for that facility were lost to the State (Citizens Council on Mental Health and Developmental Disabilities, 1986).

In 1986, federal HCFA surveyors conducted 36 direct surveys and three follow-ups. A direct survey occurred when federal auditors personally evaluated a program for its compliance with the ICF/MR regulations. These were full-blown inspections of compliance with every aspect of the ICF/MR regulations. A follow-up survey occurred when federal HCFA auditors selected three programs that had already been surveyed by the DPH, evaluating the DPH's findings. Out of the 39 surveys and follow-up surveys, they conducted in 1986, HCFA issued 18 termination recommendations, including those for the Singer Mental Health and Developmental Disabilities Center and the Howe Developmental Center. Private ICFs/MR were certainly not exempt from compliance difficulties. The Adele Karlson Center, operated by Springfield Association for Retarded Citizens, which was an ICF/DD for 70 people, was terminated from the program at a cost to the State of more than $700,000 in lost federal reimbursements (Illinois Department of Public Aid, 1988).

The Citizen's Council on Mental Health and Developmental Disabilities established a subcommittee to review the recertification process at the Howe and Ludeman Developmental Centers. Ongoing meetings and hearings were conducted in 1986 and 1987 related to this issue. In October 1987, Illinois State Sen. William Mahar wrote to Governor Thompson indicating that he and the subcommittee of the Citizens Council on Mental Health and Developmental Disabilities that he chaired had investigated this issue and concluded

that the state's Department of Public Health was not fulfilling its obligation to "accurately assess Department of Mental Health and Developmental Disabilities' ability to provide active treatment" to institutional residents (Mahar, 1987, p. 1). His position was supported by the conclusions of HCFA surveyors as well, who found the state's auditing mechanisms were not congruent with the federal standards.

A number of service providers formed the Illinois Coalition of ICF/DD providers to address the rate problems. These providers felt that Illinois' low reimbursement rates were the reason for so many of the ICF/MR compliance problems (Illinois Coalition of ICF/DD Providers, 1987). Between 1985-87, three private facilities were terminated from the program, with federal funding for a total of 327 beds eliminated (Citizens Council on Mental Health and Developmental Disabilities, 1987). In 1987, while inspecting Howe again after the facility's partial reinstatement into the ICF/MR program, HCFA surveyors again recommended termination. However, this time the facility took sufficient action which resulted in the termination decision being rescinded (Citizens Council on Mental Health and Developmental Disabilities, 1986).

At the end of the 1980s, a number of pieces of legislation were enacted relating to the developmental disabilities residential service system. In June 1987, spurred by ongoing concerns for the prevalence of abuse and neglect in the state institutions, the Citizens Council on Mental Health and Developmental Disabilities conducted an inquiry and held hearings related to these issues. These hearings led to passage of legislation that created the Office of the Inspector General within DMHDD in 1987. The Office of the Inspector General was mandated by the statute to investigate all allegations of abuse and neglect occurring in state facilities and provide an annual report to the legislature and the governor on the status of its inquiries.

In 1987, and again in 1988, Governor Thompson vetoed a Bill of Rights that had been passed by the General Assembly. This bill authorized an entitlement to services by persons with developmental disabilities. In his veto-message Governor Thompson indicated that he would not sign into law mandates that were not funded by the legislature.

In 1988, Community Integrated Living Alternatives (CILA) was authorized by statute as well. This was a new form of residential service for the State, designed after the supported living model, whereby individuals chose with whom and where they would live (Murphy, 1989). This form of housing was a radical departure from the facility-based services that had dominated the Illinois residential service system during the 1970s and much of the 1980s.

The new statute defined licensing standards for CILAs. The following year the DMHDD issued a request for proposals inviting providers to submit applications to become CILA providers (Murphy, 1989). A number of interview respondents reported that the creation of CILA was one of the first innovative service models implemented in Illinois. However, other interview respondents argued that while CILA may have been innovative for Illinois, it did not offer people with developmental disabilities true choices in living arrangements, like the practice in other states. Others stated that in some instances, group homes have just been relabeled as CILA programs, without shifting their philosophical orientation to be consumer-centered.

The Community Residence Location Planning Act passed in 1989 directed every municipality to develop a plan detailing how the locality has or will ensure adequate availability of community residential sites (Pub. Act 86-638 of 1989). These plans were to be submitted to the Illinois Planning Council on Developmental Disabilities (the Council) the following year.

Pursuant to the law, the Council reported that nearly all municipalities had submitted a plan. While these plans varied widely in quality, the Council (1991) recommended that the General Assembly not pursue passage of directive legislation related to zoning for community residences. The Council argued that the present status of zoning issues did not require new legislation, because the current status of zoning in the State seemed satisfactory and federal law prohibited zoning discrimination.

Numerous interview respondents, however, indicated that throughout the 1970s and 1980s, local opposition to the development of community homes was frequently manifested in the enactment or enforcement of restrictive zoning ordinances. The Governor's Task Force on the Future of Mental Health in Illinois (1987) also concluded that zoning problems contin-

ued to be major barriers to the ongoing development of community-based residential services. Development was widely held to be quite difficult due to restrictive zoning. Prior attempts to address zoning had failed in the legislature. House Bill 281 was introduced in 1976, and would have mandated anti-restrictive zoning; the bill did not receive a single vote in the legislature. The failure of the measure to be supported was attributed by the Illinois ARC to the power of the municipalities' lobbying group (Breslin, Ganski, Knight, O'Dell, & Unterbrink, 1980). While Illinois has never enacted legislation that would prohibit restrictive zoning practices, the federal government, in 1988, amended the Fair Housing Act to prohibit discrimination against persons with disabilities (Pub. L. 100-430). The intent of the Fair Housing Act was to specifically address zoning-related discrimination against persons with disabilities:

> The Committee intends that the discrimination against those with handicaps apply to zoning decisions and practices. The Act is intended to prohibit the application of special requirements through land-use regulations, restrictive covenants, and conditional or special use permits that have the effect of limiting the ability of such persons to live in the residence of their choice in the community (legislative history cited in Whitman & Parnas, 1999, p. 3).

In the case of Illinois, federal law preempted the state and local laws. But as one interview respondent reported, community opposition has by no means been eliminated. Some municipalities continue to use their zoning power to oppose the placement of group homes within their boundaries. This is generally accomplished by requiring permissions and variances for the establishment of new group homes. While the federal law prohibits discrimination, the law depends on having the party that has been discriminated against sue for enforcement, which can be costly.

One of the most important pieces of Illinois legislation enacted at the end of the 1980s was House Bill 69, which established monthly subsidies for families with adults and/or children with disabilities (Protection and Advocacy Inc., 1990; Pub. Act 86-921 of

1990). This subsidy was modeled after the family support subsidy program in Michigan. However, when the Illinois program began, it was funded at a low level; in 1991, its first year of funding, spending totaled $706 thousand (Braddock, Hemp, Parish, & Westrich, 1998).

At the end of the 1980s, Illinois' residential service system for persons with developmental disabilities, while having grown to serve more people, still looked much the same as it had at the end of the 1970s. The predominant form of available residential services was still state institutions, nursing homes, and ICFs/DD. *Figure 3.8* depicts the number of persons living in state-funded residential services by the type or size of the facility, in 1977 and 1990. As is evident in the figure, the setting types that grew the most, in terms of the number of people served, were nursing homes and large group homes for 7 to 15 persons. Institutional settings (those for 16 or more people) represented a major component of the state's service system in 1977 and in 1990 (Braddock et al., 2002; Lakin, 1979). Reliable data could not be found on the number of persons with developmental disabilities in privately operated residential settings before 1977, which is why the data point of 1977, and not 1970, the beginning of the study period, was selected.

Administrative Overview

Prior to 1961, facilities for persons with developmental disabilities and mental illness, along with the state's poverty programs, were administered by the Department of Public Welfare. In 1961, the Department of Mental Health was created as a separate code agency, with its director reporting to the governor. The Department of Mental Health was thereafter responsible for services to persons with mental illness and developmental disabilities. Services in 1961 were essentially institutional in nature (State Advisory Council on Mental Retardation, 1965). Psychiatric hospitals across the State, while they had been depopulating since the late 1950s, were still the main residential service available (Illinois Department of Mental Health, 1969).

The creation of the new Department of Mental Health in 1961 continued the practice of a centralized administration of both developmental disabilities and mental illness services. In subsequent years, attempts would be made to establish local or regional administration of the service system. In the 1960s, this attempt took two forms: the establishment of administrative regions termed "zones," and passage of legislation facilitating local administration of services.

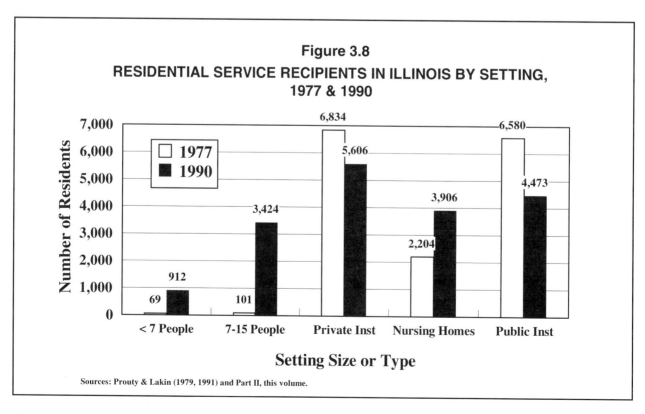

Figure 3.8
RESIDENTIAL SERVICE RECIPIENTS IN ILLINOIS BY SETTING, 1977 & 1990

Sources: Prouty & Lakin (1979, 1991) and Part II, this volume.

The development of the zone system was initiated in 1960. Concern about the state's mental health facilities led to the passage in 1960 of a $150 million bond initiative. Two thirds of this money was earmarked to improve existing institutional facilities, while the remaining $50 million was to be allocated to construct zone centers. Zone centers were intended to be the centerpiece of Illinois' community mental health plan, providing temporary inpatient and ongoing outpatient mental health and developmental disabilities services in eight regions across the State. In 1964, DMH was organized into these eight zones (Illinois Department of Mental Health, 1964, 1973c).

Three separate statutes were enacted in the 1960s, with the intent of stimulating local provision of services. In 1961, Senate Bill 377 was adopted. This allowed counties to tax citizens for "mental deficiency" programs. Counties were permitted to develop what came to be known as 377 Boards that were able to use the new taxes to provide or contract for services. Two years later, House Bill 708, the Illinois' Community Mental Health Act, was passed. This act also allowed counties to hold referenda and, if successful, to tax local residents in order to finance local mental health and developmental disabilities services. This became known as a 708 Board. In 1969, the final statute designed to facilitate local services, Senate Bill 553, was enacted. This statute allowed counties with public health departments that had previously been established by referendum to tax residents for mental health services (Ragan, 1974; Scheerenberger, 1969). This became known as a 553 Board. In spite of this new legal authority for counties to finance and provide services, the number of counties that took advantage of the law was quite limited. By 1974, seven of Illinois' 101 counties had established "377 Boards," 37 had established "708 Boards," and 36 had "553 Boards." Local spending for community mental health services totaled just $1.5 million that year (Ragan, 1974).

Through the 1960s and early 1970s, there was considerable concern among advocates, and particularly the Illinois Association for Retarded Children (IARC), that the needs of persons with developmental disabilities were not properly addressed by the Department of Mental Health, which was perceived to focus primarily on the needs of persons with mental illness. The IARC advocated for a separate develop-

mental disabilities code agency, with a cabinet-level director reporting to the governor. In 1973, largely due to IARC's advocacy efforts, the legislature passed House Bill 724, which would have separated mental illness and developmental disabilities services at the cabinet level and created a new code department for developmental disabilities services (Illinois Association for Retarded Citizens, 1973). However, Governor Dan Walker (1973) vetoed this legislation, arguing that the duplicative administrative costs were excessive and unnecessary. It is possible there were political motives behind the governor's veto as well; the IARC had vocally backed candidate Walker's opponent, incumbent Gov. Richard Ogilvie, during the 1971 gubernatorial election. One IARC interview respondent reported, "There is no doubt that we were punished for supporting Ogilvie's candidacy when Walker took office." This punishment was short-lived, however. Governor Walker actively cultivated relationships with the IARC and other mental health organizations, meeting frequently with their leadership, and touring facilities around the State (Walker, 1976). The governor went on to appoint Don Moss, the IARC's executive director, to serve on numerous task forces and committees that convened throughout his term of office (Illinois Association for Retarded Citizens, 1977).

In 1972, the State amended the Mental Health Code, and compelled the Department of Mental Health to provide an annual report to the governor and General Assembly on the status of its programs and services. The statute also mandated that the Department delineate the certification and accreditation status of all mental health facilities, including those for persons with developmental disabilities (Pub. Act 77-2722 of 1972). This codification represented legislative endorsement of an ongoing departmental objective; Joe Saxl had been hired in 1971 to assist the Division of Mental Retardation Services to obtain accreditation of the state's developmental disabilities institutions (Committee on Mental Retardation, 1971b). When the legislation was enacted in 1972, none of the state's developmental disabilities facilities were accredited (Committee on Mental Retardation, 1972).

In 1973, the Department of Mental Health became the Department of Mental Health and Developmental Disabilities (DMHDD), and the Division of Developmental Disabilities was created within it (Pub.

Act 78-992 of 1973). A deputy director was to be appointed to oversee all developmental disabilities functions. This Act also consolidated the regional system, and community placement activities were pulled from the supervision of state facility superintendents and handled by regional staff (Committee on Mental Retardation, 1973). Many interviewees felt that the regions were successful in developing community placement during this period. The regional and subregional staff worked closely with service providers, offering technical assistance in developing ew community placements. A few respondents indicated that this period was the heyday of the state system, and when the regional system was subsequently dismantled a few years later, that community placement ground to a virtual halt. One of the responsibilities of the regional staff was to assist nursing homes to convert their facilities to ICFs/MR, and to improve their programming to meet the needs of persons with developmental disabilities. During the period from 1974-78, the number of persons with developmental disabilities in community living facilities expanded from 162 to 444, and the number in ICFs/MR increased to 2,550 (DMHDD, 1983).

Many interview respondents indicated that the Department's implementation of the regional structure in the 1970s contributed to its ability to grow the community services system. Numerous interview respondents also reported that Art Dykstra's leadership in this area was very important. According to these interview respondents, Dykstra, who had been both a regional administrator and institutional superintendent, collaborated with community services providers to expand non-institutional residential services in his region. However, in a cost-cutting move implemented in 1983, the regional structure was disbanded and regional staff were laid off. Numerous interview respondents indicated that the destruction of the regional system essentially decimated the state's community placement program. Most interview respondents felt that the consolidation of placement and the centralization of the Department's administrative structure in Springfield resulted in a slowdown of the development of community services. Reliable data showing the numbers of individuals in different types of settings during this period were not available and therefore could not

be confirmed.

One interview respondent who was a national expert indicated that Illinois has never really implemented a cohesive system for developing or administering its community services, and his comments were largely echoed by many other interview respondents.

> When I'm being frank about Illinois, the thing that separates it from every other large state is that it has no organized system for delivering community services. It operates out of the central office. This is unique. Nearly all other large states have local administrative structures. I always think that this [absence in Illinois] widened the dichotomy between institutional services and community services staff… It's clearly helped to create the rift that exists.

Another structural change occurred with the passage of the Health Facilities Planning Act in 1974. This legislation created Illinois' Certificate of Need program, which was the process that controlled construction, renovation, and any modification to health-care facilities (Pub. Act 78-1156). This was enacted to establish cost controls, better management, and improve planning by health-care providers. The legislation established the state's Health Facilities Planning Board, which was a 15-member commission appointed by the governor with Senate confirmation (Health Facilities Planning Board, 1977).

This Board came to be very important to the developmental disabilities service system. It was staffed by the Department of Public Health, and conducted comprehensive needs assessments of all licensed health-care facilities in the State. When it was created in 1974, these facilities included community living facilities and ICFs/DD. Service providers interested in developing new ICFs/DD or community living facilities were obliged to apply to the Health Facilities Planning Board (Health Facilities Planning Board, 1977). As such, DMHDD did not directly control all aspects of the residential service system. After these changes were implemented, the Department's structure remained essentially the same until the mid-1990s.

Scandals

Scandals in developmental disabilities institutions have sometimes been useful for catalyzing policy changes. Perhaps the most famous example is Geraldo Rivera's exposé into conditions in New York's Willowbrook institution on Staten Island in 1972. The horrific conditions he uncovered were broadcast nationally, and provided material for a class-action lawsuit that was subsequently filed by the New York State Association for Retarded Citizens.

Numerous interviewees in Illinois felt that scandals have helped shape public policy, because they capture the public's attention and can stimulate change. Illinois has experienced many scandals in its developmental disabilities service system. A few of these warrant discussion, because of the way in which they illuminate the service system and its weaknesses, but also because of their limited impact in shaping public developmental disabilities policy.

The 1970s marked a time of many scandals involving residential facilities for people with developmental disabilities. In 1972, the Illinois Legislative Investigating Commission was authorized to investigate the beating death of a man who had been living on a developmental disabilities unit at the Peoria State Hospital (Illinois General Assembly, 1972). Before the Commission could complete its investigation, two more men with developmental disabilities died at the facility, one from a neglected ear infection. The Commission probed these two deaths as well, and found extensive evidence of systemic neglect on the developmental disabilities units at the hospital (Illinois Legislative Investigating Commission, 1973).

Another state hospital scandal occurred the same year when conditions at the Elgin State Hospital were uncovered by the Legislative Commission to Visit and Examine State Institutions' Charitable Subcommittee (1972). The Subcommittee had been investigating the suspension of a hospital doctor for practicing without a medical degree and allegations of deplorable living conditions.

At the behest of fellow Commission members, Subcommittee Chairman Sen. Frank N. Ozinga, accompanied by a member of the news media, paid an unannounced visit to the hospital to verify the allegations and possible need for full-scale Subcommittee examination of the State mental institution. (Legislative Commission to Visit and Examine State Institutions, Charitable Subcommittee, 1972, p. 1)

The senator was shocked by the conditions he found, which included sexual promiscuity, a complete lack of supervision of patients, and an array of decrepit buildings and neglectful conditions. His findings led to a full inquiry and hearings on the facility.

The Charitable Subcommittee's findings (1972) included an extensive list of recommendations related to an array of aspects of the facility's operations as well as its community placement program. At the time of the inquiry, community placement was still under the auspices and authority of state hospitals and developmental centers (Illinois Department of Mental Health, 1973b). The Subcommittee recommended strengthening institutional staffing in order to "provide a decent level of custodial care as the institution's top priority" (Legislative Commission to Visit and Examine State Institutions, Charitable Subcommittee, 1972, p. 13). Recommendations also included the

Immediate release and commitment of all funds for repair and maintenance [and] capital improvement of physical facilities at Elgin State Hospital for all projects which were not accomplished during the 1972 fiscal year and for which projects, funds have been appropriated for the current year. (p. 13)

The Subcommittee drew attention to security at the facility both with regard to drug storage and general security of the grounds. Related to the community placement program, the Subcommittee recommended that the Mental Health Code be changed to eliminate absolute discharges after placing someone outside the public facility, whereby the Department of Mental Health was completely released of its legal responsibilities for aftercare. The Subcommittee further suggested tightening treatment regulations, strengthening quality assurance in private aftercare facilities, promulgation of standards of custodial care and mechanisms to enforce such standards. Expanded monitoring functions to bolster quality assurance in private facilities was also recommended. Finally, the Subcommittee recommended that its legislative mandate be expanded to include visiting and examining private facilities; it also recommended enactment of legislation requiring private care facilities to disclose their financial records when the facilities are supported in any way by public funds.

Less than a year after the Charitable Subcommittee issued its report, the House of Representatives passed Resolution 382 (Illinois House of Representatives, 1973). The House noted the death of two patients at the Elgin State Hospital within a week of one another and under "irregular circumstances." The Resolution directed the Illinois Legislative Investigating Commission to conduct an immediate inquiry into the deaths and assess whether or not Elgin State Hospital was negligent or otherwise responsible for the deaths. Immediately after beginning its inquiry, the Illinois Legislative Investigating Commission (1974) learned that other patients had also died under unusual circumstances at the facility. As such, their investigation was expanded to include an inquiry into the causes of these other deaths.

The Commission found that medical and staff neglect of a 20-year-old patient with developmental disabilities led to his death, 30 hours after he had been admitted in good condition to the facility. A number of other patients died as a result of physical attack, possibly inflicted by fellow patients during which time they were not supervised by facility staff. In total, the six deaths at the facility were investigated, all of which were related in some way to inadequacies of care (Illinois Legislative Investigating Commission, 1974).

The Commission, in a similar fashion to the Charitable Subcommittee's work a year prior, issued an extraordinarily detailed report of its findings totaling 10 chapters and hundreds of pages. The Commission's recommendations included: enacting better safeguards for patients' protection, enhancing staffing, amending the Mental Health Code to establish minimal standards reflective of the federal court's *Wyatt v. Stickney* ruling, creating a nonpartisan human services commission, strengthening the monitoring of medical and staff services, investigating questionable practices, ending the patronage employment of superintendents, strengthening training programs, and enhancing staff certifica-

tion requirements. The Commission's recommendations also included numerous other specifications related to staffing policies, aftercare discharges, monitoring of patients, and the provision of adequate medical care (Illinois Legislative Investigating Commission, 1974).

What seems to be most relevant is the extent to which things did not change subsequent to the first investigation. The second Elgin inquiry followed immediately on the heels of the first, and had findings that were identical in many cases. This situation seems to highlight the ways in which scandals were not useful in facilitating major systems change during this period.

Limited changes did occur after the second legislative inquiry. Of particular relevance to this study were two changes that emerged in response to the situations at Elgin and Peoria. In 1973, the statutory mandate of the Charitable Subcommittee was expanded, as had been recommended, to include private facilities licensed by the State (Legislative Commission to Visit and Examine State Institutions, Subcommittee on Charitable Institutions, 1976). This statutory change did enable the Commission to provide yet another oversight mechanism as part of its role. In addition, the Peoria State Hospital was closed and community placements from state facilities were put under the jurisdiction and control of the regional subsystem. This structuring of the regions and giving them the authority to make community placements was partially designed to provide better monitoring at the local level of community placements as they occurred (Illinois Department of Mental Health, 1973b).

In spite of these changes, the scandals that faced the State would continue. Numerous interview respondents reported that DMHDD forcibly closed the Klingberg School and that Windgate, a private institution for children, was taken over by another service provider when extensive abuse and neglect was revealed in the facility. Another care facility named Winneconna in Chicago was forcibly closed by DMHDD in the mid-1970s (Legislative Commission to Visit and Examine State Institutions, Subcommittee on Charitable Institutions, 1976). In all of these situations, the care provided in these facilities was found to be totally inadequate.

Nursing home scandals involving persons with developmental disabilities emerged next as a critical issue. In 1974, the Illinois Legislative Investigating Commission was directed to conduct an inquiry into the deaths of seven patients at the Illinois Extended Care Center in Rockford (Illinois House of Representatives, 1974).

The following year the Illinois House of Representatives (1975) adopted Resolution 1277, which authorized the Illinois Legislative Investigating Commission to investigate Lake County nursing homes, and particularly the All Seasons facility. The two reports that the Commission subsequently issued relate a tale of unqualified horror. The Commission found extensive evidence of brutality, vicious sexual assaults, and extensive neglect of people with developmental disabilities living in nursing homes (Illinois Legislative Investigating Commission, 1977).

Neglectful conditions in these facilities were largely blamed for the abuses uncovered during these investigations. However, a lack of monitoring and follow-up after transferring patients to these facilities by the DMHDD, the inability of the receiving nursing homes to provide adequate care for these individuals, and the precipitous way in which individuals were transferred to the nursing homes compounded the problems. Had DMHDD conducted some type of monitoring of placements, the long-standing duration of the problems could at least have been prevented (Illinois Legislative Investigating Committee, 1977).

At the All Seasons facility, in the state's northern Lake County, residents were subjected to particularly gruesome acts and willful neglect. Facility operators committed considerable fraud and obtained reimbursements from the State for services that were never provided nor intended to be provided. In one three-week period, the facility accepted 100 individuals with developmental disabilities from Lincoln and Dixon. This occurred because the state-operated facilities were under Departmental mandates to quickly depopulate. All Seasons was interested in quickly increasing its patient census in order to receive greater levels of funding from the State (Illinois Legislative Investigating Committee, 1977).

The implications of the All Seasons case and the Commission's inquiry were really two-fold. The Nursing Home Reform Act was passed in response to the conditions that were found by these inquiries (Illinois Association for Retarded Citizens, 1979; Pub. Act 81-223 of 1979). This Act mandated stronger regulations, greater oversight of facilities, and protection of recipients' rights. The DMHDD also changed its policies to stop the practice of "dumping" individuals into nursing homes. While placement into nursing homes did not stop, the Department was required to ensure that it monitored aftercare and facilitated successful transitions into private facilities.

Another implication of the nursing home scandals was that they engendered fear on the part of the parents of Lincoln and Dixon residents. One interview respondent reported having had numerous conversations with these families, trying to allay their apprehension about the placement of their children into private facilities. The interview respondent felt that the families were quite knowledgeable about the conditions that had been uncovered in the nursing homes and were extremely fearful for their sons and daughters. There can be little doubt that the events surrounding the nursing homes helped to crystallize some portion of the parental opposition to community placement that would become such a powerful force in subsequent years.

There were many other scandals related to inadequate care in private facilities in the State, particularly in the 1970s. Several facilities, as stated previously (Klingberg, Windgate, Winneconna), were eventually closed or taken over by other service providers. Interview respondents reported other scandals that resulted in facility closures as well.

One other scandal related to a private facility merits mention. After protracted and fruitless reimbursement rate negotiations with the DMHDD, the North Aurora Center, which had been open since 1971, issued 24-hour notice of its intent to close on December 16, 1979. All of the Center's residents, nearly 500 persons with developmental disabilities, were transported by bus to the Howe, Ludeman, and Waukegan Developmental Centers in a single day (*Phillips v. Thompson*, 1983). One interviewee reported that the residents' fear and panic was palpable as DMHDD staff tried to shepherd everyone onto buses and to the public institutions:

> Everyone was screaming and crying. No one had any idea what was going on. It was an incredibly awful situation. We were terribly

lucky that the new facilities [Howe, Waukegan, and Ludeman] were available, and weren't yet full. I have no idea what we would have done otherwise with so many people on such short notice.

Several important themes related to developmental disabilities residential scandals in Illinois emerge on close analysis. The first is that scandals have generally not brought about sweeping changes in public policy. Passage of the Nursing Home Reform Act in 1979, while it grew out of the nursing home scandals, did not eliminate further nursing home placement of individuals with developmental disabilities. The scandals did not even cause close scrutiny of the practice, which was being questioned around the country at the time.

One respondent indicated that the scandals were helpful only so long as they remained a focus of the media; several respondents indicated that the amount of media time that scandals received was insufficient to transform public policy. The immediate outcome of most scandals was the closure of the facility in question. Another notable aspect of scandals in Illinois' developmental disabilities service system was that the most notorious or widely known occurred in privately operated facilities. As Illinois has defined "community" services as all privately operated facilities and "institutional" services as state-operated (Ragan, 1974), most of these scandals came to be defined as community scandals, even if they were occurring in privately operated institutions. This distinction added fuel to the schism between institutional and community advocates over the years in Illinois.

One example of the way in which a scandal received considerable attention that resulted in no major public policy was the *Chicago Sun Times* exposé on the Windgate facility, which was a private institution for children in which extensive abuse and neglect was uncovered by the reporters. In response to this exposé, Governor Walker appointed the Governor's Task Force to Investigate Abuse and Neglect in Mental Retardation Institutions in 1976, which was chaired by Don Moss, then executive director of the Illinois ARC (Illinois Association for Retarded Citizens, 1977). While the task force created by the governor subsequently released a report detailing its findings, it did not result in any significant changes in public policy or

the passage of legislation. The scandal had attracted the governor's attention to the point that he appointed a task force. However, he was succeeded by Governor Thompson in 1977, and Thompson did not follow through with the task force.

It is therefore a conclusion of this inquiry that while scandals have catalyzed public policy changes in other parts of the country, they have had a limited influence on Illinois' residential service system and its evolution.

Politics

It is impossible to disentangle the evolution of residential services in Illinois from its political system. In fact, nearly every interview respondent indicated that politics had shaped the residential service system. This section will delineate and describe the aspects of politics that have been related to the development of residential services in the State.

The Illinois Constitution and Home Rule Powers

The first important issue related to state politics is the structure of government in Illinois. The State has never passed any statewide laws that prohibit discrimination in town zoning practices. As such, the Illinois Constitution has played an important role in how residential services have developed. In 1969, when the Constitution was rewritten, it provided for home rule power for any county or municipality with a population of more than 25,000 people with an elected chief executive officer. The home rule powers conferred upon municipalities by the new Constitution enabled towns and counties to have nearly total control over the management of their own affairs. The General Assembly therefore had little authority to limit municipalities' home rule powers. This enabled towns and counties to levy their own taxes, structure their own governments, and essentially have free rein in the conduct of their administration. The Constitution is very direct in giving municipalities this authority, stating that "powers and functions of home rule units shall be construed liberally" (Constitution of 1970, Article VII, 1998).

The major implication of home rule with respect to persons with developmental disabilities was that individual municipalities could use zoning restrictions as a mechanism of prohibiting or preventing the placement of group homes within their boundaries. The Constitution (1970) did not provide for fair housing rights for persons with disabilities. As mentioned previously, many interview respondents indicated that towns frequently used their zoning laws as a means of opposing group home development.

Structure of the Legislature

In 1980, the Illinois Constitution was amended again in ways that, while dramatic for the structure of state government, would have a more subtle impact on the residential service system. Prior to the 1980 "Cutback Amendment" to the Constitution, the House of Representatives comprised 177 members. House districts each had three representatives, and each voter could allocate three votes in one of these ways: one vote each to three separate candidates, one and one half votes each to two candidates, or the "bullet" -- three votes to a single candidate. Voters could thus split their votes as they chose. Under this system, voting was cumulative, and the top three vote-getting candidates won in each district (Gove & Nowlan, 1996; Redfield, 1998). Minority party representation was assured, because parties generally fielded no more than two candidates per district. Cumulative voting resulted in a party minority representative from each district, even in traditional bastions of Democratic or Republican strength, and less partisanship (Nowlan & Gonet, 1991).

These minority party representatives often had perspectives that were quite different from the straight Democratic or Republican Party view. Since only a small proportion of their district's votes were necessary for re-election, they did not owe allegiance to the state party or even to much of their constituency. This resulted in a subset of the House that had a considerable amount of independence (Nowlan & Gonet, 1991; Redfield, 1998).

When the Constitution was changed with the Cutback Amendment in 1980, the number of representatives was reduced from 177 to 118 and cumulative voting was eliminated. This ended the system of each voter having three votes, and established new House districts with a single representative in each one. This change, of course, eliminated the minority party

representatives who had been elected under the old system (Gove & Nowlan, 1996). To understand the implications of this Constitutional change on the state's developmental disabilities residential system, it is important to first explicate the state's campaign finance system.

Campaign Finance and the Consolidation of Legislative Power

Illinois, like much of the nation following the aftermath of the Watergate scandal, enacted a campaign finance law (Pub. Act 78-1183 of 1974). However, Illinois campaign finance laws, as enacted in 1974, have remained essentially unchanged and are among the weakest in the nation from the standpoint of promoting participatory government (Palmer & Feigenbaum, 1990; Redfield, 1998).

In Illinois, the only campaign finance requirement is for full disclosure of contribution amounts, donors, and recipients. Contributors are therefore allowed under Illinois law to give any amount of money and must just submit a report declaring the amount and to whom they have made a political contribution (Palmer & Feigenbaum, 1990; Pub. Act 78-1183 of 1974).

Also note that the legislative staff in both the House and the Senate in Illinois do not report to individual legislators but to the party leadership. Democratic staffers working with legislators on the House Committee on Mental Health, for example, report to the speaker of the House or the minority leader, depending on which party is in control. During campaign season, these legislative staffers go on leave from their state jobs and become operatives in hotly contested electoral campaigns, at the behest of the party leadership (Redfield, 1998).

What has developed as a result of this system is a cadre of highly trained and experienced campaign workers who are led not by the individuals whose campaigns they run, but by the party leadership in both chambers. In addition, electoral races often receive campaign funds from the party leadership. Because there are no limits on the amount that can be given, the party leadership in each chamber has the ability to withdraw support for a campaign that is failing or infuse additional resources to a campaign that looks like it will be competitive when initially it was not. Legislators who are elected with the resources, both personnel and financial, of the party leadership are compelled to follow the leadership if they want to secure these resources for the next campaign.

The combination of the reduction in the number of representatives in the House, unlimited campaign contributions, and the control of legislative staff have resulted in a nearly complete consolidation of power among the speaker of the House, the Senate president, and the minority party leaders in both chambers (Redfield, 1998). This consolidated power, where the leadership controls a vast campaign treasury, results in many legislators owing their offices to the party leadership. It is therefore not hard to see how their independence is compromised. One political scientist has characterized this as "dancin' with the guy that brung ya" (Redfield, 1998, p. 8).

Political contributors can develop the clout to ensure their continued participation in public policy decision making, if the resources that they provide are sufficient. In Illinois, the level of campaign financing is extraordinarily high, because of laws which do not limit or restrict financing in any way. The amount of money it takes to get elected in competitive races has escalated and has exceeded $1 million in several of the most recent competitive state House races (Redfield, 1998). The high stakes for campaigns in Illinois effectively exclude from participation those individuals, like people with developmental disabilities, who lack sufficient resources to influence the service system. Influence with legislators has, however, been obtained by individuals who are service providers. The nursing home industry has been a significant contributor to Illinois campaigns (Redfield, 1994).

Another political aspect critical for people with developmental disabilities is that this type of a system tends to enforce the retention of the status quo. There is little incentive in Illinois for the elected leadership to seek innovation or to make major changes because the status quo, whereby nursing home and private ICF/MR operators contribute campaign funds, tends to be supported. The legislative powers are less likely to experiment in this system, and this has contributed to the service system in Illinois still being one of the most institutional in the country.

The Emergence of AFSCME as a Political Power

Other aspects of politics that have been important to developmental disabilities policy are worthy of brief mention as well. In the Democratic primary race for governor in 1971, Paul Simon, the choice of the Chicago political machine, was defeated by Dan Walker. In an effort to court political support, Walker sought the endorsement of the American Federation of State, County, and Municipal Employees (AFSCME), which was one of the largest unions in the nation (Derber, 1989). Candidate Walker pledged his support to their issues if he was elected. In the fall gubernatorial election, Governor Ogilvie, who had initiated the state's first income tax in 1969, was ousted by Walker (Derber, 1989).

Walker's election is important for our purposes because his support of AFSCME led him to endorse union organizing by state workers. In 1972, at the new governor's request, legislation was introduced to give state workers the right to seek union representation; it was subsequently defeated. The following year, the governor issued Executive Order 6, which by fiat allowed state workers to seek union representation (Derber, 1989). This led to the establishment of AFSCME as an important political power in the State. By 1973, AFSCME had launched a major membership drive resulting in the addition of 2,500 new members by September of the same year. AFSCME later went on to win the right to represent corrections workers and defeated the Illinois State Employee Association in the fight to determine which would represent the state's 12,000 institutional employees (Derber, 1989).

AFSCME's organizing had a profound impact on the residential service system for people with developmental disabilities because over the years, it has become an entity with considerable political clout in the State. AFSCME's support of keeping institutions open was identified by many interview respondents as a critical factor in the slow development of community-based residences. AFSCME has had continued participation in different task forces and committees (e.g., Governor's Task Force on the Future of Mental

Health in Illinois, 1987) that influence policy in the State.

Political Patronage

A final aspect of Illinois politics, patronage, has also been important to the evolution of residential services for people with developmental disabilities. Under Governor Thompson, who defeated Governor Walker and took office in 1977, political patronage reached its apex in Illinois. Political patronage was a long-standing tradition in the State, whereby many jobs were filled on the basis of political party loyalty and service.

However, Governor Thompson took this practice to new heights. By issuing Executive Order 5 in 1980, Governor Thompson instituted a comprehensive hiring freeze on all state jobs under his authority. Affecting approximately 60,000 positions, the order prohibited any hiring without the governor's express permission. In this way, the patronage system was extended to all state jobs under the control of the governor (*Rutan v. Republican Party of Illinois*, 1989). One interview respondent confirmed that after the governor's executive order was issued, the local Republican Party was required to approve a job applicant before the governor's office would consider the person for employment.

The implications for persons with developmental disabilities are clear. The state's public institutions, with their large contingents of staff, including direct service workers and crafts- and trades-people, became an important part of the web of patronage jobs in the State. Individual legislators who had facilities in their districts would often have impact on who could get a job within a facility. The facility's operations were directly linked, not to the provision of service, but to political considerations.

In 1989, the U.S. Supreme Court ruled that Governor Thompson's patronage practices were unconstitutional. To condition all state jobs on party affiliation was a violation of the First Amendment. Justice Brennan, writing for the majority, stated,

To the victor belong only those spoils that

may be constitutionally obtained…Today we are asked to decide the constitutionality of several related political patronage practices -- whether promotion, transfer, recall, and hiring decisions involving low-level public employees may be constitutionally based on party affiliation and support. We hold that they may not. (Brennan in *Rutan v. Republican Party of Illinois,* 1989, pp. 64-65)

This case had been brought by five civil service employees, who alleged that the governor's practices were a violation of their First Amendment rights. The federal district court in which the case was initially filed dismissed the case. The Seventh Circuit Court of Appeals, to which the civil service employees appealed, reversed the district court's dismissal, but stated that patronage was only inappropriate in these situations if the employment was actually terminated. The Supreme Court held that any employment action (hiring, transfer, promotion) that occurred within the patronage system could be construed as a violation of the First Amendment, if there was no "legitimate" reason for the position to be politically appointed. Since the Supreme Court's decision was not issued until October 1989, for nearly the entirety of the 1970-90 study period, patronage was an important factor in the state's operations, and particularly during Governor Thompson's administration (1976-1991).

Several interview respondents related that in the state institutions, while positions like psychologists or social workers were difficult to fill through the patronage system, nearly all other positions were filled as political appointments. Institutions became ways of rewarding the faithful for their support of a legislator or other elected official. In the community services sector, the development of group homes did not offer the opportunity for patronage jobs as they existed within the institutions. Whereas institutions offered literally dozens of opportunities for political supporters to be rewarded, community residential services represented no prize for legislators and elected officials. Institutions have been an integral part of the politics, which is another factor that has facilitated the state's retention of its institutional service system.

Politics and Developmental Disabilities: Conclusions

When asked why community-based services have not developed quickly in the State, one lobbyist flatly stated, "In Illinois, the people who have political clout bring to the table either grass roots voting power or money. Community services advocates have never done either." People with developmental disabilities and their families have often not been organized or powerful enough to have the kind of influence in the service system that other groups like the unions have exercised.

Finally, the political climate in Illinois is best understood as one that is quite conservative, not ideologically, but in the sense that the State is resistant to change and this resistance can be traced directly to its political underpinnings. The consolidation of power in the legislature at the level of the four leaders and the governor ensure a system a that is resistant to changing the status quo.

Federal Influences

During the 1970-90 study period, the most significant federal action to influence the shape of Illinois' residential service system was the authorization in 1971 of the ICF/MR program, which was created as an amendment to Title XIX of the Social Security Act. This law allowed states to receive federal Medicaid reimbursement for residential programs that met federal ICF/MR regulations (Pub. L. 92-233 of 1971). The ICF/MR program offered states the opportunity to reap major financial gains from the federal government and literally was the source of new money into service systems across the country. Illinois' financial gains from this program were considerable, totaling $61 million in 1980 alone (Braddock, Hemp, Parish, & Westrich, 1998). *Figure 3.9* depicts the annual level of federal ICF/MR funding that the State received from 1977-90, in inflation-adjusted terms. The figure also includes all other sources of funding for developmental disabilities services, in order to represent the relative importance of federal ICF/MR revenues to the state's total budget. Although the ICF/MR program began in 1974, reliable data on federal reimbursement to the State could not be found for years prior to 1977. Federal ICF/MR funds clearly were a significant portion of the state's revenues for developmental disabilities services. In 1977, federal ICF/MR funds totaled $8.3 million, and grew to $163.6 million by 1990, representing more than one fifth of the state's total DD services budget.

The impact of the ICF/MR legislation was two-fold in Illinois. To meet federal ICF/MR regulations in its public institutions and thereby receive the 50% re-

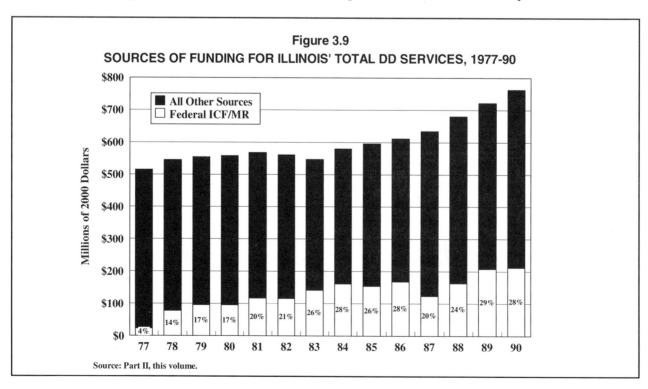

imbursement to which the State was entitled, it was necessary to downsize and improve the state's public institutions. The State poured millions of dollars into renovations aimed at improving the public institutions. Simultaneously, the facilities were compelled to accelerate their depopulation programs. This depopulation was necessary in order to meet both the minimum staffing ratios and minimum square footage requirements prescribed by the federal regulations. Extensive renovations were made to the state's developmental disabilities institutions, and to psychiatric hospitals in which developmental disabilities units were converted to ICFs/MR. Depopulation of the state's institutions therefore continued the practice of transferring residents to state psychiatric hospitals (DMHDD, 1984).

The second important implication of Illinois' participation in the ICF/MR program was the proliferation of privately operated ICFs/MR. As described previously by an interview respondent, Illinois immediately began converting existing sheltered care and nursing homes into ICFs/DD if the facility operators were willing to do so. These conversions enabled the State to obtain federal reimbursement for the services. The incentive to the providers was to boost their reimbursement rates, which were increased if they converted their facilities to ICFs/DD. The transitions in licensure that were occurring continued into the 1980s. In 1981 for instance, a number of new ICFs/DD for 15 per-

sons opened and several existing community living facilities and sheltered care facilities were converted to ICFs/DD. The early 1980s also represented a time when considerable growth of larger ICFs/DD occurred. In 1981, the Health Facilities Planning Board (1982) issued permits to construct new ICFs/DD for 35, 41, 45, and 50 persons, as well as an array of facilities for 90 to 100 people. The planned construction of large-scale private institutions was well underway in the State by the early 1980s, and these facilities would soon constitute a large portion of the state's residential service system (Health Facilities Planning Board, 1982, 1985).

The influence the federal government exhibited on Illinois' residential service system is also evident in its enforcement of the ICF/MR standards. As was discussed previously, in the mid-1980s there were ICF/MR compliance problems across Illinois in both public and private facilities. These compliance problems ultimately led to the loss of millions of dollars of federal ICF/MR revenues to the State.

Another major source of federal funds was authorized in 1981, when Congress amended the Social Security Act and allowed states to obtain federal Medicaid funds through the Home and Community Based Services (HCBS) Waiver (Pub. L. 97-35 of 1981). To obtain this funding, states had to submit Waiver applications to the HCFA and meet an array or re-

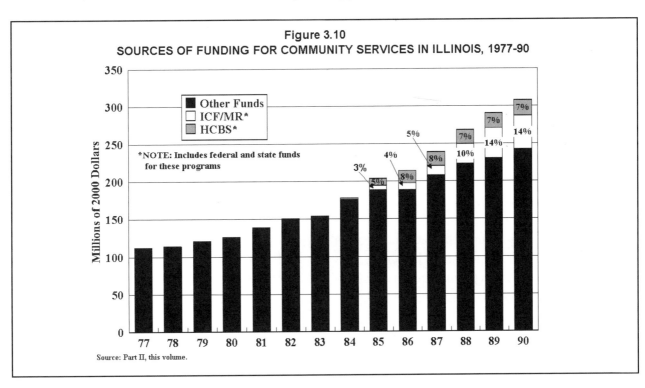

Figure 3.10
SOURCES OF FUNDING FOR COMMUNITY SERVICES IN ILLINOIS, 1977-90

Source: Part II, this volume.

quirements, including the stipulation that use of HCBS would be less costly than institutional services. The Waiver provided federal funding with a 50% state match for an array of services provided in the community including residential services, day programs and others (Braddock, Hemp, Parish, Westrich, & Park, 1998; Smith & Gettings, 1993).

Illinois was a relatively early entrant into the HCBS Waiver program. Its Waiver was approved to begin in November 1983, among the first states to receive Waiver approval. Illinois' Waiver application was initially approved for 770 residents with an expansion to 1,497 individuals by the third year. As mentioned previously, however, Illinois' use of the Waiver during the 1980s was quite limited. While federal ICF/MR funds to the State totaled $163.6 million by 1990, federal Waiver reimbursement to the State totaled just $7.9 million that year. *Figure 3.10* shows the levels of combined state-federal HCBS Waiver, ICF/MR, and other funds for Illinois' community-based services spending from 1977-90. Community-based services here include day and employment programs, case management, residential programs in settings for 15 or fewers person, and family support services.

Public Officials and Bureaucratic Leadership

The Governors

During the 1970-90 study period considered by this investigation, Illinois was led by three Governors, Richard Ogilvie (1969-73), Dan Walker (1973-77), and James Thompson (1977-91). This section will consider the role that each of these three men played with respect to the development of residential services for persons with developmental disabilities.

Governor Ogilvie's main impact on Illinois' residential service system for people with developmental disabilities came in the form of construction of new public institutions begun during his tenure. Although authorized in the 1960s, the Howe, Ludeman, and Waukegan Developmental Centers began construction during Governor Ogilvie's administration. There really was no growth in community-based residential services for people with developmental disabilities under Governor Ogilvie. Mrs. Ogilvie worked closely

with the Illinois ARC on a number of advocacy issues related to developmental disabilities and was honored by the organization. She was particularly interested in raising public awareness about developmental disabilities, but there were not many other developments under Governor Ogilvie.

Governor Walker had an impact on the residential service system in this state in several ways. By running as a maverick who courted union support to gain office, Walker supported establishing unions as collective bargaining representatives for state workers. His issuance in 1973 of Executive Order 6 gave state workers the right to seek union representation and subsequently led to the establishment of AFSCME as their representative (Derber, 1989). This began the building of a political base of power that continued throughout the 1970-90 period (Redfield, 1994).

As discussed previously, the relevance of the growth of AFSCME for people with developmental disabilities is that AFSCME represents state institutional worker. The union has actively and aggressively opposed the downsizing and closure of the state's public institutions, due to its interest in protecting union jobs in such facilities. Nearly every interview respondent in Illinois indicated that AFSCME's opposition to the downsizing of institutions has been important in maintaining them.

The other main impact that Governor Walker had on Illinois' residential service system was the construction of a number of specialized living centers across the State. These six facilities were designed for between 100 and 150 people per facility, and were part of the governor's accelerated building plan. This plan was intended to stimulate the state's economy. This program was announced in January 1975 during what the governor termed the state's worst recession since World War II (Walker, 1975). A number of respondents indicated that the governor had no particular interest in services for people with developmental disabilities and his building plan was just part of an economic package and was political in nature.

The siting of these facilities across Illinois was somewhat controversial and several respondents have suggested that facilities were constructed in areas where the governor needed to gain support from local legislators. Important for our purposes and understanding the evolution of the state's residential service system is the fact that this program represented a major infusion of state funds into the construction of facilities which were later turned over to the facility operators. The construction of the specialized living centers suggests that when it was politically expedient, money could be allocated to developmental disabilities services.

The third and final governor to lead Illinois during the 1970-90 study period was James Thompson. Governor Thompson's leadership had many implications for the residential service system in the State. As discussed previously, Governor Thompson enhanced the political patronage sy stem,which resulted in the hiring of workers at state institutions on the basis of their political service, and not necessarily due to their qualifications. The U.S. Supreme Court's patronage decision, issued in 1989 (*Rutan v. Republican Party of Illinois*, 1989), largely ended this practice, but for the majority of the time examined by this investigation, it must be understood that patronage was an important aspect of the service system.

Governor Thompson's administration also impacted the prison system. In 1977, Governor Thompson signed mandatory sentencing laws that created "Class X" felonies. This law established much stricter penalties for a set of crimes, and generally increased sentencing length (Pub. Act 80-1099). This law was passed as part of Thompson's follow-through on campaign promises during the gubernatorial race ("Class X Passes," 1978). The foundation for constructing new prisons was effectively laid with the passage of this law. When Thompson took office, there were nine state prisons. During his tenure, 10 new prisons were constructed.

The relationship of tougher sentencing laws and prison construction to the developmental disabilities service system is not precisely clear. However, under Governor Thompson, a number of state psychiatric hospitals and two developmental centers were closed and subsequently converted to prisons. Interview respondents generally concurred that there was a need for these facilities to close anyway. The psychiatric hospitals and the Dixon and Bowen Developmental Centers which were closed under Governor Thompson all were facilities in need of extensive renovations, and would have cost the State considerable sums to renovate. It is most likely that the governor and his

staff identified closing these facilities as a potential cost saving for the State and then seized upon the opportunity to convert them to prisons also in order to further save money. There is no evidence that the facilities were closed specifically to make way for the prisons. What is clear, though, is that these developmental disabilities institutions were not closed because of a philosophical commitment to the developmen of community-based residential services. In fact, the closure of the Dixon Developmental Center in 1982 did not result in the creation of any community-based residential program; all of the more than 800 Dixon residents living at the facility when the closure was announced were subsequently transferred to different institutions around the State.

In February 1982, six days after Governor Thompson announced the impending facility's closure, the Illinois State Court issued a temporary restraining order barring DMHDD from taking any further action to close the facility. The Dixon Association for Retarded Citizens had filed a lawsuit to stop the closure. The Illinois State Supreme Court eventually decided in favor of the governor, upholding his right to close that facility (*Dixon Association for Retarded Citizens et al. v. Thompson,* 1982). However, many respondents indicated that the governor did make a concession to some of the families. He agreed to construct a new institution on the grounds of Dixon for 100 individuals with deafness, blindness, and mental retardation. This facility was subsequently opened as the Mabley Developmental Center (DMHDD, 1983).

Another important aspect of Governor Thompson's leadership was his focus on cutting the costs of government. In 1977, he developed a Cost Control Task Force which was directed to find ways to improve government efficiency and cut the operating costs of government. The Task Force reported in July 1978 that there was $500 million in waste in state government (Illinois Commission on Intergovernmental Cooperation, 1979).

Not surprisingly, the media picked up on the report and gave it a good deal of attention. The report's recommendations relative to DMHDD was quite scathing. It indicated numerous administrative flaws and lack of leadership, and it issued recommendations that the DMHDD consolidate services in some areas, develop staff-to-patient ratios that were more cost effective, seek greater federal funds under Title XX of the Social Security Act, improve its recovery of Medicaid funding, and seek additional Medicare funding.

In response to the release of this report, a number of legislators were concerned with the Task Force's findings and recommendations, particularly regarding human service programs. As a result of the concern expressed by a number of legislators, the Illinois Commission on Intergovernmental Cooperation (1979) conducted an analysis of the Cost Control Task Force's report and findings and found that the Task Force was insufficiently informed about federal regulations relating to the DMHDD's program. In spite of the Commission's findings of many flaws in the Task Force report, it is clear that damage had been done by the media to the DMHDD's credibility. Furthermore, a number of editorials that deplored the waste and problems in state government certainly could not have been helpful to advocates interested in expanding the DMHDD's budget for developmental disabilities services.

Another example of Governor Thompson's interest in cost-cutting occurred in 1979, when the Purchase Care Review Board proposed a $35-a-day rate for the newly built specialized living centers. DMHDD, the IARC, and the Governor's Planning Council on Developmental Disabilities wanted the rate to be set at $47.50 a day, which was felt to more accurately represent the costs of serving the residents. This group appealed the Purchase Care Board's decision to the governor, but he upheld the Board's $35 daily rate. This level of reimbursement was widely considered to be below a rate that would allow for a decent standard of care in these facilities (Illinois Association for Retarded Citizens, 1979; Ramirez, 1979).

Later in the governor's term, the DMHDD was targeted for budget cuts. These were proposed in 1983 during the nation's recession. In response to this, the ARC held a rally in Springfield to protest the cuts (Illinois Association for Retarded Citizens, 1983), but the rally was to no avail and the governor's cuts took effect (DMHDD, 1984). One other aspect of the governor's interest in cutting the costs of government as related to the DMHDD was the appointment of Michael Belletire, the Department's first nonpsychiatrist director. Belletire was widely regarded to be a cost-

cutter who had limited understanding or knowledge of mental health or developmental disabilities services. Many interview respondents agreed that his main priorities for the DMHDD had been related to saving the State money, and he was regarded to have been particularly ineffective in establishing a service system that was responsive to the needs of the individuals being cared for.

Most interview respondents concurred that Governor Thompson's leadership resulted in poor outcomes for individuals with developmental disabilities and their families. Expansion of the community residential services program was minimal during his administration and funds to the DMHDD were barely able to maintain ICF/MR certification in many facilities (DMHDD, 1983, 1985).

The clear conclusion drawn from an analysis of the impact of these three governors on the state's developmental disabilities services is that none deemed persons with developmental disabilities to be a high priority. None provided leadership to DMHDD. And none was a champion of mental health issues or the needs of individuals with developmental disabilities.

The Legislature

The General Assembly in Illinois had two primary roles: (a) to pass legislation and send it to the governor for signature, and (b) to fulfill its watchdog function, wherein it provided oversight of state programs and investigated issues brought to its attention. These two roles will be discussed in this section, beginning with an overview of legislation or resolutions passed during the 1970-90 study period.

In response to the Developmental Disabilities Act passed by Congress in 1970, the Illinois House of Representatives passed Resolution 568 (Illinois House of Representatives, 1972). This resolution created a special House Developmental Disabilities Study Committee authorized to investigate the service system in Illinois and report on the ways in which services should be organized in order to be responsive to the requirements of the Developmental Disabilities Act. The following year the Study Committee issued its report, with strong criticisms for the Department of Mental Health and its practices. The Committee particularly argued for a complete review of the Department's plan to construct new developmental disabilities institutions. Having evaluated families' needs, the Study Committee found that most families were not interested in institutional care. The Study Committee strongly recommended a complete review and assessment of the construction plans with an eye toward providing services that were more aligned with those needs expressed by families (Developmental Disabilities Study Committee of the House of Representatives, 1973).

The impact that the Study Committee had on the Department of Mental Health and its practices is not clear, however. In the 1960s, legislation had been passed authorizing the construction of seven new developmental disabilities institutions around the Chicago area (Commission on Mental Health, 1969). By the time that the Study Committee issued its 1973 report, Ludeman Developmental Center, the first of the planned facilities, had opened. Construction was also under way for the Howe and Waukegan Developmental Centers (DMHDD, 1974).

The remaining four facilities were never constructed. Instead, the Kankakee State Psychiatric Hospital became a Developmental Center, later named Shapiro, and the Jacksonville Mental Health and Developmental Center also was eventually converted to serve only persons with developmental disabilities (Illinois Department of Mental Health, 1973b). Funds were never appropriated for the construction of the remaining four facilities, but it is unclear as to whether or not this was related to the Study Committee's report or just the ongoing lack of resources allocated for developmental disabilities services in Illinois.

In 1972, the General Assembly amended the Mental Health Code and required the Department of Mental Health to report on the accreditation and certification status of all of its public institutions. These reports were to be submitted annually to the governor and the General Assembly (Pub. Act 77-2722). In 1974, the Illinois Health Facilities Planning Board was established, which was authorized to control Illinois' Certificate of Need program. States across the country were implementing Certificate of Need systems whereby any renovation or new construction of health facilities was controlled by a single entity (Pub. Act 78-1156 of 1974). In Illinois this became the responsibility of the Health Facility's Planning Board and included in its authority was authorization for ICFs/MR.

In 1974, the legislature voted down a bill introduced at Governor Walker's behest that would have established specialized community living facilities. This bill ultimately succeeded in the legislature after being pushed by Governor Walker the next year. The authorization of six specialized living centers was part of the governor's economic stimulus program designed to combat the recession Illinois was experiencing at this time (Walker, 1975).

The Mental Health Code was amended in 1976, when action was taken to bring financial relief to families of children with developmental disabilities who needed services in a departmental or private facility. It established a schedule of fees for residential care and parents thereafter were expected to pay the same amount regardless of whether the child was placed in a public or private facility. The maximum responsibility that parents would bear for the cost of their children's care was $100 per month (Pub. Act 79-967 of 1976).

That same year the House defeated House Bill 281, a measure which would have introduced prohibitions against restrictive zoning. This bill was strongly supported by the IARC. The defeat of the bill was orchestrated by the municipalities' lobby (Breslin et al., 1980).

Legislation was also passed periodically to provide greater direction to DMHDD, particularly related to the provision of more comprehensive and coordinated leadership. In 1981, the first of these types of laws was passed, the Community Services Act. The DMHDD was directed to take steps to strengthen its services and to facilitate the independence, self-esteem, and ability to participate in and contribute to community life of individuals with mental illness, developmental disabilities, and alcohol dependence (Pub. Act 82-183). This law was intended to prevent unnecessary institutionalization and ensure that individuals had access to services that were commensurate with their individual wishes and needs. In spite of this law's passage in 1981, a great deal of growth occurred in large-scale ICFs/MR and the DMHDD's long-standing program of placing individuals with developmental disabilities in nursing homes continued (Health Facilities Planning Board, 1982, 1985). Legislation intent on directing the goals of the DMHDD was also passed in 1983, when they were mandated to establish a consistent case coordination system with the goal of meeting the full range of a service recipient's needs (Pub. Act 83-88 of 1983). The timing of this act also seems ironic, as it coincided with budget cuts to DMHDD.

In 1985, Pub. Act 84-567 directed the Governor's Planning Council on Developmental Disabilities to develop a state plan to address the needs of the population that was "aging out." Aging out is the name commonly given to individuals who are graduating or leaving the public high schools because they have reached the age at which mandatory special education is no longer required. This law again opened the door for more comprehensive planning and expressed a clear philosophical direction of meeting individuals' needs.

The General Assembly also periodically codified the existence of new residential settings. The first of these was the 1975 authorization of Governor Walker's funding of specialized living centers. The law authorized $15 million in construction funds for these new privately operated facilities, intended to serve 100 to 150 people per facility (Walker, 1976).

In the 1980s, a number of new residential programs were authorized by the legislature as well. The Community Facilities Licensing Act (Pub. Act 82-567) was passed in 1981 and authorized the Department of Public Health to develop standards and license community living facilities, which had been a part of the DMHDD network of community-based residential alternatives to institutions since 1970 (Committee on Mental Retardation, 1971a; Illinois Department of Mental Health, 1972). Passage of this law was intended to compel these facilities to conform to licensing standards and provide oversight to the services they provided. The same year, the Community Residential Alternative Licensing Act authorized the development of licensing regulations and monitoring of Community Residential Alternatives (Pub. Act 82-584). These facilities were group homes for eight or fewer individuals and were to be licensed by DMHDD. By the end of the year, eight homes with a total of 47 residents had been licensed.

In 1988, the legislature authorized community integrated living arrangements (CILA), again delineating licensing and monitoring requirements for this new service type. Much of this legislation was spearheaded or co-authored by Lee Daniels who is the current Republican minority leader in the Illinois House of Representatives and has served as speaker of the House when the Republicans were in power. In addition to being in the House of Representatives, Daniels is the parent of a person with a developmental disability. A number of interview respondents indicated that his leadership was critical in passing some of this legislation, and particularly the family support subsidy laws enacted in 1989. One interview respondent also indicated that Daniels has consistently worked to ensure that funding levels were either not cut as much as was proposed or that they remained stable. Other respondents felt that no legislator has been a true champion of aggressively developing community-based residential services in the State.

In its watchdog role, the legislature frequently reacted to scandals brought to light by the media, as discussed previously. A number of reports were generated by legislative committees comprising legislators or chaired by legislators including the Illinois Legislative Investigating Commission (1977, 1980), the Charitable Subcommittee of the Legislative Commission to Visit and Examine State Institutions (1972, 1974), and the Citizens Council on Mental Health and Developmental Disabilities (1986, 1987). A number of these different commissions were involved in investigating allegations of abuse and neglect, charges of fraud in privately operated facilities, questionable care practices, and the failure of Illinois ICFs/MR to maintain their certification status, and an array of different issues related to the administration of both public and private facilities for people with developmental disabilities.

Ad hoc committees were created as needed to investigate and evaluate different situations as they arose as well. One example was the House Developmental Disabilities Study Committee (1973) which was created in 1972, as discussed previously, in reaction to federal legislation.

In spite of the presence and activities of these committees, it is often difficult to see substantive changes that resulted in policy due to their oversight. As noted previously, scandals, and their aftermath have generally not catalyzed far-reaching changes in the state's residential service system for persons with developmental disabilities.

The Department of Mental Health and Developmental Disabilities

During the 1970-90 study, period there were many directors of the DMH and subsequently DMHDD. One of the most unfortunate findings of this study is how unsuccessful these seven directors were in advancing the community-based residential service system for people with developmental disabilities. The first four Department directors in the study period were Albert Glass, Leroy Leavitt, Robert DeVito, and Ivan Pavkovic, all of whom were psychiatrists. Michael Belletire was the first non-psychiatrist to head the Department, and by most accounts, he was appointed to the position largely as a cost-cutter by Governor Thompson. Belletire was followed by Ann Kiley and Bill Murphy.

There was tremendous consistency among interview respondents in their assessment of the leadership provided by these different directors. Interview respondents agreed that Leroy Leavitt had offered the DMHDD a strong administration and a professional way of operating the services under his charge. Interview respondents also were consistent in their assessment of Kiley's leadership. Interview respondents all stated that she had attempted to expand community-based services for persons with developmental disabilities, noting the establishment of the CILA program under her leadership. However, she attempted to close three mental health and developmental disabilities research centers at the University of Chicago at Illinois in 1986. Her tenure as director was cut short because of her death from cancer, and she was not able to implement many of the objectives that she had set for the administration.

Most interview respondents, however, felt that the DMHDD's other directors lacked vision or the ability to implement serious change in the state's system. There was some agreement among interview respondents that the reasons for directors' inability to make needed changes had more to do with Illinois' political structure and a lack of leadership from the governors.

A number of interview respondents did feel that Richard Blanton, who had been the deputy director for Developmental Disabilities from 1974-82 (DMH,1973; DMHDD, 1983), had been helpful in facilitating some of the community development that occurred during this time.

It is important to note here that it is difficult to convincingly evaluate the leadership provided by the DMHDD, given that the documentary evidence, particularly from the 1970s, is not as complete as could be hoped. In addition, many of the leaders from this time are deceased and obviously cannot share their own perspectives about what they were able to achieve. In the final analysis, there is clear and convincing evidence that the DMHDD did not offer opportunities for innovation that might have expanded the community-based residential service system.

Advocacy Groups

Advocacy efforts on behalf of persons with developmental disabilities largely came from four groups during the 1970-90 study period. The first was the Association for Retarded Citizens, which has historically been the largest advocacy organization of parents of individuals with developmental disabilities. The second advocate group in Illinois has been Voice of the Retarded, which organized families of institutional residents. A third advocacy organization, People First, is composed of individuals with developmental disabilities, which began in Illinois in 1990. A final group has advocated for services, but is primarily a trade organization lobbying on behalf of service providers: the Illinois Association of Rehabilitation Facilities (IARF).

One of the most important findings of this study is the lack of leadership provided by the IARC in championing the growth and development of community-based residential services for people with developmental disabilities. This lack of leadership during the 1970s and 1980s was related to the division in the organization between parents of children living at home and parents of institutionalized children. The lack of leadership was also related to the ARC's role representing both service providers and families (Illinois Association for Retarded Citizens, 1973; Association for Retarded Citizens of Illinois, 1985, 1986, 1987, 1988).

Prior to 1970, the Illinois Association for the Mentally Retarded (later the Association for Retarded Citizens) was recognized as the most important advocacy organization committed to obtaining services for individuals with developmental disabilities and their families (Commission on Mental Health, 1969; Illinois Department of Mental Health, 1966). In the 1960s, the ARC was largely involved with advocating for the development of community services in the State. However, community services developed in the 1960s were generally sheltered workshops and adult daycare, and did not include family-scale residential alternatives to the public institutions (Commission on Mental Health, 1969; Illinois Association for the Mentally Retarded, 1968).

In addition to seeking an expansion of workshops, schools, education, and daycare programs, the ARC pursued improvement of state institutional conditions. Specifically, the ARC sought an expansion of funding for institutions with a particular emphasis on increasing staffing levels in these facilities (Illinois Association for the Mentally Retarded, 1965, 1968; Illinois Council for Mentally Retarded Children, 1966; Illinois Department of Mental Health, 1971). Another priority of the ARC during this period was its focus on the prevention of mental retardation. This advocacy led to passage of mandatory screening of newborns for phenylketonuria (PKU), a metabolic disorder.

The ARC maintained a committee that periodically visited the state's public institutions and reported its findings to the Department of Mental Health. As the Department of Mental Health developed units within its existing psychiatric hospitals for people with developmental disabilities, the Association for Retarded Citizens sought to organize local ARC chapters for the parents of these individuals.

In the 1960s, as the Department of Mental Health began funding community services, local chapters of the ARC became service providers, often operating sheltered workshops and day programs themselves (Illinois Department of Mental Health, 1969). While it was the mission statement of the National Association of Retarded Citizens that local ARC chapters should obtain and not provide services (Illinois Council for Mentally Retarded Children, 1966), in Illinois, local ARCs became prominent service providers across the State. This direction had a profound impact on the organization in the coming decades.

A number of interview respondents revealed other major issues that emerged during the 1970s. In some cases there was considerable hostility between the parents of individuals who had been institutionalized and the parents of individuals who continued to live at home. A schism occurred in the ARC, and it was a rift that endured for decades. Parents of children who lived at home were interested in obtaining community-based residential services and were often not interested in using the state's institutional system. In many instances, they were horrified by the conditions they had seen there. Parents of individuals living in institutions were often made to feel guilty for having sought out-of-home residential placement for their children, and they sometimes objected to any effort that would have taken money from institutional services and redirected it toward the community.

As a result of these two important issues, the ARC in the 1970s and the 1980s was forced to bridge two difficult situations. Its commitment to advocating for the needs of parents and children with developmental disabilities was pitted against its role as a trade association for local units that were service providers. Inasmuch as the ARC's operating budget was derived from revenue received by local service provider chapters, the ARC pursued a path of advocacy that often involved supporting the needs of service providers. Many respondents indicated that when the ARC abandoned its fundamental commitment to individuals with developmental disabilities and their families, because it had to support service providers, it lost credibility among politicians and began to be perceived as a trade association, agitating for issues like the expansion of reimbursement rates paid to service providers.

This has been a contentious issue and interview respondents were divided in their assessments. Many strenuously objected to the notion that the ARC had a divided allegiance or that it was ineffective in its advocacy because of its representation of service providers. What is clear, however, is that the agenda that the ARC pursued did not result in serious change in the state's residential service system. The vast majority of interview respondents felt that the ARC's lack of leadership in Illinois was a primary and critical reason that the State was allowed to develop or not develop community-based residential services as it saw fit.

In many other states, ARCs have been the plaintiffs in federal class-action litigation, which sought to improve or oppose public institutions. Certainly the

Pennhurst case in Pennsylvania, Willowbrook in New York, and the Plymouth case in Michigan exemplify ARC organizations filing lawsuits that catalyzed changes in the state's service system. In Illinois, the ARC has been involved in two class-action cases. The first case, *Phillips v. Thompson,* is not well known. It was filed on behalf of the men and women who were transferred back to state institutions when the North Aurora Center closed precipitously in 1979. The ARC supported the plaintiffs in this case, which was demanding community residential placement for individuals who at one point had lived in the North Aurora Center, a privately operated institution for approximately 500 individuals. When this facility closed, all of the individuals were transferred to public institutions.

This case was dismissed after a trial before District Court, and upon appeal the judges ruled in favor of the State. Their ruling was based on the U.S. Supreme Court's *Youngberg* decision, which did not require states to provide particular types of services. The Court stated that the individuals who had been living at the North Aurora Center were voluntarily in the public institutions and did not have a right to community residential placement. *Youngberg* was the U.S. Supreme Court's decision related to the Pennhurst institution in Pennsylvania.

The second class-action lawsuit was filed by the IARC in 1988, and became known as the *Bogard* lawsuit, on behalf of 3,200 persons with developmental disabilities living in nursing homes in the State. The Public Interest Law Center of Philadelphia (PILCOP) was the attorney for the plaintiffs. By this time, PILCOP had represented plaintiffs in federal class-action institutional lawsuits in a number of states around the country.

The consent decree that was negotiated in the case allowed nursing home patients to choose where they wanted to live or to have that choice made by their guardians. *Bogard* eventually resulted in the community placement of approximately 1,300 individuals with developmental disabilities previously living in nursing homes (T. Paulaski, personal communication, August 2001). A considerable number of class members stayed in the nursing homes. The *Bogard* case was narrowly construed as representing only the class of individuals with developmental disabilities who were residing in nursing homes and as such did not have

major implications for the state's public institutional services. However, the creation of these community residential placements was an important achievement in a state that had fewer than 4,000 when the case was filed in 1988 (Braddock, Hemp, Parish, & Westrich, 1998).

The main impact of the case has been that it resulted in an expansion of financial resources, as the State was compelled to meet the dictates of the consent decree, which then created some community-based residential alternatives. These new settings were not created until the mid-1990s, however, and are therefore not a central finding of the study. It is important to reiterate that the *Bogard* case only affected individuals who were living in nursing homes and did not have any bearing of the residents in public developmental disabilities institutions.

One other outcome of the *Bogard* case for Illinois' residential system was the development of independent service coordination (ISC) agencies, which were established to provide case management or coordination for individuals with developmental disabilities, independent of provider organizations. Unfortunately, however, the independent service coordination system was not seen by many interview respondents as effectively providing a structure for residential placement. Many interview respondents indicated that the service coordination agencies are not able to effectively fulfill their mission, are inadequately funded, and lack the ability to move the service system forward or obtain appropriate services for their clientele.

An important example of the Illinois ARC's role in a national issue was its opposition to the Chafee Amendments. Senator Chafee of Rhode Island introduced the Community and Family Living Amendments (Sen. Bill 1053 of 1985), which would have authorized Medicaid funds to be used in a considerable expansion of community-based services. The bills were defeated twice, in 1984 and 1985. Voice of the Retarded, an advocacy group of families of institutional residents, opposed this and other attempts to divert Medicaid funds from institutions.

The IARC similarly opposed the Chafee Amendments. Representing some institutional families, it argued that families should have the choice of where to place their family members and choice should include institutions (Association for Retarded Citizens of Illinois, 1985, 1986). The defeat of the Chafee Amendments was a serious blow to those who were interested in ending the institutional bias of the Medicaid program, which has been used throughout the decades to fund extensive numbers of private and public institutions through the ICF/MR program. Most interview respondents indicated that on issues concerning individuals with developmental disabilities, institutional family groups like Voice of the Retarded have had more political clout in Illinois than the ARC. Self-advocacy groups like People First were not influential during the 1970-90 study period, because they did not organize in Illinois until 1990.

Two other groups in Illinois that have had advocacy missions are Equip for Equality, Illinois' Protection and Advocacy organization, and the Governor's Planning Council on Developmental Disabilities, two of the three entities funded by the Developmental Disabilities Act. The third is the University Center located at the University of Illinois at Chicago.

Most interview respondents reported that during the 1970s and 1980s, Equip for Equality was involved with individual rights issues, particularly as related to abuse and neglect incidents. Equip for Equality did not advocate for systems change, or for the expansion of community-based residential services, and has not had an impact on the residential service system in the State. In other states, federal class-action litigation directed at reforming or closing institutions has often used lawyers supplied by state Protection and Advocacy organizations; this was not the case in Illinois.

The Governor's Planning Council on Developmental Disabilities has as its statutory mandate the coordination of planning efforts on behalf of individuals with developmental disabilities. The Planning Council generally had three main modes of operation during the 1970-90 study period. It commissioned studies and investigations related to developmental disabilities services in Illinois, provided seed money for pilot projects, and provided technical assistance to legislators. Commissioned study reports have been provided to legislators and the different administrations in the hope of stimulating needed changes. The Planning Council provided funding for an array of pilot projects that were implemented across the State (Governor's Planning Council on Developmental Disabilities, 1978, 1987). However, in addition to supporting innovative

programs, the Council used its funding to facilitate the development of large, privately operated residential facilities. For example, in 1977, the Council gave a $40,000 grant to the Christian Action Ministry to start an ICF/DD for 75 people (Governor's Planning Council on Developmental Disabilities, 1978).

Less widely known is the third aspect of the Council's work in the State, informing elected officials of the impact of pending legislation or the need for legislative initiatives. Most respondents reported that the Planning Council, much like DMHDD, has not been successful in precipitating change in public policy related to the residential service system in the State. The Council was involved in crafting some legislation, most notably the creation of the family support subsidy which was passed in 1989.

In assessing the role of advocates in the State, it is clear that none succeeded in championing a transformation of the residential service system for persons with developmental disabilities. The political strength of parents of individuals living in institutions rendered them the most successful advocates in Illinois during 1970-90, as they were able to retain institutions as an important aspect of the state's service system.

Conclusions

In Illinois, a number of factors worked together to impede the development of community-based residential services. This conclusion will briefly review these factors and the interrelationships among them, answering the study's fifth research question: What were the relationships among influential factors in Illinois?

The development of community-based residential services in Illinois during the 1970-90 period occurred slowly. The evolution of the state's overall residential service system during this time was characterized by the general retention of public institutions, and the creation of private institutions, in addition to the development of community-based residences.

Figure 3.11 represents a conceptual model of the flow of influence in the State. This figure is similar to the hypothesized conceptual framework presented earlier, in that influence is shared by many parties and is dynamic. However, in Illinois, as has been discussed, different parties had varying levels of influence on the service system. In this figure, the lighter, broken ar-

Figure 3.11
CONCEPTUAL FRAMEWORK OF INFLUENCE IN ILLINOIS, 1970-90

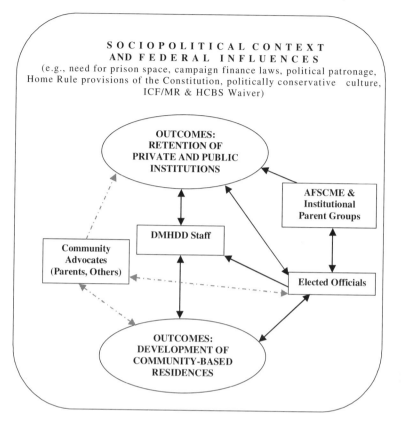

tunity for DMHDD to transfer people from developmental disabilities institutions to psychiatric hospitals. The cost-cutting motivation of Governor Thompson and a lack of creative leadership on the part of DMHDD staff impeded the adoption of innovation as well.

The larger context in which services were provided was also profoundly influential. The state's politics, and particularly the patronage system, facilitated the retention of the status quo.

Home Rule provisions of the Illinois Constitution allowed municipalities to block the development of community homes for much of the 1970s and 1980s. Given the weight of factors that either impeded innovation or fought for the retention of institutions, it is easier to understand why the growth in the state's community residences proceeded so slowly.

DISCUSSION AND CONCLUSIONS

rows represent weaker levels of influence. Dark, solid arrows represent greater levels of influence.

In Michigan, the most important factors that facilitated the development of community services were partnerships and coalitions among different leaders. In Illinois, the strongest advocacy partnerships that existed were among institutional families, institutional superintendents, and the unions, which represented institutional workers. Organizations and individuals interested in expanding community services did not form a cohesive group. The ARC was split between its allegiance to service providers, many of whom operated large-scale private facilities, and to its membership of institutional families. What was most obviously missing in Illinois was the ability of the developmental disabilities advocacy community to speak with a single voice to those in political power.

The deinstitutionalization of people with mental illness from psychiatric hospitals presented an oppor-

As the preceding sections have indicated, there were numerous factors that led Illinois and Michigan to take divergent paths in developing their residential service systems for people with developmental disabilities during the 1970-90 period, summarized in *Table 3.4*. Both states looked virtually identical in the 1960s and early 1970s, including their plans for future construction of public institutions, the dearth of available community services, and the poor conditions in their public institutions. During the 1970s and 1980s, the states were affected by factors that can be characterized within one of four domains: sociopolitical factors, leadership, litigation, and legislation. By way of answering the final research question, which was how influential factors in the two states compare, this section begins with a discussion of the each of these domains across both states, and synthesizes the findings delineated in the previous three sections. The section concludes with a discussion of the limitations of the study and recommendations for future research.

Table 3.4
MAJOR FACTORS RELATED TO THE DEVELOPMENT OF
COMMUNITY SERVICES

Factors Facilitating Community Development		Barriers to Community Development	
Illinois	Michigan	Illinois	Michigan
ICF/MR legislation	Vision and innovation of Macomb-Oakland Regional Center staff	Institutional depopulation into nursing homes & sheltered care facilities	Recession: limited resources available to community placement
Institutional accreditation goals	Advocacy and leadership of the ARC	Creation of DD units in psychiatric hospitals	Parental opposition
Regional structure in the 1970s	Legislative leadership	Legislative power is consolidated in party leadership	Union opposition
	DMH Central Office leadership	Institutional parent political clout	Legislative opposition
	Recession: excuse to cut institutional jobs & save money with community placement	Union political clout	Neighborhood opposition
	Plymouth lawsuit	Lack of DMHDD leadership	
	Michigan zoning laws	Lack of strong legislative leadership for community	
	CMH structure	Lack of gubernatorial support	
	Advocacy community support	Disorganized community parents	
	Governor Milliken support	Lack of coordinated community placement system	
		Lack of ARC leadership	
		Centralization of DMH organizational structure	

Sociopolitical Factors and the Development of the States' DD Residential Systems

Economic Factors

The first domain of factors to be considered is the sociopolitical context. During the 1970-90 period, both states' economies experienced ups and downs. The recessions Michigan experienced were much more severe than those affecting Illinois. This was due in part to the number of tax cuts that Michigan enacted during the period as well as the dominance of the auto industry on its economy. Illinois also suffered periodic economic problems, but not of the same magnitude. Understanding how the economy affected the developmental disabilities service system, however, is challenging.

In Michigan, poor economic conditions were used by advocates and the Department of Mental Health as an opportunity to justify the kinds of far-reaching changes to the service system that resulted. Community-based services were consistently lauded as being cheaper than institutional services. Economic difficulties made irresistible the substitution of cheaper community homes for more expensive institutions. This was particularly true beginning in the early 1980s, when Michigan encountered its worst economic conditions since the Depression.

The ongoing development of community-based residential services in Michigan was certainly a threat to, and did result in the loss of, institutional workers' jobs. It is possible, however, that the loss of these jobs at a time when the entire state was suffering economically made their loss seem to be a less unusual event.

In Illinois, the implications of the state's economic problems during the 1970-90 period had a more direct effect on the developmental disabilities service system. Governor Walker initiated the construction of six privately operated institutions in 1975 as part of his attempt to grapple with the recession Illinois faced at the time. Later, Governor Thompson closed a number of mental health and developmental disabilities institutions, specifically as a way of saving money.

In Illinois, hardest hit by the recession of the 1980s were the rural areas in which most of the public institutions were located. These areas of the State suffered unemployment rates considerably higher than the more urban areas; as a result, legislators most likely would not have contemplated full-scale closure of these facilities. Governor Thompson was successful in closing a number of mental health institutions during the recession, but these facilities were turned into prisons. The outcome was that state workers who lost their jobs in the public developmental disabilities institutions had the opportunity to obtain employment in the newly opened prisons.

As discussed before, some researchers have argued that economic factors are key determinants of the social policies that states adopt (Dye, 1966; Gray, 1999). These models presume that wealthier states are more likely to expend resources for social programs. Michigan and Illinois were selected for this analysis partly due to the similarities of their levels of state wealth. However, throughout the course of the 1970-90 study period, Michigan consistently was the poorer of the two states, as measured by per capita income. Michigan also endured worse unemployment during the study period (Public Sector Consultants, 2000). Yet Michigan consistently spent more of its state wealth, as measured by aggregate personal income, on developmental disabilities services than did Illinois

(Braddock, Hemp, Parish, & Westrich, 1998). This investigation, like that of other researchers in developmental disabilities policy (Braddock & Fujiura, 1987, 1991; Topper, 1997), found that state wealth did not account for differences in the development of the policy innovation of community-based residential services.

In fact, in Michigan, leaders used the ongoing economic crises that the State experienced to justify the development of community services. The presentation of this rationale was part of a successful strategy that ultimately prevailed in the State. In Illinois, there is little evidence that cost data were ever used to attempt to compel shifts in public policy. However, the budget crises the states experienced had a negative impact on developmental disabilities services, as funds were cut in both states.

Prisons

An important issue related to the two states' budgets was the significant expansion of the prison population in both states. Disentangling the relationship between prison growth and developmental disabilities institutions is difficult. In 1977, when Illinois Governor Thompson signed House Bill 1500, the Class X felony legislation, he was following through on a campaign promise that he would get tough on crime. This new law reformed the state's existing sentencing laws, and mandated stiffer sentences for a new class of crimes, so-called "Class X" felonies ("Class X Passes," 1978). During his tenure as governor, the State established 10 new prisons, a number of which were converted from mental health institutions (Illinois Department of Corrections, 2000). Mandatory sentencing clearly created a need for increased prison space, but this was true in both Michigan and Illinois. Michigan constructed 20 new prisons while Governor Blanchard was in office (Michigan Department of Corrections, 2000). *Figure 3.12* shows the growth in the number of each state's prisoners, adjusted for general population.

In 1970, Illinois had 6,341 state prisoners. This population more than doubled to 13,104 by 1980. The population doubled again during the 1980s, exceeding 27,000 prisoners by 1990. Growth in Michigan was rapid as well during this period. In 1970, the state's prison population was 9,079 inmates. By 1980,

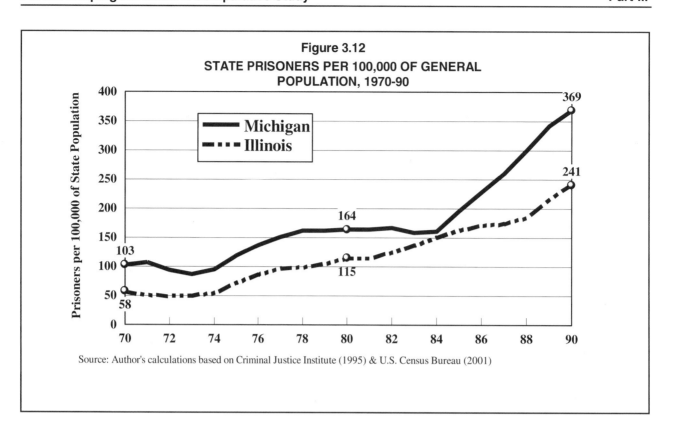

Figure 3.12
STATE PRISONERS PER 100,000 OF GENERAL POPULATION, 1970-90

Source: Author's calculations based on Criminal Justice Institute (1995) & U.S. Census Bureau (2001)

the population advanced by 67%, to 15,158 inmates. The prison population's growth during the 1980s accelerated even faster, and more than doubled to exceed 34,000 inmates by 1990 (Criminal Justice Institute, 1995; House Fiscal Agency, 1989). In Illinois, both of the public developmental disabilities institutions that closed during the 1970-90 period were converted to prisons, as were several of the state's psychiatric hospitals. In Michigan, two of the nine public institutions that closed were converted to prisons. What seems to be most widely accepted about the relationship between prisons and mental health services is that ever-expanding commitments for prison space preclude states from spending money on human service needs. A number of interview respondents in both states suggested that the prisons are increasingly being expected to fulfill the role of serving individuals with mental illness and developmental disabilities. This claim could not be substantiated by documentary evidence or existing research.

Previous researchers have found that, across the nation, a considerable number of developmental disabilities institutions that closed were subsequently converted to prisons (Braddock & Heller, 1985; Braddock, Hemp, Parish, Westrich, & Park, 1998). In Michigan and Illinois, some were as well. However, evidence was not found that developmental disabilities institutions in either state were closed just to make way for prisons, although in both states closures occurred to save money.

Governmental Structure and Politics

The other sociopolitical factors that influenced the evolution of each state's developmental disabilities service system are related to the structure of government and politics in the State. In Illinois, as has been discussed, the political culture was not conducive to the implementation of public policy innovations in the developmental disabilities field. The governmental structure and politics combined to create this political culture. The relevant aspects of the Illinois' governmental structure for our purposes are the Constitutional provisions of Home Rule, and the consolidation of legislative power in the party leadership in both the House and the Senate. Illinois' politics influenced the retention of the status quo because of the centrality of patronage to state jobs, including those in the public developmental disabilities institutions. Since institutional jobs were a way of rewarding people for their political service, institutions represented much more than simply places where people with developmental disabilities were housed. The jobs were important to the ongoing political processes of electing candidates and maintaining the loyalty of individuals who had provided political service. The importance of institutions in the patronage system cannot be minimized in Illinois, and it was one of the forces that converged to facilitate a service system in which the status quo was maintained.

In Michigan, however, politics and the structure of government did not actively bar innovation. This was the case because in the Michigan legislature power was widely distributed. Different legislators were compelled to work together if they wanted to enact any legislation, and it was not uncommon for legislators to cross party lines to pass legislation. During the 1970-90 period, legislators were quite independent. Due to the fact that patronage was not a major part of Michigan's state government, the state's institutions did not represent an important cog in the wheel of systematically rewarding party loyalty or service.

Daniel Elazar (1984) has theorized that political culture is a determinant of public policy. He evaluated an array of state traits and established three cultural classifications for the states: traditionalistic, moralistic, or individualistic. Other researchers have had mixed success applying his model to different social policy areas, and there has been almost no research of his model related to developmental disabilities policy (Gray, 1999). Braddock and Fujiura (1987, 1991) examined ARC advocacy activity, as represented by per capita membership, and found it to be a predictor of spending for community services. However, their inquiry seems to be more related to interest group activity, another sociopolitical factor, than to political culture itself.

This inquiry finds some support for elements of Elazar's theory. The political cultures in Michigan and Illinois clearly have been related to the ways in which developmental disabilities policy developed in both states. However, this investigation is hardly a test of his model, given that the study analyzed developmental disabilities policy in only two states. Instead, it is a principal conclusion of this inquiry that political culture combined with leadership explain the ways in which developmental disabilities policy developed in the states. In the concluding section, the implications of this find-

ing will be discussed for advocates.

Federal Policy Influences

Boggs and her colleagues (1988) and Braddock (1987, 2001) have argued that federal policy and the funding with which it is associated offer compelling incentives for states to pursue and provide particular developmental disabilities programs. Federal policies, like the ICF/MR and HCBS Waiver, have caused billions of federal dollars to flow to the states. There is little doubt that federal policy has had a tremendous influence on how states have structured their residential service systems. Michigan and Illinois are no exception. Both states fundamentally altered the structure of their residential service systems in response to federal stimuli; both sought to meet federal standards in order to capture federal Medicaid reimbursements. But the divergent approaches that they pursued are related to leadership and their political cultures. While federal policy offered perhaps the most powerful incentives for changing each state's service system, the larger context in each state defined the shape the changes wrought.

Federal legislation had mixed results in both states. Enactment of the federal ICF/MR program in 1971 resulted in the infusion of millions of federal Medicaid dollars into both states' developmental disabilities service systems. In the public institutions, the availability of ICF/MR funds had substantially the same impact on both states. Both states embarked upon extensive programs to renovate existing public institutions and both states were compelled to depopulate their public institutions. However, Michigan's depopulation occurred at rates that far exceeded those of Illinois. *Figure 3.13* depicts the population of both states' public institutions during the 1970-90 study period.

As is evident from the figure, both states have made considerable reductions in their public institutional population. During 1970-90, Illinois' population declined by 50% while Michigan's declined by 91%. What is important to bear in mind, however, is that this is not just a situation of one state pursuing deinstitutionalization faster than the other. In Michigan, most people who were moved out of the state's public institutions were moved into small-scale homes in the community. In Illinois, by contrast, many people

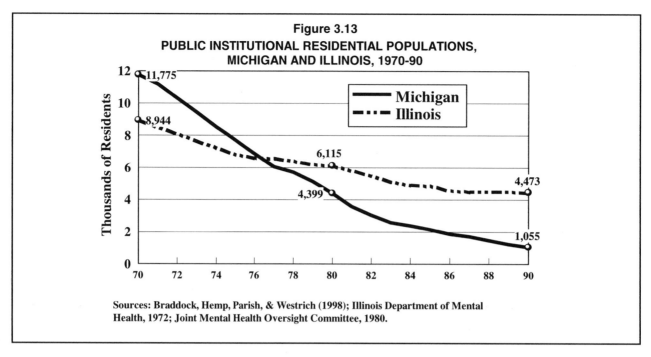

Figure 3.13
PUBLIC INSTITUTIONAL RESIDENTIAL POPULATIONS,
MICHIGAN AND ILLINOIS, 1970-90

Sources: Braddock, Hemp, Parish, & Westrich (1998); Illinois Department of Mental
Health, 1972; Joint Mental Health Oversight Committee, 1980.

moved out of the state's public institutions were placed into privately operated institutions and nursing homes. By 1990, fewer than 1,000 people with developmental disabilities were living in community settings for six or fewer people in Illinois. In Michigan there were nearly seven times that number in such small-scale community settings.

The New Federalism ushered in by the Reagan administration shifted the provision and administration of services from the federal government toward the states; this trend has accelerated in the last two decades. In our federal system of government, states have considerable latitude for the administration of social service programs, including making eligibility determination decisions, choosing funding levels, etc. Even in rigidly regulated programs like ICF/MR, states have considerable autonomy in determining how services are provided. Illinois used the ICF/MR program as a resource to create private institutions and use existing nursing homes to obtain funding from the federal government. Michigan, by contrast, was one of only a handful of states that used federal ICF/MR funds to create small-scale group homes.

At the level of implementation, the state context proved to be as important as the larger federal policy. Leaders in Michigan took advantage of the ICF/MR program to develop services that did not previously exist in the state on a large scale. Leaders in Illinois took advantage of the program to fund existing services, changing very little. The political culture facilitated the retention of the status quo in Illinois, and did not bar innovation in Michigan.

Leadership

Dimensions of Leadership

State variations in leadership exhibited in the 1970-90 period are the most important distinctions between Illinois and Michigan, and they were the most important factors in the divergent development of the two states' service systems. In Michigan, leadership in developmental disabilities services was exhibited in the 1970s by legislators, advocacy groups, particularly the ARC, and staff at DMH's Macomb-Oakland Regional Center. In the 1980s, this leadership expanded to include DMH central office staff as well. There was a convergence of leadership on the importance of developing community-based residential services and phasing out institutional services in the State.

In Illinois, what is most striking is the lack of effective leadership that emerged on behalf of the development of community-based residential services. Leaders in Illinois were not able to catalyze aggressive development of community-based residential services in the 1970s or 1980s. This is not to say that no worthwhile programs emerged, or that people were not committed to developing community services for persons with developmental disabilities. However, it is evident that the state's residential service system was not transformed; the people who attempted to do so were not successful.

The strongest leadership related to developmental disabilities services in Illinois came from proponents of institutional services. There was a convergence of leadership in support of maintaining these facilities, and its supporters were drawn from AFSCME, the parents of individuals in institutions, and institutional superintendents. Related to private facilities, nursing home operators and service providers who ran large private institutions also have been committed supporters of maintaining private institutions for people with developmental disabilities. These groups worked together to block the Chaffee Amendment, and as will be discussed in the next section, stop the closure of a public institution, build a new private institution, and limit the implications of the Supreme Court's *Olmstead* decision.

One of the most important distinctions between Illinois and Michigan was the different role played by the Association for Retarded Citizens. In Michigan, neither the statewide ARC nor its local chapters were service providers. The ARC in Michigan concentrated its efforts full-time on advocacy for people with developmental disabilities and their families. In Illinois, by contrast, most local chapters of the ARC were made up of service providers. As a result, the advocacy efforts of the ARC were on behalf of service providers as well as persons with developmental disabilities.

The actions taken by the ARCs in the two states served to illustrate the extent to which they did and did not provide leadership during this period. The Michigan ARC was instrumental in securing enactment of mandatory special education in 1971, four years before the federal government did so. The Michigan ARC also was the organization that launched the Protection and Advocacy in the State, authorized and funded by the governor to do so. The Michigan ARC subsequently filed the Plymouth class-action lawsuit in federal court, which accelerated the development of community-based residential services in that state. The Michigan ARC also worked to educate families of individuals living in institutions about the positive aspects of community placement for their sons and daughters, which worked to minimize the opposition of institu-

tional parents to community placement and subsequent institutional closure. The ARC's leadership was central to the transformation of Michigan's residential service system. Interview respondents were nearly unanimous in suggesting that the ARC was pivotal in catalyzing the development of community-based residences in Michigan.

In Illinois, by contract, the ARC never filed a class-action lawsuit seeking an improvement of institutional conditions or the closure of an institution. The Illinois ARC did not support passage of the Chafee Amendments in the mid-1980s, which would have redirected federal funds from institutions to community services. Illinois interview respondents who were not themselves affiliated with the ARC generally concurred that the ARC had not provided a level of leadership that was effective in pushing the State to develop more community-based services.

The presence of other advocacy groups in both states was less of a factor in shaping the state's evolution. These groups included Protection and Advocacy Services/Equip for Equality, the Governor's Planning Councils on Developmental Disabilities, and United Cerebral Palsy. While all of these groups were involved in some advocacy efforts during the 1970-90 period, none was perceived as critical to the evolution of either state's service systems. Self-advocacy groups, as has been mentioned previously, were not organized during the 1970-90 period, and consequently were not in a position to influence public policy.

Another key difference between the two states is the leadership exerted by the bureaucracy or staff within DMH or DMHDD. In Michigan, innovation in the 1970s began under the auspices of the Department of Mental Health at the MORC. In the 1980s, leaders at the DMH's central office in Lansing were instrumental in continuing to press for the expansion of community-based residential services. Interview respondents were again nearly unanimous in suggesting that the expansion of community-based residential services was facilitated by strong DMH leadership, first from the MORC and later at the central offices, under Ben Censoni and Patrick Babcock.

In Illinois, DMHDD staff were unable to be as effective as their counterparts in Michigan in expanding community-based residential services for people with developmental disabilities. However, a number of interview respondents stated that Art Dykstra in his capacity as Region II administrator during most of the 1973-1983 "lifetime" of the regional structure made concerted efforts to expand community-based residential services. Although Dykstra's intent and goals were admired by many interview respondents, the progress made in developing community programs in Illinois was accomplished in an overarching state context that continued to primarily construe its responsibilities in terms of institutional services. Therefore, Dykstra's ability to effect major systems change in Illinois was quite limited.

The final leadership dimension considered was that of elected officials. No governor in Michigan or Illinois during the 1970-90 study period can be characterized as having been a champion for persons with developmental disabilities. There is considerable evidence, in fact, that Illinois Governor Thompson's goals of cutting the cost of state government and his use of the patronage system were detrimental to the ongoing development of community-based residential services. Michigan Governor Milliken was not one of the main forces that facilitating change in Michigan. However, his consistent support for the development of community services in the face of considerable opposition earned him the respect of legislators, DMH staff and developmental disabilities advocates as well.

The fact that none of the governors in these two states was a champion on behalf of persons with developmental disabilities is at odds with the conclusions drawn by many Illinois interview respondents that gubernatorial leadership is necessary for public policy changes to occur. Many Illinois interview respondents felt that the residential service system was not transformed in large part because of a lack of a governor's leadership. However, in Michigan, the residential service system advanced very quickly during the administration of Governor Blanchard--a governor who was clearly not a champion, and whose leadership in developmental disabilities was not widely respected. It appears that gubernatorial leadership is not a necessary condition to facilitate changes in public developmental disabilities policy.

The other elected officials whose leadership must be considered are, of course, the legislators in both states. Michigan was particularly notable for the number and sheer will of legislators who were truly cham-

pions with the intent of developing a comprehensive community-based service system for individuals with developmental disabilities. It is important to note that these individuals were both Republicans and Democrats, with very different constituencies and from different parts of Michigan. What they seem to have shared, however, is a commitment to the value that the State must play a central role in supporting vulnerable populations like people with developmental disabilities.

By contrast, in Illinois, no legislators can properly be characterized as champions on behalf of expanding the community-based residential service system. While several interview respondents indicated that Lee Daniels, who is the parent of a person with developmental disabilities and former speaker of the House of Representatives, was supportive of developmental disabilities issues, he did not catalyze great change in the State between 1970-90. His leadership is perhaps best understood as having earned him the respect of some individuals within the system, but his effectiveness in substantively changing public policy has been limited.

Policy Entrepreneurs

This study has found clear support for research that has theorized the importance of so-called policy entrepreneurs (Kingdon, 1995). Policy entrepreneurs provide a form of leadership that is characterized by their grasp of the issues and possession of solutions, and the diligence and persistence with which they pursue their policy objectives. These entrepreneurs work many sides of policy issues, pressing for adoption of their initiatives, intervening when controversy threatens their agenda, pressuring opponents, and using the media to advance their agenda (Kingdon, 1995).

In Michigan, it is clear that much of the change that resulted in the system came directly from policy entrepreneurs. These entrepreneurs included legislators and the ARC. The ARC worked with the legislature at times to secure changes to public policy. However, they also worked independently and filed the Plymouth lawsuit, attempting to use the courts to secure their agenda. They used the media, and they also worked with institutional parents, trying to change parental attitudes from an "insider's perspective." The multiplicity of techniques and strategies that the ARC employed is a testament to their creativity and determination to facilitate change in the developmental disabilities service system.

In Illinois, as has been discussed, policy entrepreneurs did not emerge related to community services. What is less clear is the extent to which policy entrepreneurs can succeed in states with conservative political cultures like Illinois. While the findings from this investigation reveal that policy entrepreneurs were not significant in the State, this is not credible evidence that such entrepreneurs would not be able to succeed in Illinois. However, it is likely that the policy entrepreneurs would have greater difficulty in mounting successful initiatives that were transformative in nature, given Illinois' political conservatism.

Legislation

The third domain to be considered is state legislation. Federal legislation, while important, was discussed previously. State laws result either directly from legislative leadership, or because pressure brought to bear by advocacy groups is effective. State laws are, in a sense, evidence of the effectiveness of state leadership on issues. In evaluating the differences between Illinois and Michigan, there can be no doubt that the Michigan Legislature established a comprehensive legislative program that facilitated the development of community-based residential services for people with developmental disabilities.

This program came about because of the partnerships that existed between legislators, the ARC, and, beginning in the 1980s, the DMH. Legislation passed in Michigan in the 1970s included laws that prohibited discrimination in local zoning practices, that established standards of quality assurance for community-based residences, that provided for minimum distances between facilities to prevent the development of so-called mental health ghettos, and structured the entire service system itself with the 1974 passage of Michigan's Mental Health Code. While not pertaining exclusively to people with developmental disabilities, the State also passed legislation that protected the civil rights of all persons with disabilities in 1976, the Handicappers Civil Rights Act (Pub. Act 220 of 1976). One must conclude that the laws passed

in Michigan were important to the successful expansion of the state's community-based service system. Most interview respondents reported that these laws were essential in facilitating the expansion of community-based residential services.

Illinois, by contrast, had little legislation that facilitated the expansion of community-based residential services. Anti-discriminatory zoning legislation was never passed, which meant that the federal Fair Housing Amendments in 1988 (Pub. L. 100-430) represented the first time that Illinois municipalities were prohibited from using their zoning laws to discriminate against people with disabilities. Laws enacted in Illinois related to residential services included the Nursing Home Reform Act of 1979 and a number of measures enacted in the 1980s that directed the establishment of licensing guidelines for community residences. However, unlike Michigan, Illinois did not have a comprehensive legislative agenda that addressed the multiple facets of the community residential service system.

Litigation

The final domain of factors considered was litigation. Like legislation, litigation is related to leadership; to engage in filing and fighting lawsuits takes leadership and initiative. As noted previously, major litigation in Michigan consisted of the Plymouth lawsuit, which resulted in the closure of that institution and considerable acceleration in the growth of community-based residential services for people with developmental disabilities. Other important Michigan litigation included zoning lawsuits, in which towns across the State challenged the constitutionality of the 1976 Zoning Acts, hoping to have them overturned. The fact that courts consistently upheld the constitutionality of the Zoning Acts provided further support for the ongoing development of community services in Michigan.

In Illinois, no major federal class-action lawsuits were filed by the ARC or the state's Protection and Advocacy organization, Equip for Equality. In other states, either or both of these two entities have taken the lead in pursuing use of the courts to change service systems, as discussed earlier in this volume. The lawsuits fought in Illinois did not seek, or obtain, wholesale changes to the state's residential service system.

Illinois lawsuits included the *Nathan v. Levitt*

case, filed in 1974 on behalf of individuals with developmental disabilities and mental illness living in state facilities. This suit demanded improvements in the care and treatment provided to this group of institutional residents (DMHDD, 1992). Another Illinois lawsuit was *Phillips v. Thompson*, which was filed by the ARC on behalf of the individuals who were moved from a private institution to public institutions when the private facility closed in 1979. The ARC sought community placement for the individuals who had been moved to the public facilities. This case was dismissed at the trial level and again on appeal, and had no impact on the state's residential service system.

Another case was filed by the Dixon ARC, a local chapter of the Illinois ARC composed of families of Dixon Developmental Center residents. In this suit, the families attempted to stop Governor Thompson from closing one of the state's public institutions. The governor prevailed, but the case did not have an impact on the service system either, as no community placement resulted from the facility's closure.

The final lawsuits filed in both states were related to conditions for individuals with developmental disabilities who were living in nursing homes. In Michigan, this case resulted in the closure of the state's specialized nursing homes which had been constructed to serve only people with developmental disabilities (*Kope v. Watkins*, 1988). In Illinois, the nursing home case was filed by the ARC on behalf of over 3,000 individuals living in nursing hmes (*Bogard v. Patla*, 2000). The Bogard case ultimately resulted in community placement of approximately 1,300 of the nursing home residents, all of whom had the right to choose (or have their guardians choose) whether or not to remain in the nursing homes. This case did not result in a transformation of the state's residential service system, which still includes an extensive array of private and public institutional facilities as a central feature of its system.

It would be difficult to overstate the importance of the Plymouth lawsuit in shaping the development of Michigan's community-based residential service system. The suit had far-reaching implications that extended well beyond the specific needs of the Plymouth residents. Nearly every interview respondent stated that community placement began in earnest with Plymouth. Many interview respondents in Illinois also felt

that the lack of a class-action lawsuit related to institutional conditions in Illinois allowed the State to continue to maintain its public and private institutional service system.

As has been explicated in the foregoing discussion, Michigan and Illinois were different on numerous dimensions of the four domains of sociopolitical factors, legislation, leadership, and litigation. The convergence of leadership in Michigan, when coupled with other factors, catalyzed rapid changes in the state's residential service system. By contrast, in Illinois there was a convergence of factors that facilitated the ongoing dominance of institutions in the state's residential service system.

Limitations of the Study

While a number of limitations related to the study were discussed previously, the following cautions are reiterated in order to emphasize how this investigation and its findings should be interpreted. The first important limitation is related to the interviewing phase of data collection. While attempts were made to interview individuals with broadly divergent perspectives and experiences in both service systems, it is possible that the individuals who opted to participate in this study differ in significant ways from those who did not. The response rate, while high, may have been biased toward like-minded individuals with shared perspectives. For instance, a few potential Illinois respondents who declined to participate might have had significantly different perspectives on the service system. Notably, these included the political party leadership and a politically connected institutional superintendent. It is also possible that individuals whose opinions were substantially different from interview respondents did not participate because they were not nominated by others or known to the researcher from the documents that were reviewed.

A second limitation of the interview process is that in nearly all cases, questions were prioritized and not all respondents were asked to share their opinions on every question they could have answered. It would have been most beneficial to interview all of the respondents across days, not hours. The richness and the complexity of the development of public policy in these states is such that it is possible that significant issues were missed.

Given the broad array of factors that can have an impact on public policy, it is likely that this investigation did not exhaust all candidates, and some factors may remain undetected. While steps were taken to address these (e.g., all interview respondents were asked if there were any other factors that had shaped policy), one must conclude that it is possible that important factors were missed.

The other limitations of the study are related to the very important issue of recall bias. Many respondents indicated that they had not considered a particular incident or issue in literally two decades. This study was very taxing on respondents' recall abilities, and it is inevitable that important issues were forgotten. Related to this issue is the accuracy with which respondents were able to recall their own feelings and perspectives. The development of community residences and the closure of institutions were extremely contentious issues during the study period. While the social acceptability of institutional placement has waned considerably in the intervening years, it is possible that respondents who declared their support for the development of community services during the interviews were not as supportive during the 1970-90 study period. It is probably inevitable that some respondents "sanitized" their reports of what happened, and several interview respondents resorted to "politically correct" sentiments that they very well might not have felt during the 1970-90 study period.

However, a number of interview respondents expressed themselves in ways that were quite candid, revealing unflattering incidents that depicted the ways in which their thinking has changed over time. Most respondents were also very direct in stating that they did not remember certain situations.

To address these important study limitations, the investigator attempted to triangulate all major findings. Confirmatory documentary sources were sought for all findings related to the investigation. When interview respondents reported data that had not been substantiated by documentary sources, efforts were made to find documentary sources that would corroborate the interview data. When this was not possible, corroboration was required from at least two other interview respondents who were in a position to have known about the particular situation. Data that could

not be substantiated were not reported as findings. This conservative approach may have resulted in important issues being left unreported. However, it strengthens confidence in the findings that were reported.

The final way in which the findings were assessed was by member checks. As discussed previously, the study findings were reviewed with a sample of interview respondents in either state, and were reviewed with four national experts as well. These individuals all confirmed the study's findings.

Implications for Advocates

What are the ways in which advocates in these two states might catalyze changes in public policy for persons with developmental disabilities? Given the centrality of leadership and political culture to the study's findings, there are potentially different strategies that would work best in the two states.

In Michigan, considerable success resulted from coalitions that included a broad array of representatives that focused on single issues and on partnerships between elected officials, advocates, and state agency staff. Leadership that harnesses the potential of such coalitions, and successfully employs the media, provides the best strategies for changing public policy. Because Michigan's political culture is more receptive to innovation, these coalitions can be directed toward developing and advocating for truly innovative solutions to compelling problems. The element of conservatism in Michigan has presented itself as a fiscal conservatism, so solutions should be crafted in such a way that the fiscal advantages are clear, and explicitly presented. In the past, this type of approach was very successful. Community homes appealed to civil-rights-based interests because of the inherent value of integration and humane services. Community homes appealed to fiscal conservatives because of the tremendous cost savings that they represented over the state's institutions. Packaging and championing single initiatives that appeal to a multitude of diverse groups was effective in the past and should be pursued in the future in Michigan.

In Illinois, the task is frankly more challenging. Power in the system is held by service providers, as most Illinois interview respondents and this investigator concluded. Many of these providers operate institutional or community-based services that do not provide individualized services, and do not respond to service recipients' unique desires. Employing the method and tactics used so successfully in Michigan, the single-issue coalition, with broad-based representation from across the State might seem like the most logical place to begin. However, the entrenchment of the current service system, with powerful providers and a political structure that is resistant to change, makes the prospects for sweeping change doubtful. A more strategically focused approach, with a contingent of different components intended to result in incremental change over time may be most likely to succeed. While discussion of a comprehensive strategy is beyond the scope of this discussion, a brief overview will be presented.

The conservative political culture in Illinois means innovation is not actively sought, and there are strong forces working to retain the status quo. The implication of this for advocates is that targeted changes may need to be pursued incrementally, in ways that do not apparently challenge the existing structure. Pursuing major and rapid shifts in public policy may be dismissed out of hand by those in power as unrealistic alternatives. Another implication of this culture is that coalitions must be more broadly based than is traditionally the case in developmental disabilities services. For instance, organizations with a traditional interest in civil rights that have not historically been interested or involved with developmental disabilities services may need to be courted as allies on some issues. The need for the broadest possible coalitions increases as policy changes threaten aspects of the status quo.

Coalitions were an important way that change occurred in Michigan, and they offer potential in Illinois. However, given the power of service providers, and the power of unions and institutional parents, these coalitions should be structured in ways that suit the system in Illinois. A primary area that should be pursued is the improvement of the quality of services provided in community and institutional settings. This issue has less polarizing potential than pursuing institutional closures. Another strategy would be to work to improve direct care staff working conditions, including salaries, a strategy that has been pursued somewhat successfully of late and would appeal to AFSCME. The Illinois minority caucus could potentially be an ally on this front, because many direct care staff in community homes are racial minorities.

Table 3.5 suggests an array of different organizations in Illinois and the resources that each could provide. This list is not meant to be exhaustive, but

Table 3.5
POTENTIAL COALITION PARTICIPANTS IN ILLINOIS

Organization	Resources	Potential Areas of Interest
Minority Legislative Caucus	Legislative leadership	Worker issues; family issues; civil rights issues
Women's Legislative Caucus	Legislative leadership	Caregiving issues; family issues
HCFA's Chicago Regional Office	National policy information; federal clout	HCBS Waiver and ICF/MR policies; quality assurance
Internet, newspaper, and television media	Public education	Any
Feminist groups & Racial minority rights groups	Grassroots organizing, political clout	Worker issues; family issues; civil rights issues; caregiver issues
AFSCME	Political clout; grassroots organizing	Worker issues; addressing imbalance of providers' power
Better Government Association	Political strategy; public education	Any involving government
Taxpayers Rights' groups	Political clout; grassroots organizing	Cost issues in institutions; employment services for people with disabilities

to suggest ways in which a more diverse set of organizations might be induced to coalesce around developmental disabilities policy issues. Existing developmental disabilities organizations like the Center for Excellence in DD (formerly termed University Affiliated Program, UAP) could provide considerable technical expertise in policy development, building advocacy capacity, facilitating coalitions, best practices dissemination. The Illinois Civil Liberties Union or Equip for Equality, the state's DD Protection and Advocacy organization, could use its legal resources to begin litigation intended to facilitate systems change in the State. Other disability organizations like ADAPT, which advocates for a broad range of disability-related policy, are not listed because they are so obviously important to any far-reaching coalition.

Another imperative is a careful analysis of the types of policy changes that are to be pursued first. This is important because inititial successes will build advocacy capacity, facilitating advocates' respect and clout as players within the political system. The first priorities should be issues that are likely to result in success, and therefore should be more incremental. The truth is that in Illinois there is an enormous distance to be covered, and literally decades of neglect in the system must be fixed. As such, it is this investigator's recommendation that polarizing objectives, like institutional closure, not be sought as first priorities. They are unlikely to succeed without a long-term commitment of time and resources. At this point, the development of smaller successes that result in greater advocacy capacity is a very important objective.

In addition to the potential offered by coalitions, there is little doubt that a concerted public education campaign must be waged, with different goals. The first is to educate the public about the proper role of people with developmental disabilities in society, and the importance of their civil rights. Given the centralization of power within the state's government, it might be necessary for advocates to form partnerships with the media. Having joined forces with the media, a focus on "guerrilla warfare" tactics of revealing crises might be a way to successfully harangue the bureaucratic leadership into changing the service system.

Finally, the potential for successful litigation must be carefully considered. Litigation is best viewed as a long-term strategy, but it has been extremely success-

ful in shaping policy in other states, including Michigan. Traditionally, litigation has been directed at institutional conditions. Within the past decade, however, class-action lawsuits have been filed in 17 states related to improving service systems and expanding system capacity (Smith, 2002), issues that are of paramount importance in Illinois. The Illinois ARC has filed a lawsuit to address the needs of people with developmental disabilities who are waiting for services, which is a step in the right direction. Other litigation might address the lack of control people with developmental disabilities have over the services they receive. While litigation directed at reforming the service system will not result in immediate change, settlement might lay a foundation for the future.

One of the most troubling findings of this study is that persons with developmental disabilities seem to have been largely absent from the policy development process in both states. During 1970-90, people with developmental disabilities were not major players who had an impact on the servies system. Perhaps even more disturbing, however, is that the needs and desires of people with developmental disabilities and their families did not even figure into the development of policy in many ways. Decisions about institutional closures, transferring people between facilities, and creating new service types were related more to issues of political expedience than to the actual needs or desires of people with developmental disabilities themselves. One of the central themes that emerged from this investigation is that to influence public policy, particularly in Illinois, but also in Michigan, a considerable amount of political sophistication and savvy seems to be required. Not only to navigate an inordinately complex political and bureaucratic structure, but to truly participate in the ways policy decisions are made. The organizing efforts and advocacy that have emerged from groups like People First are an encouraging development. But at its core, this study suggests that self-advocates will need to grapple with an array of challenging issues.

DEVELOPMENTS IN MICHIGAN AND ILLINOIS: 1990-2000

The purpose of this section is to append an epilogue to the study, and provide an overview of the ongoing evolution of each state's residential service system during 1990-2000. It is beyond the scope of this inquiry to provide comprehensive details of the four domains (sociopolitical factors, leadership, litigation, and legislation) examined for the 1970-90 study period. However, a brief description of key events that occurred in each state's residential service system will be presented.

General Trends

During the 1970s and 1980s, Michigan aggressively depopulated its public institutions and rapidly expanded community residences for people with developmental disabilities. Illinois slowly depopulated its public institutions, and slowly expanded privately operated residences, many of which were private institutions or nursing homes. During the 1990s, both states continued along the trajectory of the prior two decades. Many differences in the two states' service systems continue to be evident, both in terms of the types of residential services available, and the ways in which services are funded.

Types of Residential Settings

In 1990, Michigan operated six public institutions for 1,055 people with developmental disabilities. That year, Illinois operated nine institutions and three units for people with developmental disabilities within psychiatric hospitals, serving a total of 4,473 persons (Braddock, Hemp, Parish, & Westrich, 1998). Michigan and Illinois had an additional 2,482 and 3,906 people with developmental disabilities living in nursing homes, respectively, in 1990. Illinois funded residential services for 5,606 people in private institutions as well. Michigan did not fund private institutions for people with developmental disabilities (Braddock, Hemp, Parish, & Westrich, 1998).

During the 1990s, Michigan continued to close its public institutions. The Oakdale, Muskegon, Newberry, and Caro centers were closed in

1991, 1992, 1992, and 1998, respectively. In May 2001, the State announced that it would close Southgate by January 2002 (Michigan Department of Community Health, 2001). The closure of Southgate will leave Michigan with a single public institution, the Mt. Pleasant Center, which served fewer than 200 people in 2000.

By contrast, Illinos did not close any of it public institutions in the 1990s, and as of September 2001 had no plans to do so. Closure of the Kiley Developmental Center in Waukegan was announced by Gov. Jim Edgar in 1995, but this decision was subsequently rescinded. The downsizing of Illinois' public institutions proceeded slowly in the 1990s. By 2000, 3,221 people were still living in state-operated institutions. Between 1990-2000, the rate of population decline in Illinois' public institutions was 28%, as compared to 77% in Michigan and 44% for the U.S. as a whole (see Part II, this volume).

Growth in the number of community-based residential settings expanded in both states during the 1990s. By 2000, nearly 12 thousand people with developmental disabilities were living in community homes in Michigan. In Illinois, the number living in community homes exceeded 11,000 people, as noted earlier in this volume. *Figure 3.14* (Michigan), and *Figure 3.15* (Illinois) depict the general course of the size of facilities in which people receiving residential services lived during 1990-2000. The number of people living in institutions does not include individuals in nursing homes,

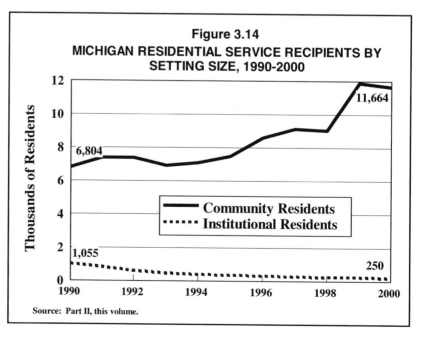

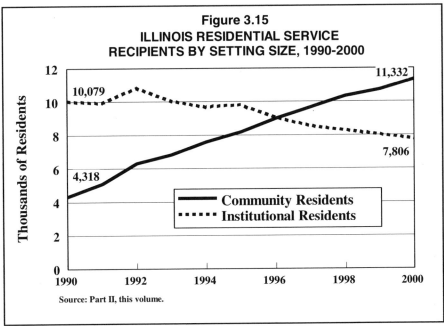

Figure 3.15
ILLINOIS RESIDENTIAL SERVICE
RECIPIENTS BY SETTING SIZE, 1990-2000

Source: Part II, this volume.

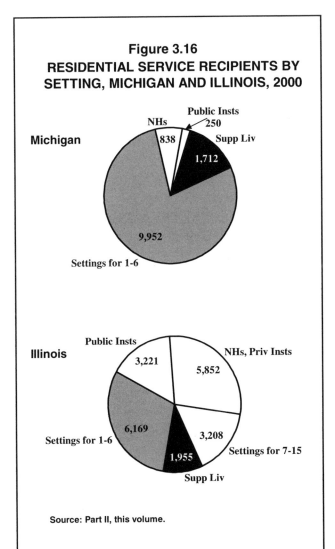

Figure 3.16
RESIDENTIAL SERVICE RECIPIENTS BY
SETTING, MICHIGAN AND ILLINOIS, 2000

Source: Part II, this volume.

but people in other privately operated institutions are included for Illinois. Community settings are defined as those for fewer than 16 people.

A seemingly similar number of persons were living in community-based residences in both states in 2000. However, these aggregate numbers mask great variability. For instance, of the more than 11 thousand people living in community settings in Illinois in 2000, nearly one third lived in ICFs/MR for 7 to 15 people. In Michigan, by contrast, no one lived in settings of more than six people, and all community ICFs/MR were closed by 1999 (see Part II, this volume). *Figure 3.16* depicts greater detail on where residential service recipients lived in 2000. As is evident from the figure, larger-scale residential settings are a dominant service type in Illinois, but have a limited role in Michigan's service system.

The states' use of supported living for people with developmental disabilities is another component of their residential service systems that evolved during the 1990s. Supported living is a residential service that can be provided in an apartment or other type of home. However, supported living is characterized by recipients choosing where and with whom they live, and receiving services that change to accommodate their changing needs. Finally, in supported living, the lease or ownership of the service recipient's housing is not supposed to be controlled by the service provider (Braddock, Hemp, Parish, Westrich, & Park 1998). Supported living represented a breakthrough in residential services for people with developmental disabilities, because, for the first time, services were intended to be individually tailored to meet recipient's unique needs. In more traditional residential service models like ICFs/MR, recipients are expected to adapt to a setting and whatever services it provides, regardless of their individual needs or desires.

In 1990, Congress authorized states to apply for Medicaid Community Supported Living Arrangement (CSLA) funds (Pub. L. 101-508). Eight states, including Michigan and Illinois, were awarded multiyear grants to initiate CSLA programs. Both states used the federal Medicaid funds to establish statewide supported living initiatives. Federal funds for CSLA to Michigan and Illinois totaled $6.9 and $7.4 million, respectively, between 1992-96, when the temporary federal funding for the program ended (Braddock, Hemp, Parish, & Westrich, 1998).

In spite of the similar source and levels of funding for CSLA, the program played different roles in each state's residential service system. In Michigan, CSLA was used as a tool to restructure much of the state's residential service system. Supported living spending in Michigan grew to exceed $100 million by 2000. According to one interview respondent:

> CSLA gave people real opportunities in Michigan to color outside the lines. They were collectively so pleased with what they accomplished with CSLA that they started to look beyond the CSLA clients and said, "Well, why aren't we doing that in the Waiver program?" which triggered changes in the Waiver program statewide. They asked "Why aren't we doing this system-wide for everyone?" And this led to their application for new Waivers. It's very interesting that the CSLA was a tiny deal and it had an enormous impact. The other key part of CSLA was that it more or less established a coalition between advocates and state people

and others around the state. The coalition helped them to collaborate with each other.

In Illinois, by contrast, the federal funds were used to expand the state's existing CILA program, and considerable expansion did occur. However, by 2000, supported living services still did not represent a major component of the state's residential system (see Part II, this volume). *Figure 3.17* depicts each state's spending for supported living services from 1992-2000.

As a result of the filing of the Illinois and Michigan nursing home lawsuits, both states were involved in nursing home litigation for much of the 1990s. The Michigan case (*Kope v. Watkins*, 1988) was finally settled in 1994, and eventually resulted in community placement for the residents with developmental disabilities who had lived in the five specialized nursing homes for people with developmental disabilities (Michigan Protection and Advocacy Service, 1994). The *Bogard* case in Illinois resulted in the adoption of a consent decree in which nursing home residents with developmental disabilities were to be given the choice of obtaining placement in the community. The consent decree allowed guardians to choose to have their family members continue to reside in the nursing homes, however. As a result, approximately 1,300 nursing home patients with developmental disabilities were eventually placed in the community (T. Paulaski, personal communication, August 2001).

The other major implication of the *Bogard* case for the developmental disabilities service system was the establishment of independent service coordination (ISC) agencies. The creation of these ISC organizations, which were not permitted to be service providers or have more than 10% of their board members as service providers, was a stipulation of the lawsuit's consent decree. Under the terms of the consent decree, Bogard class members were to be guaranteed long-term case coordination (DMHDD, 1995).

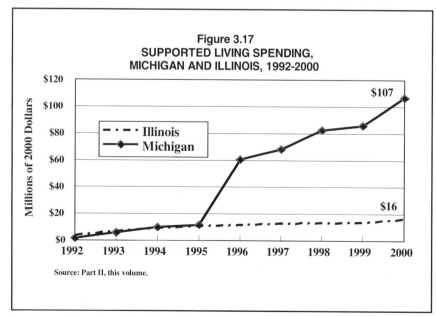

Figure 3.17
SUPPORTED LIVING SPENDING,
MICHIGAN AND ILLINOIS, 1992-2000

Source: Part II, this volume.

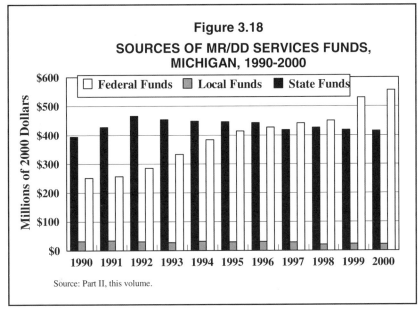

Figure 3.18
SOURCES OF MR/DD SERVICES FUNDS, MICHIGAN, 1990-2000

Source: Part II, this volume.

In spite of the litigation in both states, substantial numbers of people with developmental disabilities continued to live in nursing homes during the 1990s. By 2000, there were more than 800 people with developmental disabilities living in nursing homes in Michigan, and more than 1,200 in Illinois. The decline in the number of nursing home residents totaled 1,644 and 2,639 persons in Michigan and Illinois, respectively, during 1990-2000 (see Part II, this volume).

Financial Trends

Examining the ways in which Michigan and Illinois financed their residential service systems in the 1990s reveals several important differences between the two states. These differences influenced their residential service systems as well. Like every other state in the nation between 1990-2000, Michigan and Illinois obtained increasing levels of federal financing for developmental disabilities services (see Part II, this volume). States can increase the level of federal funds they receive in two ways. They can allocate new state funds to Medicaid services, which in turn results in increased federal Medicaid matching funds. The other alternative is to reallocate existing state funds to Medicaid services and thereby use previously unmatched state dollars to leverage federal Medicaid funds. In Michigan between 1990-2000, federal funds for developmental disabilities services increased 121% in inflation-adjusted terms. In Illinois, federal funds increased by a slower 74% during the same period (see Part II, this volume).

The expansion of federal funds in Michigan was largely facilitated by the reallocation of existing state funds. Between 1990-2000, state funds that were used to leverage federal Medicaid resources for community services expanded from 49% to 95% in Michigan. However, between 1992-2000, the actual allocation of state funds declined by 11% in inflation-adjusted terms. What this means is that even though the State was cutting state funds for developmental disabilities services, it was reallocating its existing state funds to leverage federal funds.

In Illinois, the growth in the state's expenditures for community-based developmental disabilities services came from new state dollars that were invested in the service system. Much of these new state resources were not directed at obtaining federal funds, however. Between 1990-2000, Illinois' state funds that were used to leverage federal Medicaid resources for community services expanded from 28% to 43%. In

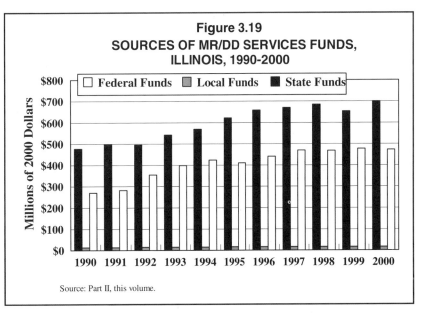

Figure 3.19
SOURCES OF MR/DD SERVICES FUNDS, ILLINOIS, 1990-2000

Source: Part II, this volume.

the state's institutional services, however, state funds used to leverage federal Medicaid funds expanded from 76% to 91% between 1990-2000. This means that Illinois was considerably more effective in using its resources to obtain federal money for institutional services (both public and private) than it was for community services. *Figures 3.18 and 3.19* depict the sources of total MR/DD spending in the two states.

The funding sources in each state are significant for our purposes because of the ways they influence the types of services that are provided. In Michigan, a concerted effort was made in the 1990s to obtain federal Medicaid funds. As a result, by 2000, for every dollar of state funds Michigan spent for developmental disabilities services, the State received $1.17 in federal Medicaid funds. For every dollar in state funds that Illinois spent for community services in 2000, it received just $0.43 in federal Medicaid funds (see Part II, this volume). Michigan's approach, whereby state funds are used to obtain the greatest amount of federal funds possible facilitates the expansion of a service system beyond the capacity that would be possible with fewer federal resources.

In Illinois, however, a different picture emerges. Because the State only uses 48% of its resources to obtain federal Medicaid reimbursement for community services, the total level of federal Medicaid funds that support community services in Illinois is considerably lower than in Michigan. In 2000, Michigan received $450 million in federal Medicaid funds; Illinois received $181 million. It is important to note that federal Medicaid funds are not capped; states can receive a level of federal funding that is limited only by the state's own Medicaid spending. The fact that Illinois uses so little of its state resources to leverage federal funds limits its community services program. For example, if Illinois reallocated just 10% of its existing state spending for community services to Medicaid services, it would capture an additional $24.2 million in federal Medicaid revenues.

The more cost effective investment Illinois makes, at least from the standpoint of using federal funds to pay for services, is institutional services. In 2000, 91% of state funds for institutions were used to obtain federal Medicaid reimbursement. This differential level of effort results in community services that are more expensive to the State. It is impossible not to conclude that there are considerable financial incentives in Illinois to maintain its institutional service system.

Family Support

Family support services are not considered to be a residential program, and thus were not a primary focus of this investigation. However, family support evolved in Michigan specifically as a way to reduce the costs of residential care, so this discussion will provide a brief overview of the ongoing evolution of family support services in both states.

Michigan passed legislation in 1983 which authorized payments to families with children with severe disabilities (Pub. Act 249 of 1983). This subsidy act was the most generous at the time that it was enacted, with payment levels set at the monthly federal SSI amount. By 2000, Michigan's subsidy program was still the largest in the nation, in terms of the total spending on families, and was among the most generous in per-family spending as well. Illinois passed legislation in 1989 that established a family support subsidy program (Pub. Act 86-921 of 1990), which was modeled on Michigan's statute.

The Illinois program is more ex-

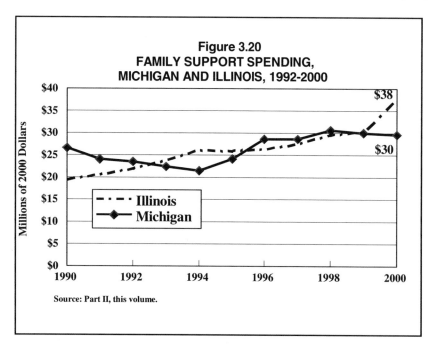

Figure 3.20
FAMILY SUPPORT SPENDING,
MICHIGAN AND ILLINOIS, 1992-2000

Source: Part II, this volume.

pansive than the Michigan program, however. Illinois provides cash subsidies to families whose children are adult-age as well as children. In Michigan, participation in the program is extended only to families in which the child with a disability is a minor. Illinois' program is also among the strongest in the country, with the nation's highest level of per-family subsidy amounts. However, the Illinois program is much more limited in the total number of families that it reaches. In 2000, Michigan's cash subsidy spending totaled $13.7 million for more than 5,000 families, and one fifth of American families receiving subsidies lived in Michigan. In 2000, Illinois' cash subsidy spending totaled $16.5 million for nearly 2,000 families (see Part II, this volume). *Figure 3.20* depicts each state's total family support spending from 1990-2000, adjusted for inflation. The spending in the figure includes cash subsidies and all other forms of family support services, including respite and other family support services.

Michigan

As discussed previously, during the 1990s, Michigan continued to transform its remaining institutions to community-based services. This section will highlight some of the key events that occurred during the 1990-2000 period, and describe factors that influenced the ongoing evolution of the service system.

Reduced Reliance on Institutions and the Ongoing Transformation to Community

During the 1970s and 1980s, Michigan led the nation in shifting its services from an institutionally based system to a statewide network of community residences. The State aggressively depopulated and then closed its public institutions, developing community homes in their place.

In the 1990s, the institutional population continued to decline in Michigan, as four public facilities were closed. However, institutions remained controversial for the State until the end of the decade. In the 1990s, the Protection and Advocacy Services organization filed a lawsuit in an attempt to close the Southgate and Mt. Pleasant institutions. However, this lawsuit was not successful. The Protection and Advocacy charged

that the State, in spite of spending considerable sums for institutional services in these facilities, was unable to provide for the residents' welfare, and protect them from harm. The case noted ongoing problems of neglect and abuse. In October 2000, a male resident at Southgate died after ingesting cleaning products; he had eaten cleaning products on numerous occasions during 2000 (Furth, 2001).

The Department of Community Health, which was responsible for developmental disabilities services in Michigan and operated the institutions, announced the closure of Southgate in May 2001 (Michigan Department of Community Health, 2001). One news article reported that the unions, which represented institutional workers, were opposed to the closure but had not taken steps to attempt to prevent the facility from closing. In addition, the media reported significant problems in maintaining adequate care in the facility (Furth, 2001).

This news report is corroborated with findings of the state's auditor general, who indicated problems in a number of areas relate to the care and treatment of residents at Southgate. These findings included failure to comply with person-centered planning requirements, use of restrictive treatment techniques without guardians' consent or appropriate oversight committee approval, ineffective communication and cooperation with community placement organizations, and failure to properly conduct investigations of recipient rights violations (Michigan Office of the Auditor General, 1999).

Changes in Elected Leadership

Michigan's developmental disabilities services system has been profoundly affected by Gov. John Engler, who took office in 1991. Governor Engler and his administration's oversight of the developmental disabilities service system in Michigan was widely reported by interview respondents to be deplorable. His cost-cutting objectives led to a 12% inflation-adjusted decline in state funds for developmental disabilities services between 1992-2000.

One main objective of his administration was the decentralization of developmental disabilities (and other) services. Many advocates argued that the push for services to be completely controlled by local Community Mental Health Boards constituted an abandonment of the state's quality assurance responsibilities. Advocates have widely reported that decentralization has been a thinly disguised attempt by the State to dump responsibility for people with developmental disabilities and their families.

One other issue related to the state's elected leadership is the enactment of term limits. Michigan voters amended the State Constitution in 1992 and established term limits for all state legislators and statewide public offices (Public Sector Consultants, 1998). Incumbents were forced off the ballot for the first time in 1998, and it is therefore not possible to assess the implications of term limits on developmental disabilities issues. One interview respondent suggested that the need to educate new legislators will become more pressing than ever before. Given the complexity of developmental disabilities services and their funding sources, and the widely divergent needs of people with developmental disabilities and their families, educating new legislators will be a daunting challenge.

Innovations

Michigan's role as an innovator in developmental disabilities services during the 1970s and 1980s has been described in some detail in this study's findings. The two main innovations that occurred in the state's developmental disabilities system will be described here: person-centered planning and the use of the HCBS Waiver for long-term care services. Other innovations, including the use of CSLA and the elimination of the state's privately operated ICFs/MR (termed AIS/MR homes), were mentioned earlier.

One particularly notable aspect of Michigan's developmental disabilities program was the implementation of person-centered planning. The State passed legislation in 1996 that amended the existing Mental Health Code and mandated person-centered planning for all individuals receiving mental health and developmental disabilities services in the State. Person-centered planning is intended to allow service recipients and their families to direct the treatment planning process, and to focus on the needs and desires of the service recipient (Michigan Department of Community Health, 1998). The amendment to the state's Mental Health Code was a watershed, in that it for-

mally empowered families to obtain the services that they desired. In addition, provisions codified to provide an appeal process, and families were to have alternatives if they were dissatisfied with the services that they were to receive (Michigan Department of Community Health, 1998).

It should be noted that person-centered planning initiatives have been pursued across the country. However, most have been piloted for small sets of persons, often from universities (e.g., Butterworth, Hagner, Heikkinen, DeMello, & McDonough, 1993) or Developmental Disabilities Planning Councils (e.g., Mount & Zwernick, 1988). However, passage of Michigan's person-centered planning legislation represented the first time a state statutorily mandated the process for its citizens with developmental disabilities.

A second major innovation that the State pursued during the 1990s was the utilization of managed long-term care services for people with developmental disabilities. In 1998, the federal Health Care Financing Administration approved Michigan's proposal to implement a Medicaid managed care program for so-called specialty services, which included mental health, developmental disabilities, and substance abuse services. The approval allowed the State to continue to solely contract with local CMH Boards, but stipulated that the State had to develop a competitive contracting system within two years (Michigan Department of Community Health, 2000). Federal regulations require open competition in managed care arrangements (Code of Federal Regulations, 1999), which precludes the CMH Boards from being the sole service contractors. In response to this requirement, Michigan worked to develop a plan to allow competition, and released a preliminary report in 1999. In response to public opposition to the plan, the Department of Community Health went back to the drawing board, and completely re-evaluated their plan and the bases for providing these specialty services. At the end of 2000, the Department of Community Health issued a final plan on procuring management of mental health services. This paper delineated plans for a system that included regional service areas across the State with single management organizations within each region.

Management organizations were to be awarded contracts for both Medicaid funds and other state funds that traditionally were allocated to the CMH Boards. These new management organizations could be any organizational entity, including proprietary firms (Michigan Department of Community Health, 2000). Advocates expressed some agreement with the structure of the new plan, but still expressed reservations about other aspects (Michigan Mental Health Association, 2000). Although intended to begin in early 2001, implementation of the program has been delayed.

Illinois

As described previously, during the 1990s, Illinois largely retained public and private institutions as central features of its residential service system. This section will highlight some of the key events that provide insight into why institutions remained significant, and discuss inroads that were made toward developing smaller-scale services.

This study found that the political structure in Illinois played a central role in maintaining the status quo, namely a commitment to residential services provided in public and private institutions. As such, a discussion of the ongoing role of politics during the 1990s is merited. Two incidents in particular have been chosen to highlight the way in which politics continued to exert major influence on the shape and context of the delivery of residential services in the State.

In 1995, Gov. Jim Edgar announced in his budget address to the General Assembly that the Kiley Developmental Center in Waukegan would be closed. According to interview respondents, the idea to close Kiley had come from staff at the DMHDD, who saw the closure as a sound budgetary strategy, as well as good for the residents, who were expected to benefit from community placement. According to several interview respondents, Kiley was selected for closure because of the number of service providers in the area, which would provide families with lots of choices in placing their children, and because the Kiley residents were perceived to be largely capable of transitioning easily into the community.

When the governor announced the closure of Kiley, it was a surprise to both the legislature and to the families of the residents of Kiley, who were not given any advance notice of the decision. In the wake of the governor's announcement, the institutional work-

ers' union, AFSCME, joined forces with the residents' families. These two groups were led by Sen. Adeline Geo-Karis, a powerful, long-time legislator, and committed supporter of Kiley. The senator, AFSCME, and families aggressively worked to fight the closure. According to interview respondents, public hearings about the facility's closure were disrupted, and a petition opposing the closure was delivered to the governor, with 33,000 signatures. Governor Edgar rescinded the closure decision, opting not to attempt to negotiate politically with Senator Geo-Karis or the unions. The closure was subsequently termed a "transition," whereby families would be given the choice of whether or not their family member living at Kiley wanted to move to a community home.

The selection of Kiley represented, at best, a great miscalculation on the part of DMHDD staff of the facility's importance to the legislature, unions, and families. The Department of Mental Health and Developmental Disabilities staff believed that the people living at Kiley were appropriate for community placement, due to their limited behavioral and medical needs. However, the fate of the facility was related to who had the clout to effect change, and not the needs of the residents. Interview respondents characterized this event as a tragedy for the State, because the way in which it unfolded effectively stopped the consideration of any further institutional closures for the foreseeable future.

Another example of the way in which politics influences the development of the state's service system is the planned construction of a new privately operated institution in an outlying suburb of Chicago. In 2000, Marklund, a service provider that operates three private institutions and hospitals for individuals with developmental disabilities, submitted an application to construct private ICFs/MR for 64 people (Illinois Department of Public Health, 2001). Marklund submitted its application to the Health Care Facilities Planning Board in accordance with state regulations regarding the development of new ICFs/MR. Total costs to construct the facility were estimated to be $13.3 million, with $6.2 million coming from governmental sources (Illinois Department of Public Health, 2001). The organization's application was not supported by the Department of Human Services, the reorganized state department that oversees developmental disabilities services in Illinois. The application was subsequently rejected by the Planning Board as well (Health Facilities Planning Board, 2001).

Marklund appealed directly to Governor George Ryan for his intervention, and by summer 2001, the provider had been issued a certificate of need (Rusco, 2001). Certificates of need are the permits that allow construction of new health-care facilities to proceed. In supporting the construction of the Marklund facility, the governor stated that parents have the right to choose institutions for their family members with developmental disabilities. To put this development in context, it is important to understand that the current development of residential services across the country is nearly always occurring at the smallest end of the continuum; most states are expanding small-scale, individualized residential services like supported living and apartment programs (Braddock, Hemp, Parish, Westrich, & Park, 1998). In the 1990s, public and private institutions alike have been downsized or closed. Illinois' development of this private institution is anachronous at best, and clearly is at odds with current research about the best home situations for people with developmental disabilities.

In spite of the governor's public statements that the new institution was a matter of choice for the parents, interview respondents disagreed that this had been the motivation behind the decision. Several interview respondents highly placed in Illinois state government stated that politically powerful friends of Marklund were the reason that the governor reversed the state's initial disapprovals for the facility's construction to proceed. The development of this facility was widely opposed by the State Arc, the self-advocacy group People First, and other advocacy organizations. Hearings on the matter proved irrelevant, however, as the decision for Marklund to proceed hinged upon the facility's political connections. A recent newsletter published by the service provider indicated that powerful U.S. Congressman Henry Hyde is among Marklund's long-time supporters (Marklund, 2001). However, it was not possible to ascertain whose influence was used to secure the Governor's permission for facility construction.

Another service provider that operates large institutions in the Chicago area recently announced that it, too, intends to pursue the development of another private institution (Connelly, 2001). This provider,

Misericordia, is widely believed to be the most politically powerful in the State, and counts as supporters Governor Ryan and the legislative leadership, particularly House Leader Michael Madigan. It is widely believed that Misericordia will be permitted to construct its new facility as well. These examples suggest that politics continue to be important to the way services are provided in Illinois.

Advocacy Efforts

One of this study's conclusions was that the state's main advocacy group, the Arc of Illinois, was unable to catalyze significant change in the residential service system during the 1970s and 1980s. This inability partly stemmed from the Arc's conflict of interest in representing service providers, and from the schism between institutional and community families that the organization represented. Most interview respondents concluded that in spite of speaking more forcefully for the need for community services during the 1990s, the Arc continued to be hamstrung in its advocacy efforts by its relationship with service providers. Some evidence of the Arc's ongoing support of service providers is evident from the reaction of the State Arc when one large service provider, Kreider Services, was successfully organized by AFSCME.

> Kreider, under the direction of Executive Director Arlan McClain, had a very strong wage/salary system with its employees. Employees start with an hourly wage of $7.00 with a shift differential and free health insurance as well. Arlan, who has been the executive director at Kreider for the past 23 years, has always provided fair and equitable wages and perks for his employees… We wish Arlan well as he moves toward working with AFSCME. (Paulaski, 1998, p. 2)

Interview respondents also widely concurred in reporting that the Arc is not regarded as a serious political power in the State, and had limited influence during most of the 1990s. Advocacy efforts by the Arc during the 1990s were directed to an array of different issues, just a few of which will be considered here. These include litigation, wage increases for direct care workers, and opposition to the construction of new institutions.

As the decade ended, the Arc was part of a coalition to increase the wages paid to direct care workers in private agencies. This coalition included service providers and, for the first time, AFSCME. AFSCME had been successful at the end of the 1990s in organizing direct care workers in privately operated residential programs. By the end of the decade, the union represented more than 3,000 of these workers (M. McMullen, personal communication, AFSCME, October 4, 2001). In 2001, the coalition of the Arc, service providers, and AFSCME successfully pushed for passage of legislation that increased the wages of direct care workers in privately operated wages by $1 per hour.

Another notable advocacy effort that the Arc undertook was the filing of class-action litigation on behalf of individuals waiting for community services in Illinois. This case, *Boudreau v. Ryan*, was filed in September 2000, and alleged that Illinois does not provide Medicaid services to eligible individuals with developmental disabilities, in violation of federal Medicaid law (Smith, 2002). This lawsuit was 1 of 17 that have been filed across the nation in attempts to compel states to address the needs of unserved people with developmental disabilities. However, in February 2002, the judge dismissed the case ruling that the plaintiffs had not demonstrated violations of Medicaid law.

Interview respondents consistently reported that the Protection and Advocacy organization, Equip for Equality, was not involved in working toward systems change in the State during the 1990s. Similarly, the Developmental Disabilities Planning Council and People First were not considered by interview respondents to be major influences in the residential service system during the 1990s.

Federal Influences

Activities by the federal government continued to play a role in shaping the state's service system in the 1990s. As discussed previously, Illinois expanded its supported living program in response to the availability of federal CSLA funds. Services in Illinois were also influenced by the regulatory authority of the federal government, and steps were taken to address the Supreme Court's *Olmstead* (1999) decision.

One prominent example of federal intervention in Illinois' residential service system occurred in 1998, when HCFA conducted a review of the state's HCBS Waiver program. In their review, HCFA auditors reviewed records, interviewed an array of service provider staff and state officials, and directly observed individuals while they were receiving services (HCFA, 1999). The report that HCFA subsequently issued was scathing, noting major problems in the administration of the program, inadequate procedures related to reporting and investigating abuse and neglect, minimal training of service recipients, limited freedom of choice for recipients, extensive problems with the provision of medical services, and numerous other problems (HCFA, 1999). As a result of the review team's findings and rampant abuse and neglect of service recipients, HCFA ordered extensive improvements in the state's program, and issued a moratorium on new admissions to foster homes.

HCFA also found that Illinois' Waiver program, instead of being consumer-centered, as is intended by federal regulations, was "provider-centered."

> Although the waiver, in theory, allows individuals freedom of choice in the delivery of services, the procedures used for enrolling and assessing, as well as managing services and service deliver, place providers in control of the service delivery structure. This has resulted in numerous problems, including inadequate assessments, inappropriate care plans, use of unqualified staff, and lack of habilitative services. Because of this, the State has failed to ensure the health and welfare of the individuals served. (HCFA, 1999, p. 16)

Another regulatory aspect of the state's residential service system in which the federal government plays a role is the ongoing certification of ICFs/MR, including state institutions. Compliance with federal ICF/MR regulations is required as a condition of participation in the ICF/MR program, which in turn results in receipt of federal Medicaid reimbursement for ICF/MR services. In Illinois, problems with institutional conditions have been an issue in the 1990s as they were in Michigan. The most recent statement of deficiencies, which is the ICF/MR certification review report, for the state's Lincoln Developmental Center revealed extensive problems complying with standards. The report noted that

> Individuals have been abused, neglected, or otherwise mistreated and the facility has not taken steps to protect individuals and prevent reoccurrence; individuals are subjected to the use of drugs or restraints without justification; and individual freedoms are denied or restricted without justification, e.g., systemic lack of privacy, of freedom of access to the community or to other individuals in use of personal possessions and money, etc. (Illinois Department of Public Health, 2000, p. 7)

The statement further reported that residents were denied opportunities for activities in integrated community settings, female residents were not given undergarments, staff did not appropriately intervene to address aggressive or self-abusive behavior of residents, insufficient direct care staff were working with residents, and noncompliance with individual program plans was frequent (Illinois Department of Public Health, 2000).

The facility's administration was required to complete a plan of correction to address all of the problems noted in the 123 pages of deficiencies, and written plans were submitted in October 2000. The extent and nature of the deficiencies found by the surveyors led to the termination of the facility from the ICF/MR program in November 2001.

A final aspect of federal influences on the state's service system is related to the Supreme Court's *Olmstead* decision (1999). Judge Ruth Bader Ginsburg, writing for the 6-3 Court majority, described the essence of the Court's ruling: "We confront the question of whether the proscription of discrimination may require placement of persons with mental disabilities in community settings rather than in institutions. The answer, we hold, is a qualified yes." In response to the *Olmstead* decision, the U.S. Department of

Health and Human Services has directed the states to assure effective implementation of the ruling by developing comprehensive plans that ensure compliance with the Americans with Disabilities Act. These guidelines encouraged states to provide services in the most appropriate, integrated setting (Westmoreland & Perez, 2000).

In Illinois, the development of the state's plan has been markedly contentious. Individuals and groups supportive of community services were at odds with parents of people who live in institutions and providers that operate large facilities. In addition, union representatives wanted to include issues related to giving direct care workers bargaining rights, which produced heated opposition from service providers. A number of planning participants filed dissenting opinions. At issue is a fundamental disagreement as to the actual mandates of the Supreme Court's *Olmstead* ruling itself. Institutional supporters argued that the ruling provides for families to continue to choose institutions, while community services supporters argued that the ruling is a mandate for closing institutions. Language in the decision is sometimes ambiguous, seeming to give credence to both sets of opinions. One dissenter, representative of the strong will of some groups to maintain institutions, wrote:

> Any language contained in the body of this document that suggests that all people can be served in the community, or that institutions serving those in need of institutional care should be closed, is not subscribed to by the Illinois League of Advocates for the Developmentally Disabled nor by me as their representative. (Burke, 2000, p. 1)

This statement is still, in 2000, at the heart of the debate in Illinois. Advocates for the retention of institutions continue to hold their ground, and there has been little success in moving the State further toward establishing more integrated community residential services for people with developmental disabilities. As of September 2001, the impact of the *Olmstead* decision on the State, beyond development of the working paper by the steering committees, has been limited at best.

Conclusions

What is most evident from this brief review of developments in Michigan and Illinois is the foundations laid in the 1970s and 1980s continued to guide each state well into the 1990s. The systemic inertia that characterized Illinois in the 1970s and 1980s remained a key feature of the residential service system in the 1990s. Evidence of this comes from the state's failure to expand supported living, and its retention of public and private institutions. Advocacy efforts of the State Arc continued to be perceived by most interview respondents as ineffective, marred by their financial reliance on service providers, whose interests they were compelled to represent. Given the ongoing importance of politics in the State, it seems unlikely that major changes to the status quo will occur soon.

In Michigan, there is little doubt the heyday of developmental disabilities community services as a civil rights struggle ended. Most interview respondents reported that the service system was eroding. This decline in the service system was attributed by most interview respondents to Gov. John Engler, and the limited effectiveness of advocates at the beginning of the 1990s. Governor Engler has been committed to reducing the size of state government, and many advocates contended that this commitment was pursued at the cost of quality services for people with developmental disabilities. One clear manifestation of these cost-cutting efforts was the reduction in state funds for developmental disabilities services, which declined 12% in inflation-adjusted terms from 1992-2000.

In spite of the financial implications of Governor Engler's administration, Michigan's developmental disabilities service system continued to be an innovator during the 1990s. The implementation of new programs included passage of legislation mandating person-centered planning, utilization of federal CSLA funds to transform part of the state's residential services to supported living, the elimination of all privately operated ICFs/MR in the State, and the initiation of managed long-term care. While a comprehensive assessment of each of these initiatives is far beyond the scope of this epilogue, it is clear that Michigan's willingness to pursue innovation in its service system is a trend that continued into the 1990s.

REFERENCES

Aday, L. A. (1996.). *Designing and conducting health surveys: A comprehensive guide.* San Francisco: Jossey-Bass.

Allard, M., Howard, A., Vorderer, L., & Wells, A. (1999). *Collected works of Gunnar Dybwad.* Washington, DC: AAMR

American Association on Mental Deficiency. (1959). *Directory of the American Association on Mental Deficiency-1958: Appendix A, Listings of state and private training schools and homes for the retarded.* Washington, DC: Author. [Archives and Library on Disability, Coleman Institute for Cognitive Disabilities, University of Colorado System]

Angelotti, S. (1997). *Closures of mental health facilities, 1980-1998.* Lansing, MI: Senate Fiscal Agency.

Association for Retarded Citizens of Illinois. (1985, March 9). *Board of Directors' meeting minutes.* Chicago: Author. [Collection of the Arc of Illinois]

Association for Retarded Citizens of Illinois. (1986, February 22). *Board of Directors' meeting minutes.* Chicago: Author. [Collection of the Arc of Illinois]

Association for Retarded Citizens of Illinois. (1987, February 7). *Board of Directors' meeting minutes.* Chicago: Author. [Collection of the Arc of Illinois]

Association for Retarded Citizens of Illinois. (1988, January 16). *Board of Directors' meeting minutes.* Chicago: Author. [Collection of the Arc of Illinois]

Babcock, C. P. (1982a, February 19). *Letter to W. Faust.* Lansing, MI: Department of Mental Health.

Babcock, C. P. (1982b, August 4). *Letter to H. Shapiro.* Lansing, MI: Department of Mental Health.

Babcock, C. P. (1983, August 3). *The need to assess the work ability of functionally limited Supplemental Security Insurance (SSI).applicants: Testimony presented to House Ways and Means Committee, Subcommittee on Public Assistance and Employment Insurance.* Lansing, MI: Department of Mental

Health. [Archives and Library on Disability, Coleman Institute for Cognitive Disabilities, University of Colorado System]

Babcock, C. P. (1985, February). *FY85-86 executive budget summary of recommendations.* Lansing, MI: Department of Mental Health. [Michigan State Archives, RG 89-498, Box 15]

Bailey, R. E, & Evans, E. S. (1996). *Descriptive inventory of the Archives of the State of Illinois* (2nd ed.). Springfield: Office of the Secretary of State, Illinois State Archives.

Bardach, E. (1977). *The implementation game: What happens after a bill becomes a law.* Cambridge, MA: The MIT Press.

Bauer, E., et al. (1988, February 2). *Letter to Governor James Blanchard.* Lansing, MI: Michigan Protection and Advocacy Service. [Archives and Library on Disability, Coleman Institute for Cognitive Disabilities, University of Colorado System]

Belcher, T. L. (1994). Movement to the community: Reduction of behavioral difficulties. *Mental Retardation, 32,* 89-90.

Benac, N. (1981, August 6). 'Home' leaders cry 'smear.' *Lansing State Journal* (pp. 3A-4A). Lansing, MI.

Berkowitz, E. D. (1995). *Mr. Social Security: The life of Wilbur Cohen.* Lawrence: University of Kansas Press.

Berry, J. O. (1995). Families and deinstitutionalization: An application of Bronfenbrenner's social ecology model. *Journal of Counseling & Development. 73,* 379-383.

Biklen, D. (1991). Small homes. In S. J. Taylor, R. Bogdan, & J. A. Racino (Eds.). *Life in the community: Case studies of organizations supporting people with disabilities* (Vol. 1, pp. 35-54). Baltimore, MD: Brookes.

Blanchard, J. (1988, March 3). Letter to Elizabeth Bauer. Lansing, MI Office of the Governor. [Archives and Library on Disability, Coleman Institute for Cognitive Disabilities, University of Colorado System]

Bogard, et al. v. Patla, et al. (2000). Modified consent decree. No. 88 C 2414.

Boggs, E. M., Hanley-Maxwell, C., Lakin, K. C. & Bradley, V. J. (1988). Federal policy and legislation: Factors that have constrained and facilitated community integration. In L. W. Heal, J. I. Haney, & A. R. N. Amado (Eds.), *Integration of developmentally disabled individuals into the community* (pp. 245-271). Baltimore: Brookes.

Boudreau, et al. v. Ryan, et al. (2001, August 21). Memorandum opinion. Case No. 00C5392, Judge John Grady, United States District Court, Northern District of Illinois.

Braddock, D. (1986a). Federal assistance for mental retardation and developmental disabilities II: The modern era. *Mental Retardation, 24,* 175-182.

Braddock, D. (1986b). From Roosevelt to Reagan: Federal spending for mental retardation and developmental disabilities. *American Journal on Mental Deficiency, 90,* 479-489.

Braddock, D. (1986c, January 21). *Deinstitutionalization in the Eighties: Trends in Georgia, the South, and the U.S. Remarks given at the University of Georgia.* Chicago: University of Illinois at Chicago.

Braddock, D. (1987). *Federal policy toward mental retardation and developmental disabilities.* Baltimore: Brookes.

Braddock, D. (1999). Aging and developmental disabilities: Demographic and policy issues affecting American families. *Mental Retardation, 37,* 155-161.

Braddock, D. (2001). *Public financial support for disability at the close of the 20th century.* Boulder: University of Colorado, Coleman Institute for Cognitive Disabilities.

Braddock, D. & Fujiura, G. (1987). State government financial effort in mental retardation. *American Journal of Mental Deficiency, 91,* 450-459.

Braddock, D. & Fujiura, G. (1991). Politics, public policy and the development of community mental retardation services in the United States. *American Journal on Mental Retardation, 95,* 369-387.

Braddock, D., & Heller, T. (1985). The closure of mental retardation institutions I: Trends in the United States. *Mental Retardation, 23,* 168-176.

Braddock, D., Hemp, R., Bachelder, L., & Fujiura,

G. (1995). *The state of the states in developmental disabilities* (4th ed.). Washington, DC: American Association on Mental Retardation.

Braddock, D., Hemp, R., Parish, S, & Westrich, J. (1998). *The state of the states in developmental disabilities* (5th ed.). Washington, DC: American Association on Mental Retardation.

Braddock, D., Hemp, R., Parish, S., Westrich, J., & Park, H. (1998). The state of the states in developmental disabilities: Summary of the study. In D. Braddock, R. Hemp, S. Parish, & J. Westrich (Eds.), *The state of the states in developmental disabilities* (5th ed., pp. 23-54). Washington, DC: American Association on Mental Retardation.

Braddock, D., Hemp, R. Rizzolo, M. C., Parish, S., & Pomeranz, A. (2002). The state of the states in developmental disabilities: 2002 study summary. Boulder: Coleman Institute for Cognitive Disabilities and Department of Psychiatry, The University of Colorado.

Brazer, H. E. (1982, Winter). Anatomy of a fiscal crisis: The Michigan case. *Public Budgeting & Finance,* 130-142.

Breslin, K., Ganski, L., Knight, A., O'Dell, D., & Unterbrink, R. L. (1980). *A report on land use regulations v. community homes for the developmentally disabled.* Chicago, IL: Association for Retarded Citizens of Illinois . [Archives and Library on Disability, Coleman Institute for Cognitive Disabilities, University of Colorado System]

Browne, W. P., & Verburg, K. (1995). *Michigan politics and government: Facing change in a complex state.* Lincoln: University of Nebraska Press.

Brundage, A. (1989). *Going to the sources: A guide to historical research and writing.* Arlington Heights, IL: Harlan Davidson.

Burke, R. (2000). *Dissenting opinion by Rita Burke, President of the Illinois League of Advocates for the Developmentally Disabled; Report on Illinois' activities in response to the Americans with Disabilities Act in light of the Olmstead Decision.* Springfield: Illinois Department of Human Services.

Burke, W. J., & Hopp, T. (1999, February 3).

Amicus curiae brief of the Voice of the Retarded, et al., In support of affirmance. Tommy Olmstead et al. v. L.C. and E.W. et al., Supreme Court No 98-536.

Burke, W. J. & Sherman, W. F. (1998, November, 11). *Petition for writ of certiorari: Parent-Guardian Association of Arlington Developmental Center v. People First of Tennessee.*

Butterworth, J., Hagner, D., Heikkinen, B., DeMello, S., & McDonough, K. (1993). *Whole life planning: A guide for organizers and facilitators.* Boston: Children's Hospital, Institute for Community Inclusion.

Calia, R. (1996). *The institutional origins of social policy in the American states.* Unpublished doctoral dissertation, University of Chicago.

Castellani, P. J. (1992). Closing institutions in New York State: Implementation and management lessons. *Journal of Policy Analysis and Management, 11,* 593-611.

Chambers, D. E. (1985). The Reagan Administration's welfare retrenchment policy: Terminating Social Security benefits for the disabled. *Policy Studies Review, 5,* 230-240.

Citizens Council on Mental Health and Developmental Disabilities. (1986). *Annual report.* Springfield, IL: Author.

Citizens Council on Mental Health and Developmental Disabilities. (1987). *Annual report.* Springfield, IL: Illinois General Assembly.

City of Livonia v. Department of Social Services, Greentrees Civic Association Inc. v. Pignatiello, 423 Michigan 466 (1985).

Class X passes as part of sentence reform law. (1978, January). *Illinois Issues, 4*(1), 27.

Code of Federal Regulations (October 1, 1999). *Title 45, Volume 1, Part 74.43, Competition.* Washington, DC: Government Printing Office.

Cohen, W. J. (1978, September 11). *Statement to the Joint Committee to Study Abuse in State Mental Health Facilities.* Lansing: University of Michigan. [Michigan State Archives, Record Group 86-6, Lot 98, Box 2]

Commission on Mental Health. (1965, April 1). *Report of the commission.* Springfield, IL: Author.

Commission on Mental Health. (1969, April 1). *Report to the General Assembly and the Governor.* Springfield, IL: Author.

Committee on Mental Retardation. (1970, July 16). *Meeting minutes.* Springfield, IL: Department of Mental Health. [Illinois State Archives, Record Group 218.009]

Committee on Mental Retardation. (1971, April 27). *Meeting minutes.* Springfield, IL: Department of Mental Health.

Committee on Mental retardation. (1971, May 19). *Meeting minutes.* Springfield, IL: Department of Mental Health. [Illinois State Archives, Record Group 218.009]

Committee on Mental retardation. (1971, July 8). *Meeting minutes.* Springfield, IL: Department of Mental Health. [Illinois State Archives, Record Group 218.009]

Committee on Mental Retardation (1972, November 16). *Meeting minutes.* Springfield, IL: Department of Mental Health [Illinois State Archives, Record Group 218.009]

Committee on Mental Retardation. (1973, March 22). *Meeting minutes.* Springfield, IL: Department of Mental Health. [Illinois State Archives, Record Group 218.009]

Connelly, S. R. (2001, May). Executive director's message. *Misericordia Newsletter.* Chicago, IL: Misericordia.

Conner v. Branstad, 839 F. Supp. 1346 (S.D. Iowa, 1993), 18 MPDLR 284.

Cook, T. D., & Campbell, D. T. (1979). *Quasi-experimentation: Design and analysis issues for field settings.* Boston: Houghton-Mifflin.

Covert, S. B., MacIntosh, J. D., & Shumway, D. L. (1994). Closing the Laconia State School and Training Center: A case study in systems change. In V. J. Bradley & B. Blaney (Eds.), *Creating individual supports for persons with developmental disabilities* (pp. 197-211). Baltimore, MD: Brookes.

Criminal Justice Institute. (1995). *Corrections yearbook.* Middletown, CT: Author.

Curtis, P. A. (1983). *Eugenic reformers, cultural perceptions of dependent populations, and the care of the feebleminded in Illinois, 1909-1920.* Unpublished doctoral dissertation, University of Illinois at Chicago.

Czaja, R., & Blair, J. (1996). *Designing surveys: A guide to decisions and procedures.* Thousand Oaks, CA: Pine Forge Press.

Davis, S. (1997, November). *A status report to the nation on people with mental retardation waiting for community services.* Arlington, TX: Arc/United States.

Dempsey, J. (1977). *Memorandum to Department of Social Services staff.* Lansing, MI: Department of Social Services. [Archives and Library on Disability, Coleman Institute for Cognitive Disabilities, University of Colorado System]

Derber, M. (1989). *Labor in Illinois: The affluent years, 1945-80.* Urbana: University of Illinois Press.

Developmental Disabilities Study Committee of the House of Representatives. (January 1973). *Report to the General Assembly.* Springfield, IL: Author.

Dilley, P. (1987). Social Security disability: Political philosophy and history. In A. T. Meyerson & T. Fine (Eds.), *Psychiatric disability: Clinical, legal and administrative dimensions.* Washington, DC: American Psychiatric Press.

Dillman, D. A. (1978). *Mail and telephone surveys: The total design method.* New York: Wiley.

Dixon Association for Retarded Citizens v. Thompson et al. (June 4, 1982). Motion for Direct Appeal to the Illinois Supreme Court, Motion For Stay, And Motion For Expedited briefing and Argument Schedule In The Supreme Court of Illinois.

Dixon Association for Retarded Citizens et al. v. Thompson et al. Opinions of the Supreme Court of Illinois. Springfield: Supreme Court of Illinois.

Dybwad, G. (1996). Setting the stage historically. In G. Dybwad & H. Bersani (Eds.), *Self-advocacy by people with disabilities* (pp. 1-17). Cambridge, MA: Brookline Books.

Dye, T. (1966). *Politics, economics, and the public: Policy outcomes in the American states.* Chicago: Rand McNally.

Elazar, D. J. (1984). *American federalism: A view from the states* (3rd ed.). New York: Harper & Row.

Flanigan, B. (1982, May 4). FBI will probe two arson cases at group homes. *Detroit Free Press,* (pp. 3A, 10A). Detroit, MI.

Franklin, C., & Ballan, M. (2001). Reliability and validity in qualitative research. In B. Thyer (Ed.), *The handbook of social work research* (pp. 273-292). Thousand Oaks, CA: Sage.

Frohboese, R., & Sales, D. (1980). Parental opposition to deinstitutionalization: A challenge in need of attention and resolution. *Law & Human Behavior, 4,* 1-87.

Furth, J. (May 11, 2001). Mental health center's planned closing cheered: But union leaders say trend betrays disabled. *Detroit News.* Detroit, MI.

Garrity v. Gallen, 522 F. Supp. 171 (D.N.H. 1981).

Glick, H. R. (1999). Courts: Politics and the judicial process. In V. Gray, R. L. Hanson, & H. Jacob (Eds.), *Politics in the American states: A comparative analysis* (pp. 232-266). Washington, D.C.: Congressional Quarterly Books.

Goldberg, S. (1985, May 16). Proposal would limit adult foster care homes. *Detroit Free Press,* (pp. 3A, 13A). Detroit, MI.

Goldman, H. H., & Gattozzi, B. S. (1988). Murder in the cathedral revisited: President Reagan and the mentally disabled. *Hospital and Community Psychiatry, 39,* 505-509.

Gove S. K., & Nowland J.D. (1996). *Illinois politics and government: The expanding metropolitan frontier.* Lincoln: University of Nebraska Press.

Governor's Interagency Community Placement Coordinating Council. (1981, June 12). *Meeting minutes.* Lansing, MI: Author. [Archives and Library on Disability, Coleman Institute for Cognitive Disabilities, University of Colorado System]

Governor's Planning Council on Developmental Disabilities. (1978). *Plan for the developmentally disabled.* Springfield, IL: Author.

Governor's Planning Council on Developmental Disabilities. (1987, April). *Data and information report on service needs and issues affecting persons who are developmentally disabled: Volume 2.* Chicago: Author. [Archives and Library on Disability, Coleman Institute for

Cognitive Disabilities, University of Colorado System]

Governor's Task Force on the Future of Mental Health in Illinois. (1987, January 15). *Report of the governor's task force on the future of mental health in Illinois.* Springfield, IL: Author. [Archives and Library on Disability, Coleman Institute for Cognitive Disabilities, University of Colorado System]

Governor's Task Force on Prevention and Investigation of Abuse in State Institutions. (1978, July 20). *Final Report.* Lansing, MI: Author.

Gray, V. (1999). The socioeconomic and political context of states. In V. Gray, R. L. Hanson, & H. Jacob (Eds.), *Politics in the American states: A comparative analysis* (pp. 1-31). Washington, D.C.: Congressional Quarterly Books.

Grimes, S. K., & Vitello, S. J. (1990). Follow-up study of family attitudes toward deinstitutionalization: Three to seven years later. *Mental Retardation, 28,* 219-225.

Griswold, P. P., & Walden, B. (1986, May 1). *Memo to Michigan Rehabilitation Community re: Supported Employment Site Applications.* Lansing, MI: Department of Education. [Archives and Library on Disability, Coleman Institute for Cognitive Disabilities, University of Colorado System]

Grosshans, W., & Chelimsky, E. (1990). *Case study evaluations.* Washington, DC: General Accounting Office.

Grumet, B. R. (1985). The changing role of the federal and state courts in safeguarding the rights of the mentally disabled. *Publius, 15,* 67-80.

Hammer, P. B., & Howse, J. (1977). Legislation. In J.L. Paul, D.J. Stedman, & G.R. Neufeld (Eds.), *Deinstitutionalization: Program and policy development* (pp. 140-165). Syracuse, NY: Syracuse University Press.

Harris, G. A. (1974, June). *A guide to services for the mentally retarded in Michigan.* Lansing: Michigan Association for Retarded Children and Adults.

Harris, G. A., and Miller, S. K. (1974). *A plan for improved services for the developmentally disabled in Michigan.* Lansing: Michigan Association for Retarded Children and Adults.

Hart, J., & Hollister, D. (1978, September 26). *Memo to interested parties.* Lansing, MI: The Senate. [Michigan State Archives, Record Group 86-6, Box 3]

Hayden, M. F. (1997). Class-action, civil rights litigation for institutionalized persons with mental retardation and other developmental disabilities. *Mental and Physical Disability Law Reporter, 21,* 411-423.

Health Care Financing Administration. (1999, January). *Management review of the Illinois Home and Community Based Services Waiver program for people with mental retardation and developmental disabilities: Control number 0205.90.* Chicago, IL: Author.

Health Facilities Planning Board. (1977). *Inventory of health facilities and needs assessment.* Springfield: Illinois Department of Public Health.

Health Facilities Planning Board (1982, May 20). *The Illinois long-term care and chronic disease facilities plan, Chapter 3B, 3rd Ed.* Springfield, IL: Illinois Department of Public Health, Office of Health Facilities and Quality of Care.

Health Facilities Planning Board. (1985). *Inventory of health care facilities and need determinations by planning area.* Springfield, IL: Author.

Health Facilities Planning Board. (2001, May 17). *Results of May 17, 2000, meeting of the Illinois Health Facilities Planning Board.* Springfield: Illinois Department of Public Health.

Heller, T., & Braddock, D. (1986). *The closure of the Dixon Developmental Center: Final report.* Chicago: University of Illinois at Chicago, Institute for the Study of Developmental Disabilities.

Hofferbert, R. I. (1966). The relation between public policy and some structural and environmental variables in the American states. *American Political Science Review, 50,* 73-82.

Holbrook, T. M., & Percy, S. L. (1992). Exploring variations in state laws providing protections for persons with disabilities. *Western Political Quarterly, 45,* 201-220.

Homeward Bound v. Hissom Mem'l Ctr., No. 85-C-437-E (N.D. Okla. Jan. 12, 1990), 14 MPDLR 133.

House Committee on Mental Health. (1983, November 8). *Meeting minutes.* Lansing, MI: Author. [Michigan State Archives, Record Group 85-25, Box 17]

House Democratic Staff. (1980, July). *1980 update survey of state residential facilities.* Springfield, IL: Author.

House Fiscal Agency. (1989, April 17). *The crisis in Michigan criminal justice system: Causes, consequences, and options.* Lansing, MI: Author.

Huberman, A. M., & Miles, M. B. (1994). Data management and analysis methods. In N.K. Denzin & Y.S. Lincoln (Eds.), *Handbook of qualitative research* (pp. 428-444). Thousand Oaks, CA: Sage.

Human Services Research Institute. (1978, June). *Michigan housing site visit report.* Washington, DC: Author.

Illinois Association for the Mentally Retarded. (1965, December). *Survey of attitudes and coping mechanisms of parents of retarded children not on waiting lists of State Schools for the mentally retarded.* Chicago, IL: Author.

Illinois Association for the Mentally Retarded. (1968, October 12). *Board of Directors' meeting minutes.* Chicago: Author. [Collection of the Arc of Illinois]

Illinois Association for Retarded Citizens. (1973, October 13). *Board of Directors' meeting minutes.* Chicago, IL: Author. [Collection of the Arc of Illinois].

Illinois Association for Retarded Citizens. (1977, June 18). *Board of Directors' meeting minutes.* Chicago, IL: Author. [Collection of the Arc of Illinois].

Illinois Association for Retarded Citizens. (1979, September 15). *Board of Directors' meeting minutes.* Chicago: Author. [Collection of the Arc of Illinois]

Illinois Association for Retarded Citizens. (1983, February 19). *Board of Directors' meeting minutes.* Chicago: Author. [Collection of the Arc of Illinois]

Illinois Coalition of ICF/DD Providers. (1987, March). *The crisis in Intermediate Care Facilities for the developmentally disabled.* Springfield, IL: Author.

Illinois Commission on Intergovernmental Cooperation. (1979, May 18). *Controlling governmental costs: A staff analysis of the Governor's Cost Control Task Force Report, Research memorandum No. 66.* Springfield, IL: Author.

Illinois Commission on Mental Health and Developmental Disabilities. (1977). *Mental Health '77: A system in transition, Annual Report, 1976-1977.* Chicago, IL: Author

Illinois Council for Mentally Retarded Children. (1966, April 2). *Board of Directors' meeting minutes.* Chicago, IL: Author. [Collection of the Arc of Illinois]

Illinois Department of Corrections. (2000). *Annual report.* Springfield, IL: Author.

Illinois Department of Mental Health. (1964). *A comprehensive planning program for mental health.* Springfield, IL: Author.

Illinois Department of Mental Health. (1966, June 1). *A statement of program and policy.* Springfield, IL: Author.

Illinois Department of Mental Health. (1969, June 1). *A statement of program and policy.* Springfield, IL: Author.

Illinois Department of Mental Health. (1971, December 27). *Policy for placement of adults in licensed community care facilities.* Springfield, IL.

Illinois Department of Mental Health. (1972, Autumn). *Reaching out: A quarterly publication of the Illinois Department of Mental Health: Annual report '72.* Springfield, IL: Author.

Illinois Department of Mental Health. (1973a). *Executive Order No. 61.* Springfield, IL: Author.

Illinois Department of Mental Health. (1973b). *Annual report for the fiscal year July 1, 1972 – June 30, 1973.* Springfield, IL: Author.

Illinois Department of Mental Health. (1973c). *Illinois state plan for the construction of Community Mental Health centers: FY 1973 addendum to the 1969 plan.* Springfield, IL: Author. [Archives and Library on Disability, Coleman Institute for Cognitive Disabilities, University of Colorado System]

Illinois Department of Mental Health and Developmental Disabilities. (1974). *Annual report for the fiscal year July 1, 1973- June 30, 1974.*

Springfield, IL: Author.

Illinois Department of Mental Health and Developmental Disabilities. (1976, November). *A five-year plan to guide the Department of Mental Health and Developmental Disabilities in its policies, operations, and administration: FY 1976-1980.* Springfield, IL: Author.

Illinois Department of Mental Health and Developmental Disabilities. (1980). *Illinois plan for state-operated developmental centers: 1980-83: Submission to HEW.* Springfield, IL: Author. [Archives and Library on Disability, Coleman Institute for Cognitive Disabilities, University of Colorado System]

Illinois Department of Mental Health and Developmental Disabilities. (1983, September). *Report to Governor James R. Thompson on the future of the mental health and developmentally disabled service system in Illinois, including specific recommendations concerning Galesburg Mental Health Center, Elgin Mental Health Center, and Manteno Mental Health Center.* Springfield, IL: Author.

Illinois Department of Mental Health and Developmental Disabilities. (1984, April). *Annual Plan: 1984-85.* Springfield, IL: Author.

Illinois Department of Mental Health and Developmental Disabilities. (1985). *Annual plan: 1985-86.* Springfield, IL: Author.

Illinois Department of Mental Health and Developmental Disabilities. (1990). *Housing development strategies.* Springfield, IL: Author.

Illinois Department of Mental Health and Developmental Disabilities. (1992). *DMHDD staff summary: Nathan v. Levitt third revised consent decree.* Springfield, IL: Author.

Illinois Department of Mental Health and Developmental Disabilities. (1995). *FY95 Bogard plan.* Springfield, IL: Author.

Illinois Department of Public Aid. (1988, January 1). *Status report on potential decertified long-term care facilities.* Springfield, IL: Author. [Archives and Library on Disability, Coleman Institute for Cognitive Disabilities, University of Colorado System]

Illinois Department of Public Health. (2000, September 28). S*tatement of deficiencies and plan of correction: Lincoln Developmental Center.* Springfield, IL: Author.

Illinois Department of Public Health. (2001). *State agency report: Marklund at Mill Creek, Project #00-080.* Springfield, IL: Author.

Illinois General Assembly. (1972, June). *House Joint Resolution 146.* Springfield, IL: Author.

Illinois House of Representatives. (1972). *House Resolution 568.*Springfield, IL: Author.

Illinois House of Representatives. (1973, June 1). *House Resolution 382.* Springfield, IL: Author.

Illinois House of Representatives. (1974, April 17). *House Resolution 785.* Springfield, IL: Author.

Illinois House of Representatives. (1975). *House Resolution 1277.* Springfield, IL: Author.

Illinois Information Service. (1970). *Press release on the groundbreaking ceremony for the Ludeman Mental Retardation Center.* Springfield, IL: Author.

Illinois Legislative Investigating Commission. (1973, February). *Peoria State Hospital.* Springfield, IL: Author.

Illinois Legislative Investigating Commission. (1974, June). *Patient deaths at Elgin State Hospital.* Springfield, IL: Author.

Illinois Legislative Investigating Commission. (1977, February). *Lake County nursing homes.* Springfield, IL: Author.

Illinois Legislative Investigating Commission. (1980, July). Illinois nursing homes. Springfield, IL: Author.

Illinois Mental Health Planning Board. (1968, December). *Comprehensive planning for mental health in Illinois: Interim report.* Chicago, IL: Author.

Illinois Office of the Auditor General. (1978, December). *Feasibility study: Use of vacant state-owned mental health and developmental disabilities facilities.* Springfield, IL: Author.

Illinois Planning Council on Developmental Disabilities. (1991, January 31). *Recommendations to the Illinois General Assembly on zoning for community residences.* Springfield, IL: Author. [Archives and Library on Disability, Coleman Institute for Cognitive Disabilities, University of Colorado System]

Interdepartmental Committee on Mental Retardation

and Illinois Association for the Mentally Retarded. (1968). *Directory of services for the mentally retarded in Illinois.* Springfield, IL: Department of Mental Health.

Joint Capital Outlay Subcommittee. (1981, July 1). *Meeting minutes.* Lansing, MI: House of Representatives. [Archives and Library on Disability, Coleman Institute for Cognitive Disabilities, University of Colorado System]

Joint Committee to Study Abuse in State Mental Health Facilities. (1978). *Report to the Michigan 79th Legislature, Regular Session of 1978.* Lansing, MI: Author. [Michigan State Archives, Record Group 86-6, Lot 98, Box 3]

Joint Mental Health Oversight Committee. (1980, July). *Interim report on community placement of mentally disabled persons in Michigan.* Lansing, MI: Author.

King, G., Keohane, R. O., & Verba, S. (1994). *Designing social inquiry: Scientific inference in qualitative research.* Princeton, NJ: Princeton University Press.

Kingdon, J. (1995). *Agendas, alternatives, and public policies* (2nd ed.). New York: Harper-Collins.

Knobbe, C. A., Carey, S. P., Rhodes, L., & Horner, R. H. (1995). Benefit-cost analysis of community residential services for adults with severe mental retardation and challenging behaviors. *American Journal on Mental Retardation, 99,* 533-541.

Kope et al. v. Watkins, Blanchard, et al. (1988, March 30).Complaint. Filed in the Third Judicial Circuit Court by Michigan Protection and Advocacy Service. Detroit, MI: Michigan Protection and Advocacy Service.

Kvale, S. (1996). *Interviews: An introduction to qualitative research interviewing.* Thousand Oaks, CA: Sage.

Lakin, K. C. (1979). *Demographic studies of residential facilities for the mentally retarded: An historical review of methodologies and findings.* Minneapolis: University of Minnesota, Developmental Disabilities Project on Residential Services and Community Adjustment.

Legislative Commission to Visit and Examine State Institutions, Charitable Subcommittee. (1972, August). *Report of the findings and recommen-*

dations after the visitation of Elgin State Hospital. Springfield, IL: Author.

Legislative Commission to Visit and Examine State Institutions, Charitable Subcommittee. (1974). *Report to the Governor and 78th General Assembly.* Springfield, IL: Author.

Legislative Commission to Visit and Examine State Institutions, Subcommittee on Charitable Institutions. (1976). *Charitable institutions report.* Springfield, IL: Author.

Leismer, J. (1983, May 31). The Plymouth Case: Implementation of a consent decree. Paper presented at AAMD Conference. Dallas, TX. [Archives and Library on Disability, Coleman Institute for Cognitive Disabilities, University of Colorado System]

Lerner, H. J. (1972). *New York Association for Retarded Children and New York State Government, 1948-1968.* New York: New York State Association for Retarded Children.

Luke, R. T. (1975). *The sources of innovation in state government: Rehabilitating the Texas mental health system.* Unpublished doctoral dissertation, Harvard University.

Lynch, P. S., Kellow, J. T., & Wilson, V. L. (1997). The impact of deinstitutionalization on the adaptive behavior of adults with mental retardation: A meta-analysis. *Education & Training in Mental Retardation, 32,* 255-261.

Mahar, W. (1987, October 8). Letter to Governor James Thompson. Springfield, IL: Author.

Malcolm, et al. v. Shamie, et al. (January 23, 1980). Final ruling. State of Michigan Court of Appeals. Judges: Burns, Cavanagh, & Holbrook.

Marklund. (2001, Summer). Marklund Care Letter, pp. 1, 3, 5. Bloomington, IL: Author.

Marshall, C., & Rossman, G.B. (1999). *Designing qualitative research* (3rd ed.). Thousand Oaks, CA: Sage.

Mazmanian, D. A., & Sabatier, P. A. (1983). *Implementation and public policy.* Glenview, IL: Scott, Foresman.

Meier, K. J. (1989). Bureaucratic leadership in public organizations. In B. D. Jones (Ed.), *Leadership and politics: New perspectives in political science* (pp. 267-288). Lawrence: University Press of Kansas.

Merriam, S. B. (1997). *Qualitative research and case study applications in education.* San Francisco: Jossey-Bass.

Michigan ARC v. Smith, 475 F. Supp. 990 (E.D. Mich. 1979), 3 MDLR 391.

Michigan Department of Community Health. (1998). *Person-centered planning practice guide.* Lansing, MI: Author.

Michigan Department of Community Health. (2000, September). *Revised plan for procurement of Medicaid specialty prepaid health plans: Final version.* Lansing, MI: Author.

Michigan Department of Community Health. (2001, May). *News release.* Lansing, MI: Author.

Michigan Department of Corrections. (2000). *Annual report.* Lansing, MI: Author.

Michigan Department of Mental Health. (1962, January). *Parents' interest in institutionalization of patients waiting admission to state home and training schools: Research report No. 38.* Lansing, MI: Author.

Michigan Department of Mental Health. (1966, July). *Progress report: A plan to combat mental retardation in Michigan.* Lansing, MI: Author.

Michigan Department of Mental Health. (1967, October). *Working patients in state hospitals.* Lansing, MI: Author. [Michigan State Archives, Record Group 80-71, Lot 49, Reel 1907

Michigan Department of Mental Health. (1973). *Macomb-Oakland Residential Center Annual Report: Transition.* St. Clemens, MI: Author.

Michigan Department of Mental Health. (1976, April). Ben and Diana will be missed. *Transition, 4* (4), 4.

Michigan Department of Mental Health. (1977). *AIS/MR and ICF/MR.* Lansing, MI: Author.

Michigan Department of Mental Health. (1978, April). Severe/profound clients placed in the community: 54% of total placements. *Transition, 6* (4), 1-2.

Michigan Department of Mental Health. (1979, March). Courts rule that MORC clients constitute a family: Decisions seen as major victory. *Transition, 7* (2), 1.

Michigan Department of Mental Health. (1980, June 2). *AIS/MR development status as of June 2,*

1980. Lansing, MI: Author.

Michigan Department of Mental Health. (1981a, July-August). News in transition. *Transition, 9* (3), 4. [Archives and Library on Disability, Coleman Institute for Cognitive Disabilities, University of Colorado System]

Michigan Department of Mental Health. (1981b). *Community placement status report.* Lansing, MI: Author.

Michigan Department of Mental Health. (1983). *FY 84-85 management plan: Summary of recommendations.* Lansing, MI: Author.

Michigan Department of Mental Health. (1985). *Fact sheet: Group homes: Alternatives to institutions.* Lansing, MI: Author. [Archives and Library on Disability, Coleman Institute for Cognitive Disabilities, University of Colorado System]

Michigan Department of Mental Health. (1987). *State of Michigan: Home and Community-Based Services Waiver for the developmentally disabled.* Lansing, MI: Author.

Michigan Department of Mental Health. (1988a). *Alternative disposition plan submitted in accordance with the provisions of the Omnibus Budget Reconciliation Act of 1987.* Lansing, MI: Author.

Michigan Department of Mental Health. (1988b). *Family support subsidy program report: FY86-87.* Lansing, MI: Author.

Michigan Department of Public Health. (1984, January). *Directory of hospitals, nursing care facilities, homes for the aged, mental health facilities.* Lansing, MI: Author.

Michigan Departments of Public Health and Mental Health. (1966). *Michigan state plan for the construction of community facilities for the mentally retarded: 1965-66.* Lansing, MI: Author.

Michigan Department of Social Services. (1980, March 5). *Bureau of Regulatory Services Licensing Manual Bulletin. Act 281, Public Act of 1979. Adult foster care facility licensing act. Effective March 27, 1980.* Lansing, MI: Author.

Michigan Departments of Social Services, Mental Health, and Education – Vocational Rehabilitation Services and State Housing Development Authority. (1976, October 12). *Memorandum of understanding.* Lansing, MI: Author. [Archives and Library on Disability, Coleman Institute for Cognitive Disabilities, University of Colorado System]

Michigan House of Representatives. (1972, March 15). House Resolution 268. Lansing, MI: Author. [Michigan State Archives, Record Group 80-71, Reel 1907, Lot 49]

Michigan Mental Health Advisory Council. (1982, December 17). *An assessment of selected issues on community placement: A report to the Governor.* Lansing, MI: Author.

Michigan Mental Health Association. (2000). April 2000 update on competitive procurement issues. *The Advocate, 24*(2), 1-3. [Published by the Michigan Mental Health Association]

Michigan Office of the Auditor General. (1981, June). *Preliminary analysis of community placement program leases and related operating issues: Interim report.* Lansing, MI: Author.

Michigan Office of the Auditor General. (1999, March). *Performance audit of Southgate Center, Department of Community Health.* Lansing, MI: Author.

Michigan Protection and Advocacy Service. (1979, April 11). *Interim P & A program performance report: Fiscal year 1978-79.* Lansing, MI: Author.

Michigan Protection and Advocacy Service. (1988, March 30). *Press release.* Lansing, MI: Author.

Michigan Protection and Advocacy Service. (1994). *Progress report.* Lansing, MI: Author.

Michigan State Planning Council on Developmental Disabilities. (1984). *Employment related activities in Michigan.* Lansing, MI: Author.

Miles, M. B., & Huberman, A. M. (1994). *Qualitative data analysis* (2nd ed.). Thousand Oaks, CA: Sage.

Miller, G. (1981). Letter to F. Kelley, Col. G. Hough, and N. Baerwaldt. Lansing, MI: Department of Management and Budget. [Archives and Library on Disability, Coleman Institute for Cognitive Disabilities, University of Colorado System]

Milliken, W. (1970a). *The Governor's budget message.* Lansing, MI: Office of the Governor.

Milliken, W. (1970b). *Governor's message to the 75th Michigan Legislature.* Lansing, MI: Office of the Governor.

Milliken, W. (1975). *Michigan state of the state message.* Lansing, MI: Office of the Governor.

Milliken, W. (1976). *State of the state message.* Lansing, MI: Office of the Governor.

Milliken, W. (1977). *State of the state message.* Lansing, MI: Office of the Governor.

Milliken, W. (1978a). *News release.* Lansing, MI: Office of the Governor. [Michigan State Archives, Record Group 86-8, Lot 98, Box 2]

Milliken, W. (1978b). *Special report to the legislature.* Lansing, MI: Office of the Governor.

Milliken, W. (1978c). Letter to Dr. John Dempsey. Lansing, MI: Office of the Governor. [Michigan State Archives, Record Group 86-6, Lot 98, Box 2]

Milliken, W. (1978d). *Michigan state of the state message.* Lansing, MI: Office of the Governor.

Milliken, W. (1979). *Michigan state of the state message.* Lansing, MI: Office of the Governor.

Milliken, W. (1980). *Michigan state of the state message.* Lansing, MI: Office of the Governor.

Milliken, W. (1982). *Michigan state of the state message.* Lansing, MI: Office of the Governor.

Moss, K. (1983). Assessing court-ordered institutional reform. *Case Analysis, 2,* 21-38.

Moss, K. (1985). The catalytic effect of a federal court decision on a state legislature. *Law & Society, 19,* 147-157.

Mount, B., & Zwernick, K. (1988). *It's never too early, it's never too late: An overview of personal futures planning.* St Paul, MN: Governor's Planning Council on Developmental Disabilities State Planning Agency.

Murphy, W. K. (1989, October 16). Memo to Department of Mental Health and Developmental Disabilities staff, facility directors, community agencies, IARF, Arc/Illinois, UCP, Autism Society, etc., RE: The Illinois Model – Community Integrated Living Arrangements for persons with developmental disabilities. Springfield, IL: Department of Mental Health and Developmental Disabilities. [Archives and Library on Disability, Coleman Institute for Cognitive Disabilities, University of Colorado System]

Nelis, T. (1995). The realities of institutions. *Impact, 9,* 1, 27.

Nelis, T., & Ward, N. (1995). Operation Close the Doors: Working for freedom. *Impact. 9,* 12.

Neugeboren, B. (1985). *Organization, policy, and practice in the human services.* New York: Longman.

Nirje, B. (1976). The normalization principle and its human management implications, in R. B. Kugel and A. Shearer (Eds.), *Changing Patterns in Residential Services For the Mentally Retarded* (pp. 231-240). Washington, DC: President's Committee on Mental Retardation.

Nowlan, J. D., & Gonet, P. M. (1991). The legislature. In J. D. Nowlan (Ed.), *Inside state government in Illinois* (pp. 65-88). Chicago: Neltnor House.

O'Brien, J., & O'Brien, C. L. (1991). Sustaining positive changes: The future development of the residential support program. In S. J. Taylor, R. Bogdan, 7 J. A. Racino (Eds.), Life in the community: Case studies of organizations supporting people with disabilities (Vol. 1, pp. 153-168). Baltimore: Brookes.

Ochberg, F. (1981, June 29). Memo to executive staff. Lansing, MI: Department of Mental Health.

Ochberg, F. (1979, October 5). Memo to Regional Directors, Hospital and Center Directors, and Community Mental Health Board Chairpersons. Subject: Consent Decree Implementation Unit. Lansing, MI: Department of Mental Health.

Office of Health and Medical Affairs. (1974, February). *Community placement program: An examination of the process and outcomes of community placement of adults and children from mental health institutions in Michigan.* Lansing, MI: Author.

Olmstead v. L. C., 119 S. Ct. 2176 (1999).

Palmer, J. A., & Feigenbaum E. D. (1990). *Campaign finance law 90: A summary of state campaign finance laws with quick reference charts.* Washington, DC: National Clearinghouse on Election Administrations.

Parish, S. L. (2001). *Comparative study of the development of MR/DD services in two midwestern states: 1970-1990.* Unpublished doctoral dissertation. Chicago: University of Illinois at Chicago.

Paulaski, T. (1998, January 16). Kreider Services unionized. *The Arc of Illinois-Today.* Homewood, IL: Arc of Illinois.

People First of Tennessee v. Arlington Developmental Ctr., 878 F. Supp. 97 (W.D. Tenn. 1992), 19 MPDLR 445.

Phillips v. Thompson, et al. (1983). 715 F. 2d 3654. (No. 82-2372).

Pomeroy, W. A. (1980, October 8). Memo to Frank Ochberg, Department of Mental Health director. Subject: Re-evaluation of Hillcrest: The deaths. Lansing, MI: Author .

Pressman, J.L., & Wildavsky, A. B. (1973). *Implementation: How great expectations in Washington are dashed in Oakland; Or, why it's amazing that federal programs work at all.* Berkeley: University of California Press.

Protection and Advocacy, Inc. (1990). *Legislative summary and analysis: The 1989 Spring session.* Chicago: Author. [Archives and Library on Disability, Coleman Institute for Cognitive Disabilities, University of Colorado System]

Prouty, R. W., & Lakin, K. C. (Eds.). (1997). *Residential services for persons with developmental disabilities: Statistics and trends through 1996.* Minneapolis: University of Minnesota, Institute on Community Integration.

Public Act 39 of 1981. (1981). Lansing, MI.

Public Act 77-2722. (1972, August 18). Springfield, IL.

Public Act 78-992 (1973). Mental Health Code Amendments. Springfield, IL.

Public Act 78-1156 (1974). Health Facilities Planning Act. Springfield, IL.

Public Act 78-1183. (1974). Act in Relation to Campaign Finance. Springfield, IL.

Public Act 79-967. (1976). Springfield, IL.

Public Act 80-1099. (1977). Springfield, IL.

Public Act 81-223. (1979, August 23). [Nursing Home Reform Act] Springfield, IL.

Public Act 82-183. (1981). Springfield, IL.

Public Act 82-567. (1981). Community Living Facilities Licensing Act. Springfield, IL.

Public Act 82-584. (1981). Community Residential Alternatives Licensing Act. Springfield, IL.

Public Act 82-921. (1982). Springfield, IL.

Public Act 83-88. (1983). Springfield, IL.

Public Act 84-567. (1985). Springfield, IL.

Public Act 86-638. (1989). Community Residence Location Planning Act. Springfield, IL.

Public Act 86-921. (1990). Developmental Disabilities Services Law. Springfield, IL.

Public Act 117 of 1975. (1975). Lansing, MI.

Public Act 151 of 1923. (1923). Lansing, MI.

Public Act 220 of 1976. (1976). Michigan Handicappers' Civil Rights Act. Lansing, MI.

Public Act 249 of 1983 (1983). Lansing, MI.

Public Act 258 of 1974. (1974). Community Mental Health Act. Lansing, MI.

Public Act 281 of 1979. (1979). Adult Foster Care Facility Licensing Act. Lansing, MI.

Public Act 360 of 1980. (1980). Lansing, MI.

Public Act 423 of 1980. (1980). Lansing, MI.

Public Acts 28-30 of 1977. (1977). Lansing, MI.

Public Acts 394-398 of 1976. (1976). Zoning Acts. Lansing, MI.

Public Interest Law Center of Philadelphia. (1988, March 23). *Frank Bogard, et al. v. Edward Duffy, et al.: A summary and explanation.* Philadelphia: Author.

Public Law 88-156. (1963). Maternal and Child Health and Mental Retardation Planning Amendments of 1963.

Public Law 91-517. (1970). Developmental Disabilities Services and Facilities Construction Act of 1970.

Public Law 92-233 (1971). Amendments to Title XIX of the Social Security Act.

Public Law 94-142. Education for All Handicapped Children Act.

Public Law 97-35. (1981). Omnibus Budget Reconciliation Act of 1981. Washington, DC.

Public Law 100-430 (1988). Fair Housing Act. Washington, DC.

Public Law 101-508. (1990). Community Supported Living Arrangements.

Public Sector Consultants. (1998, April 1). *Michigan in brief: 1998-99.* Lansing, MI: Author.

Public Sector Consultants. (2000). *Michigan in brief.* Lansing, MI: Author.

Racino, J. A. (1991). Individualized supportive living arrangements. In S. J. Taylor, R. Bogdan, & J. A. Racino (Eds.). *Life in the community: Case studies of organizations supporting people with disabilities* (Vol. 1, pp. 113-128). Baltimore: Brookes.

Racino, J. A., & Taylor, S. (1993). People first: Approaches to housing and support. In J. A. Racino, P. Walker, S. O'Connor, & S. Taylor (Eds.), *Housing, support, and community: Choices and strategies for adults with disabilities* (pp. 33-56). Baltimore: Brookes.

Ragan, J. F. (1974, November). *Mental health and developmental disabilities in Illinois: An examination.* Springfield, IL: Department of Mental Health and Developmental Disabilities.

Ramirez, R. (1979, March 26). *Memo to council members.* Springfield, IL: Governor's Planning Council on Developmental Disabilities. [Illinois State Archives, Record Group 317.01]

Rave, M. (1982). Letter to Governor-elect James J. Blanchard. Ann Arbor, MI: Mental Health Coalition of Michigan.

Redfield, K. (1994). Investing in the Illinois General Assembly: Interest group campaign contribution strategies in the 1992 legislative elections. In C. A. Roberts & P. Kleppner (Eds.), *Almanac of Illinois politics: 1994* (pp. 1-26). Springfield, IL: Sangamon State University.

Redfield, K. (1998). What keeps the four tops on top? In D. A. Joens & P. Kleppner (Eds.), *Almanac of Illinois politics: 1998* (pp. 1-8). Springfield, IL: University of Illinois, Institute for Public Affairs.

Rosen, D. (1981). Letter to the ARC/Michigan Board of Directors. Northville, MI: Office of the Master for the Plymouth Court Order. [Archives and Library on Disability, Coleman Institute for Cognitive Disabilities, University of Colorado System]

Rothman, D. J., & Rothman, S. M. (1984). *The Willowbrook wars.* New York: Harper & Row.

Rusco, J. (2001, Summer). A message from the president. *Marklund Care Letter*, p. 2. Bloomington, IL: Marklund.

Rutan et al. v. Republican Party of Illinois et al. (1989). 497 U.S. 62

Schalock, M., & Fredericks, H. D. B. (1990). Comparative costs for institutional services and services for selected populations in the community. *Behavioral Residential Treatment, 5,* 271-286.

Scheerenberger, R. C. (1968). *Mental retardation in Illinois: Progress and needs.* Springfield, IL: Department of Mental Health.

Scheerenberger, R. C. (1969). *Mental retardation in Illinois: A quarterly publication, Volune 3, No. 1.* Springfield, IL: Department of Mental Health.

Scheerenberger, R. C. (1970). *Mental retardation in Illinois: A semi-annual publication, Volume 3, No. 2.* Springfield, IL: Department of Mental Health.

Scheerenberger, R. C. (1983). *A history of mental retardation.* Baltimore: Brookes.

Scheerenberger, R. C., & Wagner, R. L. (1968). *Day programs and residential facilities for the mentally retarded in Illinois: 1967.* Springfield, IL: Division of Mental Retardation Services.

Schneider, J. (1998). *Waiting for home: The Richard Prangley story.* Grand Rapids, MI: Erdmans Publishing.

Schneider, M., Teske, P., & Mintrom, M. (1995). *Public entrepreneurs: Agents for change in American government.* Princeton, NJ: Princeton University Press.

Scott, J. (1990). *A matter of record: Documentary sources in social research.* Cambridge, MA: Polity Press.

Shafer, R. J. (1980). *A guide to historical method* (3rd ed.). Chicago: Dorsey Press.

Shapiro, H. L. (1980, June 30). Letter to Governor Milliken. Lansing, MI: Michigan Planning Council for Developmental Disabilities.

Slater, K. O. (1986). *An historical analysis of public policy for the care and treatment of people who are mentally retarded in Michigan.* Unpublished doctoral dissertation, Western Michigan University.

Sloan, K. H., & Biloon, S. (1992). Consent decrees: Policies under pressure. *Journal of State Government, 65,* 41-46.

Smith, G. A. (2002). *Status report: Litigation concerning Medicaid services for persons with developmental disabilities.* Tualatin, OR: Human Services Research Institute.

Smith, G. A., & Gettings, R. M. (1993). *Medicaid's*

ICF/MR program: Present status and recent trends. Alexandria, VA: National Association of State Directors of Developmental Disabilities Services.

Smith, G. A., & Gettings, R. M. (1994). *The HCB Waiver and CSLA Programs: An update on Medicaid's role in supporting people with developmental disabilities in the community.* Alexandria, VA: National Association of State Directors of Developmental Disabilities Services.

Smith, J. D., & Polloway, E. A. (1995). Patterns of deinstitutionalization and community placement: A dream deferred or lost? *Education and Training in Mental Retardation and Developmental Disabilities, 30,* 321-328.

Spare, P. (1999, Spring). President's message: the American Disabled for Attendant Programs Today (ADAPT). *The Voice, 1,* 1-2. [Newsletter of The Voice of the Retarded, published: Rolling Meadows, Illinois].

Spare, P. (1997; October 29). Oppose H.R. 2020: Letter sent to the entire Congress. Rolling Meadows, IL: Voice of the Retarded. Available at: http://www.naotd.org.vor2.txt.

Spitalnick, D. (1996). *Elizabeth Boggs: A tribute.* New Brunswick, NJ: University Affiliated Program of New Jersey.

Spreat, S., Conroy, J. W., & Rice, D. M. (1998). Improve quality in nursing homes or institute community placements? Implementation of OBRA for individuals with mental retardation. *Research in Developmental Disabilities, 19,* 507-518.

Spreat, S., Telles, J. L., Conroy, J. W., & Feinstein, C. (1987). Attitudes toward deinstitutionalization: National survey of families of institutionalized persons with mental retardation. *Mental Retardation, 25,* 267-274.

Stabenow, D. (1983a). *State family support/ subsidy programs* (House Committee on Mental Health minutes). Lansing, MI: House of Representatives. [Michigan State Archives, Record Group 85-25, Box 17]

Stabenow, D. (1983b). *The Family Support Subsidy Act: Questions and answers on P.A. 249 of 1983 (H.B. 4448).* Lansing, MI: House of Representatives. [Archives and Library on

Disability, Coleman Institute for Cognitive Disabilities, University of Colorado System]

State Advisory Council on Mental Retardation. (1965, July). *Patterns for planning: The Illinois approach to mental retardation: Report to Governor Otto Kerner and the Interdepartmental Committee on Mental retardation.* Springfield, IL: Author.

State of Illinois. (1970). *Constitution.* Springfield, IL: Author.

Stone, J. A. (1990). Returning to the community: A nine-year experience. *Adult Residential Care Journal, 27.*

Switzky, H. N., Dudzinski, M., Van Acker, R., & Gambro, J. (1988). Historical foundations of out-of-home residential alternatives for mentally retarded persons. In L. W. Heal, J. I. Haney, & A. R. Novak Amado (Eds.), *Integration of developmentally disabled individuals into the community* (pp. 19-36). Baltimore: Brookes.

Taylor, S. J. (1991). Toward individualized community living. In S. J. Taylor, R. Bogdan, & J. A. Racino (Eds.). *Life in the community: Case studies of organizations supporting people with disabilities* (Vol. I, pp. 105-112). Baltimore: Brookes.

Taylor, S. J., Brown, K., McCord, W., Giambetti, A., Searl, S., Mlinarcik, S., Atkinson, T., & Lichter, S. (1981). *Title XIX and deinstitutionalization: The issue for the 80s.* Syracuse, NY: Syracuse University, Center on Human Policy.

Tesch, R. (1990). *Qualitative research: Analysis types and software tools.* New York: Falmer Press.

Topper, G. (1997). *Deinstitutionalization of the mentally retarded and developmentally disabled: A statistical analysis of state variance 1977-1995.* Unpublished master's thesis, Rutgers University- Newark.

U.S. Department of Labor. (1968). *1966 Amendments to the Fair Labor Standards Act.* Washington, DC: Author.

Van Meter, M. (1980). Methodological and design issues: Techniques for assessing the representatives of snowball samples. *National Institute on Drug Abuse: Research Monograph Series, Monograph 9,* (831-43).

Visotsky, H. M. (1968). *Mental retardation and the Department of Mental Health.* Springfield, IL: Department of Mental Health .

Voice of the Retarded. (1999). Speaking out for choices. Rolling Meadows, IL: Author. Available at: http://www.vor.net/about.html

Walker, D. (1973, September 12). *Veto message.* Springfield, IL: Office of the Governor.

Walker, D. (1975, January 22). *Special message to the 79th General Assembly on the 1975-76 accelerated building program for the State of Illinois.* Springfield, IL: Office of the Governor.

Walker, D. (1976, January 14). *State of the state message to the General Assembly.* Springfield, IL: Office of the Governor.

Webb, E. J., Campbell, D. T., Schwartz, R. D., & Sechrest, L. (2000). *Unobtrusive measures* (Rev. ed.). Thousand Oaks, CA: Sage.

Wells, D. (1982, April 30). Letter to C. Simonson. Chicago, IL: Survey and Certification Operations Branch, Division of Health Standards and Quality, Department of Health and Human Services. [Illinois State Archives, Record Group 218.013]

Westmoreland, T. M., & Perez, T. (2000, January 14). *Letter to state Medicaid directors.* Washington, DC: U.S. Department of Health and Human Services.

Whitman, C., & Parnas, S. (1999). *Fair housing: The siting of group homes for the disabled and children.* Washington, DC: National League of Cities.

Wolcott, H. F. (1994). *Transforming qualitative data: Description, analysis and interpretation.* Thousand Oaks, CA: Sage.

Wolfensberger, W. (1971). Will there always be an institution? II: The impact of new service models. *Mental Retardation, 9,* 31-38.

Wolfensberger, W. (1972). *The principle of normalization in human services.* Toronto, Ontario: National Institute on Mental Retardation.

Wyatt v. Stickney, 325 F.Supp. 781 (M.D.Ala. 1971), enforced in 334 F.Supp. 1341 (1971); 344 F.Supp. 387 (1972); *Wyatt v. Aderholt,* 503 F. 2d 1305 (5th Cir. 1974).

Yin, R. K. (1994). *Case study research* (2nd ed.). Thousand Oaks, CA: Sage Publications.

Zirpoli, T. J., & Wieck, C. (1989). Economic and

political factors affecting deinstitutionalization: One state's analysis. *Journal of Special Education, 23,* 201-211.

AUTHOR INDEX

A

Adair, R. 13
Aday, L. A. 364
Agosta, J. M. 112
Albrecht, G. L. 40, 41, 42
Alexander, F. G. 8, 10, 11, 24
Allard, M. 357
Allen, E. E. 19, 20, 22
American Association on Mental Deficiency 359
American Printing House for the Blind 20, 37
Americans Disabled for Attendant Programs Today (ADAPT) 38
Andrews, J. 10, 12, 14
Angelotti, S. 383
Ansello, E. 42
Anspach, R. R. 4, 41
Arc of Illinois 89
Arc of the United States 112
Arnold, N. 38
Ashe, W. 115
Association for Retarded Citizens of Illinois 431, 433
Association of Developmental Disabilities Providers 89
Axinn, J. 13, 31

B

Babcock, C. P. 381, 383, 391, 401
Bachelder, L. 356
Bacon, F. 13
Bahl, R. 65, 120
Bailey, R. E. 369
Banks, P. D. 115
Bardach, E. 358
Barnes, C. 42
Barr, M. W. 3, 21, 27, 28
Bartlett, F. L. 27
Bassoe, P. 10
Bauer, E. 387, 393
Bauer, L. 117
Baynton, D. C. 26, 29
Beers, C. 30
Belcher, T. L. 355
Bell, A. G. 25, 29

Bell, L. V. 31
Benac, N. 380
Berger, P. 34
Berkowitz, E. D. 31, 377
Berkowitz, M. 65, 72
Berkson, G. 5
Bernstein, C. 30
Berry, J. O. 355
Bersani Jr., H. 39, 117
Bickenbach, J. E. 34
Bicknell, E. 27, 28
Biklen, D. 354
Biloon, S. 357
Birnbaum, J. 35, 41
Black, K. 8
Blair, J. 363
Blanchard, J. 394
Blanck, P. 115
Blatt, B. 25
Bliquez, L. J. 7
Bogdan, R. 27, 28
Boggs, E. M. 355, 439
Bonsall, A. 27
Boschen, K. A. 38
Bowe, F. G. 34, 37, 38
Braddock, D. 31, 32, 33, 34, 35, 36, 38, 39, 40, 65, 66, 68, 70, 72, 73, 85, 89, 91, 100, 101, 112, 115, 119, 120, 124, 126, 127, 353, 354, 355, 356, 357, 358, 376, 383, 388, 390, 396, 410, 411, 414, 416, 426, 427, 434, 439, 447, 448, 449, 450, 456, 458, 459
Bradley, V. J. 112, 355
Brazer, H. E. 382
Breckinridge, V. J. 18, 22
Bredberg, E. 3
Breslin, K. 413, 429
Brierre de Boismont, A. J. F. 24
Brigham, A. 26
British Association of the Deaf 26
Brockley, J. A. 3
Bromberg, W. 12
Brown, T. J. 22, 23
Browne, W. A. F. 24
Browne, W. P. 387

Bruininks, R. H. 89
Brundage, A. 3, 363
Bucknill, J. C. 21
Burchard, S. N. 36
Bureau of Economic Analysis 96, 97
Burke, R. 458
Burke, W. J. 357
Burleigh, M. 30
Butler, A. W. 28
Butterworth, J. 454
Button, L. A. 24

C

Caiden, N. 120
Calia, R. 355
Campbell, D. T. 367, 368
Carabello, B. J. 4
Carey, S. P. 355
Carling, P. J. 36
Carpenter, J. 28
Carrey, N. J. 20
Carrillo, H. 66
Castellani, P. J. 358
Cavallo, S. 14
Cave, A. J. E. 5
Cerletti, U. 30
Chambers, D. E. 390
Chambers, J. G. 66, 72
Charlton, J. I. 4
Chelimsky, E. 367
Chevigny, H. 34
Church, A. 29, 30
Citizens Council on Mental Health and
    Developmental Disabilities 411, 412, 430
Clay, R. M. 8
Cochrane, R. G. 25
Code of Federal Regulations 454
Cohen, W. J. 378, 379
Cole, T. 35
Colon, D. M. 12
Commission on Mental Health
    405, 406, 429, 432
Committee on Mental Retardation
    405, 406, 408, 415, 416, 430
Condillac 14
Connelly, S. R. 456
Conroy, J. W. 355

Cook, T. D. 367, 368
Covert, S. B. 38, 357, 358
Covey, H. C. 11, 16
Criminal Justice Institute 437
Curtis, P. A. 359
Czaja, R. 363

D

Dalton, A. J. 125
Daniels, M. 5, 6, 8, 18
Darlington, R. B. 33
Daston, L. 13, 28
Davenport, A. B. 28
Davidson, P. W. 125
Davies, S. P. 30
Davis, L. 3, 34
Davis, S. 126, 354
de Saint-Loup, A. 29
De Souza-Araujo, H. C. 11
Defoe, D. 15
DeJong, G. 37, 38
DeMello, S. 454
Dempsey, J. 386
DePaepe, P. 126
Derber, M. 422, 426
Developmental Disabilities Study Committee of the
    House of Representatives
    406, 407, 428, 430
Digby, A. 3, 11
Dilley, P. 390
Dillman, D. A. 363
District of Columbia Auditor 137
Dix, D. 22
Doyle, B. 39
Driedger, D. 33, 34, 37
Dudzinsky, M. 355
Dugdale, R. L. 28
Dunlap, G. 36
Dybwad, G. 39, 117, 353, 356, 357
Dye, T. 70, 355, 437

E

Earle, P. 3, 22, 23
East, E. M. 28
Eckl, C. 98
Edgerton, R. 27
Edwards, M. L. 6, 7

Edwards, P. 12, 14
Elazar, D. J. 355, 439
Elm Hill Private School and Home 26
Ely, C. W. 22
Emerson, E. 39
Enders, A. 38
Erikson, K. I. 9
Estabrook, A. H. 18
European Union 40
Evans, E. S. 370
Evans, H. C. 28, 29

F

Fabricant, S. 70
Farmer, S. 9, 10
Farrell, G. 19, 22
Fay, E. A. 22
Feigenbaum, E. D. 421
Feinstein, C. 355
Felix, R. H. 30, 33
Fenton, R. 27
Ferguson, P. M. 3
Fernald, W. E. 21, 26, 27, 28, 30
Ferster, E. Z. 29
Fessler, A. 12
Field, S. 42
Fish, W. B. 27
FitzGerald, J. F. 26
Flanigan, B. 382
Fleischer, D. Z. 36, 37
Fort, S. J. 27
Foucault, M. 11, 14
Frampton, M. E. 22
Fredericks, H. D. B. 355
French, R. S. 11, 19, 20
French, S. 37
Friedlander, H. 30
Frohboese, R. 357
Fröhlich, A. 38
Fujiura, G. T.
    70, 112, 113, 120, 124, 125, 127, 356, 358,
    437, 439
Furey, E. M. 117
Furth, J. 453

G

Galbraith, J. K. 42

Gallagher, H. G. 30
Gallaudet, E. M. 25
Gallaudet University 39
Galton, F. 28
Gambro, J. 355
Gannon, J. R. 12, 13, 18, 19, 22, 25
Ganski, L. 413
Garland, R. 6, 7, 43
Gattozzi, B. S. 390
Gaw, A. C. 6, 7, 8
Gettings, R. M. 119, 355, 425
Gill, C. J. 41
Gilman, S. L. 12, 43
Gilmore, D. S. 115
Gladstone, D. 28
Gladwin, T. 31
Glick, H. R. 357
Goddard, H. H. 28
Goldberg, S. 382
Goldman, S. 390
Goldstein, M. S. 5
Gonet, P. M. 421
Goode, D. 34
Goodey, C. F. 15
Gooding, C. 39
Gordan, J. C. 22
Gorwitz, K. 25
Gosney, E. S. 28
Gould, S. J. 28
Gove, S. K. 421
Governor's Interagency Community Placement
    Coordinating Council 380
Governor's Planning Council on Developmental
    Disabilities 434
Governor's Task Force on Prevention and Investi-
    gation of Abuse in State Institutions 378
Governor's Task Force on the Future of Mental
    Health In Illinois 413, 422
Gowman, A. G. 11, 33, 34
Grabowski, J. 36
Granfield, J. M. 117
Gray, V. 72, 355, 359, 437, 439
Greene, C. 65, 72
Greenland, C. 22
Griffin, J. D. 22
Grimes, J. M. 35
Grimes, S. K. 355

Griswold, P. P. 391
Grob, G. N. 22, 23, 25, 30, 31, 34, 35, 36
Grosshans, W. 367
Grumet, B. R. 357
Gussow 25

H

Hagner, D. 454
Hahn, H. 41
Haines, T. H. 29
Haller, B. 29
Hamburger, A. M. 33
Hamilton, S. W. 22, 24, 25, 31
Hammer, P. B. 358
Hanley-Maxwell, C. 355
Harms, E. 30, 33
Harrington, C. 66
Harris, C. C. 16
Harris, G. A. 373
Harris, P. B. 373
Hart, J. 379, 386, 396
Hatfield, A. B. 73
Hayden, M. F.
    36, 39, 72, 117, 126, 127, 353, 355, 357
Health Care Financing Administration (HCFA)
    66, 457
Health Facilities Planning Board
    409, 410, 416, 425, 429, 456
Hecht, F. 16
Hecht, I. W. D. 16
Heikkinen, B. 454
Heller, T. 38, 91, 353, 355, 358, 438
Helms, B. J. 115
Hemp, R.
    36, 65, 85, 100, 101, 115, 119, 353,
    354, 355, 356, 357, 358, 376, 383, 388,
    396, 410, 411, 414, 424, 425, 433, 437,
    438, 448, 449, 456
Henderson, C. M. 125
Herman, S. E. 113
Herr, S. S. 127
Hewitt, A. 89
Hill, M. 115
Hirad, A. 65
Hirsch, K. 3
Hoakley, Z. P. 30
Hodgson, K. W. 7

Hofferbert, R. I. 70, 355
Hoffman, A. 42
Holbrook, T. M. 355, 356, 358
Hollister, D. 379, 386, 396
Holstein, M. 35
Hopp, T. 357
Horner, R. H. 355
Houchard, B. 115
House Committee on Mental Health 383
House Democratic Staff 409
House Fiscal Agency 437
Howard, A. 357
Howard, J. 8, 11
Howe, S. G. 26
Howes, R. 85
Howse, J. 358
Huberman, A. M. 358, 366, 367
Hughes, S. L. 35
Human Services Research Institute 373
Humphrey, J. C. 42
Hurd, H. M. 22

I

Illinois Association for Retarded Citizens
    415, 419, 420, 428, 431
Illinois Association for the Mentally Retarded
    431, 432
Illinois Coalition of ICF/DD Providers 412
Illinois Commission on Intergovernmental Coopera-
    tion 427
Illinois Commission on Mental Health and Develop-
    mental Disabilities 409
Illinois Council for Mentally Retarded Children 432
Illinois Department of Corrections 437
Illinois Department of Mental Health
    405, 406, 407, 414, 415, 417, 418, 429,
    430, 431, 432
Illinois Department of Mental Health and
    Developmental Disabilities
    406, 408, 409, 410, 411, 416, 424, 427,
    428, 429, 431, 443, 450
Illinois Department of Public Aid 412
Illinois Department of Public Health 455, 458
Illinois General Assembly 417
Illinois House of Representatives 417, 418, 428
Illinois Information Service 406
Illinois Legislative Investigating Commission

417, 418, 419, 430
Illinois Mental Health Planning Board 405
Illinois Office of the Auditor General 409
Illinois Planning Council on Developmental
    Disabilities 413
Interdepartmental Committee on Mental Retardation
    and Illinois Association for the Mentally
    Retarded 405
Itard, J. M. 20

J

Jackson, M. 3
Jackson, S. W. 24
Jacobson, J. W. 36
Janicki, M. P. 42, 125
Jankauskas, R. 9
Johnson, A. 27
Joint Capital Outlay Subcommittee 380
Joint Committee to Study Abuse in State Mental
    Health Facilities 398
Joint Mental Health Oversight Committee
    375, 376, 389, 396
Jones, L. A. 34
Jørgensen, S. 38

K

Kane-Johnston, K. 115
Kanner, L. 12
Karan, O. C. 117
Kaufert, J. 38
Keith, K. 39
Kellow, J. T. 355
Kennedy, J. F. 35
Kennedy, M. J. 117
Keohane, R. O. 367
Kerlin, I. N. 26, 28
Kerney, F. 22
Kevles, D. J. 29
Key, V. O. 120
Kiernan, W. E. 115
King, G. 367
Kingdon, J. 356, 442
Kipp, R. S. 11
Kirchner, C. 37
Kirkbride, T. 22, 23
Kirshenbaum, A. 38
Knight, A. 413

Knight, G. H. 25, 27
Knobbe, C. A. 355
Koegel, L. K. 36
Koegel, R. L. 36
Koestler, F. A. 33
Koven, S. 28
Krane, N. 38
Kregel, J. 115
Kroll, J. 8, 9
Kuhlmann, F. 27
Kvale, S. 367

L

Lagomarcino, T. R. 115
Lakin, K. C. 31, 89, 126, 354, 355, 414
Lane, H. 18, 20, 25, 29
Larson, S. A. 89, 124
Lazar, I. 33
Lefley, H. 31, 34, 35, 39
Legislative Commission to Visit and Examine State
    Institutions, Subcommittee on Charitable
    Institutions 417, 418, 430
Leismer, J. 397
Lende, H. 31
Lerner, H. J. 357
Levin, H. 13, 31
Levy, R. M. 31, 35, 36
Lieberman, J. C. 66
Linton, S. 34, 41
Locke, J. 14
Longhurst, N. A. 39, 117
Luckmann, T. 34
Luke, R. T. 356
Lupton, D. 34
Lutterman, T. 65, 66, 72
Lynch, P. S. 355
Lysack, C. 38

M

MacAndrew, C. 27
MacArthur, W. 11, 25
MacDonald, M. 10, 28
MacIntosh, J. D. 38, 357
Mackelprang, R. W. 6
MadNation 31, 39
Mahar, W. 412
Maher, B. 11

Maher, W. B. 11
Marcenko, M. O. 113
Marcus, J. 8
Marklund 456
Marshall, C. 367
Martin, E. W. 36
Martin, F. 33
Martin, R. 36
Mastin, J. T. 30
Matson, F. 33
Matthews, M. A. 30
Mazmanian, D. A. 358
McDonough, K. 454
McGaughey, M. J. 115
McNally, L. C. 115
McSewyn, C. A. 115
Meier, K. J. 356
Merriam, S. B. 367
Merritt, D. J. 38
Metts, R. L. 40, 42
Meyers, J. C. 113
Michigan Department of Community Health
    448, 453, 454
Michigan Department of Corrections 437
Michigan Department of Mental Health
    371, 373, 374, 375, 376, 380, 381, 382,
    383, 386, 388, 390, 397, 399, 431
Michigan Department of Public Health 382
Michigan Department of Social Services 376, 395
Michigan Departments of Public Health and Mental
    Health 371
Michigan Departments of Social Services, Mental
    Health, and Education - Vocational Rehabilita-
    tion Services and State Housing Development
    Authority 373
Michigan House of Representatives 372, 387
Michigan Mental Health Advisory Council 375
Michigan Mental Health Association 454
Michigan Office of the Auditor General 380, 453
Michigan Protection and Advocacy Service
    377, 450
Michigan State Planning Council on Developmental
    Disabilities 391
Miles, M. 13
Miles, M. B. 358, 366, 367
Miller, G. 380, 382
Miller, S. K. 373

Milliken, W.
    372, 373, 377, 379, 383, 386, 392, 400
Minski, L. 18, 19
Mintrom, M. 356
Mitchell, D. 43, 89
Moore, S. C. 115
Mora, G. 21, 22
Moreno, J. 32
Morton, T. G. 16, 17
Moss, K. 355, 357
Mount, B. 454
Murphy, W. K. 413

N

Nagi, S. Z. 34
National Association of Protection and Advocacy
    Systems 127
National Association of State Budget Officers
    98, 99
National Association of State DD Directors
    89, 128, 129
National Association of State Mental Health Pro-
    gram Directors Research Institute 34
National Council on Disability 36, 37, 39, 41
Navon, L. 25
Neaman, J. 8
Nelis, T. 117, 353
Nerney, T. 112
Neugebauer, R. 9, 10, 16
Neugeboren, B. 356
New Jersey Department of Human Services 127
Nirje, B. 35, 374
Noll, S. 31, 33
Nowlan, J. D. 421

O

Obermann, C. E. 3, 20, 32
O'Brien, C. L. 354
O'Brien, J. 354
Ochberg, F. 379, 381, 399
O'Dell, D. 413
Office of Health and Medical Affairs 373
Oliver, M. 34, 42

P

Packard, E. P. W. 23
Palmer, J. A. 421

Pargeter, W. 24
Parish, S.
36, 65, 101, 115, 353, 354, 355, 357, 358, 376, 383, 388, 396, 410, 411, 414, 424, 425, 433, 437, 438, 448, 449, 456
Park, E. 13, 28
Park, H.
89, 355, 357, 358, 383, 425, 438, 449, 456
Parnas, S. 413
Parrish, T. B. 66
Parry, J. 31, 35, 36, 39
Parry-Jones, W. L. 14, 16
Paulaski, T. 456
Percy, S. 36
Percy, S. L. 355, 356, 358
Perez, A. 98
Perez, T. 458
Pernick, M. S. 25, 28
Peterson, D. 16, 18, 24, 30, 31, 33
Peterson, R. 37
Pinel, P. 11, 24
Pittsley, R. 117
Plann, S. 12, 21
Poindexter, B. 65
Pollock, H. M. 8, 25
Polloway, E. A. 355
Pomeranz, A. 36, 115, 354
Pomeroy, W. A. 386, 387
Popenoe, P. 28, 29
Porter, R. 4, 11, 29
Powers, G. 115
President's Panel on Mental Retardation 35
Pressman, J. L. 358
Protection and Advocacy, Inc. 414
Prouty, R. W. 126, 354
Public Sector Consultants 437, 453

Q

Quartararo, A. T. 21

R

Racino, J. A. 117, 354
Radford, J. P. 30
Rafter, N. H. 28
Ragan, J. F. 406, 408, 415, 420
Ramirez, R. 428
Ramirez-Moreno, S. 21

Ramsey, G. V. 30
Rave, M. 383
Redfield, K. 421, 422, 426
Reilly, P. R. 30
Rhodes, L. 355
Rice, D. M. 355
Rizzolo, M. C. 36, 65, 115, 354
Roberts, E. V. 34, 36, 38
Roberts, F. K. 19, 20
Roberts, J. A. F. 28
Robey, J. S. 70
Rochefort, D. A. 22
Rockey, D. 20
Roosens, E. 8
Rosen, D. 382
Rosen, G. 5, 9, 11
Rosenfeld, S. 19
Rossman, G. B. 367
Rothfels, N. 27
Rothman, D. J. 14, 21, 22, 23, 24, 25, 27, 32, 36, 355
Rothman, S. M. 32, 36, 355
Rousseau, J. J. 19, 24
Rubenstein, L. S. 31, 35, 36
Rubin, S. S. 89
Rumbaut, R. D. 8, 10
Rusco, J. 455
Rushton, P. 4, 12, 13, 14, 15
Russell, J. B. 9, 12

S

Sabatier, P. A. 358
Sacks, O. 18
Sales, D. 357
Salsgiver, R. O. 6
Sarason, S. B. 31
Savage, R. L. 70
Schafer, R. J. 3
Schalock, M. 355
Schalock, R. 39
Scheerenberger, R. C.
3, 6, 27, 28, 357, 405, 406, 407, 408, 415
Schneider, J. 402
Schneider, M. 356
Schoultz, B. 4
Schwartz, R. D. 368

Scotch, R. K. 31, 36, 38, 39, 41
Scott, J. 363
Scott, R. 34
Scull, A. 23, 24, 25, 27
Sechrest, L. 368
Seekins, T. 38
Seguin, E. 20, 27
Selesnick, S. T. 8, 10, 11, 24
Semonin, P. 28
Senese, D. 39, 117
Shafer, R. J. 363
Shapiro, H. L. 393
Shapiro, J. P. 4
Sheldon, E. W. 3
Sherman, W. F. 357
Shumway, D. L. 38, 357
Siegel, J. F. 4
Silverstein, R. 36, 41, 73
Simpson, M. K. 20
Skeels, H. M. 33
Slater, K. O. 359
Sloan, K. H. 357
Sloan, W. 28
Smith, G. A.
    73, 101, 117, 119, 126, 128, 354, 355,
    425, 447, 457
Smith, J. D. 355
Smith, S. 25
Smull, M. 117
Social Security Administration 66
Social Security Board 31
Solecki, R. 5
Spare, P. 357
Speer, G. S. 33
Spierenburg, P. 9, 13, 16
Spitalnick, D. 357
Spreat, S. 355
Stabenow, D. 383
Starr, P. 120
State Advisory Council on Mental Retardation
    405, 414
State of Illinois Constitution 420
Stevens, H. 8, 28
Stewart, J. 37, 38
Stewart, J. Q. A. 26
Stewart, T. D. 5
Stiker, H. 5, 6, 7, 11

Stone, J. A. 355
Straus, W. L. 5
Strype, J. 15
Suhr, C. 37
Summers, P. R. 66
Survey and Research Corporation 35
Suzuki, A. 12, 14
Swain, B. 11
Swayze, V. W. 30
Swinburne, H. 10, 15
Switzky, H. N. 28, 31, 355
Symonds, B. 22
Szasz, T. 24, 31

T

Talbot, M. 20
Taylor, M. 41
Taylor, S. J. 117, 354, 358
Telles, J. L. 355
Terman, D. L. 36
Tesch, R. 367
Teske, P. 356
Thiher, A. 43
Thollaug, S. C. 66
Thompson, L. 115
Thompson, T. 36
Thomson, R. G. 27, 43
Topper, G. 355, 357, 358, 437
Trent, J. W. 3, 23, 25, 26, 27, 28, 31, 33
Trombley, S. 30
Tuke, D. H. 12
Tuke, S. 23
Tyor, P. L. 25, 31

U

U.S. Bureau of the Census 26, 31, 42, 124, 125
U.S. Department of Agriculture 66
U.S. Department of Education 37, 41
U.S. Department of Health, Education, and Welfare
    35
U.S. Department of Housing and Urban
    Development 66
U.S. Department of Labor 371
U.S. Holocaust Memorial Museum 30
U.S. Office of Management and Budget 66
United Nations 40
Unterbrink, R. L. 413

Urbanavicius, A. 9

V

Valenstein, E. S. 31
Van Acker, R. 355
Van Meter, M. 365
Vaux, C. L. 33
Velche, D. 6
Verba, S. 367
Verbrugge, L. M. 41, 42
Verburg, K. 387
Visotsky, H. M. 405
Vitello, S. J. 355
Vogelsberg, R. T. 115
Voice of the Retarded 357
Vorderer, L. 357

W

Wagner, R. L. 405, 406
Wagoner, L. C. 25
Walden, B. 391
Walker, D. 409, 415, 426, 429, 430
Walker, J. L. 70
Walker, T. 33
Wallace, G. L. 30
Ward, M. J. 33
Ward, N. 4, 117, 353
Warkany, J. 6
Watkins, H. M. 28, 29, 31
Webb, E. J. 368
Wehman, P. 115
Wellin, V. 66
Wells, A. 357
Wells, D. 411
Welsford, E. 8
West, M. 115
Westmoreland, T. M. 458
Westrich, J.
    65, 353, 355, 357, 358, 376, 383, 388, 396,
    410, 411, 414, 424, 425, 433, 437, 438,
    448, 449, 456
Weymouth, A. 8, 11
Whitman, C. 413
Whitney, E. A. 13
Wieck, C. 355
Wilbur, C. T. 27
Wildavsky, A. B. 120, 358

Wilkinson, M. W. 25
Willeford, W. 8
Williams, W. 115
Wilson, V. L. 355
Winship, M. P. 16
Winspear, C. W. 28
Winzer, M. A. 7, 8, 9, 12, 15, 20
Wolcott, H. F. 367
Wolfensberger, W. 27, 30, 35, 355, 374
Wolman, J. M. 66
Wood, G. B. 22
Woodill, G. 6
Woodside, M. 29
Woodward, S. 26
Woolfson, R. C. 15
World Health Organization 34
Wright, D. 3, 12, 13, 18, 19
Wright, H. 33
Wright, L. 33

Y

Yin, R. K. 367

Z

Zames, F. 36, 37
Zandi, M. M. 98
Zirpoli, T. J. 355
Zola, I. K. 38
Zwernick, K. 454

SUBJECT INDEX

1899 Education Act (England) 28

1971 Declaration of the Rights of Mentally Retarded Persons 39

1975 Declaration of the Rights of Disabled Persons 39

1982 World Programme of Action Concerning Disabled Persons 40

377 Boards (Illinois) 415

553 Boards (Illinois) 415

708 Boards (Illinois) 415

A

A Mind that Found Itself 30

Adele Karlson Center private institution (Illinois) 412

advances in the anatomical and physiological study of hearing, vision, and the human body 12

The American Federation of State, County, and Municipal Employees (AFSCME) 361, 422, 426, 440, 446, 455, 456, 457, 458

Age of Reason 14

aging caregivers 125

aging of our society 121, 124

Alabama 113, 117, 121, 128
    profile 143-146

Alaska 86, 88, 91, 96, 97, 98, 101, 110, 112, 121, 125, 128
    profile 147-150

Aleppo 10

All Seasons nursing home (Illinois) 418, 419

almshouse 14
    the first American 14, 21

Alpine state institution (Michigan) 383

Alternative Intermediate Services for the Mentally Retarded (AISMR) 376, 382, 385, 388, 389, 399, 454

Alton psychiatric hospital (Illinois) 407

Alvarez, Bernadino 21

American Association on Mental Deficiency 375

American Asylum for the Education of the Deaf and Dumb (Hartford, CT) 22

American Coalition of Citizens with Disabilities 38

American Foundation for the Blind 33

American Journal of Insanity 23

American Printing House for the Blind 19

American Red Cross 32

Americans Disabled for Attendant Programs Today (ADAPT) 37, 447

Americans with Disabilities Act (ADA) 5, 39, 41, 357, 458

Ancient China 7

Ancient Greece 6, 7

Ancient Greece and Rome 6

Anglo-Saxons 8

Anna psychiatric hospital (Illinois) 409

annual costs of care 87

antiquity 5

Arabs 10

ARC of Illinois Archives 361

ARC of Michigan Archives 361

Archives and Library on Disability 361, 369

Arizona 86, 88, 91, 92, 96, 97, 110, 112, 113, 115, 126, 129
    profile 151-154

Arkansas 86, 91, 92, 96, 97, 100, 110, 113, 117
    profile 155-158

assistive technology 36, 101

Austria 32

B

Babcock, Patrick 381, 393, 395, 397, 398, 399, 401, 404, 441

Bacon, Francis 13, 14

Baghdad 10

Balanced Budget Act of 1997 (Public Law 105-33) 119

Barr, Martin 27

Barthelemy et al. v. Louisiana Department of Health and Hospitals (2001) 129

Barton, Clara 32

Bauer, Elizabeth 400

Beers, Clifford 30

Bell, Alexander Graham 25, 28

Bellarmine case (Michigan) 380

Belletire, Michael 411

Bethlehem Hospital (Bethel, Bethlem, Bedlam) 10, 15, 16

Beverly Farms private institution (Illinois) 410

Bicêtre 14, 20

"bidding out" 18

Bishop Nicholas 8

Blanchard, Gov. James, Michigan 383, 387, 388, 392, 393, 394, 437, 442

Blanton, Richard 431

Board of Trustees of the University of Alabama, et al. v. Garrett et al. (2001) 130

Bogard v. Patla (2000) 433, 450

Bond, Thomas 16

Bonet, Juan Pablo 12, 18

Boudreau v. Ryan (2000) 457

Bowen state institution (Illinois) 406, 411, 427

Braidwood, Thomas 18

Braille, Louis 19

British Association of the Deaf 25

British Deaf and Dumb Association (BDDA) 25

Brown, Rep. Tom, Michigan 394, 395

Buck v. Bell (1927) (sterilization) 29

Button, Lydia 23

C

Cairo 10

Califano, Secretary Joseph 36

California 97, 101, 110, 113, 119, 126, 127, 129
    profile 159-162

Calvin, John 12

canonization of St. Louis 10

Caro state institution (Michigan) 448

Catholic Church 9

Censoni, Ben 374, 379, 381, 393, 397, 398, 399, 404, 441

Center for Excellence in DD 446

Centers for Independent Living
    first center in the US 38

Centers for Medicare and Medicaid Services 66

Certificate of Need 361, 416, 429, 455

Chafee Amendment 433, 441

Chafee, Senator John (RI) 433

Chicago Sun Times 420

Christ 8

Chronological event analysis 367

City of Livonia v. Department of Social Services, Greentrees Civic Association, Inc. v. Pignatiello (1985) 382, 397

civil rights 356
    innovativeness 70

Civil War 26

"Class X" felonies 427, 437

Coding 367

Coffelt v. Department of Developmental Services (1994) 127

Cohen, Wilbur 377, 378

Coldwater state institution (Michigan) 383, 388, 402

Colorado 97, 103, 110, 115, 117, 119, 128
    profile 163-166

Columbia Institution for the Instruction of the Deaf 25

Community Facilities Licensing Act (Illinois) 430

Community Integrated Living Arrangements (CILA) (Illinois) 413

Community Living Facility (CLF) (Illinois) 408, 409, 425

Community Mental Health (CMH) Boards (Michigan) 362, 384, 385, 454

Community Mental Health Centers Act of 1963 35

Community Residence Location Planning Act (Illinois) 413

Community Residential Alternative Licensing Act (Illinois) 430

community staff wage initiatives 89

Community Supported Living Arrangement (CSLA) 449, 450, 454, 457, 459

Connecticut 18, 22, 26, 92, 97, 101, 110, 112, 113, 121
    profile 167-170

Conner v. Branstad (1993) 127, 358

Constitution of Athens 7

Copernicus 13

Cost Control Task Force (Illinois) 427

Council of World Organizations Interested in the Handicapped (CWOIH, now the International Council on Disability) 34

Crippled Children's Services National Advisory Committee 31

cross-disability
    advocacy 41
    coalitions 41
    perspective 4

The Crown in England 10

Cultural models 355

Cumulative voting (Illinois) 421
"Cutback Amendment" (Illinois) 421

D

Da Vinci, Leonardo 12
Damascus 10
Daniels, Rep. Lee, Illinois 430, 442
de l'Epée 18, 21
Deaf community organizing 25
Deaf culture 29
Deaf Institute in Paris 21
Deaf instruction
    first teacher of the deaf in the Western world 18
    oralism 21, 28
    schools for deaf and blind persons open in Europe
        18
Declaration of Independence 18
definition of intellectual disability 15
Defoe, Daniel 15
Deinstitutionalization 34, 36, 357, 358, 359, 435
Delaware 92, 97, 101, 110, 113
    profile 171-174
demonology 8
Dempsey, John 386
Denmark 19
Department of Veterans Affairs (DVA) Veterans'
    Compensation 65
des Invalides du Travail et des Invalides Civils 34
designated MR/DD units in state psychiatric
    hospitals 91
Detroit Free Press 377, 380, 386, 392, 393,
    396, 400
developmental centers 91
Developmental Disabilities Act 357
Developmental Disabilities Act (1970) 428
Developmental Disabilities Act (1975) 399
Developmental Disabilities Act (1984) 391
Developmental Disabilities Study Committee of the
    House of Representatives (Illinois) 399
developments in the American Colonies and Early
    United States 16
DeVito, Robert 430
disability
    as a social construction 3
    in literature and art 43
    in the American colonies 4
Disability Discrimination Act of 1993 (Australia)

    39, 40
disability spending
    cross-disability governmental expenditures 65
    total disability expenditure in the U.S. 72
Disabled in Action (advocacy organization) 38
Disabled Peoples' International 37
District of Columbia 25, 91, 97, 99, 101, 104,
    110, 113, 117, 121, 125, 126
    profile 175-178
Dix, Dorothea 22
Dixon Assn. for Retard. Citizens v. Thompson
    (1982) 409, 427
Dixon Association for Retarded Citizens 409, 427
Dixon State Institution (Illinois)
    405, 406, 407, 408,
    409, 419, 427, 444
Doe v. Bush (2001) 128
DVA Medical Care 65
Dykstra, Art 416, 442

E

Easter Seal Society 32
Eastern State Hospital 22
Economic models 355
economy
    record-setting growth during the 1990s 98
    slow down in momentum in U.S. 99
Edgar, Gov. Jim, Illinois 448, 455
Education of All Handicapped Children Act (EHA)
    36, 37, 357, 399
Egypt 7
electroshock 30
    right to refuse electroshock 31
Elgin psychiatric hospital (Illinois) 407, 417, 418
Elizabethan Poor Law (England) 11, 13
Elm Hill Private School and Home 26
England 12, 14, 15, 19, 20, 27, 28, 32
Engler, Gov. John 453, 459
Enlightenment 4, 14, 19
Equip for Equality (Illinois P&A) 434, 441, 443,
    447, 457
ethnocentric and class biases against immigrants 28
eugenics 28, 30, 42
    threat of the eugenicists 28
euthanasia 29, 41
exploitation of resident labor, or peonage 26
External validity 369

F

Fair Housing Act Amendment (1988)
 73, 413, 443
Fair Labor Standards Act (1966) 371
family care
 first initiated in Massachusetts 25
family, community, and consumer model
 emergence of 33
family support 98
 definition 112
Family Support Subsidy Act (Michigan) 396, 452
Fauquier, Francis 22
Fédération Internationale des Mutilés 34
feeblemindedness 29
Ferguson, Beth 380
Fernald's (1919) Waverly studies 30
Fez (Morocco) 10
finger alphabet 13
first civilian vocational rehabilitation law 32
first "workmen's compensation" law in 1902 32
fiscal effort 65
 assessing fiscal effort in the states 70, 120
Florida 92, 96, 97, 100, 101, 110, 112, 119,
 121, 125, 128
 profile 179-182
Food Stamps 65
Fox state institution (Illinois) 405, 406
France 8, 10, 14, 15, 18, 19, 32
Franklin, Benjamin 16
freak shows 28
 "caricatures of the grotesque" 27
 "taste for monsters" 28
Freedom of Information Act 361, 369
French Academy of Sciences 20
from training schools to custodial asylums 26

G

Galesburg psychiatric hospital (Illinois) 407
Galileo 13
Gallaudet, Thomas 19, 41
Gallaudet University 25
Geo-Karis, Sen. Adeline, Illinois 455
Georghospital (Elbing) 10
Georgia 86, 88, 100, 101, 110, 121, 127
 profile 183-186
Germany 8, 15, 18, 19, 29, 32, 41, 124
Gheel (Belgium) 8

Ginsburg, Judge Ruth Bader 101, 458
Glass, Albert 430
Goodwill Industries 32
Governor James Blanchard, Michigan 383, 387,
 388, 392, 393, 394, 437, 442
Governor Jim Edgar, Illinois 409, 448, 455
Governor William Milliken, Michigan 363, 377,
 378, 379, 380, 388, 392, 394, 398,
 400, 402, 404
Governor Richard Ogilvie, Illinois 406, 415,
 422, 426
Governor George Ryan, Illinois 456
Governor James Thompson, Illinois 409, 412,
 420, 422, 423, 426, 427, 428,
 435, 437
Governor Dan Walker, Illinois 406, 409, 415,
 420, 422, 426, 429, 430, 437
Governor's Task Force on the Future of Mental
 Health (Illinois) 413
Great Britain's Disability Discrimination Act of 1995
 5
Great Depression 31, 33
Greece 8, 10
gross state product (GSP) 96, 359
Grosse Hospital (Efrurt, Germany) 10
Guggenbuhl (Switzerland) 20
Guislain, Joseph 24

H

Handicappers Civil Rights Act (Michigan) 443
Hansen's Disease (leprosy) 11
Hart, Sen. Jerome, Michigan 378, 389, 396
Harvey, William 12
Haüy, Valentin 19
Hawaii 91, 110, 112, 113, 121, 126, 128
 profile 187-190
Health Care Financing Administration (HCFA)
 410, 412, 454, 457
health care programs 65
Hebrew law 5
Heinicke, Samuel 18
Hérnandez, Tiburcio 21
Herodotous 7
Heumann, Judy 36
Hillcrest state institution (Michigan) 383, 386, 387
Holland 15
Hollister, Rep. David, Michigan 378, 389,

395, 396

Home and Community Based Services (HCBS)
    Waiver 88, 99, 100, 101, 103,
    112, 119, 126, 127, 129, 353, 389,
    390, 392, 425, 426, 439, 454

Home Rule 435, 438

Home/Individual Program (H/IP) (Illinois) 410

Homeward Bound v. Hissom Memorial Center
    (1990) 89

Hôpital General 14

hospices for blind persons 8

House Bill 69 (Illinois family subsidy) 414

House Developmental Disabilities Study Committee
    (1973), (Michigan) 429

Housing and Urban Development (HUD) 65

Howe, Samuel Gridley 25, 26, 41

Howe State Institution (Illinois) 406, 411, 412,
    419, 429

humanism in art 12

Hyde, Congressman Henry 456

I

ICF/MR (Intermediate Care Facility for People with
    Mental Retardation Program) 36, 88, 98,
    101, 103, 111, 119, 126, 128,
    439, 448, 457, 458

Idaho 92, 96, 97, 110, 113, 117, 121, 126
    profile 191-194

idiocy 15

Illinois Citizen's Council on Mental Health/Develop-
    mental Disabilities 412

Illinois 23, 26, 35, 86, 88, 91, 92, 97, 110,
    113, 119, 121, 126, 128
    profile 195-198

Illinois Association of Rehabilitation Facilities
    (IARF) 431

Illinois Association for Retarded Citizens (Also Arc/
    IL and IARC) 363, 413, 415, 431, 456

Illinois Civil Liberties Union 446

Illinois Coalition of ICF/DD Providers 412

Illinois Community Mental Health Act 415

Illinois Constitution 420, 421

Illinois Department of Mental Health/Developmental
    Disabilities (DMHDD) 365, 412, 415,
    428, 431, 434

Illinois Department of Human Services 361

Illinois Department of Mental Health (DMH) 405,
    407, 408, 414, 429, 432

Illinois Department of Public Aid (IDPA) 362, 411

Illinois Department of Public Health 361, 362,
    410, 411, 412, 416

Illinois Department of Public Welfare 414

Illinois Extended Care Center private institution 418

Illinois' first institution 359

Illinois Governor's Planning Council on Develop-
    mental Disabilities 428, 434, 457

Illinois Health Facilities Planning Act (1974) 416

Illinois Health Facilities Planning Board 361,
    362, 410, 416, 425, 429, 455

Illinois League of Advocates for the Developmen-
    tally Disabled 458

Illinois Legislative Investigating Commission 418-19

Illinois Nursing Home Reform Act (1979) 419

Illinois School for the Deaf 26

Illinois State Archives 361

Illinois State Insane Asylum at Jacksonville 23

Illinois State Library 361

impairment and disability 3

income maintenance programs 65, 67

increasing longevity of persons with developmental
    disabilities 121, 125

Independent Living Movement 33, 38

Independent Service Coordination (ISC) 433

Indiana 92, 96, 97, 110, 113, 117,
    121, 126, 129
    profile 199-202

individual and family support 98, 112

Individuals with Disabilities Education Act (IDEA)
    66, 68, 73

Institute for Crippled and Disabled Men
    in 1917 32

Institutional closure in Michigan 372

Institutional closures in the U.S. 353, 357

institutional perspective 3

institutionalization 15, 19, 23, 26, 31, 41

institutions
    closures 91
    discharge 30
    privately-operated 92
    state-operated 91

Intermediate Care Facilities/Developmentally

Disabled (ICF/DD) (Illinois) 408, 409, 410
416, 425
intellectual disabilities
distinguishing between intellectual disability and
mental illness 15
intelligence tests 28
Intermediate Care Facility for People with Mental
Retardation Program (ICF/MR) 355, 362,
375, 376, 385, 388, 390, 392, 396, 408,
411, 412, 424, 426
private ICFs/MR for 15 or fewer persons 87
public ICFs/MR for 15 or fewer persons 87
Internal validity 367
International Congress on Education of the Deaf 25
International Federation of the Blind 34
Iowa 86, 91, 92, 97, 103, 110, 112, 117,
121, 126, 127
profile 203-206
Ireland 15
Italian Grand Duke Ferdinand I 15
Italy 8, 11, 18, 19, 25, 31
Itard, Jean 19, 20

J

Jacksonville state hospital (Illinois) 406, 407, 429
Japan 41, 124
Johnson, Judge Frank M. 36
Joiner, Judge Charles 379, 397
Jordan, I. King 39
Joint Legislative Committee to Study Abuse in State
Mental Health Facilities 378, 379
Judge Ruth Bader Ginsburg 101, 458
Justinian Code 7

K

Kankakee psychiatric hospital (Illinois) 407, 429
Kansas 96, 110, 112, 113, 121
profile 27-210
Kennedy, President John F. 35
Kentucky 19, 22, 26, 86, 88, 92, 97, 110,
121, 129
profile 211-214
key disability issues for developing societies 42
Kiley, Ann 431
Kiley state institution (Illinois) 406, 419, 429,
448, 455
King Charles I 16

Kirkbride, Thomas 22
Klingberg School private institution (Illinois)
418, 419
Kok, Rep. Peter, Michigan 394, 395, 396
Kope v. Watkins (1988) 384, 387, 394, 397,
444, 450

L

Laconia Developmental Center (New Hampshire)
38
Lansing Journal 380
"leaders and laggards" 65
Leavitt, Leroy 430, 431
leprosariums 11
leprosy 8, 11
spread of leprosy 11
Letter to Henry Cline 20
leveraging federal funds 103
Lewis, Jerry 38
Lincoln State Institution (Illinois) 35, 405, 406,
407, 408, 409, 411, 419, 457
litigation 127, 128
Livonia, Michigan 382
local funding 103
Locke, John 14, 15
Essay Concerning Human Understanding (1690)
15
long term care 65
Louisiana 86, 91, 97, 110, 112, 113, 121, 129
profile 215-218
Ludeman state institution (Illinois)
406, 412, 419, 429
Luther, Martin 12

M

Mabley state institution (Illinois) 409, 427
Macomb-Oakland Regional Center (MORC)
(Michigan) 374, 375, 381, 383, 384,
386, 388, 397, 398, 399, 401, 402,
404, 440, 441
madhouses 14
Madigan, House Leader Michael 456
Maine 91, 92, 97, 101, 110, 113, 121,
128, 129
profile 219-222
Makin et al. v. State of Hawaii (1999) 129
Marklund private institution (Illinois) 455, 456

marriage restriction laws 25

Maryland
22, 32, 91, 92, 96, 112, 113, 119, 121
profile 223-226

Massachusetts
22, 25, 26, 30, 31, 92, 101, 110, 112,
113, 121, 125, 128
profile 227-230

Maternal and Child Health and Mental Retardation
Planning Amendments of 1963 (Pub. L. 88-
156) 35, 405

Maternal and Child Health State Grant Program 35

Mather, Cotton 16

Mattingly Health Care private institution (Illinois)
410

Medicaid 65, 85, 99, 100, 101, 103,
117, 119, 120, 121, 127, 128, 129, 130,
396, 433, 451, 457
access to Medicaid services litigation 121
clinic/rehabilitative services 99
Community Supported Living Arrangement
(CSLA) 119
Home and Community Based Services (HCBS)
Waiver 38, 65, 70, 72, 73, 88, 99, 100,
101, 103, 112, 119, 126, 127, 129,
353, 389, 390, 392, 425, 426, 439, 454
Medicaid long term care spending 68

Medicare 65

Medieval times 8, 9, 10, 11, 27

Mendel, Gregor 28

mental asylum
the first American 21
the first North American 21

mental hygiene movement 30

mental illness 39

Mental Retardation Facilities and Community
Mental Health Centers Construction Act of
1963 (Pub. L. 88-164) 35

Mexico 15

Michigan 91, 101, 110, 112, 113, 119, 121,
125, 126, 129
profile 231-234

Michigan ARC v. Smith (1979) 400, 444

Michigan Association for Retarded Citizens (also
ARC of Michigan)
363, 381, 391, 399, 402, 441

Michigan Department of Community Health
453, 454

Michigan Department of Management and Budget
381

Michigan Department of Mental Health (DMH)
369, 375, 380, 384, 385, 386, 391,
392, 396, 397, 398, 404

Michigan Department of Public Health 396

Michigan Department of Social Services
380, 391, 396

Michigan Governor's Planning Council on Developmental Disabilities 399

Michigan Interagency Task Force on Disability
(MITF/D) 391

Michigan Joint Capital Outlay Subcommittee 380

Michigan Joint Committee to Study Abuse in State
Mental Health Facilities 396

Michigan Joint Mental Health Oversight Committee
396

Michigan Office of the Auditor General 380

Michigan Protection and Advocacy Service
377, 399, 400, 402

Michigan State Archives 369

Michigan State Housing Development Authority
(MSHDA) 373

Michigan State Library 361

Michigan Supreme Court 382

Michigan's first institution 359

Michigan's Mental Health Code 443, 454

Middle Ages 4, 8, 9, 10, 11, 13

Milliken, Gov. William, Michigan 442

Minnesota 87, 91, 92, 101, 103, 110,
112, 121
profile 235-238

Minoz, Egas 30

Misericordia private institution (Illinois) 456

Mississippi 86, 88, 91, 92, 96, 97,
100, 110, 113, 117, 121, 125, 126
profile 239-242

Missouri 91, 92, 101, 103, 115
profile 243-246

Montana 91, 97, 100, 101, 103, 110,
121, 128
profile 247-250

Montessori, Maria 20

moral treatment 23

Morocco (*See Fez*)

Moss, Don 415, 420

Mt. Pleasant state institution (Michigan) 383, 448, 453

Murphy, Bill 431

Murray state institution (Illinois) 405, 406, 411

Muskegon state institution (Michigan) 383, 448

N

Nagi, Saad 34

Nathan v. Levitt (1974) 443

National Association for Retarded Children (now The Arc) 34

National Association of State Mental Health Program Directors 34, 66

National Association of the Deaf 25

National Committee for Mental Hygiene 30

National Conference of Charities and Corrections 27

National Federation of the Blind 33

National Health Interview Survey - Disability Supplement 124

National Institute of Mental Health (NIMH) 33

National Institute on Disability and Rehabilitation Research (NIDRR) 66

National Institutes of Health (NIH) 66

National Mental Health Act 33

National Society for Crippled Children and Adults 32

Nazi Germany
    eugenic sterilization law 30
    killing of people with disabilities 30

Neanderthals
    chronic impairments in 5

Nebraska 91, 92, 97, 100, 101, 110, 121
    profile 251-254

Nepinak, John 19

Nevada 86, 91, 92, 96, 97, 110, 121
    profile 255-258

New Federalism 439

New Hampshire 91, 100, 101, 110, 117, 121, 125, 129
    profile 259-262

New Jersey 86, 88, 91, 110, 121, 126
    profile 263-266

New Mexico 100, 110, 121, 127, 128
    profile 267-270

New Testament 8

New York 21, 22, 25, 26, 27, 31, 32, 35, 91, 92, 101, 117, 121
    profile 271-274

New York Asylum at Utica 23

New York City polio epidemic in 1916 32

Newberry State Institution (Michigan) 448

Newton, Isaac 14

Normalization 353

North Aurora Center private institution (Illinois) 408, 419, 432, 433

North Carolina 29, 87, 91, 92, 97, 110, 112, 113
    profile 275-278

North Dakota 92, 97, 115, 121, 125, 126
    profile 279-282

Northville state institution (Michigan) 383

nursing facilities 66, 67, 68, 72, 86, 91, 95, 96, 112, 373, 406, 408, 411

Nursing Home Reform Act of 1979 443

O

Oakdale state institution (Michigan) 383, 448

Ochberg, Frank 379, 381, 398

Ohio 18, 26, 29, 32, 97, 101, 103, 104, 112, 115, 117, 128
    profile 283-286

Oklahoma 86, 88, 96, 97, 113, 117
    profile 287-290

Old Testament 5, 8

Olmstead v. L.C. (1999) 73, 74, 101, 103, 357, 457, 458

Omnibus Budget Reconciliation Act (OBRA) of 1981 358, 389

Oregon 91, 92, 97, 110, 112, 115, 121, 127, 128
    profile 291-294

out-of-home residential placements 86

overcrowding 23
    and the demise of the moral treatment 23

Owen, Gary, House Speaker, Michigan 380, 398

Ozinga, Sen. Frank N., Illinois 417

P

Packard, Elizabeth 23, 30

Parent advocacy groups 353

Pargeter, William 24

parole plan 30

Pattern matching 367
Pavkovic, Ivan 430
Pennhurst case 432
Pennsylvania 16, 18, 22, 26, 92, 101, 103, 112, 128
    profile 295-298
Pennsylvania Hospital for the Insane 17
Pennsylvania Provincial Assembly 16
Pennsylvania Training School for Idiotic and Feebleminded Children 26
People First 39, 356, 431, 433, 447, 456, 457
People First of Tennessee v. Arlington Development 353
people with intellectual disabilities
    as a "menace and burden" 28
Peoria psychiatric hospital (Illinois) 407, 417, 418
Péreiere, Jacob 20
Perkins Institute for the Blind 19, 22, 26
personal assistance 87
personal care 100
personal income
    aggregate statewide personal income 70
Phenylketonuria (PKU) 432
Phillips v. Thompson (1983) 419, 432, 443
Pinel, Phillipe 10, 19, 24, 41
    Treatise on Insanity 24
Pleasant Ridge, Michigan 382
Plymouth Center for Human Development (Michigan) 377, 379, 383, 386, 387, 388, 392, 393, 396, 398, 400
Policy entrepreneurs 442
Political socioeconomic models 355
Polo, Marco 13
Ponce de León, Pedro 18
Pope Innocent IV 9
poverty and disability 13
    during the Medieval period 9
Prangley, Richard 402
prehistory 5
Prerogativa Regis 10
President John F. Kennedy 356, 357, 401
President Abraham Lincoln 25
President Ronald Reagan 390, 401
President Franklin D. Roosevelt 31
President's Panel on Mental Retardation 35, 401

principle of normalization 35
Priory of St. Mary's of Bethlehem 10 (See also Behlehem Hospital)
prison population 437
Privately operated "madhouses" 14
Provencal, Gerald 374, 397, 398
psychosurgery 30
Public entrepreneurs 356
Public Interest Law Center of Philadelphia (PILCOP) 433
Pub. Act 39 of 1981 381
Pub. Act 77-2722 415, 429
Pub. Act 78-992 (Mental Health Code Amendments/Illinois) 415
Pub. Act 78-1156 (Health Facilities Planning Act/Illinois) 416, 429
Pub. Act 78-1183 (Act in Relation to Campaign Fincance/Illinois) 421
Pub. Act 79-967 429
Pub. Act 80-1099 427
Pub. Act 81-223 (Nursing Home Reform Act/Illinois) 419
Pub. Act 82-183 429
Pub. Act 82-567 (Community Living Facilities Licensing Act/Illinois) 409, 430
Pub. Act 82-584 (Community Residential Alternatives Licensing Act/Illinois) 409, 430
Pub. Act 82-921 410
Pub. Act 83-88 430
Pub. Act 84-567 429
Pub. Act 86-638 (Community Residence Location Planning Act/Illinois) 413
Pub. Act 86-921 (Developmental Disabilities Services Law/Illinois) 414, 452
Pub. Act 117 of 1975 372
Pub. Act 151 of 1923 372
Pub. Act 220 of 1976 (Persons with Disabilities Civil Rights Act/Michigan) 443
Pub. Act 249 of 1983 (Family Support Subsidy Program/Michigan) 383, 452
Pub. Act 258 of 1974 (Community Mental Health Act/Michigan) 384, 385, 394
Pub. Act 281 of 1979 (Adult Foster Care Facility Licensing Act/Michigan) 395
Pub. Act 360 of 1980 381
Pub. Act 423 of 1980 (Mental Health Code/Michigan) 380

Pub. Acts 28-30 of 1977 (Zoning Acts/Michigan) 376, 395

Pub. Acts 394-398 of 1976 (Zoning Acts/Michigan) 376, 394

Pub. L. 66-236 32

Pub. L. 88-156 (the Maternal and Child Health and Mental Retardation Planning Amendments of 1963) 35, 405

Pub. L. 88-164 (the Mental Retardation Facilities and Community Mental Health Centers Construction Act of 1963) 35

Pub. L. 91-517 (Developmental Disabilities Services and Facilities Construction Act of 1970) 375, 408

Pub. L. 92-233 (Amendments to Title XIX of the Social Security Act) 424

Pub. L. 94-142 (Education for All Handicapped Children Act) 353

Pub. L. 97-35 (Omnibus Budget Reconciliation Act of 1981) 100, 389, 425

Pub. L. 100-203 95

Pub. L. 100-407 36

Pub. L. 100-430 413, 443

Pub. L. 101-336 115

Pub. L. 101-508 119, 449

Pub. L. 105-33 112

Pub. L. 105-394 36

Pub. L. 106-170 115

Purchase Care Review Board (Illinois) 428

Q

Qualitative research 358, 367

Québec General Hospital 22

Queen Elizabeth 16

R

Reagan administration 439

Recall bias 368

Reformation 11

Rehabilitation Act 73

Rehabilitation International (RI) 37

Reliability 370

Renaissance 4, 12, 13
    and the scientific method 12

Rhode Island 22, 27, 91, 97, 101, 110, 117, 119, 121, 126
    profile 299-302

Roberts, Ed 38

Robinson Crusoe 15

Roman Emperor Claudius 6

Roman Empire 7

Rome 8, 10

Rosen, David 374, 379, 397, 398, 399

Rouse v. Cameron (1966) 35

Rousseau, Jean-Jacques 19, 23

Rush, Benjamin 18

Rushton, Edward 15, 19, 41

Rutan v. Republican Party of Illinois (1989) 423, 427

Ryan, Gov. George, Illinois 455, 456

S

Saegert (Germany) 20

Salpêtriere 14

Sampling bias 369

San Hipólito Hospital 21

Saxl, Joe 415

Scotland 15, 24

Section 504 of the Rehabilitation Act 36

segregation 4, 35, 41
    and expansion of the institutional model 29

Seguin, Edward 20, 26

selection bias 369

Self Advocates Becoming Empowered (SABE) 39

Self-advocacy groups 38, 39, 353, 402
    self-determination 41, 42
    growing strength of 115

Senator John Chafee, Rhode Island 433

Shapiro, Howard 401

Shapiro state institution (Illinois) 406, 411, 429

Sheltered care facilities 406, 425

Ship of Fools 11

shrine of St. Dymphna 8

Sicard 19, 20
    Sicard's National Institution for Deaf Mutes in Paris 19

sign language 12

Silvestri, Abba 18

Simon, Paul 422

Singer MH/DD Center (Illinois) 412

Smith, Donald 398

Snyder, Sen. Joseph, Michigan 396

social Darwinism 28

Social Model of Disability 33

Social Security Administration 390, 391
Social Security Adult Disabled Child (ADC)
    program 65
Social Security Disability Insurance (DI) 40,
    65, 390, 391
Social Services Block Grant 85, 100
Somerset House private institution (Illinois) 410
South Carolina 112, 121
    profile 303-306
South Dakota 92, 100, 101, 110, 113, 121
    profile 37-310
Southgate state institution (Michigan) 448, 453
Spain 10, 15, 18, 20
Sparta 6
special education 65, 66, 68
Specialized Living Centers (Illinois) 409, 428
St. Dymphna 8
St. Luke's Mental Hospital 15
St. Mary's Square private institution (Illinois) 410
Stabenow, Rep. Debbie, Michigan 383, 396, 401
Standard English Braille 19
Standard Rules on the Equalization of Opportunities
    for Persons with Disabilities 5, 39, 40
standpoint of professionals 3
State Asylum (Kalamazoo, Michigan) 23
state schools 91
sterilization 25, 29, 35, 41
    of institutional residents with intellectual
        disabilities 29
    of women with epilepsy and mental illness 29
stigma 41
supernatural or demonological causes 8
Supplemental Security Income (SSI) 40, 65, 67,
    355, 390, 391
supported employment 98
supported living/personal assistance 87
Swinburne, Henry 15
Switzerland 19
Syria 8
Szasz, Thomas 30

T

technology 36, 101
telethons 38
Tennessee 91, 92, 97, 110, 117, 121, 128
    profile 311-314
Texas 86, 87, 92, 97, 103, 110, 112, 121

    profile 315-318
The Life and Adventures of Mr Duncan Campbell
    15
The Right to Treatment 35
The Snake Pit 33
Thelwall, John 20
Thematic-content analysis 367
Thompson, Gov. James, Illinois 442, 444
Ticket to Work and Work Incentives Improvement
    Act 115
Title X of the Social Security Act 31
training centers 91
Tuke, William 22
Turkey 8
Turkish Ottoman Court 12

U

United Cerebral Palsy 441
United Nations 36, 39
United States v. Oregon (1987) 127
University of Illinois at Chicago's Center of Excel-
    lence 434
United States Congress 32
Utah 97, 110, 112, 113
    profile 319-322

V

variations in state commitments for MR/DD services
    104
Vermont 22, 91, 97, 101, 110, 112, 113
    profile 323-326
Versalius, Andreas 12
Veterans Compensation 67
Veterans of the Revolutionary War 18
Virginia 22, 86, 91, 97, 103, 110, 117,
    121, 128
    profile 327-330
Voice of the Retarded 431, 433

W

waiting lists 121, 126, 354
Walker, Gov. Dan, Illinois 422, 426, 430
Ward, Mary Jane 33
Washington 34, 92, 100, 110, 112, 113, 117,
    119, 128
    profile 331-334

Watkins, Thomas 393, 404
Welfare Federation of Cleveland 33
West Virginia 91, 96, 110, 113, 117, 128
    profile 335-338
Wilbur, Hervey 26
wild boy of Aveyron 20
Willowbrook State School (New York) 31, 35,
    377, 416, 432
Windgate Children's Home private institution (Illi-
    nois) 418, 419, 420
Winneconna private institution (Illinois) 418, 419
Wisconsin 97, 103, 112, 119
    profile 339-342
witchcraft
  acts 15
  as manifestations of mental illness 9
  in colonial New England 9
World Bank 42
World Council for the Welfare of the Blind 33
World Federation of the Deaf 34
World Health Organization 34
World War I 32, 33
World War II 33
Wyatt v. Stickney (1971) 35, 36, 418
Wyoming 87, 88, 91, 97, 100, 101, 103,
    110, 121, 126, 127
    profile 343-346

Y

York Retreat 22
Young, Sr., Rep. Joe, Michigan 396
Youngberg v. Romeo (1982) 433
Yudashkin, Gordon 398

Z

Zaragoza asylum 10
Zoning restrictions 376, 413, 420